Nutrition in Pregnancy and Lactation

NUTRITION IN PREGNANCY AND LACTATION

BONNIE S. WORTHINGTON-ROBERTS, *PhD*

Professor of Nutrition
University of Washington (retired)
Seattle, Washington

SUE RODWELL WILLIAMS, *PhD, MPH, RD*

President, SRW Productions, Inc.; Clinical Nutrition Consultant, Davis, California

SIXTH EDITION
illustrated

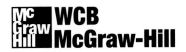

Boston, Massachusetts   Burr Ridge, Illinois   Dubuque, Iowa
Madison, Wisconsin   New York, New York   San Francisco, California   St. Louis, Missouri

WCB/McGraw-Hill

A Division of The **McGraw·Hill** *Companies*

Publisher: James M. Smith
Acquisitions Editor: Vicki E. Malinee
Managing Editor: Janet Russell
Senior Developmental Editor: Jean Babrick
Project Manager: Deborah L. Vogel
Production Editor: Mamata Reddy
Design Coordinator: Elizabeth Fett
Manufacturing Supervisor: Linda Ierardi
Cover Illustration: Jason Dowd

SIXTH EDITION

Copyright © 1997 Times Mirror Higher Education Group, In

Previous editions copyrighted 1977, 1981, 1985, 1989, 1993

Printed in the United States of America
Composition by The Clarinda Company
Printing/binding by R.R. Donnelley & Sons Company

Brown & Benchmark Publishers
2460 Kerper Boulevard
Dubuque, Iowa 52001

Library of Congress Cataloging in Publication Data

Worthington-Roberts, Bonnie S., 1943-
    Nutrition in pregnancy and lactation / Bonnie S. Worthington
-Roberts, Sue Rodwell Williams. — 6th ed.
      p. cm.
    Includes bibliographical references and index.
    ISBN 0-8151-9522-2
    1. Pregnancy—Nutritional aspects. 2. Mothers—Nutrition.
3. Lactation—Nutritional aspects. I. Williams, Sue Rodwell.
II. Title.
    [DNLM: 1. Nutrition—in pregnancy. 2. Prenatal Care.
3. Lactation. 4. Health Education. WQ 175 W933n 1997]
RG559.W67 1997
618.2′4—dc20
DNLM/DLC
for Library of Congress
                        96-32246
                         CIP

97 98 99 00/9 8 7 6 5 4 3 2

Contributors

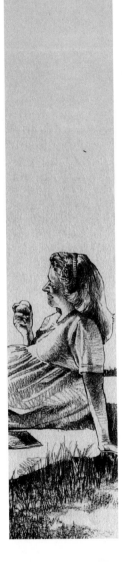

ALICIA DIXON DOCTER, MS, RD

Nutrition Education Specialist
Seattle, Washington

ANGELA M. JACOBI, RN, MSN, IBCLC

Assistant Professor, Rush University College of Nursing
Practitioner/Teacher and Lactation Consultant
Department of Maternal Child Nursing
Rush Presbyterian St. Luke's Medical Center
Chicago, Illinois

META L. LEVIN, BJ

Media Coordinator, International Lactation Consultant Association and
The Journal of Human Lactation
Lake Bluff, Illinois

JANE MITCHELL REES, MS, RD

Clinical Nutritionist, Adolescent Program,
Child Development and Mental Retardation Center,
University of Washington
Seattle, Washington

CRISTINE M. TRAHMS, MS, RD

Clinical Nutritionist, PKU Program,
Child Development and Mental Retardation Center,
University of Washington
Seattle, Washington

Preface

Nutritional support of the reproductive process and the role of nutrition in successful breastfeeding continue to be topics of major interest to clinicians and researchers. Ongoing research on these topics has led to changes in clinical practice over the years. The last several years have been particularly exciting, because of increased investigative efforts. These new findings are presented in the sixth edition of *Nutrition in Pregnancy and Lactation,* along with the fundamental information needed for a clear understanding of the subject.

AUDIENCE

Nutrition in Pregnancy and Lactation is written for health professionals in a variety of disciplines that relate to expectant families and to those who will eventually enter reproductive life. Students preparing for careers in maternal and child health will also find this text particularly helpful.

ORGANIZATION

The table of contents has been reorganized in response to users' suggestions. Chapter 1 reviews the status of maternal and child health, both in the United States and abroad. Chapter 2 examines the relation of nutrition and fertility, including the present focus on preconceptional care and counseling. The physiology of pregnancy is covered in Chapter 3, including a detailed discussion of the placenta and its vital nutritional and nonnutritional functions. This is followed, in Chapter 4, by a survey of the development of knowledge about the effect of diet on fetal development.

Chapters 5 and 6 explore, respectively, known and suspected energy and vitamin needs and mineral needs during pregnancy, including (in Chapter 5) expanded coverage of folic acid deficiency and neural tube defects. Chapter 7 discusses other dietary lifestyle components such as drug and alcohol use, which are believed (rightly or wrongly) to adversely affect pregnancy course and outcome.

After the principles of nutritional assessment are established (Chapter 8), the next two chapters cover, respectively, conditions and complications of pregnancy that may require special nutrition counseling, such as phenylketonuria (Chapter 9), and the nutritional challenges facing the pregnant adolescent (Chapter 10).

A key element in these chapters devoted to pregnancy is that they offer suggestions for the skillful application of an understanding of the relationship between nutrition and pregnancy. Considerable detail is included because the text is intended to provide practical information to be used in a clinical setting.

Moving from pregnancy to lactation, the next three chapters summarize the physiologic basis of lactation as well as economic issues relating to formula vs. human milk feedings (Chapter 11); the composition of human milk and its unique properties (Chapter 12); and practical issues related to the counseling and support of the lactating mother (Chapter 13).

The final chapter, Chapter 14, on nutrition education emphasizes the preparation of today's youth for conception before it occurs. Recommendations are given as to how, when, and where nutrition education efforts should be conducted and the impact those efforts can and do have on maternal and child health in the United States.

CHANGES IN THIS EDITION

Although the changes in the table of contents result in two additional chapters, the total length of the text has not increased appreciably. Instead, material has been reorganized into chapters of similar length, which should make reading assignments easier for the student.

This revision draws attention to recent developments in the area of nutrition and reproduction, and practical recommendations for counseling have been updated to reflect these developments.

Notable aspects of this edition include:

- Case studies, including questions in appropriate chapters that give the student practice in handling day-to-day situations in clinical settings.
- Updated vital statistics, both national and international.
- Evaluation of current weight-gain guidelines for pregnancy, as well as observations about postpartum weight loss.
- Discussion of the debate over the augmentation of nutritional needs associated with adolescent pregnancy.
- Updated management strategies for handling diabetic pregnancies
- Summary of new data on human milk composition.
- Current practical tips on lactation counseling.

ACKNOWLEDGMENTS

We are grateful to the many people who gave us their personal opinions about the book and its features. We hope that they will find this new edition a satisfactory reference or text for either professional or academic use.

The following reviewers provided many worthwhile ideas, which are reflected in the sixth edition of *Nutrition in Pregnancy and Lactation:* Joyce P. Barnett, University of Texas; Bahram Faraji, California State University/Los Angeles; Kristy Hendricks, Boston University; and Charlotte Pratt, Eastern Michigan State University.

Bonnie S. Worthington-Roberts
Sue Rodwell Williams

Contents

1 PROMOTION OF MATERNAL AND INFANT HEALTH

Bonnie S. Worthington-Roberts

Introduction, *1*
Indexes of Maternal and Infant Health, *3*
Epidemiologic Factors Affecting Mothers, *8*
Risks of Low Birth Weight, *21*
Contribution of Women, Infants, and Children's Program to Improving
    Maternal and Child Health, *25*
The Challenge Ahead—Measures to Improve Maternal and Infant Sur-
    vival and Health, *26*
Summary, *27*

2 NUTRITION, FERTILITY, AND FAMILY PLANNING

Bonnie S. Worthington-Roberts

Introduction, *31*
Fertility and Nutrition, *31*
Diet, Nutrition, and Fertility, *36*
Birth Control and Nutrition, *38*
Effect of Specific Birth Control Methods on Maternal Nutritional
    Status, *39*
A New Thrust: Preconception Care, *47*
Summary, *54*

3 PHYSIOLOGY OF PREGNANCY

Bonnie S. Worthington-Roberts

Introduction, *58*
The Length of Uncomplicated Human Gestation, *58*
Incidence of Early Pregnancy Loss, *59*
The Cardiovascular System, *59*
Blood Volume and Composition, *59*
Respiration, *63*
Renal Function, *63*
Gastrointestinal Function, *64*
Hormones, *64*

Metabolic Adjustments, *68*
Components of Weight Gain, *68*
Role of the Placenta, *85*
Summary, *90*

4   FOUNDATIONS OF RESEARCH IN PRENATAL NUTRITION

Bonnie S. Worthington-Roberts

Introduction, *94*
Early Briefs and Practices, *95*
Historical Background, *96*
Nutritional Influences on Fetal Growth, *98*
Summary, *125*

5   ENERGY AND VITAMIN NEEDS DURING PREGNANCY

Bonnie S. Worthington-Roberts

Introduction, *128*
Problems in Determining Needs, *128*
Energy, *129*
Protein, *139*
Essential Fatty Acids, *142*
Vitamins, *143*
Summary, *163*

6   MINERAL NEEDS DURING PREGNANCY

Bonnie S. Worthington-Roberts

Introduction, *167*
Minerals, *167*
Maternal and Fetal Determinants of Adult Diseases, *186*
Recommended Dietary Allowances, *188*
Summary, *188*

7   LIFESTYLE CONCERNS DURING PREGNANCY

Bonnie S. Worthington-Roberts

Introduction, *193*
Food Beliefs, Cravings, Avoidances, and Aversions, *193*
Pica, *194*
Potentially Harmful Dietary Components, *195*
Tobacco, Marijuana, and Cocaine, *206*
Rigorous Physical Exercise, *211*
Weight Management, *212*
Improving the Outcome of Pregnancy, *213*
Summary, *216*

8 NUTRITION ASSESSMENT AND GUIDANCE IN PRENATAL CARE

Sue Rodwell Williams

Introduction, *220*
Nutrition Assessment in Health Care During Pregnancy, *221*
Methods of Nutrition Assessment, *223*
Individual Nutrition Assessment, *232*
Nutrition Education and Guidance, *236*
Planning and Implementing Personal Nutrition Programs, *245*
Summary, *252*

9 MANAGEMENT OF PREGNANCY COMPLICATIONS AND SPECIAL MATERNAL DISEASE CONDITIONS

Sue Rodwell Williams
Cristine M. Trahms

Introduction, *254*
Management of High-Risk Pregnancies, *254*
Types of Anemias in Pregnancy, *256*
Hyperemesis Gravidarum, *258*
Hypertensive Disorders, *259*
Diabetes Mellitus, *264*
Maternal Phenylketonuria, *271*
Special Weight Problems in Pregnancy, *279*
Total Parenteral Nutrition During Pregnancy, *284*
Summary, *287*

10 THE PREGNANT ADOLESCENT: SPECIAL CONCERNS

Bonnie S. Worthington-Roberts
Jane Mitchell Rees

Introduction, *292*
Scope of the Problem, *293*
Is Biological Immaturity or "Environmental" Stress More Contributory to Pregnancy Outcome?, *298*
Nutritional Concerns, *302*
Assessing Nutritional Status, *308*
Dietary Patterns in the Adolescent, *309*
Improving Nutrition for Pregnant Teenagers, *310*
An International Prospective, *312*
Special Programs for Pregnant Adolescents, *313*
Summary, *315*

11 LACTATION: BASIC CONSIDERATIONS

Bonnie S. Worthington-Roberts

Introduction, *319*
Anatomy of the Mammary Gland, *319*

Breast Development, *321*
Breast Maturation, *321*
The Physiology of Lactation, *324*
Diet for the Nursing Mother, *335*
Summary, *342*

12   HUMAN MILK COMPOSITION AND INFANT GROWTH AND DEVELOPMENT

Bonnie S. Worthington-Roberts

Introduction, *345*
Composition of Human Milk, *345*
Summary, *384*

13   PROMOTION AND SUPPORT OF BREASTFEEDING

Angela M. Jacobi
Meta L. Levin

Introduction, *393*
Gastrointestinal Benefits, *395*
Antiinfective Properties, *395*
Reduced Risk of Atopic Diseases, *396*
Nutritional Properties, *397*
Cognitive Development, *397*
Other Protective Benefits, *398*
Preconception and Prenatal Period, *405*
Breastfeeding in the Postpartum Period, *409*
Assessment of Adequacy of Breastfeeding, *413*
Feeding Frequency, *414*
Assessment of Output as a Measure of Adequacy, *415*
Importance of Positioning: Comfort for Mother, *416*
Importance of Positioning: Correct for Baby, *416*
Importance of Correct Latching On, *418*
Most Frequent Breastfeeding Concerns, *419*
Physical Discomforts When Beginning Breastfeeding, *423*
Beyond Birth: Maintaining Lactation During Separations and
    Illness, *427*
Contraindications to Breastfeeding, *436*
Breastfeeding Multiples, *437*
Weaning, *437*
Summary, *439*

14   NUTRITION EDUCATION: A SUPPORT FOR REPRODUCTION

Jane Mitchell Rees
Alicia Dixon Docter
Bonnie S. Worthington-Roberts

Introduction, *446*
The Nutritional Environment, *447*

The Process of Nutrition Education, *449*
Groups in Need of Nutrition Education, *450*
Content of Education to Improve Reproduction, *452*
Techniques, *454*
Opportunities for Nutrition Education, *468*
Summary, *473*

APPENDIX   Vitamin and Minerals and Pregnancy Outcome, *479*

GLOSSARY, *487*

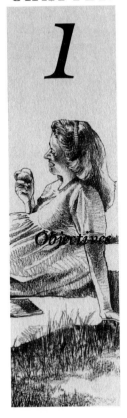

1

Promotion of Maternal and Infant Health

Bonnie S. Worthington-Roberts

✦✦✦

After completing this chapter, the student will be able to:

✓ *Define major indices of maternal and infant health.*

✓ *Describe the factors that increase risk of low birth weight.*

✓ *Discuss characteristics that increase a mother's risk of poor pregnancy outcome.*

✓ *List appropriate goals for the improvement in maternal and infant health in both developed and developing countries.*

Introduction

Of all periods in the life cycle, pregnancy is one of the most critical and is unique. When a woman becomes pregnant, all the experiences of her past join with those of the present to lay the foundations of a new life whose potential, in turn, will influence the welfare of generations to come. The critical place that pregnancy occupies in the chain of life has health and social importance for individuals, families, and society as a whole.

The unique nature of pregnancy lies in the fact that at no other time does the well-being of one individual so directly depend on the well-being of another. During the gestational period the mother and child have an intimate and inseparable relationship. The physical and mental health of the mother before and during her pregnancy has profound effects on the status of her infant in utero and at birth. It is only through efforts directed at the mother that advantages can be provided to ensure that her infant will be born well.

The vulnerability and dependence of the infant and the intergenerational significance of pregnancy in the life cycle have led all societies throughout history to recognize the special needs of pregnant women and to make provisions for their care. In a modern world the goal is no longer simply to produce a living infant from a living mother. As society struggles with problems of overpopulation and scarce resources, we are increasingly faced with the moral and social responsibility to make sure that every woman who chooses to conceive has the opportunity for a safe and successful pregnancy and the ability to deliver and care for an infant whose maximum physical and mental potential is not impaired.

Births[1]

The number of births in the United States has declined each year since 1990. A peak was reached in this year following a gradual rise since 1975. The number of births reached an all-time high in 1961, at the height of the "baby boom."

Year	Number of births
1961	4,268,326
1990	4,158,212
1992	4,065,014
1993	4,039,000 (provisional)

In 1993, the *birth rate* (number of live births per 1,000 population) decreased to 15.7 and the *fertility rate* (number of live births per 1,000 women between the ages of 15 and 44 years) declined to 68.3. Both of these rates are still higher than those that prevailed throughout most of the 1980s.

The decline in births appears to be a result of a combination of a fall in the fertility rate and a declining number of women in childbearing years. A further decrease in the number of births is expected, since it is estimated that there should be a slight decline in the number of women in their childbearing years during the mid-1990s.

Geographic differences are seen in birth rate. Consistent with the national picture, the number of births declined in 38 states and Washington, D.C. but increased in 12 states. Birth rates declined in 44 states and Washington, D.C. and rose in five states, remaining unchanged in one. The highest rates were Utah (19.6), the perennial leader, followed by California (18.9), Texas (18.3), and Arizona (18.0). Lowest were Maine (12.1), West Virginia (12.1), and Vermont (12.6).

Regarding age of the mother, a turning point was reached in 1992 for teenage pregnancies (Table 1-1). From 1986 to 1991, birth rates for women age 15 to 17 increased by 27% but declined 2% in 1992. However, the 1991 and 1992 rates were still higher than in any year since 1973.

TABLE 1-1   *Birth Rates for Young Mothers (Age 15-19), Selected Years, by Race, 1992*

Group	Birth Rate
All races	
1970	68.3
1980	53.0
1985	51.0
1990	59.9
1992	60.7
Race, 1992	
White	51.8
Black	112.4
American Indian	84.4
Asian/Pacific Islander	26.6
Hispanic origin - 1992	
All Hispanic	107.11
Mexican	108.8
Puerto Rican	110.4
Cuban	26.3
Other Hispanic	112.1
Non-Hispanic White	41.7
Non-Hispanic Black	116.0

From National Center for Health Statistics: *Vital statistics of the United States, 1992*, Hyattsville, Md, 1994, US Department of Health and Human Services.

The decline was more marked among black mothers than white; the rates for blacks continue to be substantially higher than for whites.

The leveling off of the sharp rate of increase in teenage childbearing during the 1980s may reflect a similar leveling off since 1988 in the proportion of teenagers who are sexually active, especially among the younger teenagers. In addition, other data suggest that sexually active teenagers are more likely to be using some contraception regularly. Also, according to recently published data, it appears that abortions among teenagers have also declined in recent years. Thus the decline in teenage birth rates in 1992 would indicate that the teenage pregnancy rate has declined as well, following increases from the mid-to-late 1980s.

Births to the very young are always a matter of concern. In 1992, seven "women" younger than age 15, five white, one black, and one American Indian, had their fourth child.

At the upper end of the age spectrum, rates have continued to increase, but somewhat slower than in the past decade. Related to this is the observation that in 1992, one in every five women was childless, a sharp rise from the levels of the 1970s, when the childless proportion was one in nine. In 1992, 49% of women age 30 to 49 who were having a first child were college graduates; of women in this age group in the general population, only 24% were college graduates.

There is considerable variation by race and Hispanic origin (i.e., may be of any race). The fertility rate for black mothers was higher than that for white mothers. In general, those of Hispanic origin had higher birth and fertility rates than any non-Hispanic category. Of Hispanics, the highest rates were among those of Mexican origin and the lowest among those of Cuban origin.

Births to unmarried mothers have not increased in recent years. There is a racial difference, however, with an increase among white unmarried women and further decrease among black. In 1980 the birth rate to unmarried black women was 4.5 times the rate of whites; in 1992 it was 2.5 times.

INDEXES OF MATERNAL AND INFANT HEALTH

The goal of prenatal care is so important that the extent to which it is achieved is often used as a measure of social and economic development among nations throughout the world. International comparisons of maternal and infant health statistics reveal that promoting the health of mothers and infants requires solutions to problems that still affect a sizable proportion of the population. Much of this book focuses on the contribution that nutrition can make toward solving these problems. The importance of nutrition to the course and outcome of pregnancy can be better appreciated when the incidence of reproductive casualties and factors associated with them are understood (see box above)

WHAT INFANT MORTALITY TELLS US

"Infant mortality is the most sensitive index we possess of social welfare and sanitary administration."

A. Newsholme, 1910

To what extent and through what mediating channels do social and economic conditions (as reflected by parental education, income, housing, occupation) affect infant and perinatal mortality? How much of this effect is related to the type and quality of care received, its availability and accessibility and the ability to utilize it? How much of the effect is an outcome of the mother's earlier growth experience in an underprivileged environment, manifested at conception as a reduced capacity to bear healthy children?

From Yankauer A: What infant mortality tells us, *Am J Public Health* 80:653, 1990.

Maternal Mortality and Morbidity

At the turn of the century childbearing was one of the leading causes of mortality among women in all countries of the world. It is still a major cause of death in developing countries[32] (Table 1-2 and Table 1-3), and statistics show that, even in places like the United States, an unacceptable number of women continue to have problems.[10,20,31,32,37]

In 1992, 318 women in the United States were reported to have died of maternal causes (Table 1-2). This number does not include all deaths occurring to pregnant women; rather, it includes those deaths assigned to complications of pregnancy, childbirth, and the puerperium (90 days following birth). The maternal mortality rate for 1992 was 7.8 deaths per 100,000 live births.

Black women have a higher rate of maternal death than white women. In 1992 the maternal mortality rate for black women was 20.8, 4.2 times the rate of 5.0 for white women (Table 1-2). However, this is an improvement over previous years (Fig. 1-1).

TABLE 1-2   *Maternal Mortality in Selected Areas of the World*

Area	Year(s)	Maternal Mortality/ 100,000 Live Births
Africa	1985-1987	640
Asia	1985-1987	420
Latin America	1985-1987	270
Northern and Middle Europe	1985-1987	10
United States (All races)	1992	7.8
White		5.0
All other		18.2
Black		20.8

From Report on confidential enquiries into maternal deaths in the United Kingdom, 1985-1987; and Centers for Disease Control and Prevention: Monthly vital statistics report. Report on final mortality statistics, 1992, March 22, 1995: Public Health Service.

Poverty is known to be directly related to both maternal and infant mortality. The poverty rate for whites was 11.7% in 1994; for blacks and Hispanics, it was 30.6% in the same year. This racial difference is reflected in poverty rates by state; the highest poverty rate was recorded in Louisiana (25.7%); other states with high rates of poverty are Washington, D.C. (21.2%), New Mexico (21.1%), Texas (19.1%) and West Virginia (18.6%). The lowest rate of poverty was reported in Vermont (7.6%).[26]

Maternal deaths are most often a result of complications of the puerperium, other direct obstetric causes, pregnancy with abortive outcome, **ectopic pregnancy** and **preeclampsia/ eclampsia** (Table 1-4). Most health authorities believe that at least some of these deaths are from preventable conditions whose incidence can be reduced through early and high-quality prenatal care.

The characteristics of women dying from maternal causes differ from those of women dying from nonmaternal causes. Overall, women dying

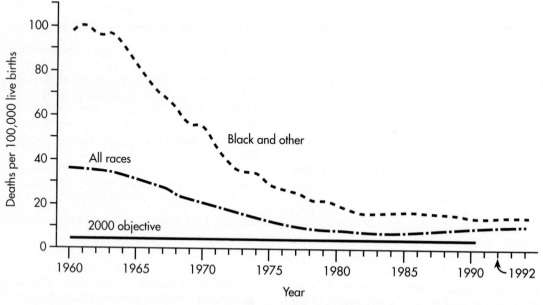

FIG. 1-1   Maternal mortality rates, by race, United States, 1960-1992.

From Centers for Disease Control: Maternal mortality; pilot surveillance in seven states, *JAMA* 255:184, 1986, and National Center for Health Statistics: *Vital statistics of the United States 1992*, Hyattsville, Md, 1995, Department of Health and Human Services.

TABLE 1-3 *Causes of Maternal Mortality in Selected Parts of the World*

Location	Year of Report	Data Source	Findings
Addis Ababa, Ethiopia	1986	Community survey	45 pregnancy-related deaths over 2 years among 9,315 pregnancies (rate: 566 per 100,000 live births); 54% of deaths from illegal abortion complications
Lagos, Nigeria	1977	Hospitals	51% of maternal deaths from abortion complications
60 developing countries	1980	Survey	Approximately 207 induced abortions per 1,000 live births; estimated total of 70,000 to 100,000 maternal deaths per year from abortion-related complications
Harare, Zimbabwe	1985	Harare Maternity Hospital	15% of all pregnancies end in incomplete or induced abortion
Lusaka, Zambia	1983	University teaching hospital	26% of 27 maternal deaths from induced abortion and ectopic pregnancy; 12,096 patients admitted with diagnosis of "spontaneous" abortion
Nairobi, Kenya	1982	Kenyatta National Hospital	Abortion-related complications accounted for 60% of acute gynecologic beds; 50 to 60 patients with induced abortions admitted daily in 1988 (about 20,000 per year in 1988 compared with 2,000 to 3,000 in mid-1970s)
Durban, South Africa	1984	King Edward III Hospital	19% of all maternal deaths from abortion
Bangladesh	1981	63 hospitals, 732 non-hospital facilities	1933 pregnancy-related deaths in 1978-1979, 26% abortion-related; overall estimate 500 to 600 deaths/100,000 live births resulting in estimate of 21,600 maternal deaths annually
Gambia	1987	Rural study	2,000 maternal deaths per 100,000 live births noted; postpartum hemorrhage and infection are leading causes
Zaria, Nigeria	1985	Urban hospital	219 maternal deaths among 7,654 women seen first time in labor vs. 19 deaths among 15,000 who had prenatal care

From Rosenfield A: Maternal mortality in developing countries, *JAMA* 262:376, 1989.

from maternal causes are older, more likely to be black, and more likely to be married than those dying from nonmaternal causes. The impact of maternal age and race on maternal mortality is illustrated in Fig. 1-2. Data from the Maternal Mortality Collaborative Study indicated that maternal mortality increased with age.[23] The maternal mortality ratio for women over 30 was 2.5 times greater than that for younger women.[31] Women are waiting longer to begin their reproductive experience (Table 1-5), therefore this observation is some cause for concern.

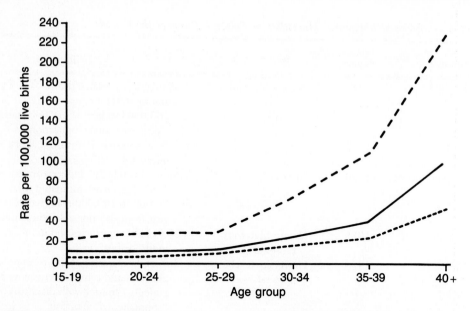

FIG. 1-2   Maternal mortality rates by age and race, Maternal Mortality Collaborative, United States, 1980-1985. Dashed line = black and other; solid line = total; dotted line = white.

From Rochat RW et al: Maternal mortality in the United States, *Obstet Gynecol* 72:91, 1988.

TABLE 1-4   *Maternal Mortality Rates by Selected Causes, United States, 1992*

Causes of Death	Rate/100,000 Live Births	Causes of Death	Rate/100,000 Live Births
Pregnancy with abortive outcome	1.3	Preeclampsia/eclampsia	2.3
Direct obstetric causes	6.1	Obstructed labor	—
Hemorrhage of pregnancy and childbirth	1.0	Complications of the puerperium	2.3
		Other direct obstetric causes	2.5

From National Center for Health Statistics. *Vital statistics of the United States, 1992,* Hyattsville, Md, 1995, US Department of Health and Human Services.

Also relevant is a report of maternal mortality in the state of Massachusetts.[33] To identify ways in which the safety of childbirth might be increased, the causes of death among 886 women who died during pregnancy or within 90 days **postpartum** were evaluated from records available from 1954 through 1985. The maternal mortality rate declined from 50 per 100,000 live births in the early 1950s to the rate of 7 per 100,000 live births in 1984 and 1985. Between one third and one half of the maternal deaths

were considered to be preventable. The leading causes of maternal death from 1954 through 1957 were infection, cardiac disease, pregnancy-associated hypertension, and hemorrhage. In contrast, from 1982 through 1988 the leading causes of death were trauma (suicide, homicide, and motor vehicle accidents) and pulmonary **embolus.**

An important observation in the Massachusetts study[33] was the rapid increase in the frequency of death among women who received

TABLE 1-5   *Birth Rates by Age of Mother*

	Age of Mother			
	15-19	20-24	35-39	40-44
All races*				
1992	60.7	114.6	32.5	5.9
1990	59.9	116.5	31.7	5.5
1985	51.0	108.3	24.0	4.0
1980	53.0	115.1	19.8	3.9
1970	68.3	167.8	31.7	8.1
Race[†]				
White	51.8	108.2	32.2	5.7
Black	112.4	158.0	28.8	5.6
American Indian	84.4	145.5	28.0	6.1
Asian/Pacific Islander	26.6	74.6	50.6	11.0
Hispanic origin[‡]				
All Hispanic	107.1	190.6	45.6	10.9
Mexican	108.8	202.3	47.7	11.8
Puerto Rican	110.4	204.9	30.0	6.5
Cuban	26.3	51.6	28.9	4.7
Other Hispanic	112.1	172.9	50.3	12.5
Non-Hispanic White	41.7	93.9	30.5	5.1
Non-Hispanic Black	116.0	163.0	29.4	5.7

*All races, United States, selected years.

†By race, United States, 1992.

‡Hispanic and non-Hispanic origin, 49 states and DC (NOTE: New Hampshire does not collect information on Hispanic origin), 1992

From National Center for Health Statistics, 1994, Hyattsville, Md

little or no prenatal care. From 1980 through 1984 the maternal mortality rate for white women was 9.6 per 100,000 live births, whereas for nonwhites it was 35 per 100,000 live births. Of the nonwhite women who died during pregnancy or within 90 days postpartum, 50% received little or no prenatal care, in contrast to only 15% of the white women.

With regard to prenatal care, 4.8% of women in the United States did not receive prenatal care in the United States in 1992. However, there were differences among the states; the percentage ranged from 0.32% in Utah to 5.63% in Washington, D.C. When compared with 1980 to 1981, during 1991 to 1992, the percentage

of women who did not receive prenatal care declined in eight states and increased in 42 states and Washington, D.C.; in nine states the increase was greater than 100%, an indication of progress.[36]

Sweden has a low maternal mortality rate, which has not declined in recent years. A recent survey described the pattern of maternal mortality by reviewing all maternal deaths in Sweden from 1980 to 1988. The maternal mortality rate in Sweden for 1980 to 1988 was 7.4 per 100,000 live births. Of the 58 deaths, 36 were direct maternal deaths. Embolism, hemorrhage, preeclampsia, and infection were the predominant causes in the direct cases. Advanced age was the most pronounced risk factor. Suboptimal standard of care was a contributing cause in almost one third of the direct maternal deaths. Accidental or incidental deaths, including suicide, accidents, and pregnancy-related deaths added six cases. There were 76 later maternal deaths, occurring 43 to 365 days postpartum. Malignancy, stroke, and heart disease were the predominant causes. After malignant disease, suicide constituted the leading cause of pregnancy-related deaths within 1 year of delivery. Modes of addressing the prevention of this unfortunate outcome are needed.[15]

A recent look at maternal mortality in the United States focused on death surveillance data from the state of New Jersey. Data were collected about all reported pregnancy-related deaths in the state from 1975 to 1989. Deaths among nonwhites were 3.6 times that for whites for the 15-year period. The causes of pregnancy-related deaths changed over this time with direct obstetrical causes playing a decreasing role. Acquired immunodeficiency syndrome (AIDS) has become the major cause of pregnancy-related mortality in New Jersey. Importantly, approximately 44% of the pregnancy-related deaths were considered to be preventable by the physician or patient or both.[21]

The U.S. Public Health Service's objective for the year 2000 for maternal mortality is a maternal death rate not to exceed 3.3 per 100,000 live births for any county or any ethnic group.[40] The relatively slow decline in the maternal mortality rate for blacks and others suggests that the year 2000 objective may not be met for this group (see Fig. 1-1).

EPIDEMIOLOGIC FACTORS AFFECTING MOTHERS

If progress is to be made in the prevention of death and disability associated with reproduction, specific factors that place women and their infants at risk must be determined. (see box above). Much has been learned about predisposing conditions by studying the distribution of reproductive casualties among population groups. Epidemiologic investigations of this type have revealed the influences of age, parity, maternal birth weight, past obstetrical out-

---

❖

> ### CHARACTERISTICS OF MATERNAL EMPLOYMENT DURING PREGNANCY
>
> **Effects on low birth weight**
> It is generally believed that maternal employment is a risk factor for low birth weight, but the manner in which employment might affect fetal growth is poorly understood. In a recent study, selected characteristics of employment during pregnancy were examined for effects on pregnancy outcomes. Results indicated that women who worked 40 hours per week or more were more likely than women working fewer hours to have a low-birth-weight delivery at ≥ 37 weeks. No physical or environmental characteristics of work were associated with low birth weight or preterm delivery.

From Peoples-Sheps MD et al: Characteristics of maternal employment during pregnancy: effects on low birth weight, *Am J Public Health* 81:1007, 1991.

---

comes, race, social class, and other variables on the course and outcome of pregnancy.[17]

Age

It has become axiomatic that the age of the mother is a determinant of her reproductive efficiency. Very young mothers may not have the physiologic maturity to withstand the additional stresses of pregnancy. Rates of low-birth-weight deliveries are significantly higher among young mothers (Table 1-6). At the other end of the spectrum, older women are beginning to show the effects of the aging process.[29] Consequently, the pattern of reproductive loss by age is a U-shaped curve, with mortality elevated in those under age 15 and over age 35. Mothers who are between 25 and 34 years of age have the best outcome of pregnancy.

Teenage mothers account for a relatively small proportion of all births, 13% in 1992. This fraction has been low in recent years for two reasons: the teenage birth rate has changed very little since 1976, and the number of teenage women declined 14% between 1976 and 1985.

TABLE 1-6 *Percent Low Birth Weight by Age and Race of the Mother (Total of 46 Reporting States and the District of Columbia, 1992)*

Age of the Mother (Years)	Percent Low Birth Weight		
	All Races	White	Black
All ages	7.3	5.9	13.4
Under 15 years	13.4	9.9	15.9
15 to 17 years	10.5	8.5	13.9
18 to 19 years	9.1	7.5	13.2
20 to 24 years	7.4	6.0	12.3
25 to 29 years	6.3	5.2	13.1
30 to 34 years	6.6	5.5	14.8
35 to 39 years	7.7	6.5	16.2
40 to 49 years	8.7	7.4	16.7

From Centers for Disease Control and Prevention: *Monthly vital statistics report*, 43:5 Supp, October 25, 1994.

The birth rates for women age 30 to 39 have increased steadily since 1976. One factor explaining the growth in this proportion is the sizable growth in the number of women in this age group (continued aging of women in the "baby boom" generation).[1]

Parity

Women often experience difficulty with their first pregnancies. First pregnancies are more often complicated by preeclampsia/eclampsia and by problems of labor and delivery. Firstborn infants also show higher rates of mortality and morbidity, but in the opinion of some investigators this may be a result of sociologic rather than physiologic factors.

Regardless of maternal age the risk of low birth weight increases with five pregnancies or more. This is evidence that birth order itself exerts an independent effect on reproductive performance.

These risks of high **parity** are further increased when the pregnancies are closely spaced. Perinatal mortality and morbidity are both greater among high-birth-order infants of mothers whose pregnancies have come in rapid succession.

Medical Risk Factors[7,8]

Adverse pregnancy outcomes, such as low birth weight, preterm delivery, and congenital malformations have been associated with several medical risk factors. The most commonly reported risk factors are anemia, (18.3 per 1,000 live births), diabetes (25.9 per 1,000 live births), and pregnancy-associated hypertension (28.5 per 1,000 live births). Mothers under age 20 are at especially increased risk of anemia (26.8), eclampsia (5.6), and renal disease (2.9). Rates for these factors tend to decrease with advancing age and then rise slightly for mothers 40 years and older.

Black mothers have disproportionately high rates for anemia, chronic hypertension, and eclampsia compared with white mothers. Among older mothers, the racial disparity for chronic hypertension widens; black mothers 30 years and older are approximately three times as likely as white mothers of the same age to have this medical risk factor. Older age of black mothers is also related to higher rates of pregnancy-associated hypertension and diabetes.

Considering other racial groups, rates of all four factors (anemia, diabetes, pregnancy-associated hypertension, and uterine bleeding) are substantially higher for Native American mothers than for any other racial or ethnic group. For example, in 1992 the anemia rate for Native Americans was 57 per 1,000 live births, 82% higher than the rate for black mothers and eight times as high as the rate of 6.8 for Japanese mothers. Among Native American mothers, the incidence of pregnancy-associated hypertension was four times as high as for Chinese mothers (42.1 compared with 9.9).

Chinese mothers have the lowest reported levels of pregnancy-associated hypertension (9.9) and uterine bleeding (4.8) of all the racial groups and comparatively low levels of anemia (10.3). However, the diabetes rate for Chinese mothers of 41.4 is comparable to the high rate for Native Americans of 42.1. Overall, diabetes rates are elevated for each of the Asian and Pacific Islanders groups in comparison with all racial groups except Native Americans.

Rates of medical complications among Hispanic mothers compare favorably with those for white non-Hispanic mothers. This may help to explain the similar levels of low birth weight in this population.

Past Obstetrical Performance

Poor performance in a prior pregnancy increases the chance of problems in subsequent ones. As long ago as 1939, clinicians noted a tendency for women who experienced specific reproductive losses to repeat them.

The chance of having a low-birth-weight infant is also greater when past pregnancy outcome is poor. The proportion of low-birth-weight infants is about one third greater among women whose previous pregnancies ended in fetal deaths. This proportion increases when the low-birth-weight infant follows the fetal death by less than 1 year.

These observations imply that reproductive casualties are not merely chance occurrences. History *does* repeat itself, suggesting underlying circumstances that place some women at continual risk of problems developing each time they are pregnant.

Race. Maternal and perinatal mortality and morbidity rates are two to three times higher among nonwhites as compared with whites in the United States. The higher percentage of low-birth-weight black infants as compared with other groups has remained constant for the past 25 years. However, as mentioned previously, the reasons for this increased risk are not completely understood. Maternal age may account for part of it; teenage mothers are at high risk for producing low-birth-weight infants, and black mothers are more likely to be teenagers than are mothers in other ethnic groups. However, neonatal mortality is higher for blacks at every maternal age; black primiparas older than 23 years of age experience higher neonatal mortality than most black and white teenagers.[11]

Low education level, often a marker of socioeconomic status, is another risk factor for low birth weight. Black mothers are generally less educated than white mothers, and when matched for both age and education, blacks are at higher risk of delivering low-birth-weight infants. Similarly, black women are more likely than white women to delay initiation of prenatal care (Fig. 1-3), but when prenatal care is held constant, black women are still at increased risk of having a low-birth-weight infant. When maternal smoking, stature, pregnancy weight gain, all combinations of age and parity, and history of previous low-birth-weight infants are controlled, black women continue to have an increased risk of low-birth-weight delivery.

In contrast, Mexican Americans of similar economic and sociodemographic characteristics as blacks have a very low incidence of low-birth-weight infants,[44] which may reflect problems of data reporting or cultural differences (e.g., lower incidence of childbearing among unmarried women, different dietary practices, and presence of family support structures). The lower frequency of low birth weight among Hispanics as compared with other ethnic minorities should not, however, diminish attention to these medically underserved women. Their higher birth-weight–specific fetal and neonatal mortality rates as compared with the white non-Hispanic suggest that, given equal access to medical care, their mortality rates could be even lower.

Social class. Social class in Western countries is usually determined by income, occupation, and education. Since social class is so confounded by race, attempts to isolate the effects of socioeconomic variables on reproductive performance must consider variations within racial groups. A number of studies from around the world have confirmed a distinct socioeconomic gradient in the course and outcome of pregnancy.

It appears unlikely that income and education by themselves account for the differences in infant mortality and birth weight. Rather, it is the social and physical environment that these factors represent that is exerting an effect. Better housing, sanitation, diet, and health care, as well as lifestyles that give greater attention to physical and mental health promotion practices, are known to vary significantly with socioeconomic status. It is difficult, however, to capture the direct effects of these conditions on pregnancy outcomes in data from national surveys.

Prenatal care. There has been improvement in the recording on birth certificates of prenatal care[43] measures: the proportion of mothers receiving such care, when it began and how many visits were made. Almost 78% of all mothers be-

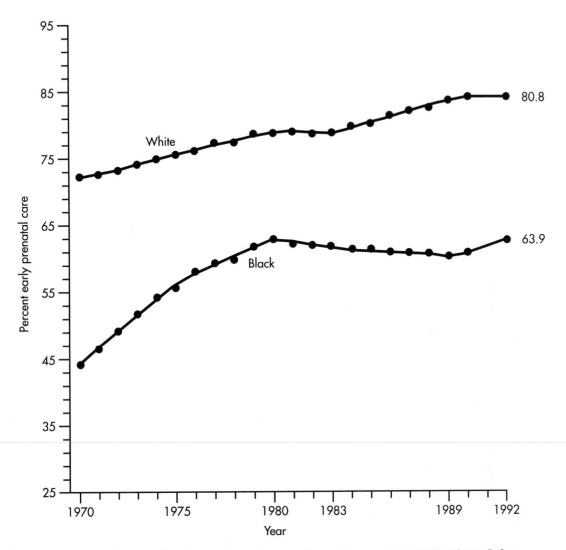

FIG. 1-3 Percent of mothers with early prenatal care, by race, 1970-1992. Note: Infant deaths are classified by race of decedents. Beginning in 1989, live births are classified by race of mother and from 1950-1990, by race of child.

From National Center for Health Statistics. Center for Disease Control: *Advance report of final natality statistics 1989 and 1992,* Hyattsville, Md, Department of Health and Human Services.

gan prenatal care in the first trimester of pregnancy in 1992; 5.2% received care too late or not at all. This represents a modest improvement over the past decade. There is, however, a fair amount of geographic variation in the timeliness of prenatal care. Maine, New Hampshire, Massachusetts, Rhode Island, and Connecticut were the highest in use, all above 87% with Ver-

mont not far behind at 84.5%. Correspondingly, these states had half the national figures for late or no prenatal care.

At the other end of the spectrum, Washington, D.C. had only 57% starting care in the first trimester and 13.9% receiving late or no care. States with high percentages in the latter category, 8% to 10%, included Arizona, New

TABLE 1-7   Timeliness of Prenatal Care by Race and Age, United States, 1992

	% Starting Care in the First Trimester			% No or Late Prenatal Care		
	All Births	15 Years	15 to 19 Years	All Births	15 Year	15 to 19 Years
All races	77.7	42.9	59.5	5.2	17.2	9.7
White	80.8	47.5	62.4	4.2	15.8	8.6
Black	63.9	39.2	53.2	9.9	18.2	12.1

From Wegman ME: Annual summary of vital statistics—1993, *Pediatrics* 94:792, 1994.

Mexico, and Texas. For the black population the geographic situation is different; Pennsylvania had the poorest record, with 16.9% of its black mothers receiving no or late care, followed by the District of Columbia, Minnesota, Nevada, New York, and West Virginia, in all of which the proportion of black mothers receiving no or late care exceeded 13%.

Age affects the timeliness of prenatal care, as is seen in Table 1-7. Attention clearly needs to be focused on the younger age groups who are more likely to suffer from lack of care and whose pregnancies are more likely to be tied to complex societal and relational problems.

Quality of prenatal care is important but hard to measure. Number of visits is one other index that appears on the new birth certificate. The National Center for Health Statistics has used the "Kessner Index", which takes into account timeliness, number of visits, and gestational age, to estimate that 70% of mothers received adequate care and 7% inadequate care in 1992. However, racial differences were great—only 54% of black mothers received adequate care and 15% inadequate care.

Scandinavia is well-known for its exemplary record of good pregnancy outcome. One difference between Scandinavia and other parts of the developed world may lie in its prenatal care strategies.[42] Table 1-8 compares components of prenatal care in Sweden and Finland with those in the United States. An overall more comprehensive approach to care may be evident from the data.

The National Commission to Prevent Infant Mortality has described effective prenatal interventions and their probable impact on infant health statistics. These include the following[25]:

If all women began prenatal care in the first trimester, the number of low-birth-weight infants would be reduced by an estimated 12,600 per year.

If all black women began prenatal care in the first trimester, 3% to 5% of low birth weight among black infants could be prevented. More visits could prevent an additional 9% to 12% of low-birth-weight infants.

If prenatal care were provided in a coordinated, comprehensive manner, with appropriate referrals to WIC programs, substance abuse treatment and high-risk maternity care, the low-birth-weight rate among the infants of high-risk women could be reduced significantly.

If smoking during pregnancy were eliminated, we could expect a 10% reduction in infant mortality and a 25% reduction in low birth weight.

If alcohol consumption during pregnancy were eliminated, we could expect a minimum of 5000 fewer cases of fetal alcohol syndrome and 50,000 fewer alcohol-affected infants.

If more pregnant women were enrolled in the Special Supplemental Food Program for Women, Infants, and Children (WIC), we could expect a decrease in low birth weight, an increase in the number of women seeking early prenatal care, and a modest reduction in the black–white infant mortality gap.

If all pregnancies were planned, infant mortality could be reduced by an estimated 10% and low birth weight by 12%.

Fetal and Infant Death and Disability[18,22]

For purposes of presenting vital statistics, prenatal and infant life are usually divided into developmental stages. These help to identify the

TABLE 1-8   *Prenatal Care in the United States, Finland and Sweden*

	Sweden	Finland	United States
Percent registered for prenatal care			
Of all pregnant women	95	90	—
In first trimester	—	99	76 (1985)
In third trimester or not at all	—	—	6 (1985)
Primary provider	Nurse-midwife	Nurse-midwife	Private physician; physician in clinic
Location	Maternity clinic	Maternity clinic	Private office, hospital, and public clinic
Screening for high risk	Routine	Routine	Yes, for some
Special care for high risk	Routine	Routine	Yes, for some
Network of maternal clinics	Full coverage	Full coverage	Scattered
All care free	Yes	Yes	Some, Medicaid
Cost paid by private or own insurance	No	No	Yes
Official directives for care	Yes	Yes	No
Continuity of care	Yes	Yes	Yes, private
Education of parents	Routine	Routine	Scattered
Maternity package	None	Routine	None
Average number of visits		15.0 (1982)	11.8 (1985)

From Wallace HM et al: Infant mortality in Sweden and Finland: Implications for the United States, *J Perinatol* 10:3, 1989.

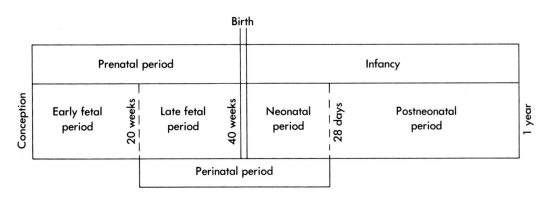

FIG. 1-4   Periods of prenatal and infant life.

periods when the developing child is particularly at risk. The stages are diagrammed in Fig. 1-4.

The 40 weeks of gestation from conception to birth are separated into two 20-week parts. These are termed the *early fetal period* and the *late fetal period,* respectively. The fetus is often referred to as the **conceptus;** during the first 8 to 12 weeks the conceptus is usually referred to as the **embryo.**

Infancy includes the time from birth to 1 year of age. The first 28 days of infant life are called the **neonatal** period. The **postneonatal** period extends from 28 days of age to the infant's first birthday.

Another period has been adopted to recognize that fetal and infant life are parts of an in-separable continuum. This is the perinatal period, which includes the two periods—late fetal and neonatal—that immediately surround birth.

Deaths in the early fetal period are difficult to estimate because loss may occur before the mother realizes that she is pregnant. Consequently, the statistic most often reported is for deaths in the late fetal period. This is called the *fetal death ratio* or sometimes the *stillbirth ratio.* In 1988, fetal deaths in the United States were 7.5 per 1000 live births.[24]

Compared with other developed countries, the United States occupies an inferior position with respect to the number of babies who die in their first year of life (Fig 1-5). Although the infant mortality rate has been steadily declining and is presently at an all-time low, 8.5 deaths per 1,000 live births, this is approximately the rate that some Scandinavian countries had more than 20 years ago. Furthermore, over the past 35 years several countries have experienced more rapid declines in infant mortality than the United States and have overtaken it in international rankings (Table 1-9). In 1950 the United States had the sixth lowest infant mortality rate in the world; by 1972 it ranked at the bottom of a list of 16 countries with vital records of sufficient quality to allow international comparisons to be made. In some parts of the United States where the recession of the early 1980s was especially serious, infant mortality rates deteriorated even further (see box on p. 16). Thus in spite of its wealth and sophisticated systems of health care, the United States has yet to discover the means of ensuring the survival of its youngest citizens. It has been suggested that if the United States had an infant mortality rate similar to that of Sweden in 1967, nearly 40,000 infant deaths could have been prevented in that year alone.[9]

As a result of Sweden's efforts to eliminate poverty and to provide comprehensive health care, there are only small social class differences in infant mortality. The wider social differences in U.S. infant mortality appear to be a consequence of less consistent and thorough attempts at social equity and universal health care. The excess infant mortality among blacks in the U.S. may partially result from racism. Public health research should examine the role of racism in infant mortality and develop interventions to

TABLE 1-9 *Infant Mortality Rates for Countries With Population Greater than 2,500,000 (Data Available September 30, 1994)*

Country	Infant Mortality Rate (1993)
Japan	4.4
Singapore	4.7
Sweden	4.8
Finland	4.4
Norway	5.9 (1992)
Canada	6.1 (1992)
Germany	6.2 (1992)
Netherlands	6.3
Hong Kong	6.4 (1991)
Switzerland	6.2
France	6.2
Denmark	5.7
United Kingdom	6.6 (1992)
Ireland	6.0
Australia	7.0 (1992)
New Zealand	7.2
Spain	7.6
Austria	6.5
Belgium	8.0
Italy	7.4
Greece	8.5
United States	8.3

Data from the United Nations Statistical Office: *Infant mortality rate per 1,000 live births,* 1994.

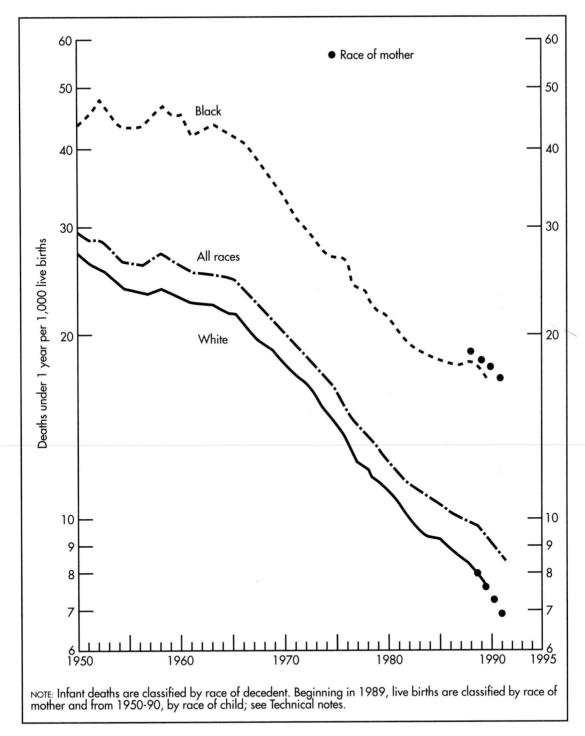

NOTE: Infant deaths are classified by race of decedent. Beginning in 1989, live births are classified by race of mother and from 1950-90, by race of child; see Technical notes.

FIG. 1-5 Infant mortality rates by race: United States, 1950-92.

❖

RATES OF MAJOR CONGENITAL MALFORMATIONS, UNITED STATES, 1992

Malformation	Rate per 1000 births
Anencephalus	0.13
Spina bifida/meningomyelocele	0.22
Hydrocephalus	0.26
Other central nervous	0.09
system anomalies	0.24
Heart malformations	1.20
Other circulatory/respiratory anomalies	1.31
Rectal atresia/stenosis	0.11
Tracheo-esophageal fistula/ esophageal atresia	0.14
Omphalocele/gastroschisis	0.24
Other gastrointestinal anomalies	0.31
Malformed genitalia	0.74
Renal agenesis	0.11
Other urogenital anomalies	1.14
Cleft lip/palate	0.85
Polydactyly, syndactyly, adactyly	0.84
Club foot	0.57
Diaphragmatic hernia	0.12
Other musculoskeletal/ integumental anomalies	1.87
Down syndrome	0.50
Other chromosomal anomalies	0.42

From National Center for Health Statistics: *Monthly vital statistics report* 43:5, October 25, 1994.

eliminate racism and its effects on the health of black Americans.[16]

Some clues to the problem of infant mortality are gained by looking more closely at when and how these infants die. By far, the largest number die within the first 28 days of life (Table 1-10). The neonatal death rate in the United States was 5.38 per 1,000 live births in 1993 compared with 2.91 in the postneonatal period.[24]

Postneonatal deaths are related to conditions in the infant's immediate environment. Rates are particularly high in poor countries without safe and hygienic conditions in the hospital and in the home. Neonatal deaths are more often associated with prenatal factors. The relatively high infant mortality rate in the United States can therefore often be traced to conditions that influence or are concurrent with the mother's state during pregnancy. To emphasize this point, it has been noted that of all infant deaths in the United States in a given year, more than half occur in the first 5 days of life, before most infants even leave the hospital and in spite of the intensive care that modern hospitals are able to provide. A large proportion of infant deaths is caused by conditions associated with immaturity (Table 1-11). Other causes include sudden infant death, congenital defects, major accidents, birth trauma, certain gastrointestinal diseases, and homicide.

The following are the facts about neonatal and postneonatal mortality in the United States: (1) Two thirds of all infant deaths occur in the neonatal period; (2) leading causes of infant deaths are congenital anomalies, disorders related to premature birth, respiratory distress syndrome, and the effects of maternal complications; (3) one third of all infant deaths occur in the postneonatal period; (4) the leading causes of death in the postneonatal period are sudden infant death syndrome (SIDS), congenital anomalies, injuries, and infection; (5) during the 1970s and 1980s, postneonatal death declined at a slower rate than neonatal mortality. This is in part a result of an increased number of unhealthy infants who survive the first 27 days after birth and later die in the postneonatal period (Figs. 1-6 and 1-7).

Despite national efforts at improving overall infant mortality, the black-to-white ratio has changed little in recent years and is still higher than in 1940 (Table 1-12), meaning that the improvement for black infants has been slower than for whites. This difference is even greater in the group younger than 28 days of age, for whom the decline in mortality for whites has been 83.5% and for blacks, 71.9%.

Differences are seen between infant mortality rates for white and black infants by cause. Congenital anomalies were the leading cause of death for white infants (25.6%). In contrast for black infants, the leading cause of death was disorders relating to short gestation and unspeci-

TABLE 1-10 **U.S. Neonatal and Postneonatal Mortality Rates (NMR and PMR) and Cause-Specific Infant Mortality Rates per 1,000 Live Births, by Maternal Race or Ethnicity, 1985 through 1987**

| Race/Ethnicity | NMR | PMR | Cause of Death* | | | | Number of Live Births |
			Perinatal Conditions	Congenital Anomalies	SIDS	Other Causes	
White[†]	5.5	3.1	3.8	2.1	1.2	1.5	1,814,669
Black	12.0	6.2	10.1	2.3	2.3	3.5	1,782,007
American Indian	6.1	7.2	4.0	2.4	3.2	3.7	103,191
Asian and Pacific Islander	4.7	2.9	3.1	2.0	1.0	1.5	327,178
Chinese	3.4	2.6	2.2	1.6	0.9	1.2	50,572
Japanese	3.9	2.7	2.6	1.7	1.3	1.0	23,919
Filipino	4.7	2.5	2.9	2.1	0.9	1.3	63,060
Other Asian[‡]	5.0	3.1	3.3	2.2	0.9	1.6	174,479
Hawaiian	7.1	4.3	5.0	2.2	1.9	2.2	15,148
Hispanic[§]	5.5	3.0	3.9	2.1	0.8	1.7	1,168,084
Mexican	5.2	2.9	3.6	2.1	0.8	1.7	740,382
Puerto Rican	7.3	3.7	5.7	2.1	1.0	2.1	109,874
Cuban	5.5	2.2	3.8	1.9	0.8	1.3	29,935
Central and South American	5.2	2.6	3.8	2.0	0.5	1.5	136,367
Other and unknown Hispanic	5.7	3.4	3.9	2.3	1.2	1.7	151,526

*ICD-9 codes 760–779 (perinatal conditions), 740–759 (congenital anomalies), and 798.0 (sudden infant death syndrome [SIDS]).
†Based on a 20% sample of live births
‡Includes Asian Indians, Koreans, Vietnamese, Cambodians, Laotians, Indonesians, and other Asian and Pacific Islanders
§Based on data from 23 reporting states and the District of Columbia
Data from National Linked Birth and Infant Death data sets, 1985-1987.

fied low birth weight (17.8%) (see box on p. 18). However, although the difference between black and white infant mortality rates varied by cause, the risk was higher for black than for white infants for all the leading causes.[1]

Researchers from Yale University examined the black-white difference in infant mortality rates from 1982 through 1986 in 38 U.S. standard metropolitan statistical areas. Infant mortality varied by a factor of almost seven (Table 1-12). Careful examination of the data showed that the most important predictor of black-white difference was an index of "segregation," independent of black-white differences in median family income and prevalence of poverty. Certain areas of California have relatively low segregation indexes and small black-white differences in infant mortality, despite considerable black-white differences in prevalence of poverty. The reasons for the apparent effect of residential segregation have not been determined.[28]

TABLE 1-11   *Infant Mortality Rates*
for Major Cause Groups
(per 1,000 Live Births, 1993
Provisional Rate)

Cause	Infant Mortality Rate
All causes	8.3
Congenital anomalies	1.7
Perinatal conditions not separately listed	2.1
Sudden infant death syndrome	1.2
Short gestation and low birth weight	1.0
Intrauterine hypoxia, birth asphyxia	0.2
Respiratory distress syndrome	0.6
Pneumonia and influenza	0.1
Accidents and adverse effects	0.2
Homicide, including child battering	0.07
Birth trauma	0.04
Certain gastrointestinal diseases	0.05
All other causes	Residual

From National Center for Health Statistics: *Vital statistics for the United States. Provisional data estimated from a 10% sample of deaths,* Hyattsville, Md, 1994, US Department of Health and Human Services.

A related observation, reported in 1992, focuses on mortality among infants of black as compared with white college-educated parents.[34] Researchers used the National Linked Birth and Infant Death Files for 1983 through 1985. In this population, the infant mortality rate was 10.2 per 1,000 live births for black infants and 5.4 per 1,000 live births for white infants. The rate of low birth weight was more than twice as high among blacks (7%) as among whites (3%). After exclusion of low-birth-weight infants, the mortality rates for black and white infants were equal. The obvious question is: why the difference in rate of low birth weight between the two groups?

BLACK–WHITE INFANT MORTALITY GAP IN THE UNITED STATES

There has been no improvement in the gap between black and white infant mortality rate in almost 40 years.

Black infants are twice as likely as white infants to die in the first year of life.

A black infant born in 1987 had less chance of living to his or her first birthday than did a white infant born in 1970; an infant born in Cuba had a better chance of surviving than a black infant born in Washington, D.C.

The infant mortality rate of Hispanics and Asians is similar to the rate in whites; the rate in blacks, on the other hand, is over 100% higher and in Native Americans 40% higher.

Black and Hispanic mothers are more likely to receive late or no prenatal care; the same applies to Native American mothers.

The western states of the United States report lower rates of black infant mortality than the rest of the country, mainly due to a lower rate of low birth weight among blacks; this suggests that improvements in black infant mortality are achievable.

Another observation relevant to this discussion was reported by researchers in Boston who studied health behaviors and birth outcome among 201 foreign-born and 616 U.S.-born black women receiving prenatal care at Boston City Hospital.[5] Foreign-born women had better prepregnancy nutritional status and prenatal health behaviors, and their infants had greater intrauterine growth. The investigators concluded that black women are not a homogeneous group and that culture and ethnicity (in addition to other variables) must be considered in the study of their birth outcomes.

Infant mortality among Hispanics in the United States is higher than that of whites but not as high as recorded for blacks. Among Hispanic groups, the neonatal mortality risk is re-

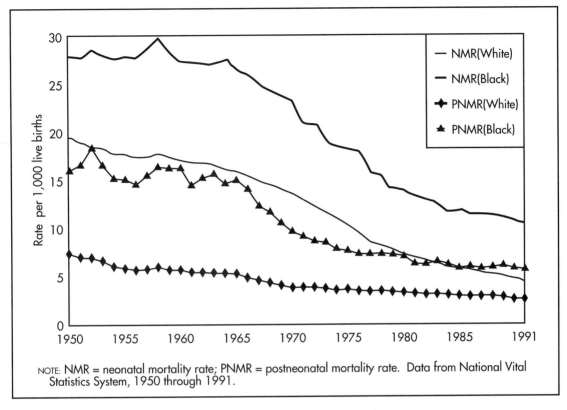

FIG. 1-6 U.S. neonatal and postneonatal mortality rates by race of child, 1950 through 1991.

From Singh GR, Yu SM: Infant morality in the United States: trends, differentials, and projections, 1950 through 2010, *Am J Public Health* 85:957, 1995.

portedly higher among Puerto Rican islanders and continental Puerto Ricans and lower among Cuban Americans and Mexican Americans. The postneonatal mortality risk in the 1980s was highest among continental Puerto Ricans and lowest among Cuban Americans. It is clear that there is much heterogeneity in the Hispanic population in the United States, and this suggests that interventions to prevent infant mortality be tailored to ethnic-group–specific risk factors and outcomes.[1,43]

Another group at high risk for infant mortality is the Native American population. Although there has been a dramatic decrease in infant mortality in this group, it remains higher than the national rate. Especially problematic is post-

neonatal mortality, which is twice as high as that in the white race. Limited data suggest that this postneonatal difference may result largely from preventable accidents, SIDS, and treatable medical conditions such as gastroenteritis. This suggests that Native American infants leave the hospital healthy but go home to unsafe environments, which decrease their chances of survival beyond 1 year. In particular, the poorer socioeconomic conditions that Native American families experience and the related problems of alcoholism, unemployment, and family disorganization contribute to the high rate of postneonatal mortality. Intervention programs to lower the postneonatal mortality of Native Americans should focus on promoting prompt health seek-

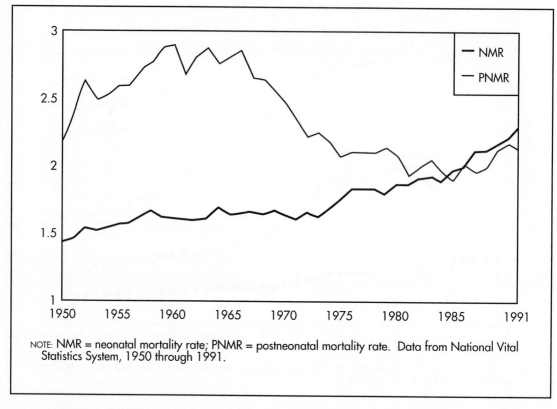

FIG. 1-7 Black/white ratios of U.S. neonatal and postneonatal mortality rates, 1950 through 1991.

From Singh GR, Yu SM: Infant mortality in the United States: trends, differentials, and projections, 1950 through 2010, *Am J Public Health,* 85:957, 1995.

ing for treatable medical conditions, and prevention of accidents and other postneonatal health problems.[35]

As a group, women born in Mexico who give birth in the United States have birth outcomes that are as good as or are better than those of white Americans or Mexican Americans (i.e., U.S.-born women of Mexican descent). Data show that Mexican immigrants have lower rates of low birth weight, intrauterine growth retardation and infant mortality. Although underregistration of infant deaths has been claimed to artificially inflate favorable birth outcomes, health advantages may be associated with improved birth outcomes.[12]

Mexican immigrants also bring with them a cultural orientation that includes many protective behaviors and values that enhance perinatal outcomes—lower consumption of alcohol, drugs, and cigarettes, particularly during pregnancy. Immigrants also tend to adhere to a traditional Mexican diet which is high in vitamins A and C, folate, calcium, iron, and protein. In addition, Americans tend to migrate away from kinship networks, whereas Mexicans migrate toward them. Such networks may assist mothers in providing adequate nutrition, child care, and support for drug-free habits, as well as provide emotional and financial support. At a time of pressure in the United States to restrict access to health care for immigrants, attention might well be given to focusing on protecting their health from the harmful effects of acculturation.[12]

TABLE 1-12   *Infant Mortality (per 1,000 Live Births) by Age and Race, Selected Years*

	1993	1990	1988	1985	1980	1960	1940	% Decline 1940 to 1991
Total	8.29	9.2	9.95	10.6	12.6	26.0	47.0	81.1
White		7.6	8.51	9.3	11.0	22.9	43.2	83.1
Black		17.6	17.62	18.2	21.4	44.3	72.9	75.9
B/W ratio		2.4	2.07	2.0	1.9	1.9	1.7	—
<28 days	5.38	5.8	6.32	7.0	8.5	18.7	28.8	80.6
White		4.8	5.37	6.1	7.5	17.2	27.2	83.5
Black		11.6	11.45	12.1	14.1	27.8	39.9	71.9
B/W ratio		2.4	2.13	2.0	1.9	1.6	1.5	—
Postneonatal	2.91	3.4	3.64	3.7	4.1	7.3	18.3	81.4
White		2.8	3.15	3.2	3.5	5.7	16.0	82.5
Black		6.4	6.12	6.1	7.3	16.5	33.0	80.9
B/W ratio		2.3	1.96	1.9	2.1	2.9	2.1	—

From National Center for Health Statistics: *Vital statistics of the United States: figures for 1993 are provisional, that is estimated from a 10% sample of deaths. Total values include races other than white and black,* Hyattsville, Md, 1993, US Department of Health and Human Services.

On the positive side, the infant mortality rate in the United States is the lowest ever recorded. Both neonatal and postneonatal components participated; however, for the first time (1992) in some years the postneonatal decline was distinctly more rapid (about 6%) than the neonatal, which was less than 1%. From 1940, when antibiotics became available, to 1980 the decline in neonatal and postneonatal mortality was about equal. Some interpreted this as an indication that advances in preventing and treating infectious and other diseases of later infancy were keeping pace with advances in neonatology. From 1980 to 1992 the decline in neonatal mortality was considerably faster (some 36%) as neonatology moved forward, whereas the postneonatal mortality rate declined about 24%. No clear explanation for the very recent difference is apparent, so it may simply be a short-term variation.[35]

The geographic variation in infant mortality in the United States is worthy of comment. By region, the lowest mortality rate in 1993 was observed in New England (6.8 per 1,000 live births); of the states, New Hampshire had the lowest rate (4.8 per 1,000 live births). In 1993, Washington, D.C. again had the highest infant mortality rate, with 18.6 deaths per 1,000 live births (Table 1-13). States with the highest infant mortality rates were Mississippi (11.9), South Dakota (10.5), Illinois (10.3), North Carolina (10.3), and Georgia (10.1).

A high rate of early infant death is the worst possible outcome of pregnancy, but the casualties of reproduction also include the thousands of children who are impaired but do not die. These children suffer from the same conditions that in their most severe forms cause death, as well as disorders such as **cerebral palsy, epilepsy,** and mental retardation. Still more have physical handicaps and developmental disabilities that may be prenatal in origin but are undetected until later in life.

RISKS OF LOW BIRTH WEIGHT

Infants who weigh less than 2500 g (5 lb 8 oz) at birth are referred to as **low birth weight.** Although the word *premature* is sometimes used to describe these infants, the term is confusing because low-birth-weight infants are really of two different types: those who are born too small because they are born too soon, and those who are born on time but are too small for their gestational age. To avoid confusion, the word

TABLE 1-13   *Infant and Neonatal Mortality, Final for 1992*

State and Region	Mortality Rate <1 Year	Mortality Rate <28 Days	State and Region	Mortality Rate <1 Year	Mortality Rate <28 Days
New England	6.8	4.7	South Atlantic—cont'd		
Maine	5.6	3.5	North Carolina	10.0	6.8
New Hampshire	5.9	3.4	South Carolina	10.4	6.9
Vermont	7.2	4.0	Georgia	10.3	6.7
Massachusetts	6.5	4.8	Florida	8.8	5.9
Rhode Island	7.4	5.4	East South Central	9.9	6.1
Connecticut	7.6	5.5	Kentucky	8.3	4.6
Middle Atlantic	8.8	5.9	Tennessee	9.4	5.7
New York	8.8	5.9	Alabama	10.5	6.9
New Jersey	8.4	5.7	Mississippi	11.9	7.5
Pennsylvania	9.0	6.0	West South Central	8.3	5.0
East North Central	9.5	6.1	Arkansas	10.3	5.9
Ohio	9.4	5.9	Louisiana	9.4	5.7
Indiana	9.4	6.0	Oklahoma	8.8	5.1
Illinois	10.1	6.5	Texas	7.8	4.7
Michigan	10.2	6.7	Mountain	7.5	4.1
Wisconsin	7.2	4.3	Montana	7.5	3.0
West North Central	8.0	4.8	Idaho	8.8	5.2
Minnesota	7.1	4.5	Wyoming	8.9	4.0
Iowa	8.0	4.7	Colorado	7.6	4.2
Missouri	8.5	5.2	New Mexico	7.6	3.9
North Dakota	7.8	5.0	Arizona	8.4	4.8
South Dakota	9.3	5.1	Utah	5.9	3.5
Nebraska	7.4	3.9	Nevada	6.7	2.9
Kansas	8.7	5.3	Pacific	7.0	4.2
South Atlantic	9.8	6.5	Washington	6.8	3.7
Delaware	8.6	5.9	Oregon	7.1	3.8
Maryland	9.8	6.7	California	7.0	4.3
District of Columbia	19.6	12.9	Alaska	8.6	4.0
Virginia	9.5	6.3	Hawaii	6.3	3.9
West Virginia	9.2	5.6			

From National Center for Health Statistics: *Vital statistics of the United States: rates per 1,000 live births,* Hyattsville, Md, 1995, US Department of Health and Human Services.

preterm is used for infants born under 37 weeks gestation; **small for gestational age** describes infants who are underweight at birth, whatever the gestational age.

On a worldwide basis, of the 127 million infants born in 1982, 16%—some 20 million—had a low birth weight. Variations between and within geographic regions remain considerable.[38] The incidence of low birth weight by region ranges from 31.1% in Middle South Asia

and 19.7% for Asia as a whole to 14.0% in Africa, 10.1% in Latin America, 6.8% in North America, and 6.5% in Europe (Table 1-14). In countries where the proportion of low-birth-weight infants is low, most are preterm; where the proportion is high, the majority of low-birth-weight infants have fetal growth retardation. The causes of fetal growth retardation are multiple and interrelated and include low maternal food intake, hard physical work during pregnancy, and illness, es-

TABLE 1-14 *Estimated Number of Births of All Live Infants and Low-Birth-Weight Infants by Region, 1982; and Estimated Proportion of Low-Birth-Weight Infants, 1979 and 1982*

Region	Live Births*	Low-Birth-Weight Infants		
		1982*	1979 (%)[†]	1982 (%)
Africa	23,148	3,233	15.0	14.0
North Africa	4,814	495	13	10
Western Africa	7,278	1,256	17	17
Eastern Africa	6,930	922	14	13
Middle Africa	2,554	398	15	16
Southern Africa	1,372	162	15	12
North America	4,402	299	7.3	6.8
Latin America	12,490	1,259	10.2	10.1
Middle America	3,669	448	12[‡]	12
Caribbean	867	102	13	12
Tropical South America	7,033	647	9	9
Temperate South America	921	62	8	7
Asia	74,885	14,750	20.3	19.7
Western South Asia	4,080	302	16	7
Middle South Asia	35,311	10,947	31	31
Eastern South Asia	12,336	2,088	18	17
East Asia	23,158	1,413	6	6
Europe	6,857	445	7.7	6.5
Northern Europe	1,010	61	6	6
Western Europe	1,819	95	6	5
Eastern Europe	1,855	140	8	8
Southern Europe	2,173	149	9	7
Oceania	507	59	12.2	11.6
Union of Soviet Socialist Republics	5,111	409	8.0	8.0
World	127,400	20,450	16.8	16.0
Developed countries	18,200	1,250	7.4	6.9
Developing countries	109,200	19,200	18.4	17.6

*In thousands
[†]Decimals are only shown for continents, since estimates for subregions are subject to a greater margin of error
[‡]Previous estimate for Middle America corrected
From United Nations, Department of International Economic and Social Affairs: *Demographic indicators of countries: estimates and projects assessed in 1980,* New York, 1982, United Nations Publications.

pecially infection. Short maternal stature, very young age, high parity, and close birth spacing are all associated factors. Although suboptimal nutritional support may be associated with all of these factors, it is impossible to quantify the significance of this variable with the etiologic factors of low birth weight in any setting.

The overall incidence of low birth weight for 1992 was 7.1%, the highest rate reported since 1978 (Table 1-15). However, the proportion of low birth weight among black infants was 13.2%, whereas for whites, it was 5.8%. The incidence of very low birth weight (less than 1,500 grams) was 1.3% but again the level for blacks was 3.0%, whereas that for whites was 1.0%. The median birth weight for babies born in 1992 was 3,360 grams; for whites, it was 3,410 grams and for blacks it was 3,170 grams.

TABLE 1-15   *Percent of Low Birth Weight and Preterm Births, by Race of Mothers; United States, 1992*

Race of Mother	% Low Birth Weight	% Very Low Birth Weight	% Preterm
All races	7.1	1.3	10.7
White	5.8	1.0	9.1
Black	13.3	3.0	18.4
American Indian	6.2	1.0	11.6
Asian and Pacific Islander	—	—	—
Total	6.6	0.9	9.9
Chinese	5.0	0.7	7.0
Japanese	7.0	0.8	7.9
Hawaiian	6.9	1.0	11.4
Filipino	7.4	1.1	10.9
Other	6.7	0.9	10.5

From Centers for Disease Control and Prevention: *Monthly vital statistics report,* 43:5, October 25, 1994.

Some reasons for the higher rate of low birth weight among black infants are that they are much more likely to be born preterm and their mothers are more likely to have a lower weight gain during pregnancy. However, even for mothers with ideal weight gain and length of gestation, the risk of low birth weight for black infants is twice that for white infants.

Infants born to Native American mothers have a relatively favorable level of low birth weight (6.2%), despite high levels of teenage childbearing and numerous other demographic and medical risk factors. This is in part a result of the comparatively modest levels of low birth weight among Native American teenagers—the lowest of any other racial or ethnic group in 1992 (6.2%).

Among Asian and Pacific Islander births,[6] low-birth-weight levels ranged from a low of 5.0% for Chinese births, the lowest level reported for any racial or ethnic group, to 7.4% for Filipino births. Japanese births recently rose to 7.0% low birth weight. There is obviously much heterogeneity among the Asian and Pacific Is-

landers with regard to this birth outcome. Among Hispanic mothers, the incidence of low birth weight in 1992 was 6.1%, ranging from 5.6% for infants born to Mexican mothers to 9.2% for Puerto Rican infants.[7]

It appears to be an anomaly that Mexican women have a very favorable pregnancy outcome as measured by percent low birth weight. The prevalence of traditional risk factors, including elevated rates of teenage childbearing, low educational levels, and inadequate prenatal care, would appear to place Mexican infants at great peril. Some possible explanations are that low levels of tobacco and alcohol use and adequate nutrition during pregnancy among pregnant Mexican women may offset sociodemographic risks. Noteworthy, however, is the observation that Mexican mothers born outside the United States have a substantially lower rate of low birth weight (5.1%) than do their US-born counterparts (6.5%). This suggests that the protective practices of Mexican mothers born abroad, which contribute to their good birth outcomes, may not be sustained in the second generation of Mexican mothers.[7]

Closely spaced births are associated with higher levels of low birth weight and other adverse outcomes. For 1992, 27% of births occurred within 2 years and about one half within 3 years. Black infants are more likely than white infants to be born at short intervals.[30] This reflects their higher fertility and younger ages at the beginning of childbearing of black mothers. When born at these shortened intervals, black infants are also more likely to be of low birth weight than white infants (16.6% compared with 6.5%).

The proportion of infants born preterm was 10.7% in 1992. (see table 1-15). This represents a small improvement over recent years and it largely occurred among preterm births to black mothers (18.4%). The incidence of preterm births for white mothers was 9.1% in 1992. The risk of early birth varied widely by age of the mother, with rates ranging from 8.1% for mothers ages 25 to 29 to 18.4% for mothers under age 15. White teenage mothers ages 15 to 19 were as likely as mothers 40 years and older to have a preterm birth (11.6%).[7,8]

New information relevent to the etiologic factors of low birth weight is now available from the revised U.S. Certificate of Live Birth for 47 states and Washington D.C. The revised certificate includes questions relating to medical risk factors during pregnancy, such as anemia and heart disease, and such factors as tobacco and alcohol use, and weight gain during pregnancy. These data combined with other socioeconomic data from birth certificates should improve the likelihood of understanding the persistent and large racial differentials in the incidence of low birth weight in the United States.

The adverse outcomes experienced by preterm and growth-retarded infants are so well-documented that low birth weight itself is considered an adverse outcome of pregnancy. Deaths of low-birth-weight infants in the neonatal period are about 30 times more common than deaths of newborns of normal weight. Data confirm that perinatal mortality varies to a much greater extent with birth weight than with the length of gestation. It is widely believed that if the birth-weight distribution could be improved, this alone would produce a substantial reduction in infant mortality.

A number of studies have also shown an increased incidence of handicapping conditions among infants who have the misfortune of being born too small. Low birth weight is a known etiologic factor in cerebral palsy, and it has been implicated in epilepsy and various forms of mental retardation as well. There is also evidence that, as a group, children who were extremely undersized at birth have more frequent hospitalizations for illness, more visual and hearing disabilities, more behavioral disorders, and more learning problems when they enter school.[13]

The Kramer Study

A Canadian study[19] researched the determinants of intrauterine growth retardation and shortened gestation. A review was conducted of the English- and French-language medical literature published from 1970 to 1984, focusing on 43 potential determinants of intrauterine growth and gestational duration. Factors with well-established direct causal impact were identified and their relative importance indicated for typical developing and developed country settings.

In developing countries, race is a determinant responsible for a large proportion of intrauterine growth retardation, particularly in countries with a high prevalence of black and Indian racial origins. The other major factors are poor gestational nutrition, low prepregnant weight, short maternal stature, and malaria. Of the five leading factors, three may be modifiable in the short term: gestational nutrition, prepregnant weight, and malaria.

The single most important factor determining intrauterine growth retardation in developed countries is cigarette smoking. This is followed by poor gestational nutrition, low prepregnancy weight, primiparity, and short stature. These are all potentially modifiable, once again with obvious implications for public health intervention.

For gestational duration, only prepregnancy weight, prior history of prematurity or spontaneous abortion, in utero exposure to diethylstilbestrol, and cigarette smoking have well-established direct causal effects. In developing countries as well as developed countries most instances of prematurity occurring in the population remain unexplained. Prematurity is a major focus of etiologic research on low birth weight in developed countries.

Interventions should be specific for the population concerned and aimed at modifiable determinants of intrauterine growth and gestational duration that are quantitatively important for that population. Public health authorities, however, also need to consider such issues as cost effectiveness, cultural acceptability, and political feasibility. Although beyond the scope of this book, these issues must be weighed in planning any intervention program.

CONTRIBUTION OF WOMEN, INFANTS, AND CHILDREN PROGRAM TO IMPROVING MATERNAL AND CHILD HEALTH

The Special Supplemental Food Program for Women, Infants and Children (WIC) was established over a decade ago to assure adequate nutrition for this high-risk population. It is funded by the U.S. Department of Agriculture and provides nutrition education for low-income women and children and vouchers for the purchase of specific supplemental foods and infant formula. Pregnant, breastfeeding, and postpartum women; infants; and children up to age 5 who are at medical or nutritional risk are eligible. WIC also refers participants to prenatal care, well-child care and other services.

A number of studies over the years have shown that maternal participation in prenatal WIC programs improves birth outcomes. However, cost-benefit studies have been few. Recently, researchers in North Carolina linked Medicaid and WIC data files to birth certificates for live births in North Carolina in 1988.[4] It was found that women who received Medicaid benefits and prenatal WIC services had substantially lower rates of low and very low birth weight than did women who received Medicaid but not prenatal WIC. Among white women, the rate of low birth weight was 22% lower for WIC participants and the rate of very low birthweight was 44% lower. Among black women, the rates were 31% and 57% lower, respectively, for the WIC participants. From these data it was estimated that for each dollar spent on WIC services, Medicaid savings in costs for newborn medical care were $2.91. A high level of WIC participation was associated with better birth outcomes. These findings strongly suggest that prenatal WIC participation can effectively reduce low birthweight and newborn medical care costs among infants born to women in poverty.

THE CHALLENGE AHEAD— MEASURES TO IMPROVE MATERNAL AND INFANT SURVIVAL AND HEALTH

The epidemiologic data provide a profile of women who have the greatest risk of problems developing in pregnancy:

Nonwhite race
Poverty
Lack of education
Under 17 or over 35 years of age
First pregnancy or high parity
Pregnancies less than 1 year apart
Prior obstetrical complications
Previous fetal/infant death or disability
Use of tobacco

Women with one or more of these characteristics are also more likely to produce a low-birth-weight infant who has physical or mental impairments or who will die in the first year of life. These women must be the targets of special intervention if recurrent tragedies of reproductive loss are to be prevented.

After a period of virtual stagnation at midcentury, the reduction in infant mortality began to accelerate and the gap between whites and nonwhites is now the narrowest it has ever been. There is evidence, however, that the picture can still be improved.

In 1979 the U.S. Surgeon General issued a report on health promotion and disease prevention entitled *Healthy People*.[14] In this report the Surgeon General pointed out that despite the progress made in reducing infant mortality, the first year of life remains the most hazardous period for all Americans until age 65. The death rate for black infants is about the same as the rate for white infants was 25 years ago. The United States must continue to try to improve maternal and infant health (see box on p. 27). Reducing the rate of low birth weight is seen as one of the most important means of reaching this goal.

This chapter has attempted to demonstrate that morbidity and mortality rates are the end results of a number of complex and interrelated factors. Any attempt to explain them in terms of a single cause or a simple solution will only confound efforts to find answers to the problems that still remain. Nonetheless, it is not unreasonable to assert that the extension of better prenatal care to disadvantaged women and the wider availability and acceptance of family planning have greatly contributed to the overall decline in reproductive casualties over the past 20 years.

These measures should continue to improve pregnancy outcomes. It is doubtful, however, that they alone can equalize the risks for white and nonwhite women and their infants. It is also unlikely that bringing the nonwhite infant mortality rate into line with that of whites will automatically move the United States from its present basement position to the top of the list of international rankings.

One implication is that if further progress is to be made in promoting maternal and infant

BORN IN THE USA: INFANT HEALTH PARADOX

Immigrants experience better perinatal outcomes than U.S.-born women. Researchers in California reported this finding after studying data from the Comprehensive Perinatal Program (CPP) at the University of California at San Diego Medical Center. Records of 1,464 low-income women who received prenatal care through the program and gave birth at the center through 1991 were studied. Overall, 61% of the babies of foreign-born women obtained the scale's optimum score, compared with 54% of the U.S.-born women's babies. Within racial and ethnic groups, 71% of Asian-born women's infants obtained the top score. Thorough review of available information led to the conclusion that US-born women are characterized as much more likely than immigrants to:

1. Have higher levels of education, employment, and income
2. Be taller, heavier, and gain more weight during pregnancy
3. Have more abortions and fewer live births
4. Consume fewer fruits and cereals but more fats and milk products
5. Experience more medical conditions, particularly sexually transmitted diseases and genitourinary problems
6. Smoke, abuse alcohol and other drugs, and have risk factors for AIDS
7. Have a history of psychosocial problems: be a victim of both child abuse and spousal abuse, and have stressful relationships with the father of the baby and their own family members
8. Experience depression, be considered at risk psychosocially, and be referred to a social worker

These characteristics illustrate that the biomedical, nutritional, and psychosocial disadvantages of some U.S.-born women may eclipse their comparative socioeconomic advantages in having healthy babies.

Becerra JE et al: Born in the USA: infant health paradox, *JAMA* 272:1803, 1994.

health, health professionals must now go beyond the obvious solutions and seek ways to identify and modify the underlying risk factors in reproduction. This is the challenge that has begun to focus increased attention on the role of nutrition in the course and outcome of pregnancy. With this perspective in mind, we can proceed to an understanding of the importance of nutrition in prenatal care.

Summary

Despite the progress that has been made during the past 50 years, the basic challenges and concerns in maternal and child health are much the same today as they were in the 1930s. The 1979 Surgeon General's report on health promotion and disease prevention, *Healthy People*, brought these challenges into sharp contemporary focus. The report stressed the high priority that disease prevention and health promotion must take as the key elements of national health strategy. The Surgeon General proposed specific objectives for maternal and child health in 1990; these objectives were not achieved and therefore were revised for the year 2000. These new goals for the year 2000 are as follows[41]:

1. Reduce the infant mortality rate to no more than 7 per 1,000 live births; specific targets:

Blacks	11
American Indians/Alaska natives	8.5
Puerto Ricans	8
Neonatal mortality	4.5
Neonatal mortality among blacks	7
Neonatal mortality among Puerto Ricans	5.2
Postneonatal mortality	2.5
Postneonatal mortality among blacks	4
Postneonatal mortality among American Indians/Alaska natives	4
Postneonatal mortality among Puerto Ricans	2.8

2. Reduce the fetal death rate (20 or more weeks of gestation) to no more than 5 per 1,000 live births plus fetal deaths; specific target:

Blacks	7.5

3. Reduce the maternal mortality rate to no more than 3.3 per 100,000 live births; specific target:

Blacks	5

4. Reduce the incidence of fetal alcohol syndrome to no more than 0.12 per 1,000 live births; specific targets:

American Indians/Alaska natives	2
Blacks	0.4

5. Reduce low birth weight to an incidence of no more than 5% of live births and very low birth weight to no more than 1% of births; specific target:
   Blacks   9% and 2%
6. Increase to at least 85% the proportion of mothers who achieve the minimum recommended weight gain during their pregnancies.
7. Reduce severe complications of pregnancy to no more than 15 per 100 deliveries.
8. Reduce the cesarean delivery rate to no more than 15 per 100 deliveries; specific targets:
   Primary (first-time) cesarean delivery   12
   Repeat cesarean deliveries   65
9. Increase to at least 75% the proportion of mothers who breast-feed their babies in the early postpartum period and to at least 50% the proportion who continue breast-feeding until their babies are 5 to 6 months old; specific targets:
   Early postpartum
   Low-income mothers   75%
   Black mothers   75%
   Hispanic mothers   75%
   American Indian/Alaska native   75%
   mothers
   At age 5-6 months
   Low-income mothers   50%
   Black mothers   50%
   Hispanic mothers   50%
   American Indian/Alaska native   50%
   mothers
10. Increase abstinence from tobacco use by pregnant women to at least 90% and increase abstinence from alcohol, cocaine, and marijuana by pregnant women by at least 20%.
11. Increase to at least 90% the proportion of all pregnant women who receive prenatal care in the first trimester of pregnancy; specific targets:
   Black women   90%
   American Indian/Alaska native women   90%
   Hispanic women   90%
12. Increase to at least 60% the proportion of primary-care providers who provide age-appropriate preconception care and counseling.
13. Increase to at least 90% the proportion of women enrolled in prenatal care who are offered screening and counseling on prenatal detection of fetal abnormalities.

If the national health objective for reducing infant mortality is to be achieved, strategies need to be considered that address the heterogeneity of factors accounting for infant mortality in the United States. Examples include the following:

1. Reducing mortality from disorders related to short gestation and unspecified low birth weight will require improved access to adequate prenatal care and understanding of etiologic risk factors for preterm delivery.
2. Reduction of deaths related to maternal complications of pregnancy will require both expansion of access to prenatal care and assessment of the adequacy of the content of care.

According to the Centers for Disease Control and Prevention, efforts to address these and other risk factors may increase the likelihood of achieving the year 2000 national health objective for reduction of infant mortality.

REVIEW QUESTIONS

1. Define the current level of maternal mortality in the United States and specify the major causes.
2. Indicate the major causes of infant mortality in the United States and relate the level of infant mortality to that in other developed countries.
3. Suggest possible explanations for the increased incidence of low birthweight among blacks as compared with others in the United States.
4. List the Surgeon General's specific objectives related to maternal and child health to be attained by the year 2000.

LEARNING ACTIVITIES

1. Investigate local sources of vital statistics data, specifically those related to issues of maternal and child health.
2. Inquire in local hospitals about the prevalence of nutrition-related problems in inpatient and outpatient units.
3. Develop an article for a local newspaper explaining why the infant mortality rate is so high in the United States as compared with other developed countries.

REFERENCES

1. Annual summary of births, deaths, marriages, United States, 1993. *Monthly vital statistics report,* Washington DC: National Center for Health Statistics, October 11, 1994.
2. Becerra JE et al: Infant mortality among Hispanics: a portrait of heterogeneity, *JAMA* 265:217, 1991.

3. Becerra JE et al: Born in the USA: infant health paradox, *JAMA* 272:1803, 1994.
4. Buescher PA et al: WIC participation can reduce low birth weight and newborn medical costs: a cost-benefit analysis of WIC participation in North Carolina, *J Am Diet Assoc* 93:163, 1993.
5. Cabral H et al: Foreign-born and U.S.-born black women: differences in health behaviors and birth outcomes, *Am J Public Health* 80:70, 1990.
6. Centers for Disease Control and Prevention: *Monthly vital statistics report. Birth characteristics for Asian or Pacific Islander subgroups, 1992,* May 11, 1995: US Department of Health and Human Services.
7. Centers for Disease Control and Prevention: *Monthly vital statistics report.* 43:5 Supp, October 25, 1994, US Department of Health and Human Services.
8. Centers for Disease Control and Prevention: *Monthly vital statistics report* 43:6 Supp, March 22, 1995, US Department of Health and Human Services.
9. Chase H: Perinatal and infant mortality in the United States and six West European countries, *Am J Public Health* 57:1735, 1967.
10. Dorfman S: Maternal mortality in New York City, 1981-1983, *Obstet Gynecol* 76:317, 1990.
11. Geronimus AT: The effects of race, residence, and prenatal care on the relationship of maternal age to neonatal mortality, *Am J Public Health* 76:1416, 1986.
12. Guendelman S: Mexican women in the United States, *Lancet* 344:352, 1994.
13. Hack M et al: School-age outcomes in children with birthweights under 750 g, *N Engl J Med* 331:753, 1994.
14. *Healthy people:* the Surgeon General's report on health promotion and disease prevention, DHEW (PHS) Publ No. 79-55071. Washington, DC, 1979, US Government Printing Office.
15. Hogberg U, Innala E, Sandstrom A: Maternal mortality in Sweden, 1980-1988, *Obstet Gynecol* 84:240, 1994.
16. Hogue CJR, Hargraves MA: Class, race, and infant mortality in the United States, *Am J Public Health* 83:9, 1993.
17. Institute of Medicine: *Preventing low birth-weight,* Washington, DC, 1985, National Academy Press.
18. Kleinman JC, Fingerhut LA, Prager K: Differences in infant mortality by race, nativity status, and other maternal characteristics, *Am J Dis Child* 145:194, 1991.
19. Kramer MS: Intrauterine growth and gestational duration, *Pediatrics* 80:502, 1987.
20. May WJ, Greiss FC: Maternal mortality in North Carolina: a forty-year experience, *Am J Obstet Gynecol* 161:555, 1989.
21. Mertz KJ, Parker AL, Halpin GJ: Pregnancy-related mortality in New Jersey, 1975-1989, *Am J Public Health* 82:1085, 1992.
22. Nakamura RM, King R, Kimball EH et al: Excess infant mortality in an American Indian population 1940 to 1990, *JAMA* 266:2244, 1991.
23. National Center for Health Statistics: *Vital and health statistics: trends and variations in first births to older women, 1970-1986,* Hyattsville, Md, 1989, US Department of Health and Human Services.
24. National Center for Health Statistics: *Vital statistics of the United States 1988,* Hyattsville, Md, 1991, US Department of Health and Human Services.
25. National Commission to Prevent Infant Mortality: Troubling trends: the health of America's next generation, Washington DC, 1995, Superintendent of Documents, Government Printing Office.
26. National Commission to Prevent Infant Mortality: Number of Americans in poverty declines in 1994. Community Nutrition Institute, October 6, 1995.
27. Peoples-Sheps MD, Siegel E, Suchindran CM, et al: Characteristics of maternal employment during pregnancy: effects on low birth weight, *Am J Public Health* 81:1007, 1991.
28. Polednak AP: Black–white differences in infant mortality in 38 standard metropolitan statistical areas, *Am J Public Health* 81:1480, 1991.
29. Prysak M, Lorenz RP, and Kisly A: Pregnancy outcome in nulliparous women 35 years and older. *Obstet Gynecol* 85:65, 1995.
30. Rawlings JS, Rawlings VB, and Read JA: Prevalence of low birth weight and preterm delivery in relation to the interval between pregnancies among white and black women. *N Engl J Med* 332:69, 1995.
31. Rochat RW, Koonin LM, Atrash HK et al: Maternal mortality in the United States: report from the maternal mortality collaborative study, *Obstet Gynecol* 72:91, 1988.

32. Rosenfield A: Maternal mortality in developing countries: an ongoing but neglected epidemic, *JAMA* 262:376, 1989.

33. Sachs BP et al: Maternal mortality in Massachusetts: trends and prevention, *N Engl J Med* 316:667, 1987.

34. Schoendorf KC, Hogue CJR, Kleinman JC, and Rowley D: Mortality among infants of black as compared with white college-educated parents. *N Engl J Med* 326:1522, 1992.

35. Singh GK Yu SM: Infant mortality in the United States: trends, differentials and projections: 1950 through 2010. *Am J Public Health* 85:957, 1995.

36. ————— State-specific trends among women who did not receive prenatal care–United States, 1980-1992. *JAMA* 273:616, 1995.

37. Syverson CJ, Chavkin W, Atrash HK et al: Pregnancy related mortality in New York City, 1980 to 1984: causes of death and associated risk factors, *Am J Obstet Gynecol* 164:603, 1991.

38. United Nations: *Demographic yearbook,* New York, 1991, United Nations Publications.

39. United Nations, Department of International Economic and Social Affairs: *Demographic indicators of countries: estimates and projects assessed in 1980,* New York, 1982, United Nations Publications.

40. US Department of Commerce: *Statistical abstract of the United States 1991,* Washington DC, 1991, Bureau of the Census.

41. US Department of Health and Human Services: Healthy people 2000, Washington DC, 1989, ODPHP National Health Information Center.

42. Wallace HM, Ericsson A, Bolander AM et al: Infant mortality in Sweden and Finland: implications for the United States, *J Perinatol* 10:3, 1989.

43. Wegman ME: Annual summary of vital statistics—1993. *Pediatrics* 94:792, 1994.

44. Williams RL, Binkin NJ, Clingman EJ: Pregnancy outcomes among Spanish surname women in California, *Am J Public Health* 76:387, 1986.

45. Yankauer A: What infant mortality tells us, *Am J Public Health* 80:653, 1990.

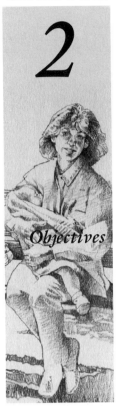

2

Nutrition, Fertility, and Family Planning

Bonnie S. Worthington-Roberts

Objectives

After completing this chapter, the student will be able to:

✓ *Define important nutritional and nonnutritional factors that affect female fertility.*

✓ *Discuss the impact of contraceptive agents on nutritional status of the female.*

✓ *Summarize the value of preconceptional interventions (especially related to diet/nutrition) in improving pregnancy course and outcome.*

Introduction

Rapid population growth and inadequate world food supplies in the areas of greatest need are two of the critical global realities facing humankind in our generation. The relationship of population growth to food supply has been known for centuries, although most of the attention has been directed at famine or starvation and the effects on mortality. We now know, however, that the much more prevalent problem of chronic malnutrition can also significantly affect birth rates.

One of the major concerns of mature women in all societies is the regulation of family size through planned contraception. Many approaches to family planning can be identified around the world, and observed practices relate largely to cultural patterns and also reflect, to some extent, socioeconomic status and availability of "modern devices." Generally, approaches to birth control differ markedly between industrialized developed countries on the one hand and malnourished developing nations on the other. In the former circumstance limitation of family size is widely accepted, but in the latter, where hunger and poverty prevail, a couple's desire for many children is a response to high infant mortality, the need for extra hands to increase family productivity and income, and the hope for security in old age.

FERTILITY AND NUTRITION
General

In many parts of the world uncontrolled fertility and malnutrition coexist. These phenomena are highly interactive. High fertility rates mean more babies to feed and more malnutrition if the availability of adequate food does not keep pace. Chronically malnourished mothers living under marginal economic conditions have a high rate of fetal loss; yet this ill-nourished group has a high pregnancy rate.[55]

Establishing the relationship between pregnancy outcome and maternal nutriture is highly problematical for the human population because both are conditioned by a number of variables. Hence poverty commonly dictates food supply and the accessibility of medical care. The level of education and cultural identity may influence the direction of prenatal care and illness management. Previous experience with child rearing and earlier pregnancies may shape maternal behavior during the current pregnancy. Some, none, or all of these factors may be important influences on maternal nutriture and pregnancy outcome for a given mother.

Maternal malnutrition adversely affects the survival of the infant. Both the short-term and long-term maternal nutritional state are independently related to infant mortality. The association of low socioeconomic status with high infant mortality largely reflects malnutrition and illness, which leads to the delivery of poorly viable infants.

Poor socioeconomic circumstances imply economic, cultural, and biological deprivation. Women of lower socioeconomic status are more likely to give birth out of wedlock or to marry early and be multiparous. They tend to be shorter, have a smaller pelvis, and generally experience poorer health. Women in poverty are likely to work more during pregnancy and delay prenatal care or receive no care at all. The care they do receive for themselves and their children is more likely to be suboptimal.

Undernutrition shortens the duration of the reproductive life span and reduces its efficiency. The undernourished woman has a later menarche and an earlier menopause than her well-nourished counterpart. The onset and maintenance of regular menstrual function depend on the maintenance of a minimum weight for height, implying that a critical fat storage may be important for human female reproductive capacity.[13] Body weight changes in the range of

10% to 15% are associated with the cessation and restoration of menstrual cycles. Menstrual cycles may become irregular or anovulatory or cease altogether if undernutrition is severe. Moreover, an underfed pregnant woman has a higher probability of miscarriage or stillbirth. If she delivers successfully, her lactation amenorrhea may be prolonged as compared with that of a well-nourished woman, resulting in longer birth intervals.[13]

Poor nutrition of the mother in her infancy and childhood may affect infant mortality in the next generation. For example, maternal height, an index of earlier nutritional history during growth, is consistently related to infant mortality in an inverse manner. The mechanism of this observation is obscure, although impaired placental nutrient supply with decreased fetal growth and obstetrical complications from a contracted pelvis are suggested. Similarly, women who were themselves low-birth-weight infants have been reported to demonstrate a higher-than-expected incidence of poor pregnancy outcome than women with higher birth weights (Figs. 2-1 and 2-2).[19,27,28] Although an explanation for this phenomenon has yet to be defined, it is possible that with reduced birth weight, the growth and development of one or more organ systems may be interfered with, including the reproductive and/or endocrine systems. This suggests that no matter how effective prenatal, perinatal, and neonatal care become, such care alone may not prevent some problems of pregnancy.

Pregnancy in Adolescence

The pregnant teenager is confronted with a number of special risks and stresses that may influence the outcome of the pregnancy and the well-being of the mother (Chapter 9). The nutritional stresses for the pregnant teenager are superimposed on the nutritional needs associated with continued growth and maturation. Although childbirth among women in their late teens has become less hazardous in "modern settings," a greater risk of difficulty persists among those under 20 years of age in developing countries. The specific reasons for the observed differences are not completely understood, but better obstetrical care and improved

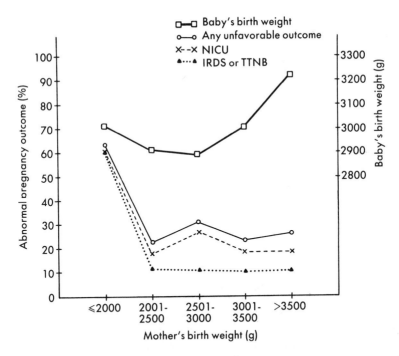

FIG. 2-1 Relationship of mother's birth weight to her own pregnancy outcome as observed in over 700 women delivering at University Hospital, University of Washington, Seattle, Washington. Unfavorable outcomes included miscarriage, stillbirth, congenital malformation, neonatal death, required neonatal intensive care (NICU), idiopathic respiratory distress syndrome (IRDS), transient tachypnea of the newborn (TTNB), and neonatal apnea. All other outcomes were considered favorable.

Modified from Hackman E et al: Maternal birth-weight and subsequent pregnancy outcome, *JAMA* 250:2016, 1983. Copyright 1983, American Medical Association.

socioeconomic conditions likely account for much of the disparity.

This adverse situation is especially prominent in less-developed countries of the world because early marriage and immediate pregnancy routinely occur. Often the family of the young couple counts the months that elapse between consummated alliance and pregnancy, which ultimately proves the bride's worth. It is even the case in some countries that pregnancy is a prerequisite to marriage, as is often observed for legitimization in modern societies. In any case, because of the obvious tendency toward early conception in many parts of the world, serious attention must be given to optimizing the nutritional status of adolescent girls. Ideally trends toward delay in the first pregnancy can be promoted so that the quality of health of both mother and infant will not be compromised by poor nutritional support.

Pregnancy in Late Maternal Age

Pregnancy in the immediate premenopausal years is correlated consistently with obstetrical complication and unfavorable outcomes. Older women may also be the women of highest parity; women of high parity are susceptible to anemia and lower weight to height ratios. High parity is associated with greater fetal wastage. Thus the late pregnancy may represent a risk for unfavorable outcome on two counts.[55]

However, new data temper these long estab-

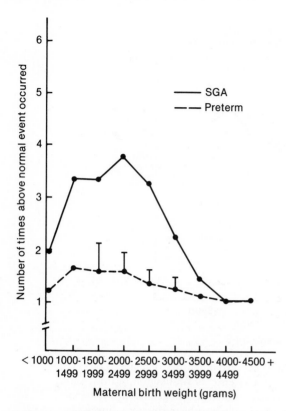

FIG. 2-2 Degree of increase in small-for-gestational age and preterm birth by maternal birth weight.

Modified from Klebanoff MA and Yip R: Influences of maternal birth weight on rate of fetal growth and duration of gestation, *J Pediatr* 111:287, 1987.

lished conclusions.[42] As mentioned previously, during the last several decades, women age 35 and older conceived in increasing numbers and represented a greater percentage of total births. There appears to be a consensus that women 35 years and older have greater risks of diabetes, spontaneous abortion, hypertensive disorders, autosomal trisomy, maternal mortality, and cesarean birth. Disagreement continues over other outcome issues. For this reason, researchers in Michigan compared pregnancy and delivery complications of first births in women 35 years and older with women 25 to 29 years old. Maternal and newborn records were studied retrospectively. The results indicated that nulliparous

women age 35 and older had significantly higher rates of antepartum, intrapartum, and newborn complications than nulliparas between the ages of 25 and 29 but not an increased perinatal mortality rate. Despite the increased risk of complications, maternal and perinatal outcomes were good. These findings are consistent with the recent literature challenging the traditional view that pregnancies in older women are fraught with hazards. They are, however, prone to complications, many of which are responsible for the increased neonatal morbidity and costs associated with neonatal intensive care admission.

In view of the increased risk of poor pregnancy outcome among older women, it may be advantageous that **fecundity** decreases with older age. A study of more than 2,000 women whose husbands were totally sterile demonstrated that successful conception after artificial insemination was lower in women over age 30 than in younger women; women over age 35 showed significantly lower conception rates than any of the other groups (Fig. 2-3).[12]

Birth Spacing

Pregnancy stimulates an adjustment of the mother, fetus, and placenta to a new physiologic state. After birth the process reverses, and readjustment takes place. It is undesirable for another pregnancy to occur before the readjustment is complete.[55,58] A reduced interval between pregnancies is one of several factors related to prematurity and low birth weight.

The interval during pregnancy and between successive conceptions can be usefully divided into three parts.[55] The first stage of the process is pregnancy. After the birth of the infant the mother enters an anovulatory period during which she is amenorrheic. With the postpartum physiological readjustment, ovulation is reestablished, and the mother is again at risk for pregnancy. Table 2-1 illustrates factors that shorten each of the components of the interconceptional interval and interventions that may lengthen the interval. Factors that foreshorten the pregnancy are those that jeopardize a favorable reproductive outcome. Measures that enhance a favorable outcome tend to restore the gestational length. The **anovulatory period**

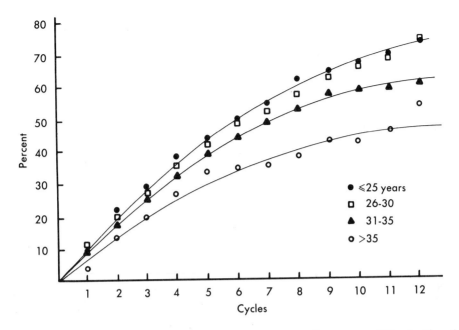

FIG. 2-3   Theoretical cumulative success rates in age groups. Four curves differ significantly. Because curves of two younger groups were similar, they are represented by single tracing. These curves differ significantly from those of two older groups. There were 371 women in the <26 group, 1079 in the 26 to 30 group, 599 in the 31 to 35 group, and 144 in the >35 group.

From Federation CECOS (Schwartz D and Mayaux BA): Female fecundity as a function of age. *N Engl J Med* 306:404, 1982. Reprinted by permission.

will be shortened if the pregnancy was shortened by a fetal death or a premature birth. Death of a young breast-fed infant or the absence or curtailment of breastfeeding eliminates the anovulatory effect of prolactin and other anterior pituitary hormones released by the stimulus of the baby's sucking. In many traditional cultures abstinence from sexual intercourse was practiced during lactation. As this practice of sexual abstinence has eroded, other effective birth control methods may not be substituted. The result may be an early conception. The encouragement of breast-feeding together with effective use of alternative birth control methods and better medical care may maximize the duration of the anovulatory period. Effective birth control techniques can prolong the pregnancy-free interval after ovulation resumes, according to the desires of the parents.

In places where high fertility prevails and modern birth control techniques are unavailable, the usual interval between children is between 2½ and 3 years.[55] This interval includes the extension of amenorrhea achieved by lactation and the traditional sexual abstinence practiced in many parts of the world during that period. When artificial feeding replaces breastfeeding and lactation, sexual taboos may also be removed, and the interval of child spacing is shortened by at least 6 months. The pregnancy-free interval is also drastically shortened after a fetal or neonatal death. Although a well-nourished, healthy woman in an affluent society may not be threatened by a shortened interconceptional period, a chronically malnourished woman in marginal socioeconomic circumstances may find her health seriously compromised by a shortened interval.

TABLE 2-1   *Three Major Components of the Interval between Conceptions*

	Major Components	Factors that Shorten the Interval	Interventions that Lengthen the Interval
Conception			
	Pregnancy	Interruption of pregnancy or premature delivery	Adequate nutrition enhances favorable outcome Improved socioeconomic status Better medical care
Delivery			
	Anovulatory period and amenorrhea	Perinatal death Absence or curtailment of breast-feeding	Breast-feeding may delay return of ovulation Birth control can replace failure to practice traditional postpartum (lactation) abstinence Nutrition education in breast-feeding Better medical care
Return of ovulation			
	Ovulating and menstruating (at risk for pregnancy)	Failure of modern birth control Failure of postpartum abstinence Infant death may motivate conception	Birth control Better medical care
Conception			

Modified from Subcommittee on Nutrition and Fertility, Food and Nutrition Board, National Research Council, National Academy of Sciences: *Nutrition and fertility interrelationships: implications for policy and action,* Washington, DC, 1975, Government Printing Office.

DIET, NUTRITION, AND FERTILITY

It has long been known that undernutrition impairs human fertility. Undernutrition is associated with progressive loss of ovulatory cycles and menstrual function. Amenorrhea is usually seen in cases of anorexia nervosa. It may also develop during the course of rigorous dieting to achieve weight loss. In fact, it may accompany the progression of any chronic disease associated with weight loss. It is easy to accept the traditional explanation of this phenomenon as one of protecting the developing embryo and fetus. That is, if the mother is nutritionally debilitated, she is in no position to support herself and a developing offspring.

The role that specific nutrients play in maintenance or interference with fertility is a subject of interest but one about which very little is known. Anecdotal reports are occasionally provided in the scientific literature but rarely have well-controlled studies been conducted.

Amenorrhea associated with hypercarotene-mia has been reported more than once and continues to be of interest in the scientific community, especially in light of the current interest in use of carotene supplements. One report suggests that high blood concentrations of carotene are directly related to loss of menstrual function.[25]

Infertility has also been reported to occur in the presence of folate deficiency.[10] In light of current interest in the role that folic acid plays in the prevention of neural tube defects, inadequate folic acid status resulting in infertility might actually protect against abnormal embryonic development. Neural tube defects, and their relation to folic acid deficiency are discussed in detail in Chapter 5.

Still controversial is whether vegetarianism is associated with ovulatory irregularity. Researchers in Pennsylvania studied 41 nonvegetarian and 34 vegetarian premenopausal women who were indistinguishable with respect to height, weight, body-mass index and menarche. The incidence of menstrual irregularities was 4.9% among nonvegetarians and 26.5% among vegetarians. The vegetarian group consumed significantly greater amounts of polyunsaturated fatty acids, carbohydrates, vitamin B-6, and dietary fiber, whereas the nonvegetarians reported greater intakes of saturated fatty acids, protein, cholesterol, caffeine, and alcohol. The results are consistent with the notion that menstrual regularity can be influenced by specific dietary components that may have direct effects or may exert their effects by modulating circulating sex steroid status.[40]

However, another comparison between vegetarian and nonvegetarian women failed to find differences in ovulatory disturbances. Mean cycle lengths were similar but vegetarians had longer luteal phase lengths. Cycle types also differed; vegetarians had fewer anovulatory cycles (4.6% vs. 15.1%). Overall, the researchers concluded that ovulatory disturbances were less common among vegetarians.[2]

Epidemiologic data suggest that dietary galactose may deleteriously affect ovarian function. Populations in which lactose intolerance is infrequent and milk consumption is high have greater dietary exposure to galactose. Researchers analyzed data from various countries to determine whether age-specific fertility rates correlate with prevalence of adult deficiency of gut lactase and per capita milk consumption. Significant correlations were found among these variables. Fertility at older ages appears to be lower, and declines in fertility with aging appear to be steeper in populations with high per capita consumption of milk and a greater ability to digest its lactose component. These findings, at the moment, are simply provocative.[7]

The same can be said about the relation of female infertility to consumption of caffeinated beverages. This issue was examined in American women—1,050 with primary infertility and 3833 controls—who had recently given birth. The infertile women were categorized by cause of infertility: ovulatory factor, tubal disease, cervical factor, endometriosis, or idiopathic infertility. After controlling statistically for confounding factors there was a significant increase in risk of infertility resulting from tubal disease or endometriosis at the upper levels of caffeine intake, indicating a threshold effect. (An upper level of caffeine intake was defined as approximately equivalent to two cups of coffee or four cans of cola per day.)[18]

Alcohol intake during pregnancy is well-known to adversely affect the developing fetus. Evidence also suggests, however, that there is a relationship between alcohol intake and fertility. In a study conducted in Boston, interviews were conducted with 3,833 women who recently gave birth and 1,050 women from seven infertility clinics; women from the infertility clinics were classified according to the most likely cause of their infertility. Statistical analysis showed an increase in infertility, resulting from ovulatory factor or endometriosis, with alcohol use. The risk of endometriosis was about 50% higher in case subjects with any alcohol intake than in control subjects. The researchers concluded that moderate alcohol use may contribute to the risk of specific types of infertility.[17]

Although smoking is not a dietary topic, it is worth several comments. An association has been reported between cigarette smoking and reduced fertility. Researchers have measured the nicotine metabolite cotinine in ovarian follicular fluid collected at the time of oocyte recovery during treatment for in-vitro fertilization. In a group of women in whom follicular fluid cotinine could not be detected, 116 oocytes were collected, of which 72% became fertilized. Among women with detectable cotinine concentrations in follicular fluid, 45 eggs were retrieved and 44% of them were eventually fertilized. These findings suggest that infertile women should be advised to stop or reduce smoking generally and especially before treatment by in vitro fertilization.[45]

A mechanism for the subfertility associated with exposure to cigarette smoke has been suggested to be inhibition by constituents of cigarette smoke of steroidogenesis. Women smokers have lower endogenous estrogen concentrations than do nonsmokers. Components of cigarette smoke inhibit an enzyme that catalyzes production of estrogens from their steroid precursors. Other abnormalities may also be induced. Nicotine interferes with cortical granule formation in the egg, which is involved in the normal block to polyspermic fertilization. Nicotine can also be concentrated in preimplantation blastocysts, so it could have a direct effect on embryogenesis and implantation. An appropriate message might be: *Smoking in the face of nutritional deficiencies may aggravate an already compromised fertility status.*

BIRTH CONTROL AND NUTRITION

Birth control achieves its greatest impact on nutrition by preventing pregnancies among women at high risk for obstetrical complications and poor pregnancy outcome. Such a high-risk group includes teenage women, women of high parity and late maternal age, and chronically malnourished women of any age. Birth control allows parents to space pregnancies at greater intervals. Longer intervals improve the prospects for a favorable pregnancy outcome and allow the mother to make a fuller physical and nutritional recovery between childbirths.

In conditions of uncontrolled fertility and chronic malnutrition the introduction of birth control can reduce the nutritional stress on the malnourished mother and her family. Under such circumstances birth control may especially enhance the nutritional status of the youngest child as yet unweaned. By delaying the arrival of a new baby who would preempt the breast milk supply, the mother protects her youngest from inferior substitute feeding and the risks of gastrointestinal-tract infections.

Birth control and nutrition impinge on the most fundamental of human social behaviors: sexual activity and eating. Limiting one's fertility and choosing well what one eats are highly personal events. They require accurate knowledge and a sustained commitment to act on that knowledge. Birth control and good nutrition are total participatory activities for which the person takes full personal responsibility.

Appropriate education and access to birth control methods and a good diet are essential but not sufficient without the motivation to act. Couples typically do not accept family planning when infant mortality is high and they see fewer of their children surviving. Moreover, as long as parents perceive a large family size as advantageous, they are not inclined to practice birth control. Large populations in many parts of the world find themselves in such a marginal economic position that even the argument of fertility control to avoid having more mouths to feed has little meaning. Their life experiences tell them that producing fewer babies does not necessarily mitigate their hunger. In this climate of hunger and concern about child mortality, protection of the pregnancy-free period is highly unlikely, and the focus of the family is typically placed on maintenance of the surviving infant at substantial risk for illness or death.

If the socioeconomic circumstances of needy families improve and if adequate educational programs are established, parents might recognize that smaller family size enhances the family's opportunities. If attitudes like this are developed, birth control may assume a level of significant acceptance. Improved maternal and child nutrition itself can encourage this acceptance by reducing infant and child mortality. If survival of offspring is noted to improve, family planning will ultimately become more desirable. Thus it can be said that better nutrition favors the adoption of fertility control.

EFFECT OF SPECIFIC BIRTH CONTROL METHODS ON MATERNAL NUTRITIONAL STATUS

Oral Contraceptives

Oral contraceptives (OCs) remain the most popular and most effective reversible contraceptives approved for use in the United States.[16,57] The oral agents typically employed consist of a synthetic estrogen (ethinyl estradiol or mestranol) and one of several synthetic progestogens. Combinations of estrogens and progesterones were first marketed in 1957 for correction of menstrual disorders, and by 1960 the drugs were approved as OC agents.

Since the early days of oral contraceptives, many unique formulations have been marketed in the United States. Most of these preparations have contained a constant amount of estrogen and progestin (**monophasic** combinations); other types are **sequential, progestion only** ("minipills") and the **multiphasic** formulations.[16]

Sequential formulations (now obsolete) contained estrogen alone during the first 14 to 16 days of use each cycle followed by an estrogen–progestin combination during the last 5 to 7 days of use. These pills were available until 1976. Minipills were first introduced in 1972 and have never accounted for more than a fraction of a percent of retail oral contraceptive prescriptions. The more recently introduced multiphasic formulations, which vary estrogen and/or progestin amounts during the cycle, were first introduced in 1982 in an attempt to emulate hormone fluctuations of the menstrual cycle and to lower overall hormone doses. These pills are available in 21-day and 28-day packs, the latter containing seven placebos.[16]

The trend over the past 25 years in Great Britain and the United States has been toward reduction in dosage of both estrogenic and progestational substances (Fig. 2-4), and with this trend has come a reduced incidence of recognized side effects and metabolic alterations. Pills now provide about 30 to 50 µg of an estrogen and 1 mg or less of a progestin.

The mechanism of action of OCs was originally assumed to be simple suppression of ovulation. Indeed, the original combination type of preparation, norethynodrel (Enovid), contained relatively high doses of both estrins and progestins and *did* suppress ovulation most of the time. Careful evaluation has shown, however, that preparations containing smaller doses sometimes do not suppress ovulation but are still effective in preventing conception. The proposed mechanisms of action of estrogens and progestins are summarized in the box on p. 41.

Side effects and general metabolic complications. Since widespread use of OCs has developed, observed side effects and metabolic complications resulting from prolonged use have received increasing attention by both basic science and clinical researchers.[47] The complications reported as a result of taking OCs can be divided roughly into those that are merely annoying and those that are serious or potentially fatal (see box on p. 42). Many of the reported problems are also seen in women during the time of pregnancy. Minor complications of OC usage include mild to moderate weight gain (3 to 6 lb. [1.3 to 2.7 kg]), fluid retention, nausea, vomiting, emotional changes, facial pigmentation, slight loss of hair, and headaches. With regard to the last, there is some evidence to suggest that women who have suffered from migraine or similar vascular headaches may be unable to use this form of contraceptive. Evidence also suggests that underweight women are more susceptible to these problems. Of considerable interest is the observation that OCs were in use for nearly 8 years before medical science presented conclusive evidence that serious and even fatal complications could result.

Major complications are of three types: hypertension and its sequelae, thromboembolic phenomena with and without premature myocardial infarction, and metabolic disorders, in particular diabetes mellitus. Hepatic hemorrhage and primary hepatic tumors have also been reported. The problem of hypertension secondary to OC use generally occurs in women who have a **familial trait** or actually have had hypertension before using OCs. The same can be said for diabetes. Deaths resulting from **pulmonary embolism,** coronary occlusion, and stroke, however, have been reported with a relatively high frequency in young women who have used OCs for at least 6 months.[54]

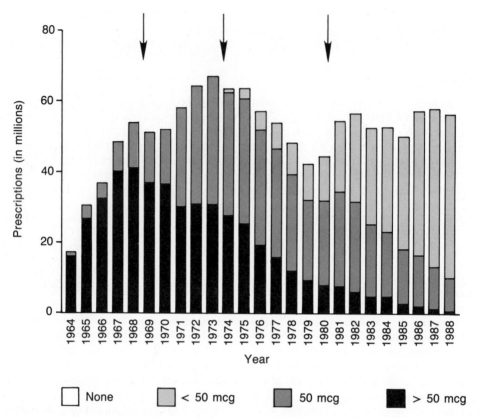

FIG. 2-4   Number of retail oral contraceptive prescriptions by estrogen dose, 1964-1988, United States. Arrows indicate points at which changes in date collection methods occurred.

From Gertsman BB et al: Trends in the content and use of oral contraceptives in the United States, 1964-1988, *Am J Public Health* 81:90, 1991.

The absolute contraindications to oral contraceptive use have remained unchanged, whereas relative contraindications have been relaxed in recent years. Absolute contraindications include **thromboembolic disorders,** cerebrovascular or coronary artery disease, breast cancer, estrogen-dependent **neoplasia,** undiagnosed abnormal genital bleeding, known or suspected pregnancy, and liver tumor.[25,36] Relative contraindications include age older than 45 years, diabetes, hypertension, smoking, gallbladder disease, gestational **cholestasis,** history of renal disease, impaired liver function, and **hyperlipidemia.**

Lipid metabolism. Repeated observations have now shown clearly that in women taking

OCs, increased coagulability of the blood develops, accompanied by an increase in concentration of triglycerides and low-density and very-low-density lipoproteins, as well as a decrease in concentration of high-density lipoproteins. Variability among women is considerable, however, and seems to depend on the type and dose of component steroids. In general, high-density lipoproteins increase with increasing doses of estrogens and decrease with increasing doses or potency of progestins. The specific formulation of the OC appears to determine its net effect on serum lipoprotein patterns.[31,47]

Carbohydrate metabolism. Since the 1960s, research has indicated that oral contraceptives disturb carbohydrate metabolism. This was first

❖

MECHANISMS OF ACTION OF ESTROGENS AND PROGESTINS IN ORAL CONTRACEPTIVE AGENTS

Estrogens

Inhibit ovulation via the effect of estrogen on the hypothalamus and the subsequent suppression of pituitary follicle-stimulating hormone and luteinizing hormone; 95% to 98% effective

Do not inhibit implantation of the fertilized egg unless doses 50 to 100 times that found in typical OCs are provided

Progestins

Promote development of "hostile cervical mucus," which hampers the transport of sperm and decreases the ability of sperm to penetrate the cervical mucus (hostile mucus is scanty, thick, and cellular)

Change character of cervical secretions such that capacitation of the sperm does not occur (capacitation is the activation of the hydrolytic spermatic enzymes that are required for the sperm to penetrate the cells surrounding the ovum)

May decelerate ovum transport

May inhibit implantation through modification of the follicle-stimulating hormone and/or luteinizing hormone peaks enough so that even when ovulation occurs, the decreased progestin production by the corpus luteum leads to inhibition of implantation

May inhibit ovulation via subtle disturbance in hypothalamic pituitary and ovarian function and a modification of the midcycle surge of follicle-stimulating hormone and luteinizing hormone

---

thought to be due to the action of the estrogenic component of OCs, but later it was shown that the progestational component is responsible.[68] However, the significance of these findings has been questioned because modern OCs contain low levels of these hormonal agents. In one study, the effect of seven low-dose OC preparations on carbohydrate metabolism was investigated in 70 healthy volunteers. An oral glucose-tolerance test was performed before and after 6 months of treatment; glucose disappearance and insulin response curve were determined. Long-term glucose homeostasis was assessed by estimating the extent of glycosylation of plasma proteins and hemoglobin A_{1c}. The area under the curve for insulin and glucose did not change during treatment with any of the preparations. In addition, the representative variables for long-term glucose control did not increase for any of the preparations during treatment. One might conclude from these results that the low-dose OCs investigated in the study do not have any adverse effects on carbohydrate metabolism.

Protein metabolism. Plasma proteins are changed in women using OCs. Albumin concentration is generally decreased as a result of decreased synthesis in the presence of unchanged plasma volume. The α- and β-globulins routinely increase along with fibrinogen, cortisol-binding globulin, thyroid-binding globulin, ceruloplasmin, and transferrin. The rise in blood pressure seen in some women taking OCs is attributed to an increase in an α_2-globulin, angiotensin I, which is converted by renin to angiotensin II, a potent vasoconstrictor.

Although amino acid metabolism in the OC user has not received in-depth consideration, some alteration appears to occur, possibly related to the rise in free cortisol concentration. Reduced circulating levels of some amino acids have been reported along with increased rates of urinary excretion. Metabolism of tryptophan has received much attention, and clearly it is altered to some degree by OC use; the conversion of tryptophan to nicotinic acid is augmented. Since vitamin B_6 is used as a cofactor for several enzymes in this tryptophan pathway, changes in parameters of vitamin B_6 metabolism are also apparent in some women using OCs.

Vitamin status. Much attention has been paid to vitamin status of OC users. A variety of

❖

KNOWN SIDE EFFECTS FROM USE OF ORAL CONTRACEPTIVE AGENTS

Possibly life-threatening

Blood clots in the legs, pelvis, lungs, heart, or brain

Headaches

Blurred vision, loss of vision, or flashing lights

Severe leg pains

Severe chest pains or shortness of breath

Serious

Acceleration of existent gallbladder disease, with upper abdominal pain, indigestion, and the development of gallstones

Hypertension

Fairly minor

Nausea

Weight gain, fluid retention, breast fullness or tenderness

Mild headaches

Spotting between periods

Decreased menstrual blood flow

Missed periods

More problems with yeast infection, vaginal itching, or discharge

Depression, mood changes, fatigue

Decreased sex drive (rare)

Acne

Chloasma (spots of darkened skin on the face)

evaluations have been reported, including those performed on serum, red cells, white cells, and urine (Table 2-2). Although most of the changes appear to be mild, some women react considerably to the compounds in OCs and as a result may eventually develop evidence of vitamin deficiency. This circumstance, however, is the exception to the rule in that the majority of OC users show minimal response.

Of interest is a report by Adams et al.[1] that OC-induced depression in women can be alleviated by vitamin B_6 therapy in depressed women with biochemical evidence of an absolute deficiency of vitamin B_6. In this study, 22 depressed women using OCs were found whose symptoms were judged to be caused by the effects of OCs.

Eleven of the women demonstrated clear-cut biochemical evidence of vitamin B_6 deficiency, as judged by lower urinary excretion of 4-pyridoxic acid (a major excretory product of vitamin B_6), increased urinary 3-hydroxykynurenine/3-hydroxyanthranilic acid ratios, and decreased activity of pyridoxal phosphate–dependent erythrocyte aspartate and alanine aminotransferase enzymes. In a double-blind crossover trial these deficient women responded favorably to the administration of pyridoxine hydrochloride; the remaining 11 women without absolute vitamin B_6 deficit demonstrated no such clinical response to the pyridoxine supplement, and placebo administration was without effect.

Possible explanations for OC-induced depression have been proposed by Adams et al.[1] and involve disturbance in brain-amine metabolism. Defective synthesis of brain 5-hydroxytryptamine (5-HT) is implicated, and low levels of 5-HT metabolite have been found in the cerebrospinal fluid of depressed patients. In addition, there is evidence of low 5-HT and 5-hydroxyindolacetic acid in the hindbrains of depressive suicide victims. Finally, the administration of the 5-HT precursor L-tryptophan may be effective in the treatment of depression.

It is proposed therefore that the administration of vitamin B_6 can correct two of the possible mechanisms whereby abnormal tryptophan metabolism develops in response to OC use. Vitamin B_6 might thus prevent the accumulation of tryptophan metabolites that inhibit tryptophan transport into the brain, and it could also restore normal activity to 5-hydroxytryptamine decarboxylase. The preliminary findings of Adams et al.[1] support the effectiveness of vitamin B_6 therapy in improving clinical symptomatology in *some* women with OC-induced depression. It seems reasonable to explore the value of supplementation in women with significant tendencies toward pessimism, dissatisfaction, crying, and tension related very clearly to OC use.

In later research, the vitamin B_6 requirements of OC users were assessed by Bosse and Donald.[5] Eight college-age women using estrogen-containing OCs were fed a low vitamin B_6 diet (0.36 mg/day) for 42 days. Following depletion, repletion was attempted using three

TABLE 2-2 **Oral Contraceptives and Nutritional Status**

Nutrient	Observed Modification in Nutritional Status
Lipids	↑ Plasma triglycerides and β-lipoproteins (very-low-density and low-density lipoproteins) ↓ Plasma α-lipoproteins (high-density lipoproteins) No consistent change in plasma cholesterol; women with familial type II hyperlipoproteinemia show marked increases in plasma cholesterol
Protein and amino acids	↓ Plasma albumin ↑ Plasma α- and β-globulins ↑ Plasma fibrinogen, cortisol-binding globulin, thyroid-binding globulin, retinol-binding protein, transferrin, ceruloplasmin ↑ Conversion of tryptophan to nicotinic acid
Carbohydrate	Small elevations in blood glucose and insulin; glucose tolerance curves shift upward, but shape of the curve is unchanged
Minerals	↓ Serum concentration of calcium, phosphorus, magnesium, and zinc ↑ Erythrocyte concentration of zinc ↑ Serum concentration of iron and copper (along with their respective carrier proteins)
Vitamins	↑ Circulating levels of vitamin A (along with retinol-binding protein) ↓ Circulating levels of carotene, folacin, vitamin B_{12}, and vitamin B_6; reports on circulating levels of vitamins C and E have varied ↑ In vitro stimulation of erythrocyte transketolase and glutathione reductase with thiamine and riboflavin, respectively; suggests availability of these vitamins may be insufficient for maximum enzyme activity in vivo, especially in women whose diets are marginal Biochemical signs of vitamin B_6 deficiency in some women (low urinary pyridoxic acid, plasma phosphate, and erythrocyte aminotransferase)

levels of vitamin B_6: 0.96 mg/day, 1.56 mg/day, and 5.06 mg/day. Vitamin B_6 status was assessed by red cell pyridoxal level, red-cell alanine aminotransferase activity, and red-cell aspartic aminotransferase activity; observations were also made of reactivity of these enzymes when presented with pyridoxal phosphate. Results were compared with data acquired from OC nonusers who consumed a similar diet. The findings tended to suggest that 0.96 mg/day of vitamin B_6 was not adequate to meet the needs of OC users. Intake of 1.5 mg/day, however, was sufficient to return almost all users to predepletion vitamin B_6 status. In line with these data the investigators recommend that an intake of 1.5 to 5 mg/day of vitamin B_6 should be satisfactory for maintenance of status of the typical OC users. Since the usual vitamin B_6 consumption of the adult American woman is between 1.5 and 2.5 mg/day, supplementation does not seem necessary as a routine procedure.

It is clear, however, that debate still exists when the data of Roepke and Kirksey are evaluated.[43] These investigators assessed the vitamin B_6 nutriture of women during pregnancy and lactation to determine whether or not previous use of OCs resulted in reduced reserves of the vitamin. Vitamin B_6 levels were measured (1) in maternal serum and urine at 5 and 7 months' gestation and at delivery, (2) in cord blood, and (3) in milk at 3 and 14 days postpartum. Long-term use of OCs (more than 30 months) resulted in significantly lower levels of vitamin B_6 in maternal serum at 5 months' gestation and at delivery as compared with short-term users and nonusers (1 to 30 months) (Fig. 2-5). Milk and cord blood levels of vitamin B_6 were also lower in the long-term OC population (Figs. 2-5 and 2-6). These results suggest that long-term use of OCs may reduce body reserves of vitamin B_6. Since the hormonal effects of pregnancy augment vitamin B_6 needs, the combined situation of reduced vitamin B_6 reserves and increased vi-

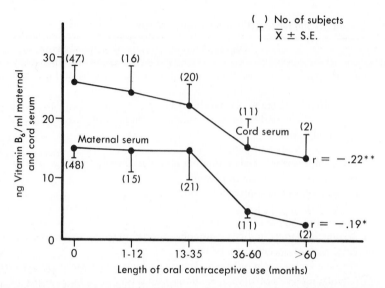

FIG. 2-5 Levels of vitamin B_6 in maternal and cord serum at delivery associated with months of oral contraceptive use. * = correlation coefficient, levels of vitamin B_6 in maternal serum, and length of oral contraceptive use ($p < 0.03$); ** = correlation coefficient, levels of vitamin B_6 in cord serum, and length of oral contraceptive use ($p < 0.01$).

From Roepke JLB and Kirksey A: Vitamin B_6 nutriture during pregnancy and lactation, *Am J Clin Nutr* 32:2257, 1979.

tamin B_6 need may place past long-term OC users and their developing offspring at increased risk of vitamin B_6 deficiency and its consequences.

In summary, these data tend to suggest a variable susceptibility among women to OC-induced vitamin B_6 deficiency. All OC users require adequate but not exceptionally large doses of pyridoxine, and megavitamin therapy is certainly not indicated as a routine preventive measure. It appears, however, that long-term use of these contraceptive agents may increase risk of depleting body vitamin B_6 reserves. This is especially true when diet is substandard, and in such cases a low level of vitamin supplementation may be advisable. For further discussion of oral contraceptive use and vitamin B_6 requirements, see the "Issues and Opinions in Nutrition" sections in recent volumes of the *Journal of Nutrition*.[33,36]

Folic acid status is also of interest with regard to the consequences of oral contraception. Although conflicting data have been published on serum folic acid levels in OC users, the majority of reports indicate a decrease in serum folate, at least in some subjects, during the early part of the menstrual cycle.[31] Red-cell folate also declines. These abnormalities may be improved or corrected following folic acid supplementation. The significance of these findings presently is unknown, especially since the above-mentioned reports are becoming outdated and new OC agents of reduced potency have not been evaluated.

Other research on vitamin status and oral contraceptive use was conducted many years ago using older versions of OCs. The results of these efforts, even using the more potent agents, provided little cause for alarm. The observation of increased serum vitamin A levels in OC users led to fears that a pregnancy following the arrest of contraception might be associated with malformation in the fetus, since vitamin A is known to be teratogenic in large doses. Attention to this possibility by Wald, Schorah, and Smithells,[60] however, revealed no significant difference in vi-

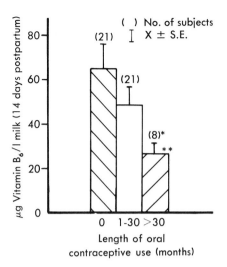

FIG. 2-6 Levels of vitamin B$_6$ in milk at 14 days postpartum in relation to months of OC use. Single asterisk denotes significant difference from mean level associated with 1 to 30 months of OC use ($p < 0.02$); double asterisk denotes significant difference on mean level associated with no OC use ($p < 0.003$).

From Roepke JLB and Kirksey A: Vitamin B$_6$ nutriture during pregnancy and lactation: II. The effect of long-term use of oral contraceptives, *Am J Clin Nutr* 32:2257, 1979.

tamin A levels in the first trimester of pregnancy between women who had never taken OCs and women who discontinued them shortly before conceiving. Women who conceived within 20 weeks of discontinuing OCs had no increase in the incidence of abortion or abnormalities in their babies. The significance of the observed effect of OCs on serum vitamin A level is unknown, but available data strongly suggest that the phenomenon is not detrimental to the health of the woman or to future offspring.

Mineral status. Plasma calcium, phosphorus, and magnesium levels are reduced by the estrogens in OCs. The reduction in plasma levels of these minerals occurs within the first 3 months of treatment and does not appear to change further by longer use of OCs. No significant changes in urinary excretion of calcium, phosphorus, or magnesium have been detected, but bone mineral concentrations may be higher in users than in nonusers.[37]

As far as trace minerals are concerned, few thorough investigations in this area have yet been completed. Early research showed that serum iron levels and iron-binding capacity are both increased by OCs, and diminution of menstrual blood loss often accompanies cyclic hormonal therapy; these observations suggest that iron needs may be slightly reduced in OC users. Estrogen is associated with a significant elevation in serum copper and ceruloplasmin without changes in urinary copper excretion; this observation, like those related to iron, is suggestive of a reduced requirement for copper while a woman is using OCs.

With regard to the effect of OCs on zinc status, conflicting data have been reported. Early reports of reduced plasma zinc concentrations provoked some concern but later research failed to detect an effect of OCs on plasma zinc levels (Table 2-3). Minor changes in postabsorptive utilization of zinc were later associated with OC use.

Thirteen long-term (>3 years) users of oral contraceptives have been followed during their pregnancies,[41] all of which began within 6 months after terminating OC use. During the first trimester and at delivery, red-cell zinc values were reduced, but these changes appeared to be subclinical in magnitude. Because no changes in maternal plasma zinc and copper levels were observed and no hematologic, biochemical, or anthropometric differences were observed in neonates, long-term OC use appeared to have little or no effect on zinc and copper metabolism in subsequent pregnancies.

In summary, as described by King,[26] OC therapy may alter the postabsorptive use of zinc. Circulating zinc levels may be reduced while some tissue levels may be increased. Also, the release of zinc from tissues may be depressed in OC users. There is no evidence, however, that these changes alter the dietary zinc requirement. Endogenous zinc losses have not been found to increase with OC use and signs of zinc deficiency are not evident; zinc-dependent functions do not appear to be compromised. One might therefore conclude that women using OCs do not require extra dietary zinc.

Implications. Although early reports of adverse nutritional consequences related to OC

TABLE 2-3   *Effect of Oral Contraceptive Agents on Plasma Zinc**

Reference	−OC (μg/100 ml)	+OC (μg/100 ml)	% Change
Studies reporting a change			
Briggs, 1971	99 + 14	83 + 16	16
Aiken, 1973	107 + 11	97 + 11	9
Prasad, 1975	119 + 16	112 + 16	6
Chooi, 1976	71 + 34	59 + 18	17
Prema, 1980	110 + 19	76 + 18	31
Studies not reporting a change			
Hess, 1977	81 + 14	85 + 11	NS
Vir, 1981	89 + 10	86 + 13	NS
Hinks, 1983	80 + 12	82 + 12	NS

Modified from King JC: Do women using oral contraceptive agents require extra zinc? *J Nutr* 117:217, 1987.
*Mean + SD. NS = not significant.

use have suggested some cause for concern, little more recent data suggest that nutritional requirements are significantly affected by these agents. The low potency of today's OCs has been associated with reduction in a number of biochemical and physiologic side effects. Reduced or augmented circulating levels of specific nutrients in OC users has not generally been associated with undesirable health consequences or measurable problems in future pregnancies. Special dietary advice for women using OCs is therefore unnecessary, at least for the majority of individuals.

However, some concern still exists for individuals who choose to use the pill for many months and simultaneously choose diets of marginal or even poor quality. The potential exists over the long term for development of suboptimal folic acid and/or vitamin B_6 status (see box on p. 47). Regardless of whether such changes in vitamin status adversely affect future pregnancies has yet to be examined in human populations.

Other Contraceptive Methods

Effects of other contraceptive "agents" on nutritional status have received relatively little attention by the scientific community. Intrauterine devices (IUDs) are still used by some women; most contain copper but some release progesterone, and none is considered ideal. The mechanisms of action are still unclear, but the following are proposed ideas:

1. Increase motility of ovum in fallopian tube
2. Promote local inflammatory responses, causing lysis of the blastocyst and/or prevention of implantation
3. Promote mechanical dislodging of the implanted blastocyst from the endometrium
4. Increase local production of prostaglandins, which inhibit implantation
5. Create competition of copper and zinc, inhibiting carbonic anhydrase and possibly alkaline phosphatase activity; copper may also interfere with estrogen uptake by the uterine mucosa or with cellular uptake of DNA in the endometrium
6. Immobilize sperm

The influence on overall nutritional status of the IUD user is minimal, with the exception of its well-known production of increased blood (and iron) loss during menstruation. Women exhibiting substantial blood loss each month (more than 50 ml) should be advised to supplement their diet with absorbable iron salts (i.e., ferrous sulfate, ferrous gluconate).

Patient Counseling

Available data suggest that OC use does not automatically mandate in-depth nutrition coun-

❖
DIETARY SOURCES OF FOLIC ACID, IRON, AND VITAMIN B₆

Folic acid (folacin)
Dark green leafy vegetables
Lettuce
Lima beans
Cauliflower
Liver
Meats
Eggs
Nuts
Iron
Meats
Egg yolk
Whole wheat (or fortified products)
Seafood
Green leafy vegetables
Nuts
Legumes
Vitamin B₆ (pyridoxine)
Liver
Meats
Cabbage
Banana
Eggs
Corn
Whole wheat
Fish
Rolled oats

seling. Many women who use OCs do so for only a short time and maintain reasonable dietary patterns. Such women should be congratulated for their dietary behavior; special emphasis on folic acid-rich and vitamin B_6-rich foods may be warranted.

Like any woman with poor dietary patterns, OC users in this category should be provided nutritional counseling, individualized to address relevant concerns. Again, emphasis on good food sources of folic acid and vitamin B_6 seems justified. Nutritional supplements should not be routinely recommended although medical conditions or lifestyle circumstances may warrant selection of an appropriate low-dosage product.

The most helpful recommendation for the woman with an IUD is to provide for iron needs in relation to menstrual blood losses. Improvement in iron intake through dietary modification can be suggested as sufficient in itself to meet iron needs, but supplementation with iron salts may be appropriate for women with excessive menstrual bleeding.

A NEW THRUST: PRECONCEPTION CARE

A major movement is under way to motivate potential new parents to participate in advance planning of their pregnancies.[22,23] This effort, now referred to as "preconception care," allows for preparation of the best possible prenatal environment for the conceptus. The components of preconception care are listed in the box on p. 48. They include risk assessment, health promotion, and interventions to reduce risk. Risks identifiable before conception may involve medical, social, psychological, or lifestyle conditions. Risk assessment provides an opportunity to identify social factors related to poor obstetric outcome, including inadequate housing, low income, less than a high school education, and problems related to being a single parent. Once risks are known, some women may benefit from counseling and referral to social, mental health, and substance abuse treatment programs or vocational training.

Preconception assessment of nutritional status should identify individuals who are underweight or overweight; conditions such as bulimia, anorexia, pica, or hypervitaminosis; and special dietary habits such as vegetarianism. Nutrition counseling may prove useful; this may include information about dietary control of chronic diseases such as diabetes mellitus. The same applies to phenylketonuria; strict control of maternal serum phenylalanine levels is essential to optimizing chances for normal development of the offspring.[34]

It is hoped that eventually preconception care will be shown to yield such positive results that insurance coverage will routinely be provided and clinicians will urge their clients of reproductive age to prepare for conception in every possible way. This preparation should include a formal preconception evaluation to determine (1)

❖

COMPONENTS OF PRECONCEPTION CARE AS PART OF PRIMARY CARE SERVICES

Risk assessment

Individual and social conditions (age, diet, education, housing, and economic status)

Adverse health behaviors (tobacco, alcohol, and illicit drug abuse)

Medical conditions (immune status, medications, genetic illness, illnesses including infection, and prior obstetric history)

Psychological conditions (personal and family readiness for pregnancy, stress, anxiety, and depression)

Environmental conditions (workplace hazards, toxic chemicals, and radiation contamination)

Barriers to family planning, prenatal care, and primary health care

Health promotion

Promotion of healthy behaviors (proper nutrition, avoidance of smoking, alcohol, teratogens, and practice of "safe sex")

Counseling about the availability of social, financial, and vocational assistance programs

Advice of family planning, pregnancy spacing, and contraception

Counseling about the importance of early registration and compliance with prenatal care, including high-risk programs if warranted

Identification of barriers to care and assistance in overcoming them

Arrangements for ongoing care

Interventions

Treatment of medical conditions, including changes in medications, if appropriate, and referral to high-risk pregnancy programs

Referral for treatment of adverse health behaviors (tobacco, alcohol, and illicit drug abuse)

Rubella and hepatitis immunization

Reduction of psychosocial risks that may involve counseling or referral to home health agencies, community mental health centers, safe shelters, enrollment in medical assistance, and assistance with housing

Nutrition counseling, supplementation or referral to improve adequacy of diet

Home visit to further assess and intervene in the home environment

Provision of family planning services

From Jack B, Culpepper L: Preconception care: risk reduction and health promotion, *JAMA* 264:1147, 1990.

if reproduction is associated with high risk that is not modifiable and thus suggests that serious consideration should be given to avoiding pregnancy and (2) if modifiable risks are identified and addressed, can it be expected that there will be a marked increase in the likelihood of good pregnancy outcome?

Underweight

Numerous studies have clearly shown that underweight women are at increased risk for reproductive problems.[11] Not only is fertility compromised but the likelihood of premature delivery and intrauterine growth retardation is increased; Apgar scores of offspring are more frequently low (Table 2-4). The condition of underweight is potentially modifiable since it is often related to abusive dieting practices and/or

exercise programs. A woman motivated toward improvement of her body-weight-for-height status may successfully and healthfully achieve her goal within a relatively short time (3 to 6 months).

Obesity

Women who exceed their desirable body weight by more than 35% are at greater risk than normal-weight women for an unsatisfactory pregnancy course and outcome. Numerous studies have shown that obese women are at higher risk for antenatal complications, especially pregnancy-induced hypertension, gestational diabetes, urinary tract infections and pyelonephritis[15]; they also are more likely to demonstrate prolonged labor followed by difficult vaginal delivery and thus more frequently

TABLE 2-4 *Infant Morbidity in Underweight Women and Normal-Weight Controls*

Infant Morbidity	Low Prepregnancy Weight (% of Births)	Normal Weight Controls (% of Births)
Low birth weight	15.3	7.6
Prematurity	23.0	14.0
Low Apgar score	19.0	12.0

From Edwards LE, et al: Pregnancy in the underweight woman: course, outcome and growth patterns of the infant, *Am J Obstet Gynecol* 135:297, 1979.

deliver by cesarean section.[29] Perinatal mortality is likewise higher. Surviving babies of obese mothers may present more treatment challenges during the neonatal period since they often demonstrate difficulty in regulating blood glucose.[30] Theoretically, reducing the degree of maternal obesity before conception should improve pregnancy progress and outcome. Attempts along this line are worth making if time allows and the woman appears to be properly motivated. Unfortunately, such motivation may not exist, or if it does, the ability to follow a prescribed program may be limited. In any case, attempts should be made throughout the reproductive period (if not before) to prevent the development of excessive adiposity.

Micronutrient Imbalances

If deficiencies or excesses of either vitamins or minerals are associated with congenital malformations and/or spontaneous abortion, then correction of such imbalances is most likely to improve outcome if it is accomplished prior to (or at least by) the time of conception. Unfortunately, our understanding of the role of nutrient deficits and excesses in the etiology of early-pregnancy problems is very poor.

Folic Acid Deficiency

Maternal folic acid deficiency[9] in experimental animals has long been associated with increased incidence of congenital malformations in the offspring. Malformations have also been described in the offspring of women who used drugs that are folate antagonists. Limited evidence in humans also suggests that deficiency of this vitamin may be associated with spontaneous abortion. Recently, the importance of folic acid in the prevention of neural tube defects (NTDs) in human infants has been well-established, but this came only after many years of observation and experimentation.[61]

Clinicians in Northern Europe suggested in the 1960s that folic acid might prevent neural tube defects. Limited evidence was available at that time and little attention was paid to the idea. However, Smithells et al,[49,50,51] Sheppard et al[48] and Laurence et al[32] examined the impact of vitamin supplementation (or specifically folic acid) on the recurrence of NTDs among women who had previously given birth to such offspring. Their findings yielded favorable outcomes with supplementation positively associated with reduction in risk of recurrence. However, these researchers were criticized for methodological errors in study design and execution. Only after the British Medical Research Council issued its impressive study did the world take notice.[39] This randomized prevention trial began in July 1983 and was stopped in April 1991. It involved 33 centers, 17 in the United Kingdom and 16 in six other countries. Study participants were women who had a previous pregnancy that resulted in an infant with a neural tube defect and who were planning a subsequent pregnancy. Each participant was randomly assigned to one of four supplementation groups (A, B, C, and D). Group A received 4 mg of folic acid daily; Group B, a multivitamin preparation plus 4 mg folic acid; Group C, neither the multivitamin nor folic acid; and Group D, the multivitamin preparation without folic acid. All capsules contained two mineral supplements.

CDC RECOMMENDATIONS FOR FOLIC ACID SUPPLEMENTATION FOR WOMEN— AUGUST 1991

1. Women who have had a pregnancy resulting in an infant or fetus with a neural-tube defect should be counseled about the increased risk in subsequent pregnancies and should be advised that folic acid supplementation may substantially reduce the risk for neural-tube defects in subsequent pregnancies.

2. Women who have had a pregnancy resulting in an infant or fetus with a neural-tube defect should be advised to consult their physician as soon as they plan a pregnancy. Unless contraindicated, they should be advised to take 4 mg per day of folic acid starting at the time they plan to become pregnant. Women should take the supplement from at least 4 weeks before conception through the first 3 months of pregnancy.

3. The 4-mg daily dose should be taken only under a physician's supervision. Tablets containing 1 mg of folic acid are available as a prescription item. The dose of folic acid should be obtained from pills containing only folic acid. Multivitamin (over-the-counter and prescription) preparations containing folic acid should not be used to attain the 4-mg dose because harmful levels of vitamins A and D could also be taken. Prescribing physicians should be aware of the potential for high doses of folic acid to complicate the diagnosis of vitamin B_{12} deficiency. Anemia resulting from vitamin B_{12} deficiency may be prevented with high doses of folic acid; however, the neurologic damage that can result from vitamin B_{12} deficiency could continue.

4. These recommendations are provided only for women who previously have given birth to an infant or had a fetus with a neural-tube defect; they are not intended for (1) women who have never given birth to an infant or had a fetus with a neural-tube defect, (2) relatives of women who have had an infant or fetus with a neural-tube defect, (3) women who themselves have spina bifida, or (4) women who take the anticonvulsant valproic acid—a known cause of spina bifida.

From *MMWR* 40:515, 1991.

During the study period, complete information was available on 1,195 pregnancy outcomes. Folic acid supplementation was associated with a 71% reduction in the recurrence of neural tube defects. Use of the multivitamins without folic acid was not associated with a protective effect. Because of the substantial protective effect, the study data monitoring group recommended halting the study early so that all women at risk could receive the potential benefits of supplementation. The Centers for Disease Control and Prevention in the United States now recommends the use of folic acid supplementation (4 mg/day) for women who previously have had an infant or fetus with spina bifida, anencephaly, or encephalocele (see box above).[6]

Concurrent with and following the above-mentioned research activity, effort was under-way to test the value of folic acid supplementation periconceptionally on the *occurrence* of NTDs. Czeizel and colleagues[8] in Hungary recruited women who were planning a pregnancy and assigned them randomly to receive (before and during early pregnancy) a 0.4 mg folic acid supplement or a placebo containing trace elements. None of the women had previously delivered an abnormal offspring. The results of the study were very impressive—a markedly reduced incidence of NTDs in the folic acid supplemented group.

This landmark study was accompanied by a series of observational studies, many of which were conducted in various parts of the United States. Here, groups of women were interviewed about their vitamin supplementation patterns around the time of conception. Patterns of vitamin use among women who had delivered babies with NTDs were compared with patterns of women who had delivered normal infants. Of nine studies conducted, only one was negative. That is, eight of the studies showed that taking vitamins around the time of conception was associated with a significantly reduced risk of delivering an infant with NTDs.

With this abundance of data in hand, the Centers for Disease Control and Prevention and the U.S. Public Health Service recommended that "all women of childbearing age who are capable of becoming pregnant should consume 0.4 mg of folic acid per day for the purpose of reducing their risk of having a pregnancy affected with spina bifida or other neural tube defects." This recommendation was followed by several other countries.[9]

The subject of folic acid deficiency and pregnancy course and outcome will be discussed further later in this text. Fortification of grain products with folic acid was approved in 1996. This practice will take effect in 1998 and should improve folic acid status of the women who use these foods.

Vitamin A Teratogenesis

Excessive consumption of vitamin A appears to be teratogenic. A number of case reports of adverse pregnancy outcome have been associated with a daily ingestion of 25,000 IU or more.[56] These data derive from Adverse Drug Reaction Reports filed with the Food and Drug Administration (FDA) concerning the use of vitamin A during pregnancy. Almost all of the FDA cases are brief retrospective reports of malformed infants or fetuses exposed to supplements of at least 25,000 IU/day of vitamin A during pregnancy. In addition, epidemiologic evidence indicates that the drug isotretinoin (used for treatment of cystic acne) causes major malformations involving craniofacial, central nervous system, cardiac, and thymic changes[3]; isotretinoin is a vitamin A analogue. The Teratology Society[56] urges that women in their reproductive years be informed that the excessive use of vitamin A shortly before and during pregnancy could be harmful to their babies. They further support the practice of labeling products containing vitamin A to indicate that consumption of excessive amounts of vitamin A may be hazardous to the embryo or fetus when taken during pregnancy and that women of childbearing age should consult with their physicians before consuming these products.

Proof of the potential hazards of excessive doses of vitamin A came recently from researchers at Boston University.[46] They interviewed more than 20,000 pregnant women who were identified by their scheduling of prenatal amniocentesis or α-fetoprotein screen for birth defects. Among other things, questions were asked about diet and supplement use, specifically focusing on retinol (the preformed variety of vitamin A). Pregnancy outcome data were obtained from managing obstetricians or the mothers themselves. Results indicated that retinol intake in excess of 15,000 IU daily was associated with a significantly increased risk of birth defects, specifically those that related to development of the neural crest (Table 2-5). Among the babies born to women who took more than 10,000 IU of preformed vitamin A

TABLE 2-5   *Teratogenicity of Vitamin A: Defects Related to Cranial Neural Crest Development*

	# Defects	% Defects
Daily retinol intake (IU)		
0-5000	33	0.51
5001-10,000	59	0.47
10,001-15,000	20	0.63
>15,001	9	1.8
Retinol intake from food (IU)		
0-5000	114	0.52
5001-10,000	5	0.62
10,001-15,000	2	1.06
Retinol intake from supplements		
0-5000	51	0.46
5001-8,000	54	0.51
8001-10,000	9	1.18
>10,001	7	2.21

From: Rothman KJ et al: Teratogenicity of high vitamin A intake, *N Engl J Med* 333:1369, 1995

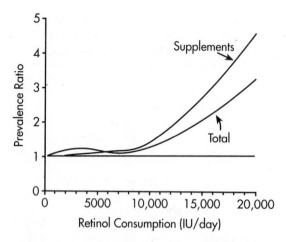

FIG. 2-7 Estimated prevalence ratio for birth defects related to the cranial neural crest, according to retinol intake during the first trimester of pregnancy.

From Rothman KJ et al: Teratogenicity of high vitamin A intake, *N Engl J Med* 333:1369, 1995.

per day in the form of supplements, about one infant in 57 had a malformation attributable to the supplement (Fig. 2-7).

Zinc Deficiency

Considerable interest has developed in the significance of zinc deficiency in adversely affecting pregnancy outcome. Zinc deficiency is highly teratogenic in rats. Nonhuman primates are also affected; abnormal brain development and behavior have been described in offspring of zinc-deficient monkeys.

Limited epidemiologic evidence suggests that the malformation rate and other poor pregnancy outcomes may be higher in populations in which zinc deficiency has been recognized. In addition, (1) Jameson has observed that women with low serum levels of zinc demonstrated high incidence of abnormal deliveries, including congenital malformations[24]; (2) women with acrodermatitis enteropathica (a genetic disorder of zinc metabolism treated effectively with supplemental zinc) show much-improved pregnancy outcomes than in the past when supplemental zinc was not employed[20]; and (3) plasma zinc concentrations were significantly lower in the blood of 54 women who gave birth to congeni-

tally malformed babies as compared with control mothers.[52]

Although the potential value of zinc supplementation has been examined in several populations, to date, the data are judged to be insufficient to mandate the institution of preconceptional zinc supplementation practices. However, since the zinc intake of premenopausal women is marginal at best (9 to 11 mg/day), prenatal nutrition counseling might appropriately include guidelines for optimizing zinc intake.

Substance Use/Abuse

Alcohol. Research has confirmed that excessive consumption of alcohol adversely affects fetal development. In 1973, researchers described a unique set of characteristics of infants born to women who were chronic alcoholics. These infants exhibited specific anomalies of the eyes, nose, heart, and central nervous system that were accompanied by growth retardation and mental retardation. This condition is now recognized as the "fetal alcohol syndrome" (FAS). It occurs in 1 to 2 infants per 1,000 live births in the United States.

The impact of more moderate levels of alcohol consumption on fetal development has also been the focus of much research. It is now appreciated that moderate drinkers may produce offspring with "fetal alcohol effects" (more subtle features of FAS); such women also demonstrate a higher rate of spontaneous abortion, abruptio placentae, and low-birth-weight delivery.

Possible fetal alcohol effects (PFAE) is a term used to describe individuals who have been prenatally exposed to alcohol and present with cognitive and behavioral problems, but who do not have all of the facial characteristics of FAS. As put simply by one researcher, PFAE is "FAS without a face." In the absence of the characteristic facial features, the cognitive/behavioral dysfunction in an individual cannot be directly and exclusively linked to the prenatal alcohol exposure. Therefore FAE is not a medical diagnosis at this time, and it is more accurate to use the term *possible* fetal alcohol effects. PFAE is also not a "mild" form of FAS. In fact, individuals with PFAE can be just as severely affected cognitively and behaviorally as those with FAS. The needs of individuals with PFAE and their families may be just as acute as those with full FAS; however, it is more difficult for individuals with PFAE to access services because they do not have a medical diagnosis.

The bottomline is that alcohol consumption during pregnancy may adversely affect pregnancy outcome. The effects may be dramatic or subtle. In either case, *all women planning for conception should be advised to avoid alcoholic beverages. Women with a known addiction to alcohol should be strongly encouraged to enroll in a treatment program and abstain from unprotected sexual activity if treatment is unsuccessful.*

Caffeine. The possible danger of caffeine to the developing fetus has been examined in several animal models. Massive doses appear to be teratogenic in rats and mice,[4] but the effects of smaller quantities have not been satisfactorily examined. During the past 15 years, a number of studies have dealt with the incidence of birth defects in children and caffeine consumption by their mothers. No associations have been found. In one study, more than 12,000 women were questioned soon after delivery about their coffee and tea consumption.[35] No relationship was found between coffee and tea consumption and excess malformations among their babies. Another study published the same year[61] involved 2,030 infants, examined for a relationship between their mother's caffeine intake during pregnancy and six specific birth defects (inguinal hernia, cleft lip with and without cleft palate, isolated cleft palate, cardiac defects, pyloric stenosis, and neural-tube defects). The findings were negative, and the authors concluded that maternal ingestion of caffeine in tea, coffee, and cola has a minimal, if any, effect on incidence of those six birth defects.

However, a prospective cohort study involving over 3000 women in Connecticut is provocative.[53] Almost 80% of these pregnant women used some caffeine daily and 28% consumed 150 mg or more of caffeine each day. This latter group of moderate to heavy users of caffeine was significantly more likely to experience late first- and second-trimester spontaneous abortion when compared with nonusers and light users (0 to 149 mg daily) of caffeine. Although this report does suggest some cause

for concern, the authors point out that confirmation of these findings through additional research is essential before implicating caffeine in the etiology of spontaneous abortion.

Overall, data obtained from human populations do not provide *convincing* evidence that caffeine affects embryonic development. Even so, common sense should prevail, and women considering pregnancy might legitimately be advised to use caffeine in moderation if they choose to use it at all.

Aspartame. Since the approval of aspartame for use in carbonated beverages (1983), there has been debate about the safety of this sweetener in the diets of pregnant women. Major concern has been voiced about the added phenylalanine load, because high circulating levels of phenylalanine (as are seen in women with poorly controlled phenylketonuria, or PKU) are known to damage the fetal brain.[34] However, individuals who do not have PKU have plenty of phenylalanine hydroxylase activity in the liver to prevent any substantial and sustained rise in serum phenylalanine after consuming aspartame-rich beverages or foods. Because no data exist to suggest that use of aspartame-containing products is associated with adverse pregnancy outcome, it seems unreasonable to direct women to avoid this alternative sweetener.

Control of Chronic Disease

Data are now abundant supporting the value for the fetus of preconceptional or very early prenatal control of certain chronic diseases. Good examples of the effectiveness of these early interventions are maternal PKU and insulin-dependent diabetes mellitus (IDDM). Metabolic control of both diseases involves conscientious dietary manipulation well before the critical period of embryonic development. In the case of the women with PKU, restriction of dietary phenylalanine is mandatory, while satisfying the protein and other nutrient requirements of mother and fetus; data indicate that the IQ of the offspring is inversely related to maternal serum phenylalanine concentration during pregnancy.[34]

The woman with IDDM must control blood glucose levels through careful food selection and scheduled meal timing in concert with the administration of insulin. In a nonrandomized study of diabetic women in Europe, preconceptional control was associated with a reduction in the incidence of congenital malformations in comparison with that of the nondiabetic control population[14]:

	Malformation rate (by %)
Nondiabetic women (n = 420)	1.4
Women with IDDM (n = 420)	5.5
With early counseling (n = 128)	0.8
Counseling after 8 weeks gestation (n = 292)	7.5

In a large multicenter study in the United States during the early 1980s, very early prenatal intervention for management of IDDM was associated with a marked reduction in the congenital malformation rate but not to the low level of the nondiabetic women.[37]

	Malformation rate (by percent)
Nondiabetic women (n = 468)	3.5
Women with IDDM who had late counseling (n = 296)	13.0
Women with IDDM who had counseling at 15 to 21 days post conception (n = 409)	6.0

The incidence of spontaneous abortion was also significantly reduced in this early-counseled population, presumably a result of the improved metabolic control.[38]

It makes sense, therefore, that efforts should be made preconceptionally to motivate women with controllable diseases to prepare themselves for conception by initiating dietary and other necessary lifestyle changes to allow the optimal maternal metabolic state. This can certainly be said for women with IDDM and PKU, but it also applies to women with other chronic diseases. Not only will such efforts reduce morbidity and mortality of offspring, but they may also improve the health and well-being of the mother during the prenatal period.

The Negative Pregnancy Test: An Opportunity for Preconception Care

Nearly half of the pregnancies in the United States are unplanned or unintended; it logically follows that many women seek professional health care to determine whether they are pregnant. If pregnancy is confirmed, preconceptional counseling is not possible. However, if the test is negative, it is possible for the health care provider to "slip in" some preconceptional care.[21]

To examine the value of such an approach, a survey was administered during a structured interview to 136 women who had a negative pregnancy test visit in a family practice residency ambulatory practice. The survey solicited the presence of self-reported risk variables associated with maternal conditions related to poor obstetric outcome, risk factors for poor obstetric outcome, and risks for developing these conditions. Results indicated that more than 50% of the women reported a medical or reproductive risk that could adversely affect pregnancy; 50% of women reported a genetic risk; 29% reported a risk for human immunodeficiency virus (HIV) infection; and more than 25% reported recent use of illegal substances. It therefore appears that a negative pregnancy test visit provides an opportunity for preconception risk assessment and counseling.

Summary

It is clear that nutrition, fertility, and family planning are issues with considerable interrelationship in developed as well as developing societies. Future planning with regard to nutrition policy and programs must focus on specific needs in given communities. Integrated programs involving birth control strategies/services and nutritional maintenance should be developed with special attention to the protection of adolescent, pregnant, and lactating women, as well as the young children they care for. Oral and other methods of birth control seem safer today than ever before; continued monitoring of the side effects and nutritional consequences is reasonable. In the meantime, much progress will be made in the next several decades with preconception intervention. While this seems difficult to those who are young and not very anxious to "plan," common sense dictates that much effort should be expended in this direction. Many health care dollars are spent in solving problems that could have been lessened or ameliorated; a major focus of reproductive services should be in this direction.

REVIEW QUESTIONS

1. Discuss ways in which the diet of a woman might affect her fertility.
2. Diet is not the only factor that may influence fertility in women. What else will affect it?
3. How might today's contraceptive agents affect nutritional needs of women?
4. Outline the diet/nutrition-relevant preconceptional interventions that are likely to improve pregnancy outcome.

LEARNING ACTIVITIES

1. Determine the local use of various contraceptive agents and assess the type of "nutrition" advice given to users.
2. Ask regional health care providers for young women about the incidence of amenorrhea and the consequences they have seen.

REFERENCES

1. Adams RW et al: Effect of pyridoxine hydrochloride (vitamin B_6) upon depression associated with oral contraception, *Lancet* 1:897, 1973.
2. Barr SI, Janelle KC, Prior JC: Vegetarian vs nonvegetarian diets, dietary constraint, and subclinical ovulatory disturbances: prospective 6-mo study, *Am J Clin Nutr* 60:887, 1994.
3. Benke PJ: The isotretinoin teratogen syndrome, *JAMA* 251:3267, 1984.
4. Bertrand M, Schwan E, Frandon A et al: Systematic and specific teratogenic effects of caffeine in rodents, *CR Soc Biol* 159:2199, 1965.
5. Bosse TR, Donald EA: The vitamin B_6 requirement in oral contraceptive users: I. Assessment of pyridoxal level and transferase activity in erythrocytes, *Am J Clin Nutr* 32:1015, 1979.
6. Centers for Disease Control: Interim recommendations for folic acid supplementation for women—August 1991, *MMWR* 40:515, 1991.
7. Cramer DW, Xu H, and Sahi T: Adult hypolactasia, milk consumption and age-specific fertility, *Am J Epid* 139:282, 1994.
8. Czeizel AE: Controlled studies of multivitamin supplementation on pregnancy outcomes, *Ann NY Acad Sci* 678:266, 1993.
9. Czeizel AE: Folic acid in the prevention of neural tube defects, *J Pediatr Gastroent Nutr* 20:4, 1995.
10. Dawson DW: Infertility and folate deficiency: case reports, *Br J Obstet Gynaecol* 89:678, 1982.
11. Edwards LE, et al: Pregnancy in the underweight woman: course, outcome and growth patterns of the infant, *Am J Obstet Gynecol* 135:297, 1979.
12. Fédération CECOS, Schwartz D, Mayaux BA: Female fecundity as a function of age: results of artificial insemination in 2193 nulliparous women with azoospermic husbands, *N Engl J Med* 306:404, 1982.
13. Frisch RE: Nutrition, fatness and fertility: the effect of food intake on reproductive ability. In Mosley WH, editor: *Nutrition and human reproduction*, New York, 1978, Plenum.
14. Fuhrmann K, Reiher H, Semmler K et al: Prevention of congenital malformations in infants of insulin-dependent diabetic mothers, *Diabetes Care* 6:219, 1983.
15. Garbaciak JA, Richter M, Miller S et al: Maternal weight and pregnancy complications, *Obstet Gynecol* 152:238, 1985.
16. Gerstman BB, Gross TP, Kennedy DL et al: Trends in the content and use of oral contraceptives in the United States, 1964-88, *Am J Public Health* 81:90, 1991.
17. Grodstein F, Goldman MB, Cramer DW: Infertility in women and moderate alcohol use, *Am J Public Health* 84:1429, 1994.
18. Grodstein F et al: Relation of female infertility to consumption of caffeinated beverages, *Am J Epid* 137:1353, 1993.
19. Hackman E et al: Maternal birth weight and subsequent pregnancy outcome, *JAMA* 250:2016, 1983.
20. Hambidge KM, Neidner KH, Walravens PA: Zinc, acrodermatitis and congenital malformations, *Lancet* 1:577, 1975.
21. Jack BW: The negative pregnancy test: an opportunity for preconception care *Arch Fam Med* 4:340, 1995.
22. Jack B, Culpepper L: Preconception care. In Merkatz I, Thompson J, Mullen P et al, editors: *New perspectives on prenatal care*, New York, 1990, Elsevier.
23. Jack B, Culpepper L: Preconception care: risk reduction and health promotion, *JAMA* 264:1147, 1990.
24. Jameson S: Effects of zinc deficiency in human reproduction, *Acta Med Scand* 5(Suppl 593):64, 1976.
25. Kemmann E, Pasquale SA, Skaf R: Amenorrhea associated with carotenemia, *JAMA* 249:926, 1983.

26. King JC: Do women using oral contraceptive agents require extra zinc? *J Nutr* 117:217, 1987.

27. Klebanoff MA et al: Low birth weight across generations, *JAMA* 252:2423, 1984.

28. Klebanoff MA, Yip R: Influence of maternal birth weight on rate of fetal growth and duration of gestation, *J Pediatr* 111:287, 1987.

29. Kleigman RM, Gross T: Perinatal problems of the obese mother and her infant, *Obstet Gynecol* 66:229, 1985.

30. Kleigman R, Gross T, Morton S et al: Intrauterine growth and postnatal fasting metabolism in infants of obese mothers, *J Pediatr* 104:601, 1984.

31. Krauss RM, Burkman RT: The metabolic impact of oral contraceptives, *Am J Obstet Gynecol* 167:1177, 1992.

32. Laurence KM, James N, Miller MH et al: Double-blind randomized controlled trial of folate treatment before conception to prevent recurrence of neural-tube defects, *BMJ* 282:1509, 1981.

33. Leklem JE: Vitamin B_6 requirements and oral contraceptive use—a concern? *J Nutr* 116:475, 1986.

34. Levy HL and Waisbren SE: Effects of untreated maternal phenylketonuria and hyperphenylalaninemia on the fetus, *N Engl J Med* 309:1269, 1983.

35. Linn S, Schoenbaum SC, Monsen RR et al: No association between coffee consumption and adverse outcomes of pregnancy, *N Engl J Med* 306:141, 1982.

36. Miller LT: Do oral contraceptive agents affect nutrient requirements—vitamin B_6? *J Nutr* 116:1344, 1986.

37. Mills JL, Knopp RH, Simpson JL et al: Lack of relation of increased malformation rates in infants of diabetic mothers to glycemic control during organogenesis, *N Engl J Med* 318:671, 1988.

38. Mills JL, Simpson JL, Driscoll SG: Incidence of spontaneous abortion among normal women and insulin-dependent diabetic women whose pregnancies were identified within 21 days of conception, *N Engl J Med* 319:1617, 1988.

39. MRC Vitamin Study Research Group: Prevention of neural tube defects: results of the Medical Research Council vitamin study, *Lancet* 338:131, 1991.

40. Pedersen AB et al: Menstrual differences due to vegetation and nonvegetarian diets, *Am J Clin Nutr* 53:879, 1991.

41. Powell-Beard L, Kei KY, Shenker L: Effect of long-term oral contraceptive therapy before pregnancy on maternal and fetal zinc and copper status, *Obstet Gynecol* 69:26, 1987.

42. Prysak M, Lorenz RP, Kisly A: Pregnancy outcome in nulliparous women 35 years and older, *Obstet Gynecol* 85:65, 1995.

43. Roepke JLB, Kirksey A: Vitamin B_6 nutriture during pregnancy and lactation: II. The effect of long-term use of oral contraceptives, *Am J Clin Nutr* 32:2257, 1979.

44. Rosenberg L, Mitchell A, Shapiro S, Stone D: Selected birth defects in relation to caffeine-containing beverages, *JAMA* 247:1429, 1982.

45. Rosevear et al: Smoking and decreased fertilization rates in vitro, *Lancet* 340:1195, 1992.

46. Rothman KJ et al: Teratogenicity of high vitamin A intake. *N Engl J Med* 333:1369, 1995.

47. Shaw RW: Adverse long-term effects of oral contraceptives: a review, *Br J Obstet Gynaecol* 94:724, 1987.

48. Sheppard S, Nevin NC, Seller MJ et al: Neural tube defect recurrence after 'partial' vitamin supplementation, *J Med Genet* 26:326, 1989.

49. Smithells RW, Nevin NC, Seller MD et al: Further experience of vitamin supplementation for prevention of neural tube defect recurrences, *Lancet* 1:1027, 1983.

50. Smithells RW, Sheppard S, Schorah CJ et al: Apparent prevention of neural tube defects by periconceptional vitamin supplementation, *Arch Dis Child* 56:911, 1981.

51. Smithells RW, Sheppard S, Schorah CJ et al: Possible prevention of neural-tube defects by periconceptional vitamin supplementation, *Lancet* 1:339, 1980.

52. Soltan MH, Jenkins MH: Maternal and fetal plasma zinc concentration and fetal abnormality, *Br J Obstet Gynaecol* 89:56, 1982.

53. Srisuphan W, Bracken MB: Caffeine consumption during pregnancy and association with late spontaneous abortion, *Am J Obstet Gynecol* 154:14, 1986.

54. Stergachis A: Epidemiology of the noncontraceptive effects of oral contraceptives, *Am J Obstet Gynecol* 167:1165, 1992.

55. Subcommittee on Nutrition and Fertility, Food

and Nutrition Board, National Research Council, National Academy of Sciences: *Nutrition and fertility interrelationships: implications for policy and action*. Washington, DC, 1975, Government Printing Office.

56. Teratology Society: Teratology Society position paper: recommendations for vitamin A use during pregnancy, *Teratology* 35:269, 1987.

57. Trussell J, Vaughan B: Contraceptive use projections: 1990 to 2010, *Am J Obstet Gynecol* 167:1160, 1992.

58. Tyson JE, Perez A: The maintenance of infecundity in postpartum women. In Mosley, WH, editor: *Nutrition and human reproduction*, New York, 1978, Plenum.196

59. Vakil DV, Ayiomamitis A, Nizami N: *Nutr Res* 5:911, 1985.

60. Wald J, Schorah CJ, Smithells RW: Vitamin A, pregnancy, and oral contraceptives, *BMJ* 1:57, 1974.

61. Wald NJ: Neural tube defects and vitamins: the need for a randomized clinical trial, *Br J Obstet Gynaecol* 91:516, 1984.

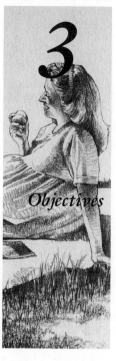

3

Physiology of Pregnancy

Bonnie S. Worthington-Roberts

Objectives

✦✦✦

After completing this chapter, the student will be able to:

✓ *Describe the major anatomical and physiological changes that occur during the course of human pregnancy*

✓ *Discuss maternal weight gain patterns in normal women*

✓ *Discuss the role of the placenta in the maintenance of a normal pregnancy*

Introduction

Normal pregnancy is accompanied by anatomic and physiologic changes that affect almost every function of the body. Many of these changes are apparent in the very early weeks.[12] This indicates that they are not merely a response to the physiologic stress imposed by the fetus but are an integral part of the maternal-fetal system, which creates the most favorable environment possible for the developing child. The changes are necessary to regulate maternal metabolism, promote fetal growth, and prepare the mother for labor, birth, and lactation.

The changes that occur in pregnancy are too complex to be given full treatment here, but a look at some that have effects on general metabolism will lay the foundation for interpreting nutritional requirements and dietary allowances.

THE LENGTH OF UNCOMPLICATED HUMAN GESTATION

It was proposed in the 1800s that pregnancy lasts 266 days. To examine the accuracy of this estimate, researchers in Boston studied uncomplicated spontaneous-labor pregnancy in a group of private care white mothers.[48] The historical belief that human gestation was 10 menstrual cycles in duration was not confirmed. For primiparas, the median duration of gestation from assumed ovulation to delivery was 274 days, significantly longer than the predicted 266 days. For multiparas the median duration of pregnancy was 269 days, also significantly longer than the prediction. This study suggests that when estimating a due date for private-care white patients, a practitioner should count back three months from the first day of the last menses, then add 15 days for primiparas or 10 days for multiparas.

INCIDENCE OF EARLY PREGNANCY LOSS

There has always been uncertainty about the frequency of early pregnancy loss. In an effort to assess this phenomenon, researchers studied 221 women by collecting daily urine specimens and measuring human chorionic gonadotropin (HCG) levels.[72] Pregnancy was diagnosed in 198 women by an increase in HCG level near the expected time of implantation. Of these, pregnancies, 22% ended before pregnancy was detected clinically. The total rate of pregnancy loss after implantation including clinically recognized spontaneous abortions was 31%. Most of the 40 women with unrecognized early pregnancy losses had normal fertility since 95% of them subsequently became clinically pregnant within 2 years. This study demonstrates the long-suspected high incidence of "occult abortion" following implantation.

THE CARDIOVASCULAR SYSTEM

Extensive anatomic and physiologic changes occur in the cardiovascular system during the course of pregnancy. These adaptations protect the woman's normal physiologic functioning, meet the metabolic demands pregnancy imposes on her body, and provide for fetal development and growth needs.

The slight cardiac hypertrophy or dilation is probably secondary to increased blood volume and cardiac output. As the diaphragm is displaced upward, the heart is elevated upward and to the left. The degree of shift depends on the duration of pregnancy and the size and position of the uterus.

Auscultatory changes accompany the changes in heart size and position. Increases in blood volume and cardiac output also contribute to auscultatory changes common in pregnancy: a third heart sound and an ejection murmur. Between weeks 14 and 20, pulse increases slowly up to 10 to 15 beats per minute, which persists to term. Palpitations may occur, and bradycardia may begin after delivery and persist for 1 week. Arterial blood pressure varies with age, and blood pressure readings vary with the position of the woman. Blood pressure is highest in the sitting position, lowest when lying in the left lateral recumbent position, and intermediate when supine. During the first half of pregnancy, there is a decrease in both systolic and diastolic pressure of 5 to 10 mm Hg. The decrease in blood pressure is probably the result of peripheral vasodilation from hormonal changes during pregnancy. During the third trimester, maternal blood pressure should return to the values obtained during the first trimester (Fig. 3-1).

Cardiac output increases from 30% to 50% by week 32 of pregnancy; it declines to about a 20% increase at week 40. The elevated cardiac output is largely a result of increased stroke volume and in response to increased tissue demands for oxygen (normal value is 5 to 5.5 L/min). The cardiac output decreases with the woman in the supine position and increases with any exertion such as labor and delivery. The circulation time decreases slightly by week 32. It returns to near normal near **term.**

Inadequate adjustment in maternal hemodynamics may adversely affect pregnancy outcome. Underweight women provide a good example. Rosso et al[60] studied 12 normal-weight (control group) and 12 underweight women to test whether fetal growth retardation in underweight gravidas is related to inadequate maternal hemodynamic adjustments. Underweight mothers had significantly smaller infants than did the control group and six infants of the underweight mothers were considered growth-retarded. The results strongly suggested that underweight mothers are at higher risk of fetal growth retardation because of smaller plasma volume and lower cardiac output.

There is a greater tendency for coagulation during pregnancy because of increases in various clotting factors. Fibrinolysis (splitting up or dissolution of a clot) is depressed during pregnancy and the **postpartum** period, and the woman is more vulnerable to thrombosis.

BLOOD VOLUME AND COMPOSITION

Plasma is the fluid component of blood, whereas serum is the part of plasma that remains after its coagulation factors have been removed. Total plasma volume in a nonpregnant woman

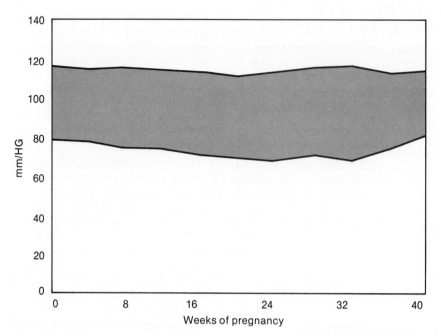

FIG. 3-1   Change in blood pressure during the course of human pregnancy.

averages 2,600 ml. Near the end of the first trimester of pregnancy, plasma volume begins to increase, and by 34 weeks it is about 50% greater than it was at conception.

There is considerable variation from these averages. Women who have small volumes to begin with usually have a greater increase, as do **multigravidas** and mothers with multiple births.

Researchers have shown that the increase in plasma volume is correlated with obstetrical performance. They found that women who have a small increase as compared with the average are more likely to have **stillbirths, abortions,** and low-birth-weight babies. This is seen in women with hypertension, renal disease, low maternal weight gain, diuretic treatment, preeclampsia, smoking and undernutrition.[41] Clearly the restriction of a normal expansion of plasma volume is undesirable in pregnancy.

If the availability of nutrients or the synthesis of normal blood constituents does not keep pace with the expansion of plasma volume, their concentrations per 100 ml of blood will decrease, even though the total amounts may rise.

This is apparently what happens with red blood cells, serum proteins, minerals, and water-soluble vitamins.

Red-cell production is stimulated during pregnancy so that their numbers gradually rise, but the increase is not as large as the expansion of plasma volume (Fig. 3-2). The hematocrit, which is normally around 35% in women, may be as low as 29% to 31% during pregnancy. The amount of hemoglobin in each red blood cell does not change, but because there are fewer red blood cells per 100 ml of blood, hemodilution occurs. Nonpregnant values of 13 to 14 gm/100 ml can drop as low as 10 or 11 gm/100 ml in the early months. In a nonpregnant woman this level of hemoglobin would indicate anemia, but in pregnancy the red blood cells are normochromic and normocytic.

Serum Levels of Nutrients

Serum levels of the major nutrients typical for pregnant and nonpregnant women are compared in Table 3-1. The values for pregnant women must be interpreted with caution. Investigators have obtained different values depend-

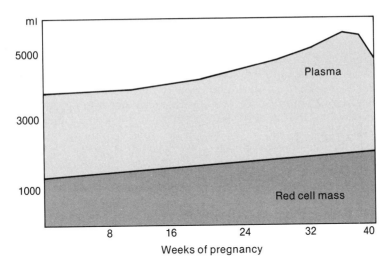

FIG. 3-2 Increase in plasma volume and red-cell mass during the course of human pregnancy.

TABLE 3-1 *Serum Nutrient Levels in Pregnant and Nonpregnant Women*

Nutrient	Normal Nonpregnancy Range	Values in Pregnancy
Total protein	6.5-8.5 g/100 ml	6.0-8.0
Albumin	3.5-5.0 g/100 ml	3.0-4.5
Glucose	<110 mg/100 ml	<120
Cholesterol	120-190 mg/100 ml	200-325
Vitamin A	20-60 μg/100 ml	20-60
Carotene	50-300 μg/100 ml	80-325
Ascorbic acid	0.2-2.0 mg/100 ml	0.2-1.5
Folic acid	5-21 ng/100 ml	3-15
Calcium	4.6-5.5 mEq/L	4.2-5.2
Iron/iron-binding capacity	>50/250-400 μg 100 ml	>40/300-450

Modified from Aubry RH, Roberts A, Cuenca V: The assessment of maternal nutrition, *Clin Perinatol* 2:207, 1975.

ing on the laboratory methods used. Moreover, levels of certain nutrients can be influenced by a number of maternal factors such as age, parity, smoking, and the use of various medications before or during pregnancy. Even the sex of the fetus can influence the mother's blood levels of some nutrients. The levels will also fluctuate at different times during gestation.

Total serum protein gradually decreases during pregnancy, leveling off at about 28 weeks. Most of the reduction in serum proteins is a result of a sharp decline in the albumin fraction. Alpha and beta globulins show a progressive increase. The reduction in serum albumin changes colloidal osmotic pressure of the blood. This, in conjunction with the expanded plasma volume, is another factor responsible for the tendency of pregnant women to accumulate extracellular fluid.

In contrast to the water-soluble nutrients, those that are fat soluble show increased serum concentrations during pregnancy. There are progressive increases in serum triglycerides, cholesterol, free fatty acids, and vitamin A. These higher lipid levels are what maintain the concentrations of alpha and beta globulins, since to circulate, triglycerides and cholesterol must be protein-bound.[37]

These changes are associated with alterations in the endocrine system, particularly the substantial rise in estrogen and progesterone from the gradually growing placenta. The concentration of all lipoprotein fractions increases during pregnancy. Very low-density lipoprotein (VLDL) cholesterol and triglyceride increase

250% over prepregnancy levels, and low-density lipoprotein (LDL) cholesterol increases 160%, all with peak levels at term. High-density lipoprotein (HDL) cholesterol is maximally increased in the middle of pregnancy by about 150% and substantially declines to a little over 100% at term. At least one study has demonstrated that the elevation in HDL during gestation is confined to the HDL_2 fraction.[22]

The mechanisms of these lipoprotein changes have not been studied in humans but the hypertriglyceridemia in animal models is related to enhanced VLDL entry into the circulation.[37] In addition, diminished adipose tissue lipoprotein lipase (LPL) activity in late gestation may cause a rerouting of triglyceride fatty acids to other tissues[29] such as muscle, mammary gland, placenta, and uterus for oxidation, rather than storage, since triglyceride transport is not reduced in pregnancy. All of these changes appear to be sex hormone related.

Effect of Changes in Lipid Metabolism

Overall, major changes occur in lipid metabolism in the pregnant woman, especially during the second half of gestation.[29] Greater adipose tissue lipolysis improves the availability of the liver of substrates for triglyceride formation; along with endogenous changes, the end result is the movement of triglycerides into the circulation in the form of VLDLs. This pool of triglycerides is augmented by chylomicron triglycerides from dietary lipids, the production of which is also increased (at least to some degree) by maternal hyperphagia and efficient gut lipid absorption. Serum triglyceride levels remain elevated until late gestation as a result of reduced LPL activity in the extrahepatic tissues (especially adipose tissue); this phenome-non does not permit removal of triglycerides at a rate that keeps up with the enhanced production. These changes contribute to fulfill maternal and fetal metabolic needs. If food is scarce, the use of glycerol released from adipose tissue helps maintain normal blood glucose levels through gluconeogenesis; ketones generated from maternal fat may also serve as an energy source for the fetus. As parturition approaches, an increase in mammary gland LPL activity occurs; this facilitates

the circulating triglycerides to be taken by mammary cells and a reduction in circulating triglyceride ultimately is seen.

With regard to the hypercholesterolemia of pregnancy, it presumably occurs from metabolic and endocrine influences. To what extent this characteristic of pregnancy can be modified by diet is a question of interest, since pregnancy is the most common cause of hypercholesterolemia in premenopausal women. In one study, the hypercholesterolemia of pregnancy was greatly ameliorated by the removal of cholesterol from the diet.[46] This was seen not only in normal subjects but also in women with familial hypercholesterolemia. These results are in contrast to two previous studies reporting unsuccessful attempts to modify the hypercholesterolemia of pregnancy using different approaches. One research group concluded that the use of a fat-modified diet, decreased in saturated fat and increased in polyunsaturated fat, failed to prevent the rise in serum cholesterol in seven outpatient pregnant women.[28] Another group of investigators could not produce an exaggerated hypercholesterolemia by adding 2 g crystalline cholesterol to the usual diet of pregnancy women.[50]

Although it is somewhat unclear how dietary change may modify the hypercholesterolemia of pregnancy, it is recognized that this phenomenon occurs in all cultures surveyed including those whose habitual diets are high in cholesterol and in those who typically consume a diet low in cholesterol. However, the customary dietary cholesterol and fat intakes of the various populations would appear to determine the baseline serum cholesterol concentration from which the increase in pregnancy occurs. McMurray et al[46] maintain that in countries like the United States, where dietary intake of saturated fat and cholesterol is high, restriction in consumption of these substances may ameliorate the usual hypercholesterolemia of pregnancy. The risks and benefits of a general recommendation along this line are not known where the pregnant woman is concerned. However, there is little reason to suspect a health risk. Saturated fats and cholesterol are not essential nutrients for humans. Worldwide, normal infants are born to mothers who vary widely in plasma cholesterol concentrations because there are wide ranges in the cholesterol and fat contents of diets and genes from different cultures.

With this in mind, one might suggest that there are several benefits of recommending a diet low in cholesterol and reduced in saturated fat content during pregnancy. A low cholesterol diet may reduce the high incidence of gallstones in multiparous women, since diet is known to influence the cholesterol-to-bile acid ratio in bile and thus may affect stone formation.[19] Women with previously diagnosed hyperlipidemia who become pregnant could reduce their even more pronounced hyperlipidemia of pregnancy by consuming a diet low in cholesterol and controlled in other dietary constituents. A diet low in cholesterol and saturated fat and composed of foods widely available in our culture could be adequate in protein, vitamins and minerals for pregnant women.[17] In addition, this diet could be rich in fiber, high in nutrient density and consistent with current recommendations for dietary prevention of atherosclerosis and other chronic diseases common in the United States.

RESPIRATION

Respiratory adaptations occur during pregnancy to provide for both maternal and fetal needs. Maternal oxygen requirements increase in response to the acceleration in metabolic rate and the need to add to the tissue mass in the uterus and breasts. The fetus requires oxygen and a way to eliminate carbon dioxide.

In response to elevated levels of estrogen, increased vascularization also occurs in the respiratory tract. As the capillaries become engorged, edema and hyperemia develop within the nose, pharynx, larynx, trachea, and bronchi. This congestion within the tissues of the respiratory tract gives rise to several conditions commonly seen in pregnancy. These conditions include nasal and sinus stuffiness, epistaxis (nosebleed), changes in the voice, and marked inflammatory response to even a mild upper respiratory infection. Increased vascularity swells tympanic membranes and eustachian tubes, giving rise to symptoms of impaired hearing, earaches, or a sense of fullness in the ears.

As mentioned previously, the level of the diaphragm is displaced by as much as 4 cm during pregnancy. With advancing pregnancy, thoracic breathing replaces abdominal breathing and descent of the diaphragm with inspiration becomes less possible.

The pregnant woman breathes more deeply (greater tidal volume, the amount of gases exchanged with each breath) but increases her respiratory rate only slightly (about two breaths per minute). There is a more efficient exchange of lung gases in the alveoli; the oxygen-carrying capacity of the blood is increased accordingly.

RENAL FUNCTION

In normal pregnancy, renal function is altered considerably. The woman's kidneys must manage the increased metabolic and circulatory demands of the maternal body as well as excretion of fetal waste products. Changes in renal function are caused by pregnancy hormones, an increase in blood volume, the woman's posture, and nutritional intake.

To facilitate the clearance of creatinine, urea, and other waste products of fetal and maternal metabolism, blood flow through the kidneys and the glomerular filtration rate are increased during pregnancy. The change in glomerular filtration is partially caused by the lower osmotic pressure, which results from the fall in serum albumin. This is one adaptation that appears to be purely mechanical, since no effects of hormones on this aspect of kidney function have been shown. However, there are consequences for nutrition.

According to Hytten and Thomson,[33] "The kidney during pregnancy shows an astonishing profligacy with nutrients." Normally, most of the glucose, amino acids, and water-soluble vitamins that are filtered by the kidneys are reabsorbed in the tubules to preserve the body's balance. However, in pregnancy, substantial quantities of these nutrients appear in the urine. The most satisfactory explanation at present is that the high glomerular filtration rate offers the tubules greater quantities of nutrients than they can feasibly reabsorb. Because the change in filtration rate is largely mechanical, there may not be an accompanying mechanism by which the tubules can readjust.

GASTROINTESTINAL FUNCTION

The functioning of the gastrointestinal system undergoes a number of interesting changes during the course of pregnancy. The appetite increases and nausea and vomiting may occur, motility is diminished and intestinal secretion is reduced, and sense of taste is altered and absorption of nutrients is enhanced (see box at right).

Increased progesterone production causes decreased tone and motility of the smooth muscles of the gastrointestinal tract. This leads to esophageal regurgitation, decreased emptying time of the stomach, and reverse peristalsis. As a result, the pregnant woman may experience heartburn. The decreased smooth muscle tone also results in an increase in water absorption from the colon, and constipation may result. In addition, constipation is secondary to hypoperistalsis, unusual food choice, lack of fluids, abdominal pressure by the pregnant uterus and displacement of intestines with some compression. Hemorrhoids may be everted or may bleed during straining at stool.

Decreased emptying time of the gallbladder is typical. This feature, together with slight hypercholesterolemia from increased progesterone levels, may account for the frequent development of gallstones during pregnancy.

Intraabdominal alterations that can cause discomfort include pelvic heaviness or pressure, flatulence, distention and bowel cramping, and uterine contractions. In addition to displacement of intestines, pressure from the expanding uterus increases venous pressure in the pelvic organs. Although most abdominal discomfort is a consequence of normal maternal alterations, occasionally bowel obstruction or an inflammatory process may be present.

Insofar as taste is concerned, one study[10] examined the ability of pregnant women to discriminate among different concentrations of salt and sucrose solutions. Results of tests with salt solutions showed that pregnant women were significantly less able to correctly identify concentration differences and preferred significantly stronger salt solutions than did nonpregnant women. The researchers suggest that these observations may reflect a physiological mechanism for increasing salt intake during pregnancy.

IMPROVED LACTOSE DIGESTION DURING PREGNANCY[70]

The presence of lactose maldigestion was examined in a group of 114 pregnant women early in pregnancy and near term. Women tested before the 15th week of gestation showed indications of lactose maldigestion in 54%. By term, 44% of those originally classified as maldigesters had become digesters. This apparent adaptive improvement in intestinal handling of milk lactose during gestation has implications for calcium intake and potentially improved absorption of calcium.

From Villar J et al: Improved lactose digestion during pregnancy: a case of physiologic adaptation? *Obstet Gynecol* 71:697, 1988.

HORMONES

The pregnant woman secretes more than 30 different hormones throughout gestation. Some, like those just mentioned, are present only in pregnancy, whereas others that are normally present have altered rates of secretion that are modified by the pregnant state.

Most hormones are proteins or steroids that are synthesized from precursors such as amino acids and cholesterol in endocrine glands throughout the body. Their production is influenced by the mother's general health and nutritional status. Under normal circumstances they are controlling factors in a complex feedback system that maintains homeostasis between cellular and extracellular constituents and metabolism. During pregnancy many of these homeostatic mechanisms are "reset" so that changes occur in the retention, utilization, and excretion of nutrients. Some of the hormones that exert important effects on nutrient metabolism are summarized in Table 3-2. Only those that have more general implications for nutritional management are singled out for discussion here.

Progesterone and Estrogen

Progesterone and estrogen are two hormones that have major effects on maternal physiology during pregnancy. The chief action of proges-

TABLE 3-2 *Hormonal Effects on Nutrient Metabolism in Pregnancy*

Hormone	Primary Source of Secretion	Principal Effects
Progesterone	Placenta	Reduces gastric motility; favors maternal fat deposition; increases sodium excretion; reduces alveolar and arterial PCO_2; interferes with folic acid metabolism
Estrogen	Placenta	Reduces serum proteins; increases hydroscopic properties of connective tissue; affects thyroid function; interferes with folic acid metabolism
Human placental lactogen (HPL)	Placenta	Elevates blood glucose from breakdown of glycogen
Human chorionic thyrotropin (HCT)	Placenta	Stimulates production of thyroid hormones
Human growth hormone (HGH)	Anterior pituitary	Elevates blood glucose; stimulates growth of long bones; promotes nitrogen retention
Thyroid-stimulating hormone (TSH)	Anterior pituitary	Stimulates secretion of thyroxine; increases uptake of iodine by thyroid gland
Thyroxine	Thyroid	Regulates rate of cellular oxidation (basal metabolism)
Parathyroid hormone (PTH)	Parathyroid	Promotes calcium resorption from bone; increases calcium absorption; promotes urinary excretion of phosphate
Calcitonin (CT)	Thyroid	Inhibits calcium resorption from bone
Insulin	Beta cells of pancreas	Reduces blood glucose levels to promote energy production and synthesis of fat
Glucagon	Alpha cells of pancreas	Elevates blood glucose levels from glycogen breakdown
Aldosterone	Adrenal cortex	Promotes sodium retention and potassium excretion
Cortisone	Adrenal cortex	Elevates blood glucose from protein breakdown
Renin-angiotensin	Kidneys	Stimulates aldosterone secretion; promotes sodium and water retention; increases thirst

terone is to cause a relaxation of the smooth muscles of the uterus so that it can expand as the fetus grows, but it also has a relaxing effect on other smooth muscles in the body. Relaxation of the muscles of the gastrointestinal tract reduces motility in the gut, allowing more time for the nutrients to be absorbed. The slower movement is also a cause of the constipation commonly experienced by pregnant women. General metabolic effects of progesterone are to induce maternal fat deposition, reduce alveolar and arterial PCO_2, and increase renal sodium excretion.

The secretion of estrogen is lower than that of progesterone during the early months of pregnancy, but it rises sharply near term. Its role is to promote the growth and control the function of the uterus, but it too has generalized effects on nutrition. One effect that has caused some difficulties for clinicians is the alteration of the structure of mucopolysaccharides in connective tissue. This alteration is beneficial because it makes the tissue more flexible and therefore assists in dilating the uterus at birth, but it also increases the affinity of connective tissue to water. The hydroscopic effect of estrogen and the sodium-losing effect of progesterone produce a confusing clinical picture of the pregnant woman's fluid and electrolyte balance. Because of estrogen, many pregnant women complain of excess fluid retention in the skin. Their faces and fingers become puffy, and there are other indications of generalized edema. In addition, changes in cardiovascular dynamics cause extracellular fluid to accumulate in the feet and legs.

Since excess fluid retention is one of the hallmarks of preeclampsia, some clinicians view these changes with alarm. Rather rigorous treatment with diuretics and a sodium-restricted diet may be initiated to promote water loss. The evidence, however, weighs against this practice. It is now appreciated that while the incidence of generalized and peripheral (ankle) edema is high, it is not associated with an increase in perinatal mortality when the two other symptoms of preeclampsia—hypertension and proteinuria—are absent. In fact, women with mild edema have slightly larger babies and a lower rate of prematurity.

The propensity of women to lose sodium from the action of progesterone is compensated by an increased secretion of aldosterone from the adrenal glands and renin from the juxtaglomerular apparatus of the kidneys. If sodium restriction is imposed, this system must work harder to maintain normal sodium concentrations in the body. Pushed beyond the stress naturally induced by pregnancy, the system could become exhausted so that, in the long run, less aldosterone and renin are produced. The sodium and water depletion that would result is more dangerous than the mild degrees of edema that the treatment is supposed to prevent. This has been demonstrated in pregnant rats that are placed on sodium-restricted diets that would be equivalent to 1 gm sodium or a "no added salt" diet in humans.

Although hormonal effects on fluid and electrolyte balance need more research, the mechanisms that are understood to date suggest that a mild degree of edema is physiologic in pregnancy and that the measures commonly used to prevent it impose an unnecessary risk.

Thyroxine

The iodine-containing hormone thyroxine is secreted by the thyroid gland. Circulating levels of thyroxine regulate the rate of oxidation reactions that are involved in the production of energy. The hormone therefore has a major role in metabolism and influences caloric requirements.

The secretion of thyroxine is a good example of how hormonal interactions control homeostatic mechanisms during pregnancy. Normally the manufacture and release of thyroxine are under the influence of thyroid-stimulating hormone (TSH), a pituitary hormone that in turn is regulated by the hypothalamus. The hypothalamus appears to be sensitive to changing rates of nutrient use in the tissues. High rates of utilization send two kinds of messages through the hypothalamus. One stimulates appetite and the desire to eat; the other stimulates TSH and thyroxine release so that nutrients in food can be used.

In pregnancy, progesterone and estrogen enter into this feedback and control system. Progesterone increases the sensitivity of the respiratory centers and causes the pregnant woman to "overbreathe." The reduction of P_{CO_2} that results depresses the circulating levels of thyroxine. Ordinarily this would excite the pituitary to secrete TSH so that levels of thyroxine can increase, but estrogen acts as a break to prevent overtaxation of the thyroid and keeps the process under control. The net effect is an overall rise in thyroxine with TSH maintained in the nonpregnant range (Fig. 3-3).

Although the picture is complex, it has implications for clinical management. The adaptive mechanisms under hormonal control are set to respond to increased rates of oxygen and nutrient utilization during pregnancy. These have an effect on oxygen requirements and caloric needs. Hyperventilation occurs spontaneously so that sufficient oxygen is available for the production of energy. When a pregnant woman is allowed to "eat to appetite," an adequate intake of the raw materials for energy production found in food is also ensured.

Insulin

There are a number of hormones concerned with maintaining the concentration of nutrients in the blood. Insulin affects blood glucose levels, and its action is critical in normal pregnancy. The fetus can use only glucose to meet its energy needs. Maternal metabolism is therefore keyed to make sure that adequate amounts of glucose are supplied.

The specific mechanisms of insulin secretion and glucose regulation in pregnancy are not fully understood. Normally, insulin is secreted by the β-cells of the pancreas when blood glu-

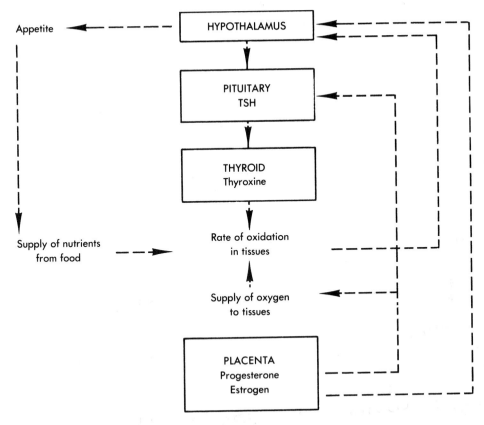

FIG. 3-3   Hormonal regulation of energy metabolism in pregnancy.

cose levels are high. Insulin facilitates the transport of glucose to the cells, where it is used to produce energy or synthesize fat. The adequacy of insulin secretion is measured by the rate at which glucose disappears from the blood after an oral load.

Pregnant women have normal insulin responses to glucose in early pregnancy, but in the later months, it takes more insulin to remove the same amount of glucose from the blood. Reasons for this are speculative. One explanation is simply that the increased needs for glucose by the growing fetus put a considerable strain on the system so that by the end of pregnancy the action of insulin becomes less efficient. However, there are indications that other hormones of pregnancy are also involved. Those known to have an antagonistic relationship to insulin include human placental lactogen

(HPL), human growth hormone (HGH), and cortisone.

Human Placental Lactogen, Human Growth Hormone, and Cortisone

HPL and HGH antagonize insulin by continuing to feed glucose into the blood from the breakdown of glycogen. It is also possible that HPL increases the rate of insulin destruction in the placenta.

Cortisone also favors the elevation of blood glucose levels by stimulating its synthesis from amino acids that come from the breakdown of protein tissues. Cortisone levels are usually at or below normal in early pregnancy, but they rise steeply at term. This rise is induced by estrogen to help the mother through labor. High cortisone levels may increase the destruction of insulin in the liver.

Whatever specific mechanisms are involved, the effects of altered insulin efficiency in the face of other hormonal antagonists place a stress on the beta cells of the pancreas. Prediabetic women may show frank indications of impaired glucose tolerance. If diabetes exists before pregnancy, the condition may become worse. The diet of pregnant women must be managed to minimize this stress. As will be shown, there is a danger to both the mother and the fetus if impaired glucose metabolism results in **ketoacidosis.**

METABOLIC ADJUSTMENTS

The basal metabolic rate (BMR) usually rises by the fourth month of gestation, although small increments may occur before that time. It is normally increased by 15% to 20% by term.[20] The BMR returns to nonpregnant levels by 5 to 6 days postpartum. The elevation in BMR reflects increased oxygen demands of the uterine–placental-fetal unit as well as oxygen consumption from increased maternal cardiac work. Peripheral vasodilation assists in the release of the excess heat production, though some women may continue to experience heat intolerance. Lassitude and fatigability after only slight exertion are described by many women in early pregnancy. These feelings may persist along with a greater need for sleep.

A complex series of adjustments in carbohydrate, protein, and fat metabolism occur during gestation to ensure that the fetus receives a continuous supply of fuel when the needs are maximal in late pregnancy. These adjustments are induced by changes in the endocrine milieu and by development of new endocrine tissue, the placenta.[5]

Approximately 50% to 70% of the kilocalories required daily by the fetus in the third trimester (43 kcal/kg/day) are derived from glucose[3]; about 20% of the kilocalories are derived from amino acids and the remainder from fat. When maternal blood glucose levels fall, the rate of glucose transfer to the fetus declines and fatty acids may become a more dominant fuel source. The net effect of maternal fuel adaptations is to increase the use of fat as a fuel source by the mother to conserve glucose for the fetus. During the second trimester, the mother prepares for the anticipated fetal glucose demand by storing fat; in the third trimester, when the fetal glucose demand causes maternal plasma glucose levels to fall, lipolysis increases in the maternal compartment.[4]

During a brief fast, such as overnight, maternal plasma glucose concentrations in pregnant women fall significantly below that of nonpregnant women because of continual placental uptake of glucose and impaired hepatic gluconeogenesis. The reduced capacity for gluconeogenesis is related in part to the reduced availability of alanine; the latter is the result of increased placental alanine uptake and restrained maternal muscle breakdown. Lipolysis is enhanced and mild ketosis may occur.[11] In the postprandial period, maternal glucose uptake is lower than in nonpregnant women, despite increased plasma insulin concentrations. More of the glucose removed by the liver is converted to triglycerides; these are stored in maternal adipose tissue to be available for later fasting periods.

Overall, the major adjustment in energy utilization during pregnancy is a shift in the fuel sources. Fat becomes the major maternal fuel whereas glucose is the major fetal fuel. Because the size of the maternal tissue is considerably greater than the size of the fetal mass, lipolysis dominates, causing the respiratory quotient to fall in fasting women. Pregnant women gain weight readily without appreciable changes in energy intake; this is because water normally comprises about 65% of the weight gain, not because energy is utilized more efficiently. However, there is still some question about the efficiency of energy utilization, especially in the pregnant woman exposed to severe food deprivation.[20]

COMPONENTS OF WEIGHT GAIN

The weight gained in a normal pregnancy is the result of physiologic processes designed to foster fetal and maternal growth. Much of the weight gain can be accounted for by the products of gestation.

The total number of pounds gained in pregnancy will vary among individual women. Young mothers and **primigravidas** usually gain more than older mothers and multigravidas. A normal gain for most healthy women is about 25 to 35 lb (11 to 15 kg).[34]

Although women vary in the composition of the weight they gain during pregnancy, a general picture can be described. Less than half the total weight gain resides in the fetus, placenta, and amniotic fluid; the remainder is found in maternal reproductive tissues, fluid, blood and "stores."

Composition of weight gain in pregnancy

Component	Weight gain (kg)	Weight gain (lb)
Fetus	3.2-3.6	7-8
Placenta and amniotic fluid	1.4-1.8	3-4
Tissue fluid	2.3-2.7	5-6
Maternal blood	1.4-1.8	3-4
Enlargement of the uterus	0.9-1.8	2-3
Maternal "stores" (mostly fat)	2.3-3.6	5-8
TOTAL		25-35

Observations of pregnant women have shown that there is a variable level of tissue fluid accumulation. This likely relates to the relative balance of specific hormones associated with fluid and electrolyte balance. Several recent studies have focused on total body water in pregnancy. Determinations were made using two sophisticated methodologies—deuterium dilution and bioelectrical impedance. These methods appear to yield relatively similar results. Overall, total body water increased significantly during pregnancy, then decreased postpartum (Table 3-3).[45]

The weight component labeled "maternal stores" is largely composed of body fat, although some increase in lean body mass (other than reproductive tissues) may also occur. The action of progesterone in the pregnant woman dictates that the fat pad be produced to serve as a caloric reserve for both pregnancy and lactation. Fatfold measurements during gestation have shown gradual increases in subcutaneous fat at the abdomen, back, upper thigh, and above the triceps muscle (Fig. 3-4 and 3-5). Fat is deposited mostly in the thigh and subscapular region.[71]

There has been interest in the notion that birth weight might be predicted from the pattern of fat deposition in the pregnant mother. In

TABLE 3-3 *Total Body Water Changes During and After Human Pregnancy*[45]

	Total Body Water (kg)	Water Weight/Body Weight (%)
Prepregnancy	31.8	50.4
First Trimester	32.5	51.1
Second Trimester	35.1	49.5
Third Trimester	39.6	50.0
Postpartum (8-10)	34.2	50.3

Data from Lukaski HC et al:
Total body water in pregnancy: assessment by using bioelectrical impedance, *Am J. Clin Nutr* 59:578, 1994.

a large prospective study involving predominantly black pregnant women, the effects of three skinfold measurements (triceps, subscapular, and suprailiac) on newborn birthweight was evaluated.[54] The mother's triceps skinfold measurement was found to correlate most strongly with the newborn's birth weight. However, this study does not address changes in fat pad thickness during pregnancy, which may relate to later pregnancy outcome.

The potential value of monitoring changes in body fatness during pregnancy was assessed by British investigators.[69] Anthropometric indicators of nutritional status were examined systematically in 81 Asian women living in the city of Birmingham. Results indicated that mothers who increased their triceps skinfold by ≥ 20 μm during the second trimester were nutritionally at risk for having a small baby (Fig. 3-6). The researchers speculate that this measurement reflects the balance of energy intake minus energy expenditure during the critical second trimester when the mother would normally be laying down extra fat in anticipation of later fetal needs. Whether or not measurement of triceps skinfold will become a useful tool in prenatal care in the future remains to be seen.

The Gambian Study

Little is known about the pattern of fat deposition in pregnant women who are chronically undernourished. One report has addressed this

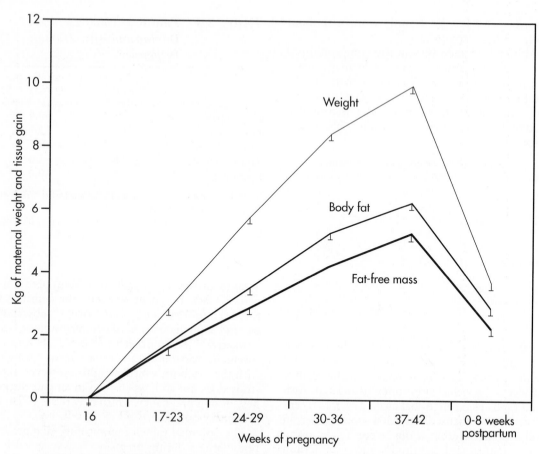

FIG. 3-4 Absolute changes in weight and body composition during pregnancy and post partum. One hundred five pregnant women prospectively monitored from the tenth week of gestation. All term deliveries (≥37 weeks) and first prenatal visit <17 weeks. Body fat represents largest component of tissue gain during pregnancy. *Bars* indicate standard errors.

From Villar J. et al. Effect of fat and fat-free mass deposition during pregnancy on birth weight. *Am J Obstet Gynecol* 167:1344, 1992.

issue by monitoring body fat gain in 50 rural Gambian women exposed to seasonal energy demands of subsistence farming and to annual preharvest food shortages.[40] Of these, 28 women received dietary supplements in amounts previously shown to increase birth weight.[58] In women not taking supplements, fat gain was profoundly affected by the seasons through which the pregnancy progressed, ranging from an estimated loss of 4.7 kg to a net gain of 3 kg at various times of the year (Fig. 3-7). Supplementation increased fat gain during pregnancy by about 2 kg and gave protection against the

worst effects of the season on energy balance.

In women taking supplements, the tendency to deposit fat during the first and second trimester of pregnancy counterbalanced any tendency toward fat loss at certain times of the year. These women entered the third trimester with additional reserves of fat that could be drawn from to support the needs of fetal growth. In contrast, women not taking supplements were unable to build up additional adipose tissue stores early in pregnancy and, consequently, fetal growth was more exposed to the effects of food shortage and increased total energy expen-

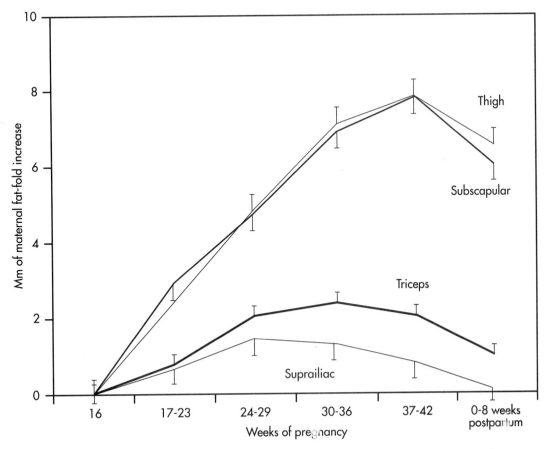

FIG. 3-5 Absolute changes in skin-fold thickness during pregnancy and post partum. One hundred five healthy pregnant women prospectively monitored from the tenth week of gestation. All term deliveries (≥37 weeks) and first prenatal visit <17 weeks. Most fat deposition during pregnancy occurs in thigh and subscapular regions. *Bars* indicate standard errors.

From Villar J et al: Effect of fat and fat-free mass deposition during pregnancy on birth weight, *Am J Obstet Gynecol* 167:1344, 1992.

diture during the rainy season. This helps explain the well-known selective effect of supplementation in increasing birth weight during the rains in this region.

The Pattern of Weight Gain[34]

What should be noted is that weight gain in the first 10 weeks is small and that much of it is caused by growth of the uterus and expansion of the mother's blood. At this time the fetus weighs only about 5 gm (0.17 oz), but toward the end of pregnancy, growth of the fetus accounts for the largest portion of the weight increment. The mother's rate of weight gain should parallel these trends. If she eats to appetite, the mother should gain a total of 2 to 4 lb (0.9 to 1.8 kg) by the end of the first trimester and about 1 lb (0.45 kg) each week thereafter. If pounds gained are plotted over the weeks of gestation, the curve would resemble that shown in Fig. 3-8.

Although most pregnant women demonstrate a gradual rate of weight gain during the course of pregnancy, others deviate from this pattern by gaining more or less during specific gestational periods. Researchers in California defined such

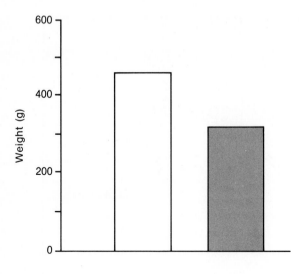

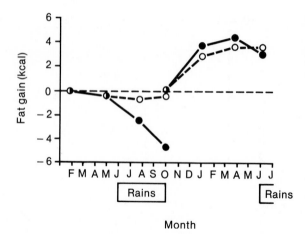

FIG. 3-7   Fat gain during pregnancy in rural Gambian women conceiving at worst and best times of year. ●——● = unsupplemented; ○——○ = supplemented.

From Lawrence M et al: Fat gain during pregnancy in rural Gambian women conceiving at worst & best times of year, *Am J Clin Nutr* 45:1442, 1987.

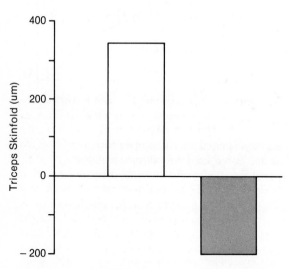

FIG. 3-6   Changes in weight (g) and triceps skinfold (μm) between weeks 18 and 28 of gestation. ▬▬▬ = nutritionally at-risk mothers (triceps skinfold increment less than or equal to 20 μm/wk); ▭▭▭ = adequately nourished mothers (triceps skinfold increment greater than 20 μm/wk).

From Viegas OAC, Cole TJ, Wharton BA: Impaired fat deposition in pregnancy: an indicator for nutritional intervention. *Am J Clin Nutr* 45:23, 1987.

differences in a large population of women (10,418) who delivered in the San Francisco area between 1980 and 1990.[1] As was expected, the group demonstrated the lowest rate of weight gain in the first trimester, the highest rate of weight gain in the second trimester and a slightly slower rate of weight gain in the third trimester. Maternal height, hypertension, cesarean delivery, and fetal size correlated positively with the rate of weight gain in each trimester. The most important maternal predictors of weight gain per trimester were age and Asian origin in the first trimester; prepregnancy body mass, parity, and height in the second trimester; and hypertension, age, and parity in the third trimester. This can be summarized as follows:

Maternal characteristic	Impact on rate of weight gain	During which trimester
Age	Increased	1
	Decreased	3
Asian origin	Decreased	1
Prepregnancy body mass	Decreased	2
Parity	Decreased	2,3
Height	Increased	2
Hypertension	Increased	3

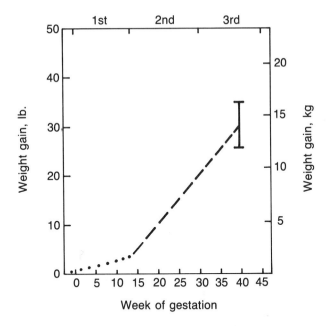

FIG. 3-8 Prenatal weight-gain grid for normal-weight women. Assumes 1.6-kg (3.5-lb) gain in the first trimester and remaining gain at a rate of 0.44 kg (0.97 lb) per week.

From Institute of Medicine: *Nutrition during pregnancy: weight gain and nutrient supplements,* Washington DC, 1990, National Academy Press.

Maternal attitude toward weight gain during pregnancy might be expected to influence actual weight gain during pregnancy. This issue was evaluated in a recent study of 1,000 women who completed an 18-item questionnaire administered at a mean of 20 weeks' gestation.[18] Results indicated that maternal attitude regarding weight gain is strongly influenced by prepregnancy body size; thin women tend to have positive attitudes and obese women tend to have negative attitudes about weight gain. Within body mass index groups, a positive attitude did not predict appropriate weight gain or birth weight of the baby. The researchers speculate that this may explain in part why nutritional counseling programs often are associated with only minimal increases in birth weight.

Determining the reasons for low prenatal weight gain provides a challenge to the health care provider. Although explanations may relate to maternal illness or dietary deprivation, they may also be associated with psychosocial status. This possibility was addressed by researchers in Alabama who administered a tool to assess depression, anxiety, stress, self-esteem, and social support.[30] The self-administered questionnaire was completed in midpregnancy by 536 black and 270 white low-income, nonobese, multiparous women who subsequently delivered at term. All of the women had one or more risk factors for fetal growth retardation. Associations were looked for between low prenatal weight gain and scores for psychosocial status while controlling for sociodemographic and reproductive variables. Interestingly, none of the scale scores was associated with low gain among black women, but for white women, four of the scale scores were associated with low gain.

This intriguing difference between black and white low-income women deserves further evaluation. Since all had BMIs of less than 26, fat content of the body was not an issue. Other explanations are possible. First, black and white women may differ in their perceptions of what constitutes psychosocial stress. Second, there may be variations in biological and behavioral responses to specific stressors. Third, there may be variation in the availability of stress mediators. Fourth, there may exist entirely separate mechanisms for low prenatal weight gain among black women. The Alabama researchers propose that these observations, along with recent reports of wide individual variability in the energy costs of pregnancy together suggest the following: attempts to manipulate pregnancy weight gain through dietary means will meet with variable success until psychosocial and other factors affecting prenatal energy intake and/or utilization are delineated further.[30]

Recommendations for Weight Management

The goal of weight management during pregnancy should be to promote optimal nutrition for the mother and the child.[67] Weight gain is considered a satisfactory measure of adequacy of prenatal nutrition. Although the Committee on Maternal Nutrition in 1970 recommended an optimal weight gain during pregnancy of 24 pounds,[16] that recommendation was based on data from a longitudinal study of only 60 pregnant women in the mid-1950s. Data from the Perinatal Collaborative Study, which described over 50,000 women and their pregnancies between 1959 and 1965, suggest that the best obstetrical outcomes occur among normal-weight women who gain 27 lb ($\pm20\%$)[52]; using perinatal mortality rate as an index of pregnancy outcome, optimum weight gain for underweight women was about 30 lb and for overweight women it was about 15 lb. Newer data from the 1980 National Natality Survey and the 1980 National Fetal Mortality Survey indicate that the lowest fetal mortality rate and the lowest rate of low birth weight occur with a weight gain of 26 to 35 lb.[53] Data provided by Brown in 1986 support these findings.[8]

A committee appointed by the National Academy of Sciences (NAS)[35] has undertaken a thorough review of available data related to weight gain and pregnancy outcome. Most of the literature reviewed pertained to women living in developed nations and a majority of the reports involved white women. Thus the conclusions of this expert panel relate to women in the United States and may not apply to women

TABLE 3-4 *Recommended Relative Weight-for-Height Categories for Pregnant Women*

Prepregnancy Weight-for-Height Category	Ideal BMI* Range	Weight-for-Height Range† (%)
Light or low	<19.8	<90
Normal	19.8-26	90-120
Heavy or high	>26-29	120-135
Extreme obesity	>29	>135

*Body-mass index [weight (in kilograms) divided by height (in meters) squared].

†Percent of the 1959 Metropolitan Life Tables ideal weight for height.

From National Academy of Sciences: *Nutrition during pregnancy: weight gain and nutrient supplements,* Washington, DC, 1990, National Academy Press.

living in less-developed countries or recent immigrants from developing countries to the United States. Overall, few studies were identified that provided direct evidence of the most desirable patterns of weight gain for women of different weight or height, and how such weight gain might be achieved through diet. However, the subcommittee concluded that gestational weight gain has an important relationship to fetal growth and that this relationship appears to vary according to prepregnancy weight for height. Recommended relative weight-for-height categories for pregnant women are defined in Table 3-4. Recommended total weight gain ranges for pregnant women are summarized in Table 3-5.

The NAS Committee on Nutritional Status in Pregnancy and Lactation[36] recommended that health care providers adopt and implement standardized procedures for obtaining and recording anthropometric measurements to serve as a basis for classifying women according to weight for height, setting weight-gain goals, and monitoring weight gain over the course of pregnancy.[81] Clinicians are advised to direct attention to the following: (1) During health care prior to conception, accurately measure and record in the medical record the woman's weight and height without shoes, using stan-

TABLE 3-5 *Recommended Total Weight-Gain Ranges for Pregnant Women*

Weight-for-Height Category*	Other	Recommended Total Gain (lb)
Low	≥62″ tall	28-40
Normal	≥62″ tall	25-35
High	Any height, any age	18-30
Extremely obese	Any height, any age	15-30
Low	Short† (<62″ tall)	20-35
Normal	Short†	18-30
Low	<2 yr postmenarche	30-40
Normal	<2 yr postmenarche	28-40

*Assumes the woman is at least 2 years post menarche unless otherwise indicated.

†The lower end of the range is most appropriate for very short women.

From National Academy of Sciences: *Nutrition during pregnancy: weight gain and nutrient supplements,* Washington, DC, 1990, National Academy Press.

dardized procedures. (2) Measure weight and height at the first prenatal visit using rigorously standardized procedures. (3) Use standardized procedures to measure weight at each visit. (4) Record weight on a table and plot it on a grid in the obstetric record. Since a tested grid has not yet been produced, no specific grid is recommended over another.

The NAS Committee recommended[35] that a weight-gain goal be set, preferably beginning at the comprehensive initial prenatal examination, by the gravida and the professional mutually. A range of desirable total gestational weight gain and rate of weight gain should be identified and accompanied by appropriate counseling. The recommended range for total weight gain and pattern of gain should be based mainly on relative prepregnancy weight for height and height,[34] as summarized in Table 3-4. Adjustments are recommended for women within 2 years of menarche and for short women. Women carrying twins

should probably have a goal in the range of 35 to 45 lb. The literature provides no basis for special recommendations for women of different ethnic backgrounds or for older mothers. It is likely that differences in prepregnancy weight-for-height and height account for most differences among ethnic groups. In the case of black women, shorter gestational duration may account for part of the lower mean weight gain.[32]

By monitoring weight gain throughout the pregnancy, abnormal patterns of gain may be identified and appropriate interventions chosen. Reasons for marked or persistent deviations from the expected pattern of gain should be investigated. When abnormal gain does not appear to be a result of measurement error, care provider and patient should jointly develop and implement appropriate actions.[35]

Special Subgroups of Women

Although underweight and overweight women represent two major subgroups deserving special consideration during pregnancy, other subgroups such as morbidly obese women (>135% of ideal body weight), adolescents, and women carrying more than one fetus (multiple gestation) are also of interest.[51] With morbidly obese women, adverse pregnancy course and outcome are very common,[39] and preconceptional weight loss is highly desirable. However, since this is often not accomplished, prenatal care must include especially careful monitoring. Some data suggest that no ideal weight gain can be recommended for this population; these women tend to produce big babies at all levels of gain (Fig. 3-9). The goal in nutrition counseling should be to emphasize food choices of high nutritional quality with avoidance of unnecessary calorie-rich foods. Ideally, the present pregnancy will not be associated with further augmentation in the already abundant fat pad.

Adolescent pregnancy is discussed in Chapter 10 and therefore will not be considered in depth here. However, several reports have suggested that as a group, healthy pregnant teens should gain about 35 lb during pregnancy.[25,27,44,47] Recommendations obviously should be individualized to include attention to prepregnancy weight and gynecologic age (years since menarche).

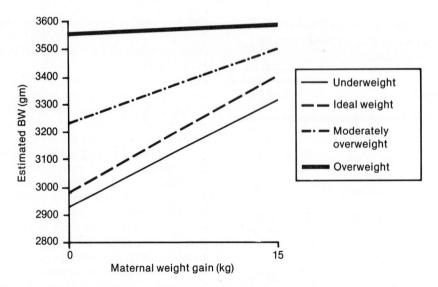

FIG. 3-9 Birth weight of live-born infants at term by prepregnancy body mass and weight gain, adjusted for maternal age, race parity, socioeconomic status, cigarette smoking and gestational age ($n = 2964$).

From Abrams BF, Laros RK: Prepregnancy weight, weight gain and birth weight, Am J Obstet Gynecol 154:503, 1986.

Women pregnant with twins, triplets, or greater numbers of offspring should obviously gain more weight than women undergoing single pregnancies.[9,23] Observations of large numbers of such women, however, have not been reported such that standards of weight gain can be recommended. A study in Seattle,[57] however, addressed weight gain patterns in women pregnant with twins; women with optimal outcome were used to define the weight gain curve. Optimal outcome of pregnancy was defined as: both babies weighed at least 2,500 gm at birth, gestational age exceeded 37 weeks, and Apgar scores at 5 minutes were 7 or greater. A mean weight gain in this population was 44 lb (Fig. 3-10, *A*). Mean weight gain in pregnancies associated with less than optimal outcome was 37 lb; this group showed a slowing of weight gain during the last 10 weeks of pregnancy (Fig. 3-10, *B*).

Weight-gain Charts

A variety of usable weight-gain charts are now available that reflect the current guidelines. In most cases, prepregnancy weight status is determined by use of body mass index (weight in kg/h in m^2); charts for determining body mass index are provided in Fig. 3-11. The Institute of Medicine provided its official chart in 1992; it is available in measures of either kilograms or pounds (Fig. 3-12).

Efforts have been made to evaluate the most recent weight gain recommendations for pregnant women, which were developed in the early 1990s by the Institute of Medicine (IOM) of the National Academy of Sciences (NAS). Evaluations of these recommendations have sought to determine if the recommended weight gains are associated with the least perinatal mortality and morbidity. To date, the follow-up studies indicate that the relatively new standards are appropriate for the general population of U.S. women.[2,14,30,56,64] In addition, limited weight gain during specific periods of pregnancy may be predictive of later outcome. For example, weight gain during the second trimester was related in one study to fetal birth weight.[2]

Parenthetically, a sudden weight gain that greatly exceeds the expected rate is likely to be

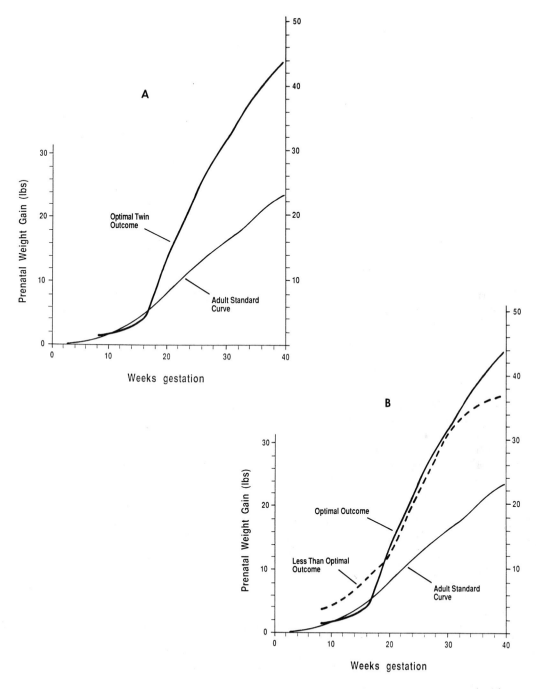

FIG. 3-10 **A,** Weight gain during twin gestation with optimal outcome as compared with standard curve. **B,** Weight gain during twin gestation (optimal outcome and less than optimal outcome) compared with standard curve.

From Pederson A, Worthington-Roberts B, Hickok D: *J Am Diet Assoc* 1989.

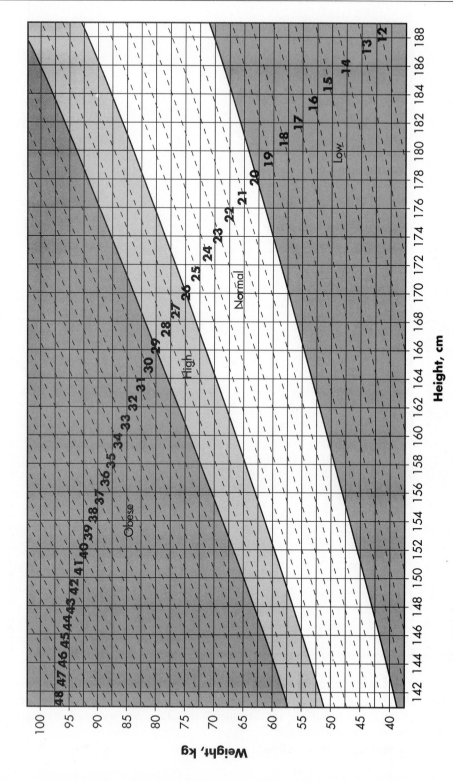

FIG. 3-11   Chart for estimating body mass index (BMI) category and BMI. A, Metric units.

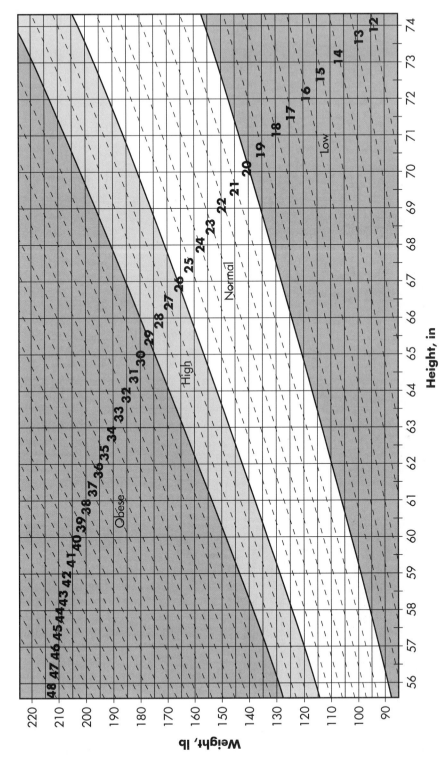

FIG. 3-11,B   Pounds and inches. NOTE: To find BMI category (e.g., obese), find the point where the woman's height and weight intersect. To estimate BMI, read the bold number on the dashed line that is closest to this point.

From Food Nutrition Board, Institute of Medicine, 1992.

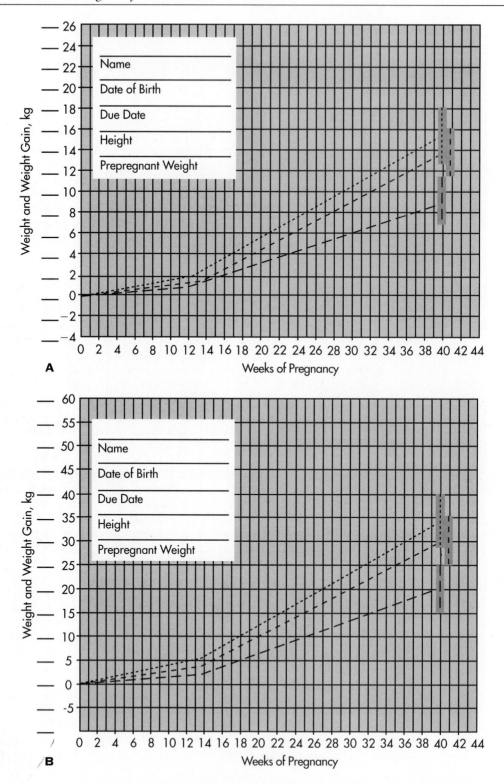

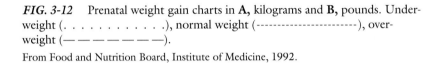

FIG. 3-12   Prenatal weight gain charts in **A,** kilograms and **B,** pounds. Underweight (. . . . .), normal weight (-----------------------), overweight (— — — — — — —).

From Food and Nutrition Board, Institute of Medicine, 1992.

caused by excess fluid retention. Although mild generalized edema is physiologically normal and some women can gain as much as 9 L of fluid and still have clinically normal pregnancies, this fluid accumulation is gradual. A large shift in water balance reflected by a sudden increase in weight is usually an indication of preeclampsia, particularly if it occurs after the twentieth week.

Much of the past confusion about weight gain during pregnancy and the misguided attempts to restrict it are the results of the failure to appreciate that the components and rate of weight gain are more important than the actual number of pounds a woman puts on. Pregnancy should be a positive period of growth in which most of the gain is in lean body (protein) tissue. A gain from too much fluid or too much fat is not conducive to good health.

Postpartum Weight Retention

In evaluating the adequacy of current weight gain recommendations for pregnant women, attention has been drawn to the consequences of level of prenatal weight gain on postpartum weight retention. Since weight gain recommendations today exceed those proposed in the past, concern has been expressed about the potential of the new guidelines contributing to the growing level of obesity in the United States. Since obesity increases the risks of problems developing during later pregnancies as well as in the postreproductive period, any factor seen to be contributing to our "adiposity" is of concern. Thus, a number of studies in the last few years have attempted to assess the contribution of pregnancy weight gain to postpartum weight retention in different populations.

Gradual weight loss generally occurs during the year following delivery. Rates of weight loss vary considerably among women but in general, the majority of the postpregnancy fat pad is lost during the first 6 months postpartum. In a study

of nearly 800 women,[61] the average total weight loss was 27 lb, corresponding to an average weight retained from the first obstetric visit to the last weight retained at 6 months postpartum of 3.1 lb. Of these women 22% had returned to their prepregnancy weight or less by 6 weeks and 37% by 6 months postpartum. Fig. 3-13 illustrates the cumulative weight loss pattern of this population.

Recent research focused on evaluating body composition change during this time by use of magnetic resonance imaging (MRI).[66] This technique allows for the approximation of changes in in adipose tissue volume (ATV). Fifteen Swedish women were assessed before pregnancy and at intervals after delivery (5 to 10 days, 2 months, 6 months, and 12 months). The women had more ATV postdelivery than before pregnancy. Of the ATV gained during pregnancy, 76% was placed subcutaneously, and the postpartum decrease was due to a loss of subcutaneous ATV. During pregnancy, 68% of the increased ATV was located in the torso and 16% in the thighs. Postpartum adipose tissue was mobilized more completely from the thigh than from the trunk. The results also indicated that women with a high weight gain during pregnancy retained lean tissue in their bodies (Fig. 3-14). The variability, however, among women was substantial (Fig. 3-15).

Pregnancy-related weight gain and postpartum retention were also evaluated by researchers in the United States. In the 1988 National Maternal and Infant Survey,[36] one group observed weight retention 10 to 18 months following delivery in selected women who had live births. The actual weight gains of these women during pregnancy were retrospectively classified according to the Institutes of Medicine guidelines. The results indicated that weight retention following delivery increased as weight gain increased; black women retained more weight than white

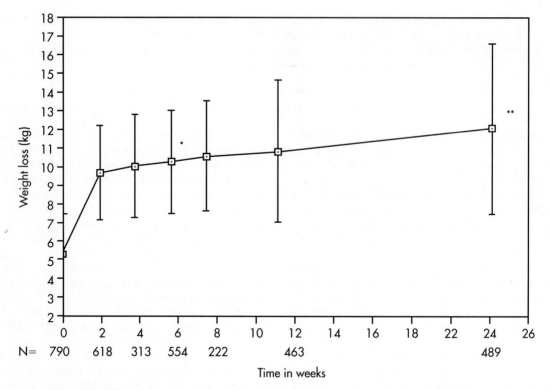

FIG. 3-13   Cumulative weight loss from last antepartum visit to 6 months postpartum.

From Schauberger CW, Rooney BL, Brimer LM: Factors that influence weight loss in the puerperium, *Obstet Gynecol* 79:424, 1992.

women with comparable weight gain. The mean retained weight was 1.6 lb for white women who gained the amount of weight currently recommended, whereas it was 7.2 lb for black women. These researchers conclude that if pregnant women gain weight according to the institute's guidelines, they need not be concerned about retaining a substantial amount of weight postpartum. However, black women are in need of advice about how to lose weight following delivery.

Comparison of postpartum weight retention between black and white women was also reported by other investigators. Again, using data from the 1988 National Maternal and Infant Survey, analysis focused on retention of 20 lb or more among 990 black and 1,129 white women who began pregnancy at normal weight for height.[55] In this case, black mothers were twice as likely to retain at least 20 lb than white moth-

ers. This difference between races did not differ substantially by socioeconomic status. Interestingly, many factors affecting postpartum weight retention differed by maternal race. For example, unmarried status was associated with weight retention among white mothers, whereas high parity was associated with weight retention among black mothers. Low socioeconomic status and high prenatal weight gain were associated with an increased risk of weight retention for both black and white mothers. The suggestion made by these researchers is that population-specific strategies may be needed to help mothers return to their prepregnancy weight.

One further observation along this same line compared gestational weight gain, pregnancy outcome, and postpartum weight retention.[63] Rate of gestational weight gain was measured prospectively in a sample of 274 young, low-income and primarily minority women (ages 12 to

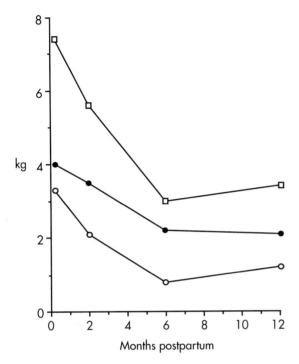

FIG. 3-14 Body weight (□), total body fat (●), and fat-free body weight (○) of Swedish women throughout the first year postpartum. The figures given are averages and represent differences from the corresponding prepregnant figures.

From Sohlstrom A, Forsum E: Changes in adipose tissue volume and distribution during reproduction in Swedish women as assessed by magnetic resonance imaging, *Am J Clin Nutr* 61:287, 1995.

29) with pregravid body mass indices in the normal range (19.8-26.0). Excessive weight gain was defined as one greater than 1.5 lb/week. Follow up was conducted at 4 to 6 weeks and 6 months postpartum. Results indicated that weight gained at an excessive rate by women with normal weight-for-height did not greatly enhance fetal growth and gestation duration but contributed instead to postpartum overweight.

It would be nice to explain the differences that are seen in rate and degree of postpartum weight loss among women. An effort was made recently to define factors that influence weight loss in the puerperium. A sizable group of women (*n* = 795) were followed up with frequent weight measurements and questionnaires about their activities for 6 months postpartum.[61] The mean net weight gain from the first prenatal visit to 6 months postpartum was 3.1 lb. Weight gain during the prenatal period was the variable most highly correlated to weight loss. Breastfeeding, exercise, season of the year, age, and marital status were not correlated. Average retained weight was not significantly different by absence or presence of another young child, nor did it differ by length of time since the last delivery. An early return to the workplace was associated with greater weight loss at 6 months, possibly because of increased caloric expenditure or greater restriction of access to food during the week. These data do provide some insight into relevant factors to variability in postpartum weight loss among women.

Does experiencing one or more pregnancies have any direct bearing on percent body fat later in life? In a project entitled the *Cardia Study*,[65] this question was evaluated in a group of 2,788 white and black women who participated in a prepaid health care plan. Women who remained nulliparous were compared with those who had been pregnant at least once. The women were followed up at 5 years after initial evaluation; those that had been pregnant had maintained at least 12 months of postpartum experience. Overall, those women who had experienced pregnancy during the 5-year interval weighed 4.5 to 7 lb more than those who had never been pregnant. Multiparas did not differ from nulliparas in adipose tissue change in either racial group. At each level of parity, black women demonstrated greater adverse changes in percentage of adipose tissue than did white women. These data suggest that women tend to experience modest increases in body weight after a first pregnancy and that these changes are persistent. However, this study does not address the association between pregnancy experience and percent body fat many years after reproductive life is over.

However, another study from the University of Minnesota reports that the more children a woman has, the higher her weight is likely to be at age 50.[7] This study from the Iowa Women's Health Study included 41,184 postmenopausal women, who reported their weight at ages 18,

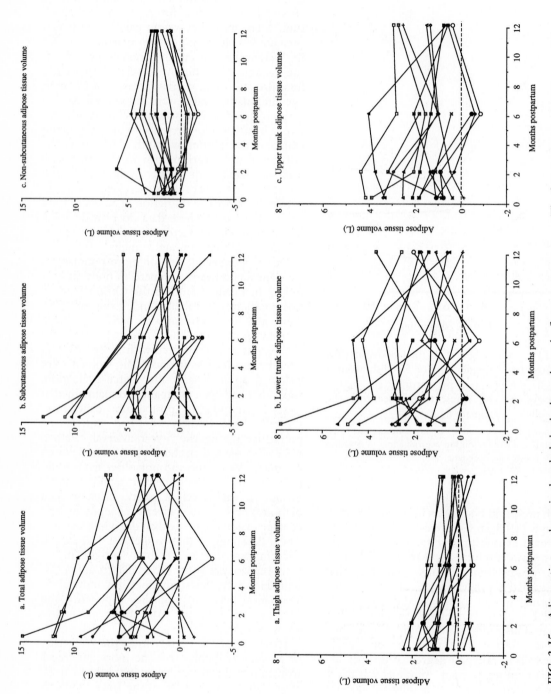

FIG. 3-15 Adipose tissue volume in the whole body throughout the first year postpartum. The figures represent differences from the corresponding prepregnant figures. Each line represents one woman.

From Sohlstrom A, Forsum E: Changes in adipose tissue volume and distribution during reproduction in Swedish women as assessed by magnetic resonance imaging, *Am J Clin Nutr* 61:287, 1995.

30, 40, and 50, and the number of children each had. At each age, women with lifetime parity of one or two live births had lower weight and were less likely to be overweight than those with three or more births, or those with none. A steady increase in body mass index was seen as parity increased from three to eight live births. Parity was associated with an increase of 1.21 lb per live birth.

It was also found that women gained 0.77 lbs per year between the ages of 18 and 50 for a total of 24 lb. A difference of 2.3 lb less was recorded, as education increased from less-than-high-school to high school and another 2.2 lb for greater than high school. Never-married women gained nearly 4.4 lb less than married women, and smokers gained 7.3 lbs less than nonsmokers. Parity was related to 3% of the increase for women with one live birth, 6% for women with two live births, and 31% for women with nine or more births.

These findings derive from a population of women living in an affluent society; the weight-gain scenario may be different in other societies. The tendency for increased percent adipose tissue with reproductive experience may be a preventable circumstance in the United States. Until more data are available, this question cannot be answered satisfactorily.

ROLE OF THE PLACENTA[50]

The placenta is not a passive barrier between mother and fetus; it plays an active role in reproduction. The placenta is the principal site of production for several of the hormones responsible for the regulation of maternal growth and development. For the fetus it is the only way that nutrients, oxygen, and waste products can be exchanged.[26,50]

Structure and Development

Evolving from a small mass of cells in the first weeks of pregnancy, the placenta becomes a complex network of tissue and blood vessels weighing about 1.4 lb (650 gm) at term. The vital role it plays as a link between mother and child is represented by the two principal parts of the placenta—one uterine and the other fetal.

On the maternal side the placenta is part of the uterine mucosa. When the tiny blastocyst implants in the uterus 6 or 7 days after fertilization, the uterine tissue and blood vessels break down to form small spaces called lacunae that fill with maternal blood. These spaces are eventually bound on the maternal side by the decidua or basal plate. Blood begins to circulate in the spaces at about 12 days' gestation.

Meanwhile the **trophoblast** grows and sends out rootlike villi into the pools of maternal blood. The villi contain capillaries, which will exchange nutrients and waste products between the mother and the fetus. In the early weeks of pregnancy the villi are thick columns of cells, but as they subdivide throughout gestation the villi become thinner and produce numerous branches. Some branches of the villi become anchored to the maternal tissue, and others remain free or floating in the intravillous spaces. The multiple villous branches provide a large surface area for efficient exchange of nutrients and waste products between mother and fetus (Fig. 3-16). Even though the uterine and embryonic tissues are extremely interdigitated, the blood of the mother and the embryo never mix because they are always separated by the placental membrane (Fig. 3-17).

Mechanisms of Nutrient Transfer

The efficiency of placental nutrient transfer is a determinant of fetal well-being. Reduced surface area of the villi, insufficient vascularization, or changes in the hydrostatic pressure in the intervillous space can limit the supply of nutrients available to the fetus and inhibit normal growth.

Nutrient transfer in the placenta is a complex process.[4,15,21] It employs all the mechanisms used for the absorption of nutrients from the gastrointestinal tract: simple diffusion, facilitated diffusion, active transport, and **pinocytosis**. The difference, however, is that in the placenta, two completely separate blood supplies are maintained. The maternal circulation remains in the intervillous space. The fetal capillaries are separated from the maternal blood by two layers of cells. Their thickness is approximately 5.5 μm (Fig. 3-17).

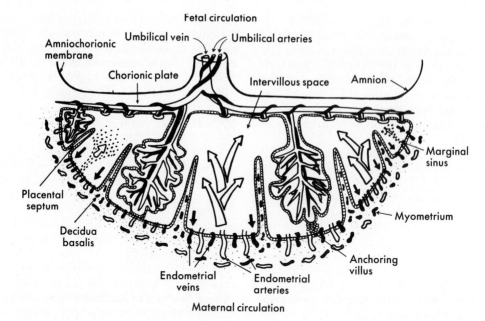

Fetal circulation

Amniochorionic membrane

Umbilical vein

Umbilical arteries

Chorionic plate

Intervillous space

Amnion

Marginal sinus

Placental septum

Myometrium

Decidua basalis

Anchoring villus

Endometrial veins

Endometrial arteries

Maternal circulation

FIG. 3-16 Section through a mature placenta showing relationship of fetal placenta (villous chorion) to maternal placenta (decidua basalis), fetal placental circulation, and maternal placental circulation. Maternal blood is forced into intervillous space, and exchanges occur with fetal blood as maternal blood flows around villi. Incoming arterial blood pushes venous blood into endometrial veins, which are scattered over surface of maternal placenta. Umbilical arteries carry deoxygenated fetal blood to placenta, and umbilical vein carries oxygenated blood to fetus.

Although the same nutrient may be simultaneously transferred by more than one mechanism, the major means of transport can be determined by comparing nutrient concentrations in maternal and cord blood. If the concentrations are equal, the transfer has most likely occurred by simple or facilitated diffusion. Simple diffusion is a passive process in which nutrients move from high concentrations in the maternal blood to lower concentrations in the fetal capillaries until equilibrium is reached. Facilitated diffusion differs from simple diffusion in that the rate of transfer is faster than would be expected; the mechanism of facilitated diffusion is not established, but it is thought that a carrier in the membrane is employed. Active transport requires both a carrier protein and metabolic energy to move a nutrient against an electrochemical gradient. The following substances are believed to cross the placenta via the specified mechanisms.[31]

Transport mechanism	Substance transported
Passive diffusion	Oxygen
	Carbon dioxide
	Fatty acids
	Steroids
	Nucleosides
	Electrolytes
	Fat-soluble vitamins
Facilitated diffusion	Sugars
Active transport	Amino acids
	Some cations (calcium, iron, iodine, phosphate)
	Water-soluble vitamins*
Solvent drag	Electrolytes

*At very high concentrations vitamin C has been shown to cross the placenta via diffusion.

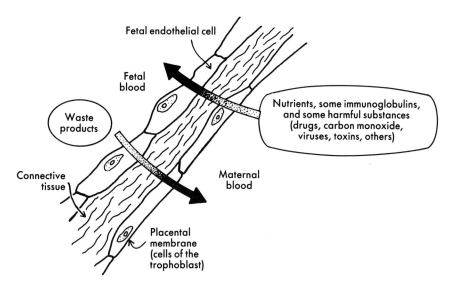

Fetal endothelial cell

Fetal blood

Waste products

Nutrients, some immunoglobulins, and some harmful substances (drugs, carbon monoxide, viruses, toxins, others)

Connective tissue

Maternal blood

Placental membrane (cells of the trophoblast)

FIG. 3-17 Nutrients, waste products, and other transportable compounds must cross two layers of cells in process of movement through placenta.

Most proteins do not cross the placenta since their molecular size is too large to allow penetration through the cells of the villi. This protects the fetus from acquiring harmful agents of high molecular weight, but it also means that the fetus must synthesize its own proteins from its supply of amino acids. An exception is the maternal immunoglobulin IgG. It is not known why this particular protein crosses the placenta, but it appears that the selectivity is related to the structure and not to the size of the molecule. IgG is probably transported by pinocytosis. The benefit to the fetus is that it has the same resistance to infectious diseases as the mother. This resistance lasts from 6 to 9 months after birth, until the infant can manufacture antibodies.

The placenta also acts to ensure that once nutrients are transported to the fetus, they do not "slide back down" the concentration gradient into the mother's blood. Ascorbic acid, for example, crosses the placenta in its reduced form as dehydroascorbic acid. Once inside the fetus, it is converted back to active L-ascorbic acid, which is impermeable to the placenta. Calcium transport is subject to similar protection through the mediation of hormones. Active transport of calcium makes the mother hypocalcemic as compared with the fetus. Her response is to secrete parathyroid hormone (PTH) to favor bone resorption and increase serum calcium levels. If PTH reached the fetus, the effect would be to reverse the normal process of bone development. The relative impermeability of the placenta to maternal PTH prevents this from happening. Instead, the fetus responds to its own high blood calcium levels by secreting endogenous calcitonin, the hormone that enhances the deposition of calcium in bone. Meanwhile the placenta is freely permeable to vitamin D, favoring calcium retention in both the mother and the fetus.[42]

These mechanisms of placental transport have implications for the nutritional treatment of pregnant women. Since vitamins A and D are both transported by simple diffusion, they will continue to accumulate in the fetus as long as maternal blood levels are high. Both vitamins A and D are toxic in excessive amounts. Administration of high doses of vitamin A to pregnant animals has produced cleft palate, abnormalities of the urinary tract, and malformations in other organs of the fetus arising from the mesoderm. The effects in humans are now well documented.[68]

Excessive doses of vitamin D can result in fetal hypercalcemia. Friedman and Mills[24] have induced aortic stenosis and abnormal skull development in rabbits by feeding their mothers high levels of vitamin D during pregnancy. Premature closure of the fontanel from excessive vitamin D has been reported in newborn humans as well.[16]

Megadoses of water-soluble vitamins are not generally toxic, since the fetus can excrete unneeded amounts, but high doses given to the mother may have other undesirable consequences. Malone[43] suggests that the physiologic competition for transport carriers may become pathologic when certain nutrients are in excess. If essential amino acids are forced to compete with unnecessarily large quantities of vitamin C or the B vitamins, the result could be impaired or defective growth. In addition, prolonged high maternal intake of a vitamin may increase the metabolism of this vitamin by the offspring after birth; this has been shown for vitamin C, and several cases of scurvy in the neonatal period have been reported to be associated with excessive supplementation with vitamin C by the mother during pregnancy.[13]

The placenta not only transports nutrients but also in some cases has been shown to store them.[62] The placenta can store most vitamins increasingly, depending on their availability and sequestration to the mother. Heightened release of these vitamins to the fetus generally depends closely on saturation of vitamin reserves in the placenta. Much remains to be learned about modifiability of placental vitamin transfer by placental abnormalities. However, it appears that adequate vitamin nutrition of the fetus is ensured only when placental vitamin binders are saturated.

Respiratory and Excretory Exchange

Besides serving as a lifeline for nutrients, the placenta functions in the exchange of respiratory gases and waste products between the mother and fetus.

The delivery of oxygen to the fetus is just as important to proper metabolism as an adequate supply of nutrients. The mother makes adjustments in her breathing to meet fetal oxygen needs, but the amount ultimately depends on the blood flow through the uterus to the placental villi. Near term the rate of flow through the intervillous space is 375 to 560 ml/min. Exchange is made between maternal red cells, which characteristically have a lower affinity for oxygen during pregnancy, and fetal red cells, which have a high affinity.

Maternal nutrition can influence oxygen exchange through the production of hemoglobin. Each gram of hemoglobin carries 1.34 ml of oxygen. In normal concentrations, it can deliver up to 16 ml of oxygen per 100 ml of blood to the placenta. If maternal hemoglobin levels are depressed from iron deficiency, the supply of oxygen per 100 ml of blood is reduced. Since the fetus can tolerate little variation in the rate at which oxygen is supplied, the mother must compensate by increasing her cardiac output.

Another function of the placenta is to rid the fetus of metabolic waste. The placenta is freely permeable to carbon dioxide, water, urea, creatinine, and uric acid. Hyperventilation on the part of the mother reduces her P_{CO_2} so that carbon dioxide exchange from the fetus is accomplished by simple diffusion. Urea, creatinine, and uric acid, which are the wastes of fetal amino acid metabolism, move through the placenta by diffusion and active transport.

Placental Hormones

The production of hormones to regulate the activities of pregnancy is one of the most interesting special functions of the placenta. From the earliest days of pregnancy the cells of the trophoblast and their successors in the placenta manufacture a large variety of hormones. The first to be manufactured in appreciable amounts is the protein HCG. Early in the differentiation of the trophoblast this hormone is found coating the trophoblast's outer cell surfaces, where it is believed to act as an immunologically protective layer, preventing the rejection of the blastocyst and thereby facilitating implantation. HCG also stimulates the synthesis of estrogen in the placenta. Synthesis of estrogen actually begins in the free-floating blastocyst where it acts to facilitate implantation. The fact that the cells of the small, primitive blastocyst are already equipped to conduct complex steroid manipulations is a measure of the importance of these hormones at this early stage.

As pregnancy proceeds, large amounts of progesterone are synthesized in the placenta, principally from maternal cholesterol. In addition to sustaining pregnancy, this hormone serves as a raw material for the production of estrogens (mainly estrone, estradiol, and estriol), which in turn act on many organs and tissues of both the mother and fetus. Interestingly, the human placenta lacks the enzymes needed for converting the large amounts of progesterone it makes into certain essential estrogens and other steroids. Consequently, these synthetic events are carried out in "the fetal zone" cells, which are clusters of transient cells found in the developing adrenal glands of the fetus; these cells lack the enzymes necessary to manufacture progesterone but possess the requisite ones for its conversion. In this way the fetal and placental tissues complement each other. When the fetus' endocrine glands become sufficiently mature to take over the manufacture of steroid hormones, the fetal zone cells gradually diminish and eventually disappear. Presumably, this sophisticated collaboration is organized and timed by precise genetic instructions and is regulated by equally precise releasing hormones.

Because a great variety of regulatory hormones are synthesized in the placenta, including HCG, human placental lactogen (HPL), chorionic somatomammotropin, and human chorionic thyrotropin (HCT), the control exercised by the placenta during pregnancy must be as comprehensive as that maintained by the pituitary gland throughout life. By means of these hormones the placenta not only carries out the functions of the fetus's pituitary until the organ is ready to perform on its own but also conducts the entire "endocrine orchestra of pregnancy," which performs largely in the placenta itself.[6]

Immunologic Protection

During pregnancy, it is absolutely vital that the embryo be protected from immunologic rejection by maternal tissue. One of the mechanisms that seems to play a part in this task is the nonspecific suppression of lymphocytes, the cells that normally mediate the rejection of a graft. Experiments have shown that lymphocytes can be suppressed by HCG, HPL, prolactin, cortisone, progesterone, the estrogens, and a variety of proteins and glycoproteins.[6]

It is also likely that the embryo is protected by the large, tightly packed decidual cells that enclose it soon after the implantation of the blastocyst. This protective barrier prevents the drainage of lymphocytes to maternal tissues. In addition, the maternal blood vessels do not invade the trophoblast of the placenta, so this potential means of graft rejection is blocked. In the

TABLE 3-6 *Morphological Characteristics of Placentas from Two Socioeconomic Groups**

	Boston	Guatemala
Mass components (g per placenta)		
Fresh placental weight	571.4 ± 21.20	485.4 ± 18.34
Effective placental mass	338.8 ± 16.34	274.6 ± 13.86
Peripheral villous mass	167.6 ± 8.80	124.9 ± 7.64
Peripheral trophoblastic mass	57.4 ± 2.97	42.3 ± 2.71
Villous surface analysis (m^2)		
Peripheral villous surface	16.09 ± 0.51	12.62 ± 0.64
Peripheral villous capillary surface	12.04 ± 1.29	8.06 ± 0.68

*Values given as means $\pm$ SEM. All differences are statistically significant ($p < 0.01$).
From Laga EM, Driscoll SG, Munro HN: Comparison of placentas from two socioeconomic groups: II. Biochemical characteristics, *Pediatrics* 50:33, 1972; Rosso P: Placental growth, development and function in relation to maternal nutrition, *Fed Proc* 39:250, 1980.

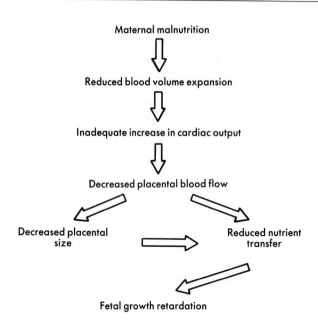

Maternal malnutrition

Reduced blood volume expansion

Inadequate increase in cardiac output

Decreased placental blood flow

Decreased placental size

Reduced nutrient transfer

Fetal growth retardation

FIG. 3-18   Postulated mechanisms responsible for placental and fetal growth retardation as seen with maternal malnutrition in animal models and in human subjects.

Modified from Rosso P: Placental growth, development and function in relation to maternal nutrition, *Fed Proc* 39:250, 1980.

early days of the development of the trophoblast further protection is afforded by the absence of the expression of antigens. So even though the embryonic tissue is foreign, it manages to conceal the fact, at least for a while.[6]

Effects of Malnutrition

Maternal malnutrition has also been found to interfere with normal placental growth and function.[38,59] This is reflected by lower placental weight, smaller placental size, and reduced deoxyribonucleic acid (DNA) content; affected placentas also have a reduced peripheral villous mass and villous surface (Table 3-6). Biochemical studies have revealed a reduced polysome:monosome ratio, as well as reduced ash, hydroxyproline, fat, and glycogen. The functional implications of some of these changes are still unclear. In malnourished women reduced estriol and pregnanediol excretion has been reported. Malnourished rats near term have a reduced maternal-fetal transfer of α-amino-isobutyric acid and glucose, but it is still unclear to what extent the reduced transfer is caused by placental factors or preplacental factors such as reduced placental blood flow, which is also known to be present in malnourished animals (Fig. 3-18).

Summary

During a normal pregnancy, substantial changes take place in the anatomy, physiology, and endocrinology of the woman. These changes support the growth and development of the fetus while maintaining the health of the mother. Weight gain during pregnancy is a gross measure of the adequacy of nutritional support during this time. "Overnutrition" does not benefit the fetus but may leave the mother with an excessive postpregnancy fat pad. Adaptations occur in the face of food shortage such that available kilocalories may aid in supporting fetal needs at the expense of maternal fat deposition. However, poor diet combined with limited maternal energy reserves invariably reduces the birth weight of the infant. The importance of the placenta cannot be overemphasized, and any circumstance that interferes with placental growth or destroys placental tissue will have a potentially devastating impact on the course and outcome of pregnancy.

REVIEW QUESTIONS

1. Describe major functional changes that occur during pregnancy, as associated with the cardiovascular, respiratory, renal, and gastrointestinal systems.

❖ ❖ ❖

CASE STUDY

Physiology of Pregnancy

Marcia Nahikian-Nelms PhD, RD, Southeast Missouri State University

Clarice Johnson is a 35-year-old African-American woman who at 25 weeks gestation is referred to you for nutritional evaluation. She is para 3 gravida 1. This pregnancy is considered to be high-risk because of her previous pregnancy outcomes. Her first pregnancy ended in a fetal death at 24 weeks gestation, and her second pregnancy produced a viable infant who was born at 32 weeks gestation weighing 4 lbs 11oz and is now 36 months old. You obtain the following data from her outpatient chart:

Height 5'6" Weight 120 lbs; prepregnancy weight: 125 lbs

Biochemical indices: Chol 289 mg/100ml LDL 140, HDL 38; Hgb 9.9 gm/100ml.

You also note in the medical record that she has complained to the nurse practitioner about severe heartburn, that has made eating difficult. She has been prescribed iron supplementation in addition to her prenatal vitamins. The client admits that both types of supplements tend to make her constipated.

1. (a) Evaluate her current weight status. The following is the weight gain record in her chart: 1/9/96 - 127 lbs, 2/11/96 - 116 lbs, 3/7/96 - 115 3/4 lbs, 4/12/96 - 122 lbs, and today's visit - 120 lbs. Plot this information on a maternal weight gain curve. (b) Has she gained adequate amounts of weight? How can the plotting of her weight history assist you in making a clinical assessment? (c) How may her weight status affect fetal outcome? (d) What should be her optimal weight gain at this stage of pregnancy? (e) How would you explain these components to her?

2. When evaluating her biochemical indices, which should be a concern to you? Explain why or why not for each.

3. Heartburn and constipation are common symptoms experienced during pregnancy. How are they related to the physiological changes of pregnancy? How would you explain these changes to her?

---

2. Discuss the major endocrine changes during pregnancy.
3. Outline important metabolic adjustments during pregnancy.
4. Identify the functions of the human placenta.

LEARNING ACTIVITIES

1. Interview a pregnant woman with the intent of learning more about her physiologic and psychological responses to her pregnancy.
2. Speak to her spouse/partner about his perceptions of the physiologic changes he perceives in her.
3. Arrange to speak with a clinician who deals regularly with pregnant women to determine what are the common issues raised by patients and what are the routine monitoring procedures conducted during pregnancy.

REFERENCES

1. Abrams B, Carmichael l S, Selvin S: Factors associated with the pattern of maternal weight gain during pregnancy, *Obstet Gynecol* 86:170, 1995.
2. Abrams B, Selvin S: Maternal weight gain pattern and birth weight, *Obstet Gynecol* 86:163, 1995.
3. Adam PJ, Felig P: Carbohydrate, fat, and amino acid metabolism in the pregnant women and fetus. In Falkner F, Tanner JM, editors: *Human growth, Principles and prenatal growth,* vol 1, New York, 1978, Plenum.
4. Battaglia FC: Placental transport and utilization of amino acids and carbohydrates, *Fed Proc* 45:2508, 1986.
5. Battaglia FC, Meschia G: Principal substrates of fetal metabolism, *Physiol Rev* 58:499, 1978.
6. Beaconsfield P, Birdwood G, Beaconsfield R: The placenta, *Sci Am* 243:95, 1980.

7. Brown JE, Kaye SA, Folsom AR: Parity-related weight changes in women, *Intern J Obesity* 16: 627, 1992.

8. Brown JE: Prenatal weight gains related to the birth of healthy-sized infants to low-income women, *J Am Diet Assoc* 86:1679, 1986.

9. Brown JE, Schlosser PT: Prepregnancy weight status, prenatal weight gain and the outcome of term twin gestations, *Am J Obstet Gynecol* 162: 182, 1990.

10. Brown JE, Toma RB: Taste changes during pregnancy, *Am J Clin Nutr* 43:414, 1986.

11. Chez RA, Curcio FD: Ketonuria in normal pregnancy, *Obstet Gynecol* 69:272, 1987.

12. Clapp F, Seaward BL, Sleamaker RH et al: Maternal physiologic adaptations to early human pregnancy, *Am J Obstet Gynecol* 159:1456, 1988.

13. Cochrane WA: Overnutrition in prenatal and neonatal life: a problem? *Can Med Assoc J* 93: 893, 1965.

14. Cogswell ME et al: Gestational weight gain among average-weight and overweight women—What is excessive? *Am J Obstet Gynecol* 172:705, 1995.

15. Coleman RA: Placental metabolism and transport of lipid, *Fed Proc* 45:2519, 1986.

16. Committee on Maternal Nutrition, Food and Nutrition Board: *Maternal nutrition and the course of pregnancy,* Washington DC, 1970, U.S. Government Printing Office.

17. Connor WE et al: The Alternative Diet Book, Iowa City, IA, 1976, Iowa City Press.

18. Copper RL et al: The relationship of maternal attitude toward weight gain during pregnancy, *Obstet Gynecol* 85:590, 1995.

19. DenBesten L, Connor WE, Bell S: The effect of dietary cholesterol on the composition of human bile, *Surgery* 73:266, 1973.

20. Durnin JVGA: Energy requirements of pregnancy: an integration of the longitudinal data from the five-country study, *Lancet* 2:1131, 1987.

21. Faber JJ, Thornburg KL: Fetal nutrition: supply, combustion, interconversion and deposition, *Fed Proc* 45:2502, 1986.

22. Fahraeus L, Larsson-Cohn ULF, Wallentin L: Plasma lipoproteins including high density lipoprotein sub-fractions during normal pregnancy. *Obstet Gynecol* 66:468, 1985.

23. French K, Ford DA, Fairchild MM: Maternal weight gain in twin pregnancy, *Topics Clin Nutr* 6:45, 1991.

24. Friedman WF, Mills LF: The relationship between vitamin D and the craniofacial and dental anomalies of the supravalvular aortic stenosis syndrome, *Pediatrics* 43:12, 1969.

25. Frisancho AR, Matos J, Flegel P: Maternal nutritional status and adolescent pregnancy outcome, *Am J Clin Nutr* 38:739, 1983.

26. Giroud A: *The nutrition of the embryo,* Springfield, Ill, 1970, Charles C Thomas.

27. Garn SM et al: Are pregnant teenagers still in rapid growth? *Am J Dis Child* 138:32, 1984.

28. Green, J.G. Serum cholesterol changes in pregnancy. *Am J Obstet Gynecol* 95:387, 1966.

29. Herrera E et al: Role of lipoprotein lipase activity on lipoprotein metabolism and the fate of circulating triglycerides in pregnancy. *Am J Obstet Gynecol* 158:1575, 1988.

30. Hickey CA et al: Relationship of psychosocial status to low prenatal weight gain among nonobese black and white women delivering at term. *Obstet Gynecol* 86:177, 1995.

31. Hill EP, Longo LD: Dynamics of maternal-fetal nutrient transfer, *Fed Proc* 39:239, 1980.

32. Hulsey TC, Levkoff AH, Alexander GA: Birth weights of infants of black and white mothers without pregnancy complications, *Am J Obstet Gynecol* 164:1299, 1991.

33. Hytten FE, Thomson AM: Maternal physiological adjustments. In Committee on Maternal Nutrition, Food and Nutrition Board, National Research Council, National Academy of Sciences: *Maternal nutrition and the course of pregnancy,* Washington, DC, 1970, Government Printing Office.

34. Institute of Medicine: *Nutrition during pregnancy: weight gain and nutrient supplements,* Washington DC, 1990, National Academy Press.

35. Keppel KG, Taffel SM: Pregnancy-related weight gain and retention: implications of the 1990 Institute of Medicine guidelines, *Am J Public Health* 83:1100, 1993.

36. Knopp RH et al: Lipoprotein metabolism in pregnancy, fat transport to the fetus and the effects of diabetes. *Biol Neonate* 50:297, 1986.

37. Laga EM, Driscoll SG, Munro HN: Comparison of placentas from two socioeconomic groups: II. Biochemical characteristics, *Pediatrics* 50:33, 1972.

38. Larsen CE, Serdula MK, Sullivan KM: Macrosomia: influence of maternal overweight among a low-income population, *Am J Obstet Gynecol* 162:490, 1990.

39. Lawrence M et al: Fat gain during pregnancy in rural African women: the effect of season and dietary status, *Am J Clin Nutr* 45:1442, 1987.

40. Lederman SA, Rosso P: The pattern of plasma volume changes in well-nourished and in food- or protein-restricted pregnant rats, *J Am Coll Nutr* 8:215, 1989.

41. Lester GE: Cholecalciferol and placental calcium transport, *Fed Proc* 45:2524, 1986.

42. Malone JI: Vitamin passage across the placenta, *Clin Perinatol* 2:295, 1975.

43. Loris P, Dewey KG, Poirier-Brode K: Weight gain and dietary intake of pregnant teenagers, *J Am Diet Assoc* 85:1296, 1985.

44. Lukasi HC et al: Total body water in pregnancy: assessment by using bioelectrical impedance. *Am J Clin Nutr* 59:578, 1994.

45. McMurry MP, Connor WE, Goplerud CP: The effects of dietary cholesterol upon the hypercholesterolemia of pregnancy, *Metabolism* 30:869, 1981.

46. Meserole LP et al: Prenatal weight gain and postpartum weight loss patterns in adolescents. *J Adolesc Health Care* 5:21, 1984.

47. Mittendorf R, Williams MA, Berkey CS et al: The length of uncomplicated human gestation, *Obstet Gynecol* 75:929, 1990.

48. Moses C et al: Effect of cholesterol feeding during pregnancy on blood cholesterol levels and placental vascular lesions, *Circulation* 6:103, 1952.

49. Munro HN: Role of the placenta in ensuring fetal nutrition, *Fed Proc* 45:2500, 1986.

50. Naeye RL: Maternal body weight and pregnancy outcome, *Am J Clin Nutr* 52:273, 1990.

51. Naeye RL: Weight gain and the outcome of pregnancy, *Am J Obstet Gynecol* 135:3, 1979.

52. National Center for Health Statistics: *Maternal weight gain and the outcome of pregnancy*, 1980, Series 21, No 44, Washington DC, 1986, Government Printing Office.

53. Neggers Y et al: Usefulness of various maternal skinfold measurements for predicting newborn birth weight, *J Am Diet Assoc* 92:1393, 1992.

54. Parker JD, Abrams B: Differences in postpartum weight retention between black and white mothers, *Obstet Gynecol* 81:768, 1993.

55. Parker JD, Abrams B: Prenatal weight gain advice: an examination of the recent prenatal weight gain recommendations of the Institute of Medicine, *Obstet Gynecol* 79:664, 1992.

56. Pederson AL, Worthington-Roberts B, Hickok DE: Weight gain patterns during twin gestation, *J Am Diet Assoc* 89:642, 1989.

57. Prentice AM et al: Prenatal dietary supplementation of Africa women and birth-weight, *Lancet* 1:489, 1983.

58. Rosso P: Placental growth, development and function in relation to maternal malnutrition, *Fed Proc* 39:250, 1980.

59. Rosso P et al: Hemodynamic changes in underweight pregnant women, *Obstet Gynecol* 79:908, 1992.

60. Schauberger CW, Rooney BL, Brimer LM: Factors that influence weight loss in the puerperium, *Obstet Gynecol* 79:424, 1992.

61. Schneider H: The role of the placenta in nutrition of the human fetus, *Am J Obstet Gynecol* 164:967, 1991.

62. Scholl TO et al: Gestational weight gain, pregnancy outcome and postpartum weight retention, *Obstet Gynecol* 86:423, 1995.

63. Siega-Riz AM, Adair LS, Hobel CJ: Institute of Medicine maternal weight gain recommendations and pregnancy outcome in a predominantly Hispanic population, *Obstet Gynecol* 84:565, 1994.

64. Smith DE et al: Longitudinal changes in adiposity associated with pregnancy. The Cardia Study, *J Am Med Assoc* 271:1747, 1994.

65. Sohlstrom A, Forsum E: Changes in adipose tissue volume and distribution during reproduction in Swedish women as assessed by magnetic resonance imaging, *Am J Clin Nutr* 61:287, 1995.

66. Susser M: Maternal weight gain, infant birth weight and diet: causal sequences, *Am J Clin Nutr* 53:1384, 1991.

67. Teratology Society: Teratology Society position paper: recommendations for vitamin A use during pregnancy, *Teratology* 35:269, 1987.

68. Viegas OAC, Cole TJ, Wharton BA: Impaired fat deposition in pregnancy: an indicator for nutritional intervention, *Am J Clin Nutr* 45:23, 1987.

69. Villar J et al: Improved lactose digestion during pregnancy: a case of physiologic adaptation? *Obstet Gynecol* 71:697, 1988.

70. Villar J et al: Effect of fat and fat-free mass deposition during pregnancy on birth weight. *Am J Obstet Gynecol* 167:1344, 1992.

71. Wilcox AJ et al: Incidence of early loss of pregnancy, *N Engl J Med* 319:189, 1988.

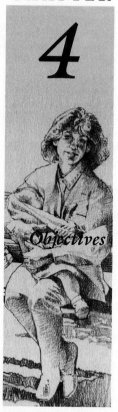

4

Foundations of Research in Prenatal Nutrition

Bonnie S. Worthington-Roberts

Objectives

✦✦

After completing this chapter, the student will be able to

✓ *Characterize the known nutritional influences on fetal growth*

✓ *Trace the development of knowledge about the role of nutrition in affecting pregnancy outcome*

✓ *Describe several human nutrition supplementation trials conducted with pregnant women*

✓ *Describe the WIC program and provide support for its continuation*

Introduction

Food is essential to life and growth. Without an adequate supply of food and the nutrients it contains, an organism cannot grow and develop normally. Eventually it dies.

In spite of these simple and well-established facts, the role that nutrition plays in the course and outcome of pregnancy has not always been appreciated. In the controlled conditions of the laboratory, researchers have been able to demonstrate harmful effects of deficient diets on pregnant animals and their offspring in a number of species. However, when studies are made on free-living human populations, direct relationships between what a mother eats during the 9 months of gestation and the course and outcome of her pregnancy have not always been shown. Consequently, the emphasis that nutri-

tion has received in prenatal care has varied over the years. At times, when researchers have been able to show positive effects, nutrition has received a great deal of attention. At other times, when studies produced equivocal results, nutrition has slipped to a position of indifference and neglect.

Part of the problem is that the changes that occur during pregnancy, their influence on nutritional needs, and the effects of long-term nutritional status on reproductive performance are not fully understood. As a science, the application of nutrition principles to pregnancy has had to depend on progress in a knowledge of reproduction itself, and as in any science, one of the most important advances is simply learning to ask the right questions. By reviewing how the emphasis of research has changed as more has become known about nutrition, reproduction, and human growth, health professionals can gain a sense of perspective that helps in understanding why different dietary recommendations for pregnant women have been made.

EARLY BELIEFS AND PRACTICES

During the 19th century much of what was known and recommended about diet during pregnancy was based on empiricism, that is, on casual observation rather than controlled studies. Since little information was available on the nutrient composition of foods or their biologic values, dietary advice was influenced by beliefs that obvious physical properties of different foods could produce specific effects on the mother or child. The beliefs were often colored by the emotional and mystical aura surrounding the pregnant state. For example, pregnant women were sometimes forbidden to eat salty, acidic, or sour foods for fear the infant would be born with a "sour" disposition. Eggs were sometimes restricted because of their association with the reproductive function. On the other hand, certain foods were encouraged for their presumed beneficial effects. Pregnant women were often advised to eat broths, warm milk, and ripe fruits to soothe the fetus and ease the birth process.

At this time dietary recommendations for pregnancy were also influenced by problems current in obstetrical practice. In the days of the industrial revolution, children in Europe had poor diets and worked long hours in dark factories. Rickets was a common nutritional disorder that impaired normal bone formation during the growing years. When women became pregnant, contracted pelvis presented a major obstetrical risk. Physicians did not have the means of delivering infants from these mothers that are available today. Mortality of both mother and child during childbirth was very high.

Experience with his own patients in the 1880s led a German physician, Prochownick, to advocate a fluid-restricted, low-carbohydrate, high-protein diet for women with contracted pelvis to be followed for 6 weeks before the birth.

Women using such a diet produced smaller infants who were easier to deliver. The diet may have had some justification in the 1880s, but it later gained in popularity and became a standard recommendation for women throughout pregnancy even when the original rationale for it no longer applied. Remnants of the Prochownick diet, restricting fluid or carbohydrate, persist today.

The importance of a pregnant woman's diet for the health of her infant has long been emphasized in customs and practices. However, there is little specific information available about diet and pregnancy before the 1930s, other than the reports on effects of food shortages during and after World War I. After the war there was a great deal of evidence that attempted to relate food shortages to the size of the baby, although much of it was considered to be inconclusive and even contradictory.

Early Research

Studies on diet in pregnancy were initiated in the 1930s, and the findings began to appear in the 1940s. Even without such data there was no lack of strong opinions. For example, the obstetrical position was stated by Danforth in 1933.[7] He began by warning pregnant women against two frequent advices "which so constantly emanate from the self-constituted obstetrical authorities of which every neighborhood possesses its quota. First, that she should eat largely because she is eating for two, and second, that she should eat sparingly because if she does not, her baby will be too large. She should be assured that neither of these dicta has any value." He goes on to note that she may be told that "it is quite impossible to influence the weight of the unborn child except within very narrow limits." By contrast, Parmelee, in the same 1933 monograph, noted that the size of the newborn child is influenced by many factors, such as heredity, race, health and nutrition of the mother, and the length of intrauterine life. He pointed out that "the clinical behaviour of a newborn infant depends to no small degree on the state of maturity to which it has developed at its birth." This divergence of viewpoint between the obstetrical and pediatric communities was to continue until the mid-1970s.

The studies begun in the 1930s* were reported in the 1940s but tended to be overshadowed by the findings that stemmed from famines and other abnormal nutritional conditions created by World War II.

Smith,[38] in his study on maternal undernutrition and birth weight in Holland, found a striking birth-weight decline that was statistically significant but was only apparent when data were examined in terms of birth weight by percentiles. He found that crude average figures can be misleading and further believed that the failure to express birth-weight data in percentiles may account for some of the discrepancies in earlier reports.

The complexity of the problem was emphasized by Toverud, Stearns, and Macy[46] in their 1950 comprehensive worldwide survey of the relationship between nutrition of the mother and the health and vigor of her infant at all stages of development: "Investigations have confirmed that prematurity is attributable to a combination of various factors, including those of nutritional, mental or social character, which influence the general well-being of the mother."

A period of disillusionment and disinterest set in after the publication of a series of reports whose chief conclusions appeared to contradict the earlier more enthusiastic concepts. Interest all but disappeared following the controversial presentations of a major clinical trial conducted at the Philadelphia Lying-In Hospital by Tompkins, Mitchell, and Wiehl.[45] Between disputes about the nature of the study as to if it really was research and reservations about the accuracy of estimates of dietary intakes, that major effort was discredited, despite its clearly beneficial outcomes for both mother and infant.

The mood of the period was well-presented by authorities on antenatal care who in 1955 presented the findings of Burke et al as "claims" that infants born at term to women receiving a diet low in protein were shorter and weighed less than those born to women whose protein intake was high. They next stated that these "claims" were "denied" by others, concluding, "It may therefore be said that claims that it is possible to reduce the baby's birth size by modifying the mother's diet in pregnancy are without foundation."[1] Along these same lines, in 1962 FAO/WHO[17] published observations that appeared to show that pregnancy could have a successful outcome in women subsisting on seemingly inadequate diets. As late as 1968, another authority wrote, "It seems fair to conclude that in normal circumstances maternal nutrition is not a limiting factor to fetal growth."[8]

HISTORICAL BACKGROUND*

The attention given to diet in pregnancy in the past decade is an outgrowth of the persistent concern about the relatively high neonatal and infant mortality rates in the United States, rates that continue above those of many industrialized countries. This concern arises, in turn, from the realization that low birth weight is a major contributing factor in two thirds of all infant deaths. Thus, reducing the number of low-birth-weight infants has been emphasized as a specific national goal.

The challenge of reducing the incidence of low-birth-weight infants arose from the realization of the relationship between low birth weight and later mental retardation. More recently the frequent findings of intraventricular hemorrhage in infants weighing less than 1500 gm (3.2 lb) at birth have been highlighted. That even lesser degrees of birth-weight deficiencies (as seen in small-for-gestational-age infants) present subsequent hazards is suggested by the findings of the frequent associations of learning disabilities and small-for-date infants.

---

*The findings of the Burke, Harding, and Stuart study[2,3] were presented in such a way that it gave the impression of a linear relation between average protein intake and infants' birth weight and length. Burke was certain that protein intake was an index figure and not a measure of a single variable (protein), since the study was conducted during the Depression on patients who were recent immigrants from Ireland and Italy. Since her study involved observations only and no counseling or dietary advice, women with good diets during pregnancy probably had equally good diets in their preconception period. In short, protein was probably a marker for income, motivation, and long-term health habits.

---

*With much-appreciated input from Howard N. Jacobson.

The need to reduce the incidence of infants of very low birth weight has been further reinforced in recent years by the fuller public realization that these infants may spend weeks or months in the hospital, a situation that adds to parental stress and to the costs of care.

A major result of the earlier (1962) landmark report of the President's Panel on Mental Retardation was the establishment of the federal Maternal and Infant Care Program, with its heavy emphasis on maternal nutrition. From the outset, however, there was great uncertainty about whether or not prenatal care, including nutrition services, could favorably modify the outcome of a high-risk pregnancy as measured by increased birth weight.

In the intervening years, a great deal of knowledge about the influence of nutritional factors on pregnancy outcomes has been acquired. Nevertheless, the uncertainties about the effectiveness of dietary interventions remain to this day. In this connection one group of investigators,[35] influenced by their experiences, was obliged to conclude that in their particular situation:

. . .high-protein supplements, gross measures had shown no improvement in outcome at birth and adverse effects on fetal growth, prematurity, and newborn survival; with balanced protein-calorie supplements, there was a nonsignificant rise in birth weights and longer gestation.

This, then, is the background against which this material is presented on the state of current knowledge concerning nutrition and pregnancy.

Follow-up Guidelines and Programs

It was not until the mid-1960s that renewed interest in infant mortality and morbidity led to a reappraisal of the influences of diet and pregnancy. Once attention was redirected toward this problem, a number of significant steps were taken. The resulting progress has been so rapid, it is nearly impossible to grasp it. A brief description of developments in the field of diet in pregnancy follows.

The White House Conference on Food, Nutrition, and Health (WHCFNH) was held in Washington in December 1969.[34] The immediate stimulus was the nationwide shock at the disclosures of widespread hunger and malnutrition in the United States. The determination to do something about it produced the WHCFNH as the first organizational step.

Many of us involved with the conduct of the Panel on Pregnancy and Very Young Infants were also involved with the soon-to-be published National Research Council (NRC) report on *Maternal Nutrition and the Course of Pregnancy*. The 1969 WHCFNH was a priceless opportunity to address the applied issues of diet and pregnancy within the context of their needed health services.

The recommendations of the WHCFNH are broad and comprehensive. They remain the only set of guidelines for use on a national basis that was formulated by representatives convened for that purpose.*

The NRC report on *Maternal Nutrition and the Course of Pregnancy* was issued in 1970, and it remains the major source of research information on the role of nutrition in human reproduction. One of the principal findings of that report was the limited and fragmentary nature of studies on diet in pregnancy. The report singled out the need for long-term longitudinal studies on women and their families. This problem still remains to be addressed.

Two sets of guidelines appeared in 1973[4,6] as a direct outgrowth of the stimulus given to nutrition services at the 1969 WHCFNH. The American Public Health Association publication[6] presented guidelines and standards primarily for use by public health workers as an aid to program planning and assessments. The NRC guidelines[4] were aimed at indicating the uses and limitations of supplementary food provided during pregnancy. The technical issues, practical problems, and political realities were explored, along with the inherent difficulties involved in multidisciplinary and multifactorial studies.

---

*One admonition that it is impossible to target food for one member of a family who takes meals with others has been borne out by the repeated findings of widespread food sharing in the Federal Special Supplementary Food Program for Women, Infants, and Children (WIC program).

The Special Supplementary Food Program for Women, Infants, and Children (WIC) was initiated under court order in 1973. The expressed purpose of the WIC program was to provide food as an adjunct to health care during critical times of growth and development. WIC has grown from a pilot program costing $40 million in 1973 to one costing well over $2.5 billion in 1995.

A milestone was reached in 1978 with the publication of *Guidelines for Assessment of Maternal Nutrition,* prepared jointly by the American College of Obstetricians and Gynecologists and the American Dietetic Association.[43] The report produced the first national consensus on the relevant nutritional risk factors at the onset of and during pregnancy. This original listing has been superseded by the more current material in the 1981 NRC report.[5]

The Society for Nutrition Education produced a teaching film and reference manual for the March of Dimes that were distributed in 1981.[5,14] This package was designed to address the inconsistent teaching of diet and nutrition to physicians and other health professionals.

The NRC produced the highly useful *Guidelines for Nutrition Services in Perinatal Care* that was distributed in 1981.[5] This report was particularly timely because it was designed for use with the rapidly growing regional networks for maternal and perinatal services. It is most helpful because it addresses the nutritional issues of infant feeding and the increasingly important issues of substance abuse.

That the place of diet in pregnancy has become more firmly established can be seen in the 1982 *Standards for Obstetric-Gynecologic Services.*[41]

There is increasing realization of the seamless web of variables that together influence the outcome of a pregnancy. Within the constellation of income, health, education, family, and fertility, food and nutrition are just one part, but an important and modifiable one. As one observer has stated, "Special efforts to improve prenatal, child, and maternal health showed clear evidence that the services did make a difference. . . . No one yet has teased out the relative effects of different variables." This is the clearest statement of the nature of the problems that need to be addressed in the years ahead.

NUTRITIONAL INFLUENCES ON FETAL GROWTH

It is not possible, for obvious ethical reasons, to examine maternal-fetal relationships directly at the cellular and molecular levels in humans. Consequently, work toward understanding how maternal nutrition influences growth and development in utero must be done on animals. The technique has usually been to manipulate the diets of pregnant animals and study the effects of cellular morphology and physiology in the offspring at various stages of gestation. Over the past few years, much information has accumulated from studies of this type. These findings have contributed to a revival of interest in the importance of nutrition in prenatal care.

Experiments in Animals

Two types of dietary restrictions have been imposed on laboratory animals to study the effects of maternal nutrition on fetal growth and development. One restriction is simply not giving the animals enough food so that the diet is low in calories. The other restriction holds calories at an adequate level but reduces or completely eliminates one or more essential nutrients. The effects of deficiencies of almost all the known nutrients have been studied this way, but restrictions of protein and calories have more relevance to humans than restrictions of vitamins or minerals. All animals need energy and use protein in essentially the same way, but the need for vitamins and minerals and their specific functions differ from species to species.

A number of investigators have demonstrated what can happen to fetuses when pregnant animals are fed calorie- or protein-restricted diets. Maternal malnutrition can interfere with the ability of the mother to conceive, it can produce death and resorption or abortion of the fetuses, and it can produce malformations or retard growth. Of course, the more severe the dietary restrictions are the more serious the effects will be.

Biochemical studies give evidence of why this occurs. One effect of protein-calorie malnutrition is an impairment of energy metabolism in the cells by interfering with the synthesis of deoxyribonucleic acid (DNA) and enzymes involved in glycolysis and the citric acid cycle.

Without adequate supplies of amino acids and energy, cell functions break down, and normal processes of growth cannot occur. The effects would be most damaging when cells are normally undergoing rapid division. This implies that the timing of the dietary deficiency, as well as its severity, is important.

Stages of cell growth. Basically all animals grow in one of two ways. They get larger because their cells increase in number or because the number of cells they already have increases in size. In the 1960s, techniques were developed to determine how these two kinds of growth take place. The method is based on measurements of DNA content of organs and tissues. In a given species all cells of a certain ploidy contain the same amount of DNA. For example, all diploid cells in the human body contain 6 picograms (pg) of DNA. For the rat, it is 6.2 pg of DNA per diploid cell. Cells of other ploidy have different amounts of DNA, but it has been shown that the DNA content is proportional to the total amount of cytoplasm. So for practical purposes the amount of DNA in an organ or tissue sample divided by the amount of DNA per

cell gives an estimation of the number of cells present. Once this is known, the total weight of the organ or, alternatively, the total protein content, can be divided by the number of cells to give an indication of the average cell size.[48]

By using this technique with rats, a sequence of cell growth common to all organs of the body has been found (Fig. 4-1). In the first stage of this sequence growth takes place only by an increase in the number of cells; that is, cells are replicating, and all are approximately of equal size. This stage of cell proliferation is called *hyperplasia.* In the second stage new cells continue to be made, but the ones already present now begin to increase in size, which is called *hypertrophy;* thus the second stage is both hyperplastic and hypertrophic. The third stage is totally hypertrophic. Growth in this stage is taking place only by increases in cell size, and no new cells are being made. The fourth stage is maturity, in which all cell growth stops. In this stage there is further development as enzyme systems are elaborated and cell functions are integrated.

The stages of cell growth are not really discrete processes but merge into one another. The

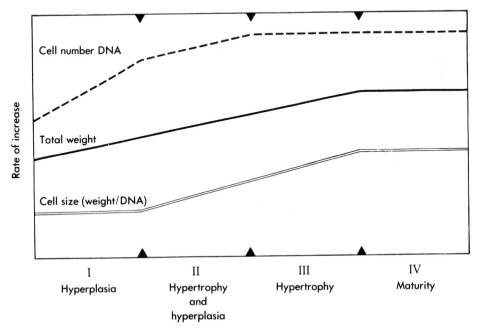

FIG. 4-1   Stages of cell growth.

length of each stage and the periods of maximum cell proliferation differ according to species and in various parts of the body. In most regions there is a continuous increase until equilibrium is reached as old cells die and new ones are made. However, in nonregenerating organs such as the brain, the number and size of cells present at maturity must last a lifetime. For this organ in particular any interference with normal cell growth may have consequences that cannot be repaired.

The rat has a normal gestational period of 21 days. Hyperplastic growth of the placenta is complete by 17 days. Throughout gestation all fetal tissues are increasing in cell number. Most continue to proliferate postnatally until weaning, but certain types of cells, such as neurons of the central nervous system, stop dividing before birth.

The consequences of any interference with normal cell growth would depend on the time at which it occurs. Interference in the hyperplastic phase would result in a decrease in the number of cells produced. If interference occurs when cells are undergoing hypertrophy, cells would be reduced in size. Both types of interference would cause the animal to experience growth failure.

Types of growth failure. It is now clear that a number of things can produce growth failure in utero. The cause can be either "intrinsic" or "extrinsic." The difference may be determined by the condition of the placentas of animals born small-for-gestational-age. In intrinsic intrauterine growth failure, placentas are usually of normal size, which implies that retardation of fetal growth was not caused by inadequate maternal-fetal transport but was the result of other factors. Some examples include chromosomal abnormalities, certain drugs that cross the placental barrier, and maternal infections. Extrinsic intrauterine growth failure is usually manifested by placentas that are reduced in size, which indicates that they were incapable of supplying the fetus with adequate nutrition.

Extrinsic intrauterine growth failure can be produced experimentally in a number of ways. One way is to ligate one of the uterine arteries of the mother rat so that blood supplies to one whole side of the uterus are cut off. The procedure is usually applied at 17 days' gestation in the rat, that is, after hyperplastic growth of the placenta is complete. Another way of producing extrinsic growth retardation is to impose a severe protein restriction on the mother's diet at different times during pregnancy to reduce the supply of nutrients available for the synthesis of placental and fetal cells.

The techniques for measuring cell number and cell size have made it possible to compare changes that occur in the placenta and fetal organs from these different types of intrauterine growth failure. Results from such comparisons are summarized in Table 4-1.

The principal feature of intrinsic growth failure is the presence of multiple malformations in the fetuses. These are absent in growth failure produced by ligation and are variable in maternal malnutrition, depending on the timing of the restriction.

In both vascular and nutritional growth failure, placentas are reduced in proportion to fetal weight. In the ligated animals and in late maternal malnutrition the reduction is caused by a decrease in the average size of the cells. Maternal protein restriction maintained throughout most of gestation, however, decreases both the number and size of placental cells.

The fetuses themselves also show different patterns of growth retardation. Those subjected to vascular insufficiency show an asymmetrical retardation. The fetuses have relatively normal brain sizes and head circumferences, but their livers are greatly reduced, by as much as 50%, and glycogen reserves are completely absent. Proportionally these animals have bigger brains and heads as compared with the rest of their bodies; they are extremely hypoglycemic at birth.

When maternal protein restriction is limited to the last few days of gestation, the fetuses exhibit a pattern of growth retardation that is similar to that produced by vascular insufficiency—proportionally big heads and small bodies. However, when the restriction is imposed throughout most of the gestational period, the pattern of fetal growth retardation becomes more symmetrical. There is a decrease in cell number of approximately 15% to 20% in all organs, including the brain; head circumference is

TABLE 4-1 **Types of Intrauterine Growth Failure**

| | Intrinsic | Extrinsic | |
		Asymmetrical	Symmetrical
Placenta			
Cell growth	Normal	Reduced 20%-30%	Reduced 20%-30%
Fetus			
Malformations	Multiple	Absent	Absent
Weight	Reduced	Reduced 20%	Reduced 20%
Head circumference	Variable	Normal	Reduced 20%
Brain			
Cell growth		Normal	Reduced 20%
Liver			
Cell growth		Reduced 50%	Reduced 20%
Glycogen		Reduced 100%	Reduced 20%

From Winick M, Brasel JA, Velasco EG: Effect of prenatal nutrition on pregnancy risk, *Clin Obstet Gynecol* 16:184, 1973.

also reduced. The reduction in cell number is greatest in the regions of the brain that are undergoing the most rapid rates of cell division.

Consequences of growth failure. These findings make it obvious that fetuses are *not* perfect parasites that can survive intrauterine insults without adverse effects. Data suggest that inadequate maternal nutrition can affect the fetus in ways that are coincident with the stages of cell growth and that the bodily reserves of the mother cannot always insulate the fetus from dietary deficiencies. What happens to animals whose mothers were nutritionally deprived during pregnancy depends to a great extent on how they are fed after birth.

Nutrition of the neonate can be manipulated by altering the number of pups a mother rat must nurse. If the typical litter is reduced from ten to three and the pups are nursed by foster mothers whose diets were not restricted during pregnancy, there is evidence that the deficits in cell numbers can be entirely made up by the time of weaning. Other studies have shown, however, that prenatally malnourished pups nursed in normal litter sizes do not catch up.

Perhaps the finding of most concern is the effect of continued deprivation on the growth of brain cells. If prenatally malnourished pups are restricted after birth by feeding them in litters of 18 pups per dam, they demonstrate a 60% re-

duction in brain cell number by the time they are weaned. This is in contrast with the 15% to 20% reduction that is seen in either prenatal or postnatal malnutrition alone. Thus it seems as though malnutrition that is continued throughout the entire time that brain cells are dividing will produce deficits that are much greater than would be expected if the separate effects were simply added together. Experiments completed in the 1960s have shown that nutritional rehabilitation will not enable these animals to recover their normal size once the period of cell proliferation is passed. They will continue to be small no matter how well fed they are after weaning. Other data suggest that maternal malnutrition may even have intergenerational effects; researchers have found that brain cell numbers were reduced in rats whose mothers were prenatally malnourished, even though these mothers had adequate diets after weaning and during gestation.

These studies would not be so disturbing if size were not related to function. The fact is, however, that alterations in normal biochemical and developmental processes have been shown to accompany fetal and neonatal malnutrition in several species of animals. Changes in the usual constituents of cells are observed, as well as the delayed appearance of specific enzyme systems. Depending on the timing of the dietary deficiency, degeneration of the cerebral cortex, the medulla, and the spinal cord can be produced. Muscular development is also impaired because of a reduced number of muscle cells and fibers.

Some investigators have associated these changes with abnormal neuromotor and mental development. For example, malnourished rats do not respond normally to stimuli in the environment and have abnormalities in gait; rat pups whose mothers had protein-restricted diets in pregnancy do not learn to run a rat maze as quickly as adequately nourished controls and are slower in avoidance conditioning.

What has been learned from animal research? Much can still be learned from experiments with animals about the processes of fetal growth and development and the consequences of maternal malnutrition, but the work to date has produced important results. The general conclusions can be summarized as follows:

1. Although a number of prenatal influences affect fetal growth, maternal malnutrition can be one cause of growth failure that results in small offspring of low birth weight.
2. Animals that are malnourished from restrictions of their mothers' diets throughout most of gestation are characterized by (a) reduced number and size of cells in the placenta, (b) reduced brain cell number and head size, (c) proportional reductions in the size of other organs, and (d) alterations in normal cell constituents and biochemical processes.
3. The consequences of malnutrition for the fetus depend on the timing, severity, and duration of the maternal dietary restriction. These consequences may be reversible if the restriction primarily affects growth in cell size, but a reduction in the number of cells may be permanent if the restriction is maintained throughout the entire period of hyperplastic growth.

Human Experience

In view of the risks of early death or permanent disability associated with low birth weight, it is apparent that the research on intrauterine growth failure in laboratory animals may have great implications for human problems. Of the annual incidence of low-birth-weight infants, it has been estimated that from 10% to 20% are the result of intrauterine growth failure. This means that between 80,000 and 120,000 infants who have experienced malnutrition in utero are born each year in the United States. An important thing to understand when interpreting these statistics is that a number of factors can retard fetal growth. When the term *fetal malnutrition* is applied to human infants, it simply means that there was a reduction in the maternal supply or placental transport of nutrients so that fetal growth is retarded significantly below genetic potential. It does not necessarily mean that the mother's own nutrition was at fault. At present there is no way to judge how many growth-retarded infants are the result of maternal malnutrition.

Although the animal experiments are highly suggestive, caution must be exercised in making direct applications to humans. A primary reason for doing research on animals is to find out what can *possibly* happen when certain conditions are imposed. The findings do not guarantee that these things *actually* happen in the normal course of human events. There are a number of reasons why the dramatic results of maternal malnutrition demonstrated in animals may not occur as readily in human beings. In effect the consequences of maternal malnutrition on fetal growth and development are all magnified in the animal studies. This is because (1) relative rates of growth and development are much slower in humans as compared with laboratory animals, (2) the timing of maximum growth also differs, (3) the number and size of fetuses a mother must nourish in utero compared with her own body size and nutrition reserves are much smaller in humans than in laboratory animals, and (4) the magnitude of dietary deprivation used for experimentation is rarely encountered in human populations under ordinary circumstances.

Human Fetal Growth

The techniques for measuring cell number and cell size are now being used to determine the stages of maximum cell growth and development in humans. Although data are presently limited, a picture that generally parallels the sequence outlined for animals is beginning to emerge (Fig. 4-2, *A* and *B*).

The human placenta grows rapidly throughout gestation. By 34 to 36 weeks it has completed cell division. From that time until term, growth continues only by an increase in the size of existing cells.

It is known from studies of **embryology** that growth of the fetus can be divided into three periods. The first is the period of **blastogenesis** in which the fertilized egg cleaves into cells that fold in on one another. These evolve into an inner cell mass, which gives rise to the embryo and an outer coat, the trophoblast, which becomes the placenta. The process of blastogenesis is complete at about 2 weeks after fertilization.

The second period is the embryonic stage, the critical time when cells differentiate into three germinal layers. The **ectoderm** gives rise to the brain, nervous system, hair, and skin. The **mesoderm** produces all the voluntary muscles, bones, and components of the cardiovascular and excretory systems. The **endoderm** differentiates to form the digestive system, respiratory system, and glandular organs of the body. By 60 days' gestation all of the major features of the human infant have been achieved.

The fetal stage is the period of most rapid growth. From the third month until term, fetal weight increases nearly 500-fold from about 6 gm (0.2 oz) to 3000 to 3500 gm (6.5 lb to 7.6 lb) at birth. Fig. 4-3 shows the average weight curve from 10 weeks until term.

Measurements of DNA and protein in embryonic and fetal tissues show that growth in the embryonic stage occurs only by an increase in the number of cells. During the fetal stage, growth in cell number continues, but it is now accompanied by an increase in cell size.

Cells of most organs continue to proliferate after birth. Data derived from cases of therapeutic abortions and accidental deaths indicate that cell division in the normal human brain is linear throughout gestation, slows after birth, and reaches a maximum around 18 months of age. It is believed that growth in cell size begins at about 7 months' gestation and may continue into the third year of life. These estimates are for the whole organ and do not identify patterns in specific cells and regions of the central nervous system. There is evidence that growth in cell number stops earlier in the cerebellum. Neuronal cell number is probably complete at birth, whereas growth of glial cells peaks near birth and continues through the first year of life.

Brain and nerve cells are not only composed of protein but also have considerable amounts of lipid materials. These include fatty acids, cholesterol, phospholipids, glycolipids, and other esters. Most lipids in brain and nerve cells are used for the synthesis of myelin, the substance that insulates the cells and aids in the conduction of nerve impulses. Changes in lipid composition are used to measure the rate of **myelination** occurring at different times.

Lipid deposition is fairly constant in the early part of gestation, but it begins to increase rapidly during the last trimester. In gray matter of the brain adult composition is reached by about 3 months of age. Myelination is slower in white matter. It attains about 90% of adult composition by 2 years of age and is not completed until the child is approximately 10 years old.

The other organs of the body grow prenatally and postnatally at varying rates. DNA measurements show that cell numbers in all organs studied to date increase from 13 weeks' gestation until term. There are continued increases in cell numbers in the heart, liver, kidney, and spleen throughout the first year of life.

No change is observed in the size of cells during the prenatal period in the heart, kidney, spleen, thyroid, thymus, tongue, esophagus, stomach, and intestines. There is a slow increase in cell size beginning at about 7 months' gestation in the liver, lungs, adrenal glands, and diaphragm.

Muscle, bone, and adipose cells exhibit patterns similar to the growth of other organs. Cells begin to proliferate rapidly at 3 to 4 months' gestation and continue to divided in postnatal life. Growth in the size of cells shows the most rapid increase beginning at about 7 months' gestation.

Growth-Retarded Infants

From the sequence of growth that has been described, it is possible to theorize the effects of malnutrition at different stages of gestation. In the early months of pregnancy a severe limita-

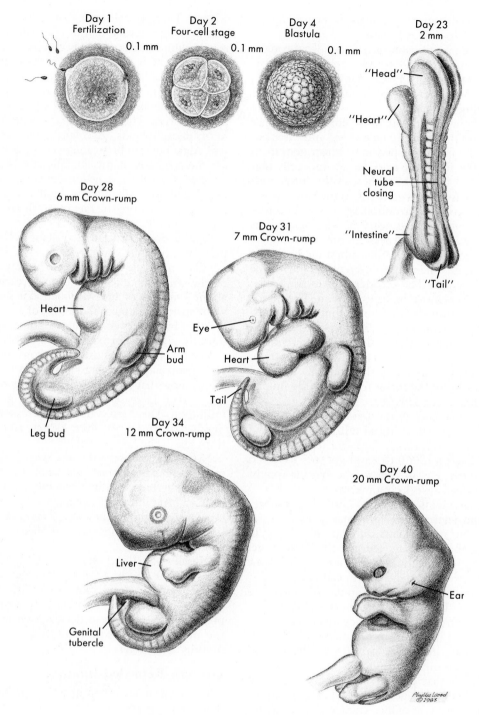

FIG. 4-2   Stages of fetal development

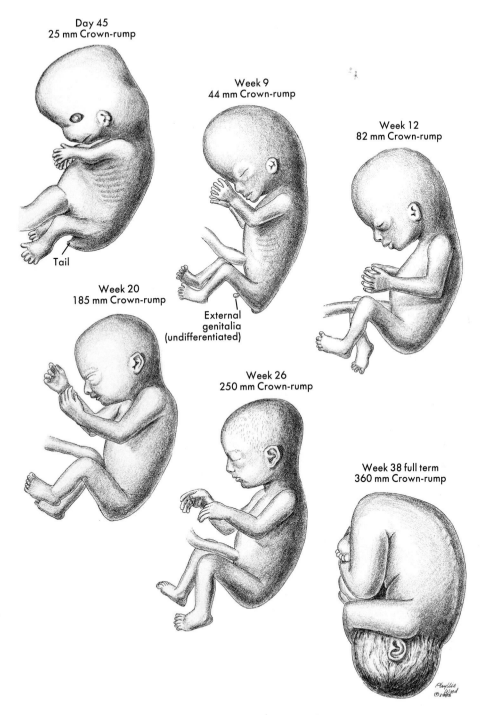

Day 45
25 mm Crown-rump

Tail

Week 9
44 mm Crown-rump

External
genitalia
(undifferentiated)

Week 12
82 mm Crown-rump

Week 20
185 mm Crown-rump

Week 26
250 mm Crown-rump

Week 38 full term
360 mm Crown-rump

FIG. 4-2, cont'd. Stages of fetal development.

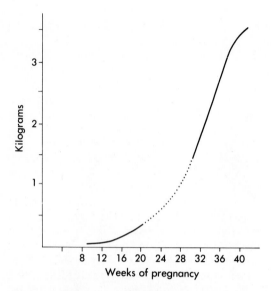

FIG. 4-3   Average curve of fetal growth.

From Hytten FE, Leitch I: *The physiology of human pregnancy*, ed 2, Oxford, 1971, Blackwell Scientific.

tion on the supply or transport of nutrients would have to occur because the quantitative requirements of the embryo are extremely small. Nevertheless, a restriction of materials and energy needed for cell synthesis and cell differentiation could produce malformations or cause the embryo to die.

Malnutrition after the third month of gestation would not have teratogenic efects, but it could interfere with fetal growth. Nutrient requirements are greatest in the last trimester of pregnancy, when cells are increasing both in number and in size. Even a relatively mild restriction could be a serious impediment at this time.

The theoretical effects of fetal malnutrition are reflected in the characteristics of small-for-gestational-age infants. Their conditions are variable, suggesting the multiple causes and importance of timing shown in animals. Among those small-for-gestational-age infants who do not have birth anomalies, there are two patterns of growth retardation. One type affects weight more than length; the other affects weight and length equally.

In the first type of retardation head circumference and skeletal growth are about normal, but the infants have poorly developed muscles and almost no subcutaneous fat. The fact that these infants have characteristics similar to the large-head, small-body features of animals malnourished during the last weeks of gestation from maternal dietary restrictions or **uterine ligation** is remarkable.

In the type of growth retardation that affects weight and length equally, the size of all parts of the body, including head circumference and skeleton, is proportionally reduced. The physical characteristics of these infants are similar to those of rat pups whose mothers were maintained on deficient diets throughout most of gestation.

Effects of Maternal Malnutrition

These observations provide fertile grounds for speculation, but is there any evidence that maternal malnutrition really is a cause of fetal malnutrition in human populations? Of necessity, much of the information is circumstantial, but there have been three kinds of studies that have addressed this question with highly significant results: (1) natural experiments in which birth statistics before, during, and after periods of acute famine are studied and compared; (2) measurements of organ size and cell numbers in stillbirths and neonatal deaths in which all causes not related to maternal malnutrition have been ruled out; and (3) **epidemiologic studies** of the nutritional correlates of birth weight.

Natural experiments. The hardships of war afford researchers an opportunity to study the effects of severe dietary restrictions during pregnancy under conditions that fortunately are seldom duplicated. Throughout most of Europe at various times during World War II, food shortages were commonplace. Reports were made on the effects of these shortages during the 1940s, but they are being considered with renewed interest today in light of the findings from animal research.

An 18-month period of acute starvation was experienced in Russia during the siege of Leningrad in 1942. Researchers compared statistics for infants born before, during, and after the siege. They found that during the famine period there was a twofold increase in fetal mortality and an increase in the number of infants weighing less than 2,500 gm (5.4 lb) at birth.

Similar findings were reported from Holland. Here the statistics are more insightful because the famine was of sharp onset and limited to approximately 6 months during the winter of 1944 and 1945. It was not accompanied by other deprivations as severe as those experienced during the siege of Leningrad, and the women of Holland were considered to have had fairly good diets before the food shortage. During the famine, dietary intake dropped to less than 1,000 cal/day, and protein was limited to 30 or 40 gm. Since the famine lasted only 6 months, babies conceived before and during it were exposed for varying lengths of time, but none were exposed for the entire course of gestation. This situation set up natural conditions that are similar to the animal experiments. When the statistics were evaluated, it was possible to consider how the timing of maternal dietary restrictions might affect fetal growth.

On the average, birth weights of infants exposed to the famine were reduced by 200 gm (7 oz). Weights were lowest for babies exposed to the famine during the entire last half of pregnancy. Added exposure before that time did not reduce birth weights further. In fact, babies who were exposed to the famine during the first 27 weeks of gestation but finished their terms after the famine ended had higher average birth weights than those who were only exposed during the last 3 weeks of gestation.

The data for stillbirths and congenital malformations followed a different pattern. The rates were lowest for infants conceived before the famine and highest for those conceived during it.

The findings are in line with what is hypothesized from knowledge of the stages of human growth. Poor nutrition in the latter part of pregnancy affects fetal growth, whereas poor nutrition in the early months affects development of the embryo and its capacity to survive.

At age 19, no mental disorders were recognized as having obvious relation to the Dutch famine experience regarding prenatal malnutrition exposure. However, in the same birth cohorts near the age of 50 years, there was evidence of more schizophrenia and an intergener-

ational effect, that is, the problems transferring to future offspring.[42a]

It is interesting to note that, in contrast with the experiences in Russia and Holland, the perinatal mortality rate in Great Britain, which had been fairly constant before the war, actually declined between 1940 and 1945 despite poor environmental conditions and no discernible improvements in prenatal care. One possible explanation is that pregnant and lactating women were given priority status for food rationing in Britain as a matter of national policy.

Organ studies. Studies that attempt to relate the size of organs in human infants to maternal nutrition must control for other conditions known to affect fetal growth. Naeye, Diener, and Dellinger[28] looked at the organs of 252 U.S. stillborn infants and infants who died in the first 48 hours of life, excluding all multiple births, maternal complications, and congenital defects. The infants were categorized as coming from poor or nonpoor families according to income. Comparisons of organs between the two groups showed that the mass of adipose tissue and the size of individual fat cells were smaller in the poor infants. These infants also had smaller livers, adrenal glands, thymuses, and spleens. Heart, kidneys, and skeleton were also reduced, but the differences were not as great. The ranking in organ sizes is consistent with reductions noted in animals who have been prenatally malnourished and in humans who have experienced uterine or placental disorders. Since the last two were ruled out, Naeye concluded that undernutrition could be responsible for prenatal growth retardation in infants from low-income families.[28]

The organs in infants who survive intrauterine malnutrition cannot be studied to see if cells are reduced in number or in size, but one organ that is available is the placenta. Winick[48] reported that the size of placentas and the number of placental cells are 15% and 20% below normal when infants experience intrauterine growth failure. By comparing placentas from different sources, he has shown that those from indigent populations in developing countries have reductions in cell numbers similar to the reductions noted in placentas from U.S. infants with intrauterine growth failure. In one interesting case in the United States a mother who was severely undernourished from anorexia nervosa during pregnancy gave birth to an infant weighing less than 2,500 gm (5.4 lb). When the placenta was examined, it was found to have only 50% of the normal number of cells.[48]

Lechtig et al[23] have also looked at human placentas. The 49 women in their study all came from Guatemala City. Their socioeconomic status was evaluated according to family income, education, and sanitary conditions in the home. Measurements of height, postpartum weight, skin folds, and the ratio of nonessential to essential amino acids in serum all showed significant differences indicative of chronic protein-calorie malnutrition in the low socioeconomic group. The average weight of placentas from women in the low socioeconomic group was 15% below the average weight of placentas from the high socioeconomic group. On microscopic examination it was found that low placental weight was associated with reduced surface area of the placental peripheral villi. The peripheral villi are responsible for the transport of nutrients to the fetus. The reduction in surface area may be what accounts for the observed association between placental weight and the size of the infant at birth.

Nutritional correlates of birth weight. Studies of the relationship between maternal nutrition and the birth weight of the infant have tended to focus directly on the nutrient composition of the diet during pregnancy. Because of variations in the nutritional requirements of individuals, these studies have produced conflicting results. However, there are two indicators of long-term and immediate nutritional status that have shown consistent associations with birth weight. These are maternal body size (height and prepregnancy weight) and the amount of weight gained by the mother during pregnancy itself.

It should not be surprising that big mothers have big babies. What is less often appreciated is that the size of the infant at birth largely depends on the size of the mother and is not influenced to a great degree by the size of the father. This was shown years ago in a classic experiment in which Shire stallions were bred with Shetland mares and Shetland stallions with Shire mares.

The newborn foals were always of a size appropriate to the mothers' breeds, and no intermediate sizes were ever produced. The same effects have since been demonstrated in a number of animals, and there is indirect evidence for the same phenomenon in humans.

It has been further demonstrated in humans that height and prepregnancy weight of the mother have independent and additive effects on the birth weight of the child. In an analysis of 4,095 mothers in the Scottish communities of Aberdeen, Thomson, Bellewicz, and Hytten[44] found that, on the average, the tallest and heaviest mothers had babies who weighed 500 gm (1 lb) more at birth than babies of the shortest and lightest mothers. It is postulated that maternal size is a conditioning factor on the ultimate size of the placenta and thus controls the blood supply of nutrients that will be available to the fetus.

The idea has support in findings from the Collaborative Perinatal Project sponsored by the National Institutes of Health. Naeye[30] analyzed data from nearly 60,000 pregnancies to discover causes of fetal and neonatal mortality among different racial groups. One finding was that Puerto Ricans experience a higher rate of placental growth retardation than whites. However, this difference disappears when women with prepregnancy weights of 101 lb (45 kg) or less are excluded from the analysis. Naeye concludes that the high rate of placental growth retardation in Puerto Ricans is a result of the greater proportion of women who enter pregnancy with low body weights. Further data from Naeye's laboratory show that, regardless of race or ethnic origin, mothers with low prepregnancy weights have much lighter placentas than heavier mothers.

Luke et al.[24] also assessed the relationship between infant birth weight and weight status of the mother. Maternal "nutrient pool" was estimated by recording postpartum weight for height; 294 uncomplicated term pregnancies were studied, and each gravida was categorized by height and postpartum weight as underweight, normal weight, or overweight. Results are summarized in Fig. 4-4. In underweight women mean infant birth weights increased 214 gm (7 oz) with each 10% increase in maternal

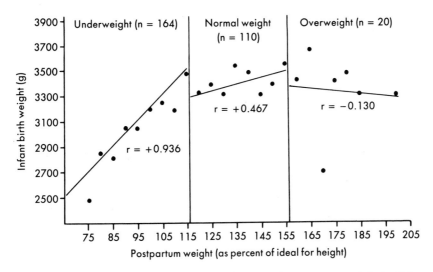

FIG. 4-4 Relationship of infant birth weight and maternal postpartum weight in 294 normal term pregnancies.

Modified from Luke B, Petrie RH: Intrauterine growth: correlation of infant birth weight and maternal postpartum weight, *Am J Clin Nutr* 33:2311, 1980.

postpartum weight. In normal weight subjects the same increase in maternal postpartum weight paralleled an increase of 41.9 gm (1.4 oz) in infant birth weight. Among overweight mothers, a negative relationship was shown between increasing maternal postpartum weight and birth weight, since for each increase of 10% in maternal postpartum weight there was a decrease of 29.8 gm (1 oz) in infant birth weight. The investigators suggest that maternal metabolic needs must take preference over fetal requirements at the extremes of the maternal nutrient pool. Only when the maternal nutrient pool is brought into the normal range can optimal intrauterine growth be realized. In clinical terms these data suggest that in the underweight gravida the pregravid weight deficit should be corrected, and in the obese gravida the excessive and endogenous reserve should be reduced before conception.

The importance of satisfactory prepregnancy weight and/or prenatal weight gain in short women was nicely illustrated by Luke et al. in 1984.[24] The influence of height and delivery weight (prepregnancy and gestational gain), expressed as percent ideal weight for height, on

birth weight was examined in 696 uncomplicated term pregnancies. Each gravida was classified by delivery weight as short, average or tall. Mean infant birth weight paralleled increasing maternal delivery weight percent in all three height groups, although the effect was most pronounced in gravidas of short stature. In that group, a 10% increase in delivery weight was associated with an increase of 127 gm in mean infant birth weight as compared with increases of 74 and 87 gm in the average and tall groups, respectively. The results of this study show that adequate pregravid weight and satisfactory gains augment optimal fetal growth in all gravidas but particularly benefit the offspring of short women.

Data available tend to suggest that underweight women may reduce their risk of adverse pregnancy outcome by establishing a higher prepregnancy weight and/or gaining extra weight during the prenatal period. The value of the latter has been shown by Naeye,[29] who evaluated data from the United States Collaborative Perinatal Project. Fig. 4-5 illustrates the results of the study with the term **net pregnancy weight gain** referring to the mother's preg-

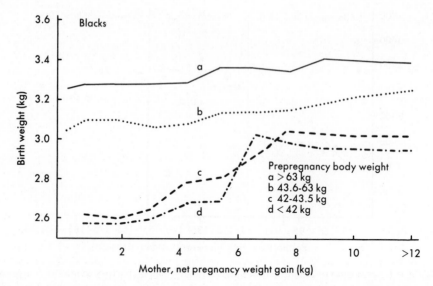

FIG. 4-5   Relationship between net pregnancy weight gain of mother and birth weight of infant.

Modified from Naeye RL: Nutritional/nonnutritional interactions that affect the outcome of pregnancy, *Am J Clin Nutr* 34:727, 1981.

nancy weight gain minus the weight of her neonate and placenta. It can be seen in the figure that mothers' pregravid body weights and net pregnancy weight gains had only a modest influence on birth weights when the mothers weighed 96 lb (44 kg) or more before pregnancy. When mothers weighed less than 96 lb at that time, fetal growth retardation appeared rather abruptly at net pregnancy weight gains under 13 lb (6 kg); whites, like blacks, showed a similar response.[29] One can speculate that the efficiency of the fetus' competition for nutrients decreases markedly below a certain threshold of maternal stores.

Naeye[29] has also proposed that hemodynamic factors may have a role in this threshold effect. He found that peak diastolic blood pressure recorded during pregnancy increased with increases in both pregravid body weights and net pregnancy weight gains. Relative fetal undergrowth associated with low prepregnancy body weights progressively disappeared as maternal peak diastolic blood pressures increased to a level of 90 to 99 mm Hg during pregnancy. Birth weights became independent of blood pressure as mothers' pregravid body weights increased; birth weights decreased only when peak diastolic pressure exceeded 99 mm Hg.

It may very well be, as Naeye[29] suggests, that the fetal growth effects attributed to nutrition are mediated through maternal blood pressure and uteroplacental perfusion. Animal studies favor this theory. This notion is further supported by Grunberger, Leodolter, and Parschalk,[16] who reported that uteroplacental perfusion is much lower with maternal blood pressures of 110/65 mm Hg and below than with higher pressures. When blood pressures of some of Grunberger's patients were increased with the administration of **deoxycorticosterone,** average birth weight at term in this treated group was 3,308 gm (7.2 lb), as compared with 2,860 gm (6.2 lb) in the untreated group. One might speculate that a homeostatic mechanism exists involving maternal nutrition, blood pressure, and uteroplacental perfusion. In times of food shortages a reduction in blood pressure might reduce the level of fetal drain on maternal nutritional stores and augment the chances that the mother may endure the crisis.

Supplementation Trials in Humans[27,31]

It is also apparent from the research on infant birth weight that special dietary management for low-income women and others who are known to be at risk for reproductive problems could produce highly beneficial results. Representative supplementation studies are outlined in Table 4-2. Results are mixed but in general, benefits are observed. Two examples of interesting endeavors include those conducted in Guatemala and Canada.

The study in Guatemala is one of the most comprehensive investigations of the relationship between maternal nutrition and the outcome of pregnancy that has ever been undertaken. It involved all women of childbearing age in four villages in a long-term, prospective study to see what effects nutrition has on physical growth and mental development of their offspring.[22] Before beginning their study the investigators collected a great deal of information about birth statistics, dietary practices, and nutritional status of the women in the four villages. They found evidence of chronic but moderate malnutrition by measuring heights, weights, and head circumferences. During pregnancy, women averaged a weight gain of about 15 lb (6.7 kg). They typically consumed about 1500 kcal and 40 gm of protein per day. This protein/kcalorie ratio is adequate. The moderate degree of malnutrition was primarily the result of insufficient food consumption. Mean birth weights in the population were between 3,000 and 3,200 gm (6.5 and 7 lb), but about one third of the infants carried to term were of low birth weight.

The plan of the study included the provision of dietary supplements to all pregnant women who would voluntarily accept them. In two of the villages the supplement Atole contained both protein and calories. The supplement Fresco was given to women in the other two villages. It contained calories but no protein. Both supplements had approximately equal amounts of vitamins and minerals.

Intakes from the supplements and home diets were recorded in each trimester of pregnancy to make sure that the women were not substituting the supplements for their usual food. The records showed that the supplements did, in fact, increase total intake by an average of 26,820 kcal during the entire course of pregnancy. However, since consumption of the supplements was voluntary, there were wide ranges of intakes. The investigators were therefore able to divide the women into a low-supplement group and a high-supplement group according to the total number of additional calories they consumed. The level of 20,000 kcal was chosen as the dividing line because this was the median value for all of the women. When the women were divided this way, there was a difference of 34,000 kcal between the mean supplemental intakes of the high and low groups.

During the first 4 years of the study complete data on maternal supplementation and birth weight were available for 405 infants born in the four villages. The first thing to be noted in the results is that for full-term infants there was a consistent increase in birth weight as the total supplemental calories of the mother increased. The distribution was such that for each 10,000 kcal ingested by the mother during pregnancy, birth weight of the infant increased 50 gm (1.7 oz). The greatest difference in birth weight was observed between infants whose mothers consumed less than 20,000 supplemental kcal and those whose mothers consumed 20,000 supplemental kcal or more. The significance of this is shown by the percent of low-birth-weight babies born to high- and low-supplemented mothers (Fig. 4-6). The rate of low birth weight was roughly two times lower when the mothers consumed 20,000 supplemental kcal or more throughout gestation.

The investigators also examined weights of the placentas. They found, on the average, that the group with low maternal supplementation had placentas weighing 11% less than the group with high maternal supplementation. Further analysis showed that most of the association between maternal supplementation and birth weight could be explained statistically by the difference in placental weight. This finding supports the earlier observation that the size of the placenta may be the means by which maternal nutrition affects birth weight (see box on p. 117).

An interesting aspect of these findings is that there was no difference in placental weight,

TABLE 4-2   Major Supplementation Studies Involving Pregnant Women

	New York	Montreal	Birmingham	Mexico	India
Type of study	Random distribution, double-blind	Food given at dispensary	Not random; supplement given to Asian mothers of 1 maternity	Supplement to pregnant women; analysis done by matching by weight, height, parity, health, SES	Poor women hospitalized only for supplement; ↑ SES and ↓ SES; used as control
Sample size (supplement + nonsupplement)	768	2,426	142	80	32
Population	Poor black; previous LBW; protein-intake <50 gm day	Low SES; inadequate diet	Supplement given independent of nutritional status	Supplement women ate more than unsupplement after controlling for supplement: diet before supplement $\overline{X}$ 1950 kcal/50 gm protein	Poor, low SES; diet before supplement 1400-1800 kcal/40 gm protein
Anthropometry	<110 lb; low weight gain in pregnancy		±155 cm ht, 54 kg weight (50th percentile)	144-156 cm height	45 kg without clinical signs of malnutrition
Supplement	Flavored drink to 2 groups + medical attention to all; real ↑ in intake: (1) 27 gm protein/275 kcal, (2) 4 gm protein/212 kcal, (3) no kcal, no protein; all received vitamins + minerals	Eggs, milk, oranges	(1) 30 mg vitamin C + 30 mg Fe; (2) 1 + 273 kcal; (3) 1 + 2 + 26 gm protein	300 kcal/20 gm protein	At hospitalization women were given 2300 kcal/ 80 gm protein + bed rest

NOTE: Offered supplements should not be completely added to habitual diet, because this decreases slightly as a result of the supplement (substitution effect). Some studies report the increment is the result of the supplement. This table contains the available information from the studies. SES = socioeconomic status; NS = not significant; BW = birth weight; LBW = low birth weight.
Modified from Villar I, Cossio TG: *Clin Nutr* 5:78, 1986.

Bogota	Guatemala	Taiwan	The Gambia	Thailand
Random assignment to pregnant women	Supplement to women of 4 communities, attendance voluntary; ad libitum intake (measured)	Random, double-blind	Supplement to all pregnant women of community	Random distribution
385	405	506	274	43
Poor; women with at least 50% of children with <85% wt/age; diet before supplement 1600 kcal/35 gm protein	Poor; endemic malnutrition in community; ↑ infection; previous diet: 1500 kcal/40 gm protein	Poor woman with at least 1 son; previous diet: 1200 kcal/40 gm protein	Rural population; previous diets: 1480/1300 kcal during dry/wet season	Rural nonsmoking women of similar socioeconomic class
149.9 cm	149 cm	—	—	In apparently good health
Dry skim milk; enriched bread; vegetable oil; vitamins + minerals for the whole family; net ↑ 155 kcal/20 gm protein	Ad libitum intake (measured) of calories and protein or of calories only	3 groups: (1) 800 kcal/40 gm protein, (2) 80 kcal/0 gm protein, (3) nothing: medical attention to all	Groundnuts, biscuits, tea with vitamins; approx. 1,000 kcal.; 431 kcal net ↑	(1) Formula providing 13 gm protein and 3 kcal per day; (2) no supplement

	New York	Montreal	Birmingham	Mexico	India
Duration of supplement	Before wk 30 of pregnancy		Supplement offered from wks 18 to 20 of gestation	From last menstruation	From wk 36 of gestation
Effect on:					
Mother	↑ Weight gain in supplemented mothers; greater if early enrollment	↑ Weight gain in supplemented mothers (0.3 lb; NS)	↑ Weight gain in 2nd trimester (fat); ↑ increment in lighter mothers	↑ Increment in supplemented mothers (3.4 kg)	Not reported
Birth weight	High-protein group: ↓ BW by 32 gm; Low protein group: ↑ BW by 41 gm (both $p > 0.05$)	40 gm (3251 vs. 3,291 gm) ($p < 0.05$)	No = between 3 groups; among the lightest supplement vs. unsupplemented = in BW was 310 gm	↑ 180 gm; 29.6% ↓ LBW	↑ 458 gm
Prematurity	↑ Premature births in high-protein group	5.7% in supplement; 6.8% in control (NS) (≠ in gestational age 0.4 days; NS)	Not reported	Not reported	Not reported
Differential impact depending on sex	Not detected	No	No	Not reported	Not reported
Adverse effects	↑ Preterm; IUGR and neonatal mortality in high-protein group	None	None	Not reported	Not reported
Others		↑ Effect on 1st birth; ↑ effect on BW if pregestational weight was <140 lb (≠ 53 gm vs. 40 gm)	No effect on well-nourished women		

Bogota	Guatemala	Taiwan	The Gambia	Thailand
1st or 2nd trimester of gestation	Any trimester (measured)	Pregestational and during entire pregnancy	Started before wk 16; lasted least 1 mo	Supplement offered from wk 28 of at gestation (±2 wks) until term
↑ Weight gain only in those bearing male fetuses	↑ Weight gain: ↑ placental weight: ↑ RNAse activity; ↓ postpartum/amenorhea: ↓ interval between birth	None (same weight gain)	↑ Weight gain when supplemented	↑ Weight gain in supplemented mothers
↑ 51 gm ≠ NS; only males: 95 ≠ ($p <$ 0.05); no ≠ in females	Positive effect; dose response; 29 gm ↑ 10,000 kcal supplement; 10% ↓ LBW; (<20,000 vs. > 20,000 kcal = 111 gm)	↑ 42 gm in males; ↑ 63 gm in females; ↓ % LBW unsupplemented	224 gm ≠ mean pre-post supplement (controlling for gestational age) in the wet season	↑ BW in supplement group (244 gm)
No effect	Yes; no effect if enrollment only during 3rd trimester; ↑ relationship with 1st trimester; 1.1 day/ 10,000 kcal; 1st vs. 3rd tercile of ingested supplement: ≠ 1.4 wk	No effect	After vs. before supplement: −0.33 wk in males; + 0.65 wk in females (both NS)	Not reported
Selected effect only for males; no effect on females	Not reported	No clear tendency	No difference	Not detected
None	Not detected (authors report underregistration and there could be bias)	None	None	None
↓ Neonatal and perinatal mortality in supplemented mothers (NS)			Effect only during wet season; no effect during dry season; 6 times ↓ in % LBW	

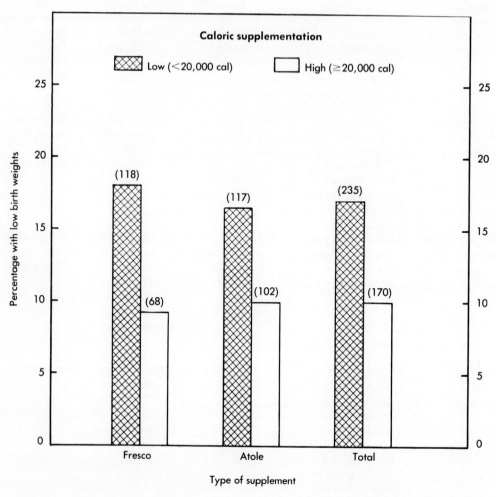

FIG. 4-6   Relationship between supplemented calories during pregnancy and proportion of low-birth-weight babies (≤2500 gm). Numbers in parentheses indicate number of cases.

From Lechtig A et al: Effect of food supplementation during pregnancy on birth weight, *Pediatrics* 56:508, 1975. Reprinted with permission.

mean birth weight, or the percent of low-birth-weight babies associated with the *type* of supplement used. As long as the calories were equivalent, it did not matter whether the supplement contained protein. This may seem surprising in view of the emphasis people tend to place on the importance of protein in the diet and the research that has been done on the effects of protein restriction in animals. The authors of the study concluded that in a population experiencing chronic but moderate malnutrition the limiting factor in the diet is calories, not protein. The amount of protein may actually be higher than that needed to maintain tissue synthesis, but the women simply do not consume enough calories to spare protein from meeting energy needs. For infants of these women the increment in birth weight from the consumption of additional calories is caused mostly by the accumulation of fetal adipose tissue. The benefits are that the entire birth-weight distribution is shifted upward. Low-birth-weight infants still

ADDITIONAL STUDIES OF NUTRITIONAL SUPPLEMENTATION DURING PREGNANCY

Protocol and results	*Researchers*
Rural Gambian women ($n = 197$) received an energy-rich prenatal dietary supplement over a 4-year period (net intake = 430 kcal/day) as compared with control women ($n = 182$). Birth weights, maternal weight gain and percent low birth weight were evaluated. Supplementation was ineffective during the dry season but highly effective during the wet season. The proportion of low-birth-weight babies decreased from 23.7% to 7.5%.	Prentice et al[32]
Powdered milk or a milk-based fortified product was distributed to pregnant underweight Chilean women for use during pregnancy. Women in the latter group had greater weight gain and greater mean birth weights; iron status was also superior.	Mardones-Santander et al[25]
One hundred sixty-nine mothers were enrolled during two consecutive pregnancies and the intervening lactation period in the Guatemalan Nutritional Supplementation Study. Women were grouped according to the level of caloric supplementation they received (high or low). The adjusted mean birth weights of the second offspring of the women with high supplementation during two pregnancies (about an extra 180 kcal/day) and the in-between lactation period (about an extra 245 kcal/day) were up to 301 gm greater than that of the low-supplementation group.	Villar, Rivera[47]
The effect of two levels of energy supplementation in the last trimester of pregnancy was tested in a controlled randomized trial in three villages in Madura, East Java. Supplementation at either level was associated with an increase in birth weight of 100 gm and a reduction in low birth weight from 12.2% to 9.5%. Anthropometric measures of maternal nutrition did not improve.	Kardjati et al[19,20]
An intervention program was undertaken to assess dietary habits and the impact of nutrition education among pregnant women in the rural county of Florina in northern Greece. The women were, in general, healthy. Nutrition counseling was associated with improvements in dietary intake and significantly improved maternal weight gain. Mean birth weight was slightly higher in the intervention group; however, incidence of low birth weight and preterm delivery were minimally affected. The results indicate that nutrition counseling during pregnancy can improve dietary intake and maternal weight gain but the mediating influence on low frequency adverse pregnancy outcomes is indeterminate in a population that is not nutritionally at risk.	Kafatos et al[18]

Continued

❖

ADDITIONAL STUDIES OF NUTRITIONAL SUPPLEMENTATION DURING PREGNANCY—cont'd

Perinatal outcomes were compared between 354 twins "treated" with the Higgins Nutrition Intervention Program and 686 "untreated" twins. After controlling for confounding variables, it was found that the twins in the intervention group weighed an average of 80 gm more than the nonintervention twins; their low birth weight rate was 25% lower and their very-low-birth-weight rate was almost 50% lower. The rate of preterm delivery was 30% lower in the intervention and early neonatal mortality was fivefold lower. Maternal morbidity was significantly lower in the intervention group and there was a trend toward lower infant morbidity in the intervention group. These results suggest that nutritional intervention can significantly improve twin pregnancy outcome.

Dubois et al[11]

In a controlled, randomized trial in Madura, East Java, pregnant women received a high energy (HE) or low energy (LE) supplement that provided 465 kcals or 52 kcals, respectively. The effect of this intervention on the children's growth was assessed longitudinally for the first 5 years of life. Only the children of mothers who had complied at least 90 days were included. Up to the age of 24 months, HE children were significantly heavier than LE children. HE children were also taller throughout the first five years. Weight-for-height by age was similar in both groups, but stunting was less prevalent in the HE children. These results suggest that energy supplementation of women for the last 90 days of pregnancy is effective in the promotion of postnatal growth and reduction in malnutrition of preschool children.

Kusin et al[21]

have greater risks, but the fact that fewer of them are born causes a reduction in the overall rate of neonatal death.

The experiences of Primrose and Higgins[33] at the Montreal Diet Dispensary in Canada show that the benefits of extra calories and special dietary management during pregnancy are not confined to chronically malnourished women in developing countries but can also improve the pregnancy performance of high-risk mothers in more affluent nations. Knowing the risk of reproductive problems associated with low income, these investigators selected the hospital handling the highest percentage of poor patients in Montreal. All patients from two of the hospital's public maternity clinics were enrolled—a total of 1,544 women between 1963 and 1970. A unique feature was that dietary needs for calories and protein were individ-

ually calculated for each woman based on her body weight-for-height with adjustments for protein deficiency, underweight, and other stress conditions. Women whose family incomes fell below specified levels—70% of all women in the study—were given supplies of milk, eggs, and oranges every 2 weeks. All of the women received counseling on food selection to meet their individual needs every time they visited the clinic, and nutritionists visited all patients at home at least once during their pregnancies.

Such intensive nutritional care enabled the women to average 93% of their total caloric needs and 96% of their total protein requirements throughout gestation. Since the majority started out with large average daily deficits, they all showed significant improvements in the quality of their diets.

Birth statistics indicate how the mothers and their infants benefited from these measures. The incidence of low birth weight in this high-risk study group was brought down to the all-Canada rate and was lower than the rate for Quebec province. Stillbirths, neonatal mortality, and perinatal mortality were also lower than the rates prevailing in Canada and Quebec.

Primrose and Higgins[33] found a direct relationship between maternal weight gains and birth weights, which were, in turn, directly related to the length of time the women had received Diet Dispensary service. No such relationship between birth weights and service was observed for other public patients who were not part of the Montreal Diet Dispensary study but who received prenatal care and gave birth at the same hospital.

It is impossible to know how much of the improvements in pregnancy performance and outcome demonstrated in this study can be attributed to the diets of the women, the food supplements, or the special attention they received. What is important about the study is that it shows how high-risk mothers, against all odds, can experience successful pregnancies when superior nutritional guidance is a part of their prenatal care.

The WIC program. * In the United States the major food program for pregnant women is the Special Supplemental Food Program for Women, Infants, and Children, better known as WIC. This program is sponsored by the Food and Nutrition Service of the Federal Department of Agriculture. WIC was originally authorized in 1972. Current legislation lists the target population as pregnant and postpartum women (up to 6 months after delivery if not breast-feeding and up to 12 months if breast-feeding), and infants and children up to 5 years of age. To be eligible, women, infants, and children must be nutritionally at-risk and members of low-income families, that is, gross family income cannot exceed 185% of the nonfarm poverty income defined by the Office of Management and Budget.

Recently enacted legislation mandates that applicants are automatically income-eligible for WIC if they receive benefits under Medicaid, Aid to Families with Dependent Children (AFDC) or the Food Stamp Program. Applicants are also income-eligible if they are members of a family that includes an AFDC recipient, or a pregnant woman or infant receiving Medicaid assistance. The program is administered by state health departments and regulations require that eligible women, infants, and children receive nutrition education and health services as well as food.

Congress appropriates a fixed amount of program funds each year and the states cannot always serve all eligible applicants. Therefore, federal regulations provide for a participant priority system to ensure that program benefits are directed to persons at greatest nutritional risk when the demand for program benefits exceeds available resources. When a local agency has filled all available caseload slots, it places applicants on a waiting list. As slots are vacated, eligible applicants from the waiting list are enrolled in the program in accordance with the priority system. This system recognizes that pregnant and breastfeeding women and infants with documented nutritionally related medical conditions are the highest-risk groups of the WIC population.

In 1984 the General Accounting Office (GAO) published an analysis of 54 evaluations of WIC,[15] starting with the first one commissioned by the Department of Agriculture.[12] The GAO examined these studies for evidence of the effectiveness of WIC in reducing the incidence of low birth weight; preventing miscarriages, stillbirths, and fetal and neonatal mortality; improving the health and nutrition of pregnant and lactating women; and reducing the incidence of mental retardation in infants and children. It was also interested in whether WIC's effectiveness varied by differential nutritional and health risks or by the length of participation, and which of the three WIC services—food supplementation, nutrition education, or health care—was the most effective.

The GAO conclusions of interest were

1. The six birth-weight studies of high or medium quality gave "some support, but not conclusive evidence" that WIC in-

---

*Information drawn in part from the federal document entitled, *Evidence of the Effectiveness of Recommended Antepartal Care Components* from the Office of Technology Assessment, Congress of the United States, 1987.

creased infant birth weight. About 7.9% of the WIC mothers bore infants who were less than 2500 gm as compared with about 9.5% of the control mothers. Average birth weights were between 30 and 50 gm greater for WIC than for mothers in the control group.

2. The studies of fetal and neonatal mortality were insufficient to support claims about WIC's effectiveness in this area.
3. WIC appeared to have a greater positive effect on the birth weights of mothers who were teenagers, blacks, or who had several health- and nutrition-related risks.
4. Participation in WIC for more than 6 months was associated with increases in birth weights and decreases in the proportion of low-birth-weight infants.

In 1986, the Department of Agriculture issued a five-volume report on the latest and largest evaluation of WIC.[36] The principal investigator was David Rush, who had been a severe critic of earlier nutritional supplementation studies.[35,36] The evaluation was based on three contemporary studies (a longitudinal study of pregnant women, a study of infants and children, and a food expenditure study) and a historical study of pregnancy outcomes.

For the longitudinal study of pregnant women, more than 5,000 pregnant women at 174 WIC sites who were first-time registrants became the experimental subjects. Only 1,358 control women were entered into the study, although the goal was 2,000. The controls were low-income women receiving antepartal care for the first time in hospital or health department clinics in countries where WIC programs served less than 30% to 40% of eligible women. Experimental women were interviewed first at the time of entry into the WIC program and control women at entry into prenatal care. They were reinterviewed at about the eighth month of pregnancy. Hospital records were abstracted for 75% of the sample. In addition to the smaller-than-desired size of the control group and the incomplete record survey, the evaluation suffered from major differences between the socioeconomic characteristics of the WIC and the control group. The latter were more often white, had higher incomes, were more likely to

be married, and had higher-status occupations. In general, these differences would minimize program effects. Rush believed he could adjust for these differences in his statistical analyses.

The historical study was undertaken to determine the effectiveness of the program over its entire history and to permit a sample size large enough to study fetal and infant death rates. It related WIC participation during pregnancy to both extent and quality of prenatal care and perinatal outcome for the WIC program from 1974 to 1980 and for the 2 years prior during which the Commodity Supplemental Food Program operated. This study was conducted in 1,392 counties in 19 states that could provide the necessary information. Specifically, the proportion of eligible pregnant women served by WIC each year in each county (penetration) was linked to the level of maternal antepartal care and to perinatal outcome rates for the same county and year, as determined by linked birth and infant death certificates. This county-level analysis was done on the entire group of women and on four subgroups: black and white and less than or equal to or more than 12 years of education.

In terms of birth weight, the longitudinal study showed no significant effect of WIC on mean birth weight or percent of low-birth-weight or very-low-birth-weight infants. Rush suggested that this absence of effect might be a result of the lower health risks and greater social privilege of control group women, differences that could only partially be accounted for by statistical adjustment.[36] The historical study, however, showed a significant increase in mean birth weight of 23 gm. In the total population, WIC penetration was not significantly related to the proportion of low-birth-weight or very-low-birth-weight infants. A substantial, but not statistically significant, reduction in low birth weight, however, was found among less-educated whites and more-educated blacks. In addition, a special study of the quality of local WIC programs, as perceived by state WIC directors, showed a relationship between quality and increased mean birth weight and reduced frequency of low birth weight.

In terms of duration of gestation, the longitudinal study showed no significant effect of WIC on either mean duration of pregnancy or frequency of prematurity. In the historical study, however, mean pregnancy duration was significantly longer for those served by the WIC program (1.4 days). WIC participation also reduced preterm delivery in the total population by 9 per 1,000 births. There were also statistically significant reductions in very preterm (under 33 weeks) delivery in the white, less-educated group, in preterm delivery among less-educated white and black women, and longer mean pregnancy duration among less-educated whites.

The longitudinal study also measured head circumference, which none of the earlier studies had examined. Infants of women enrolled in WIC had significantly larger head circumferences than controls.

In terms of mortality, in the longitudinal study there were 31 fetal deaths (after 20 weeks' gestation) among WIC participants and 12 in the control group (9.7/1,000 vs. 14.8/1,000). Although the magnitude of difference was substantial, the numbers were not large enough to reach statistical significance. The historical study, however, showed a statistically significant reduction of 2.3 fetal deaths per 1,000 births. The estimated reduction in the neonatal death rate was of considerable magnitude, but not statistically significant. The postneonatal mortality rate reduction was of low magnitude.

Rush concluded that WIC had a significant effect on duration of pregnancy, birth weight, head growth, fetal mortality, and, perhaps, neonatal mortality.

It is believed that among the most positive effects of WIC are related directly to the nutrition education that all participants get as a part of WIC benefits. Each participant receives assessment and counseling geared to individual needs and problems. Monthly contacts allow for reinforcement of education and recommendations.

Because of the success of WIC in reaching out to large numbers of low-income women and children, several special activities have been piggybacked on the WIC staff; these include immunization outreach, drug and alcohol screening, cholesterol screening, and food stamp and Medicaid eligibility determination (see box on p. 124). These activities support the principle of one-stop social services. Hopefully, this diffu-

sion of effort will not adversely affect the proven merits of the original WIC program.

WIC provides selected foods, nutrition education, counseling and support and referral to or coordination with health care. In so doing, it has become an extremely important program for fostering food security and increasing access to health services for the youngest and most vulnerable members of society.[39]

Costs and cost-benefit of nutrition services.[45] With the increasing focus on demonstrating that federally funded services are cost effective, researchers have approached prenatal nutrition care services with this goal in mind. Studies have ranged widely in their objectives (Table 4-3); cost of care only has been reported but others have evaluated the care in terms of economic outcomes or benefits. When outcomes have been judged, the most frequent ones have been: lives saved, low birth weight averted, and effects of birth weight on cost of care.

There is little argument that the greatest costs are associated with the consequences of low birth weight. Neonatal intensive care is very expensive. The Office of Technology Assessment (OTA) estimated the admission rate to these specialized units to be 6% of all live births, and the typical (or average) length of stay was about 13 days. In 1978 dollars, the average estimated expenditure per patient was $8,000; this obviously would be much greater if calculated in 1992 dollars.

Disbrow[9,10] and Splett et al[40] have made an effort to estimate the direct costs of nutrition services in prenatal settings. Disbrow calculated costs of personnel, space, materials, transportation, and child care. This undertaking showed that the direct costs of nutrition services throughout pregnancy for a low-income prenatal population are about $41 per client. Splett et al reported the 1987 costs of prenatal nutrition care delivered at a city health department to be $72 for 3.9 visits and $121 for six visits at the county hospital.*

---

*Indirect costs of care have rarely been evaluated. Disbrow[10] estimated indirect costs for prenatal nutrition services to be $21.37 per client.

TABLE 4-3   *Cost and Cost-Benefit Studies of Prenatal Nutrition Care*

Author (year)	Study Perspective	Sample Size I	Sample Size C	Infant	Difference	Mother	Difference
Schramm (1985)[37]	I = WIC C = non-WIC	1883	5745	I = $574 C = $672	−$98	I = $1,063 C = $1,067 Medicaid costs	−$4
Ershoff et al. (1983)[13]	I = nutrition counseling + smoking cessation C = standard prenatal care	57	333	I = $466 C = $649 Standardized cost/delivery	−$183		
Splett et al. (1987)[40]	*Direct* costs for nutrition services 1 = county hospital 2 = city health dept.	(1) 196	(2) 357			1 = $72 2 = $20	−$52
Disbrow (1987)[9]	*Direct* costs for nutrition counseling	96	—			$36.48 (clinic cost) Total = $3,501.82	
Disbrow (1988)[10]	*Indirect* costs for nutrition counseling	96	—				

Stockbauer (1987)[42]	I = WIC at 3 levels:
	  <3 mo
	  3-6 mo
	  >6 mo
	C = non-WIC
		9411	8861				

Mathematica (1990)[26]	60 day saving in Medicaid costs from prenatal WIC participants in 5 states						
	I = births to WIC participants	105,000		$1,733 to $3,822 (cost for newborns + mother)	$277 to $598		
	C = Medicaid births to women not participating in WIC in 5 states (FL, MN, NC, SC) in 1987 and Jan-June 1988 (TX)						

I = intervention; C = control; BC = benefit-cost; LBW = low birth weight.

Information used with permission from Trouba PH, Okereke N, Splett PL: Summary document of nutrition intervention in prenatal care, *J Am Diet Assoc* (Suppl) S-21, 1991.

Health Services Costs

Program	Visit	Benefit-cost	Comments
$122 WIC per subject		$.83 saved per $1.00 spent	Medicaid cost differences compared BC sensitive to WIC food cost As WIC costs increased, LBW decreased
		2:1	I group had 11.6% more quit smoking vs. C group 91% of I group made diet changes vs. 68% of C group
	1 = $18 2 = $20		Cost/successful outcome for diet: 1 = $82, 2 = $130 for weight gain: 1 = $231, 2 $170 Direct costs only
$40.87 (nutrition services cost) Total = $3,923.18			
		$7.12	Indirect cost/initial visit = $7.85 Indirect cost/follow-up visit = $13.51 Includes travel costs, waiting time
	$37/month		>6 mo duration for 50 gm increase in birth weight and 18% reduction in LBW
<$110 $110-$219 $220+			Birth weight and LBW outcomes greater in blacks
		$1.77 to 3.13 newborns + mothers	Estimated Medicaid savings are independent from the effects of prenatal care
		$2.84 to 3.90 newborns only	The report notes self-selection of WIC participants

❖

THE NATIONAL WIC EVALUATION— MAJOR FINDINGS RELATED TO WOMEN AND NEWBORN INFANTS

- A significant increase in first trimester registration for prenatal care, and a significant reduction in the proportion of women with inadequate numbers of visits for prenatal care (Historical Study).
- The significant disparity in early pregnancy weight gain among WIC women was reversed during program enrollment (Longitudinal Study). There was an unexpected, but consistent and significant negative relationship between WIC benefits and maternal fat stores in late pregnancy (Longitudinal Study).
- The duration of gestation was 1.4 days longer among WIC recipients (Historical Study). There were significant decreases in the rate of preterm delivery associated with WIC benefits, but only among less-educated women (under 12 years; Historical Study).
- There were significant increases in birth weight associated with WIC benefits, with estimates ranging from 23 to 47 gm (Historical Study). While in the Longitudinal Study there was no significant difference in birth weight between infants whose mothers received WIC benefits and control women, birth weight was significantly related to the quality of the local WIC program's operation as judged by state WIC directors.

- In general, effects were greatest among pregnant women assumed to be at greater need (women with less education, or ethnic minority women; Historical Study).
- The head circumferences of infants whose mothers received WIC benefits were significantly greater than those of controls.
- Participation in WIC was associated with significantly reduced late fetal death (2.3 per 1,000 births; Historical Study). The estimated magnitude in reduction of neonatal (early infant) mortality was similar, but not significant.
- WIC was associated with improved intake of (protein, iron, calcium, and vitamin C, as well as for energy, magnesium, phosphorus, thiamine, riboflavin, niacin, vitamin B_6, and vitamin B_{12} (Longitudinal Study).
- WIC had no apparent effect on smoking or alcohol consumption, which are known to be harmful during pregnancy.
- WIC had no effect on the intention to breast-feed or on breast-feeding at discharge.

The studies that have addressed cost issues and cost-benefit ratios have generally found an increase in birth weight along with an increase in weight gain of the mother. Reduction in low-birth-weight percentage is associated with the greatest cost savings. A study of the impact of WIC participation on Medicaid costs[45] further verified net benefits attributable to nutrition intervention in pregnancy.

Not all intervention/supplementation programs provided to high-risk pregnant women have demonstrated a strong positive impact. This varied response should certainly be expected given the different populations served,

the different supplements employed, the various methods of supplement administration, and a variety of other differing variables. Overall, the findings appear to suggest that *the worse the nutritional condition of the mother entering pregnancy, the more valuable the prenatal diet and/or nutritional supplement will be in improving her pregnancy course and outcome.*

A general conclusion that can be drawn after review of all published reports on prenatal supplementation studies is that although poor women in developing countries often suffer some degree of malnutrition before and during pregnancy, only a minority of women from low socioeconomic groups in developed countries are truly undernourished. Dietary counseling and nutritional supplementation of the latter will clearly yield less dramatic measurable improvements in outcome. As-yet undefined improvements in outcome may actually occur, but existing methods prevent their definition. In developed countries it would seem, however, that nutrition intervention should focus on women whose prepregnancy status is judged to be inferior. Refined processes of clinical evaluation and monitoring may allow for the establishment of a nutritional milieu supportive of optimal pregnancy course and outcome in the majority of these women.

Summary

Over the past 100 years, efforts have been made to determine the specific roles that nutrition plays in embryonic and fetal development. Much information has been gleaned from animal models where clear-cut adverse impacts on pregnancy course and outcome can be reproduced when nutrient deficiencies or excesses are studied. Data from human populations derive from observational efforts since frank experimentation is rarely possible. Epidemiologic data support the concept of detrimental pregnancy course and outcome when nutritional conditions are suboptimal. However, it is clear that a biological force is in place that tends to protect the fetus (to some extent) when maternal diet is inadequate. Nutritional interventions prove to be effective when employed in circumstances of obvious need. We have much to learn about the more subtle effects of poor prenatal nutrition on development of the human fetus.

REVIEW QUESTIONS

1. Identify historical landmarks in attention to the importance of maternal nutrition in pregnancy course and outcome.
2. Summarize the value of nutritional supplementation during the course of human pregnancy in both developed and developing countries.
3. Describe the WIC program and cite data to justify its existence.

CASE STUDY

Carol is a 26-year-old woman with phenylketonuria, identified by newborn screening and started on treatment by 8 days of age, who has been followed by the PKU clinic since that time. She graduated from college, teaches at an elementary school, and got married 2 years ago. She and her husband Bill had premarital counseling around the reproductive concerns of women with PKU. They came to PKU clinic to meet with the team about pregnancy planning. Carol's blood phenylalanine levels have been consistently 360-480 µmol/L (6-8 mg/100 ml). She and Bill understand that these levels are reasonable for adult management of the disorder but pose a risk of maldevelopment for a fetus. They plan a period of pregnancy preparation before they make a final decision about conception. If Carol can reduce her plasma phenylalanine levels to 180 µmol/L (3 mg/100 ml) or less and maintain these levels while also maintaining her weight, positive attitude and energy, they will attempt conception. If she is not able to achieve this, she and Bill, as a couple, will consider other options for starting a family.

On her now more rigorous diet, Carol has found it somewhat difficult to increase her daily ingestion of phenylalanine-free formula enough to lower her blood phenylalanine levels. She also needs to emphasize planning family menus, maintaining her employment, her social life, and her sports activities. Bill is very supportive.

After 5 months of faithful efforts, Carol's blood phenylalanine levels have been 180 µmol/L (3 mg/100 ml) or less for 6 continuous weeks. She feels very healthy and her iron status is normal. She has established a relationship with an obstetrician who specializes in high risk pregnancy management. After significant discussion, Carol and Bill decide to attempt conceiving a child.

LEARNING ACTIVITIES

1. Explore available information on prenatal development of mammals other than humans.
2. Visit a local WIC program site and observe its operation.

3. Make a trip through the supermarket and determine what kind of "nutritional menu" you can afford for one week with $20.
4. Talk to women on the WIC program to gain a sense of how they feel about it.

REFERENCES

1. Browne FJ, McClure Browne JC: *Antenatal and postnatal care,* ed. 8, London, 1955, J & A Churchill.
2. Burke BS et al: The influence of nutrition upon the condition of the infant at birth, *J Nutr* 26:569, 1943.
3. Burke BS, Harding VV, Stuart HC: Nutrition studies during pregnancy. IV. Relation of protein content of mother's diet during pregnancy to birth length, birth weight, and condition of infant at birth, *J Pediatr* 23:506, 1943.
4. Committee on Maternal Nutrition, Food and Nutrition Board: *Nutritional supplementation and the outcome of pregnancy,* Proceedings of a workshop, Nov. 3-5, 1971, Sagamore Beach, Mass, Washington, DC, 1973, National Academy of Sciences.
5. Committee on Nutrition of the Mother and Preschool Child: *Guidelines for nutrition services in perinatal care,* Washington, DC, 1981, National Academy Press.
6. Cristakis, G, editor: Maternal nutritional assessment, *Am J Public Health* 63(Suppl):1, 1973.
7. Danforth WC: The management of normal pregnancy (prenatal care). In Curtis AH, editor: *Obstetrics and gynecology,* vol. 1, Philadelphia, 1933, W.B. Saunders.
8. Dawes GS: *Foetal and neonatal physiology,* Chicago, 1968, Year Book Medical Publishers.
9. Disbrow DD: The economic costs of nutrition service for a low-income prenatal population: I. direct costs, *J Pediatr Perinatal Nutr* 1:35, 1987.
10. Disbrow DD: The economic costs of nutrition service for a low-income prenatal population: indirect and intangible cost, *J Pediatr Perinatal Nutr* 2:17, 1988.
11. Dubois S et al: Twin pregnancy: the impact of the Higgins Nutrition Intervention Program on maternal and neonatal outcomes, *Am J Clin Nutr* 53:1397, 1991.
12. Edozien JC, Switzer BR, Bryan RB: Medical evaluation of the special supplemental food program for women, infants, and children, *Am J Clin Nutr* 32:677, 1979.
13. Ershoff DH, Aaronson NK, Danahar BG et al: Behavioral, health and cost outcomes at an HMO-based prenatal health education program, *Public Health Rep* 98:536, 1983.
14. Gordon AN: *Nutrition management of high-risk pregnancy—reference manual,* Berkeley, Calif, 1981, Society for Nutrition Education.
15. Government Accounting Office: *WIC evaluations provide some favorable but not conclusive evidence on the effects expected for the special supplemental program for women, infants, and children.* Washington, DC, January 30, 1984. Government Accounting Office.
16. Grunberger W, Leodolter S, Parschalk O: Maternal hypertension: fetal outcome in treated and untreated cases, *Gynecol Obstet Invest* 10:32, 1979.
17. Joint FAO/WHO Expert Committee on Nutrition: *Sixth report,* Geneva, 1962, World Health Organization.
18. Kafatos AG, Vlachonkolis IG, Codrington CA: Nutrition during pregnancy: the effects of an educational intervention program in Greece, *Am J Clin Nutr* 50:970, 1989.
19. Kardjati S, Kusin JA, De With C: Energy supplementation in the last trimester of pregnancy in East Java: I. Effect on birthweight, *Br J Obstet Gynaecol* 95:783, 1988.
20. Kardjati S, Schofield WM, de With C: Energy supplementation in the last trimester of pregnancy in East Java, Indonesia: effect on maternal anthropometry, *Am J Clin Nutr* 52:987, 1990.
21. Kusin JA et al: Energy supplementation during pregnancy and postnatal growth. *Lancet* 340:623, 1992.
22. Lechtig A et al: Effect of food supplementation during pregnancy on birth weight, *Pediatrics* 56:508, 1975.
23. Lechtig A et al; Effect of moderate maternal malnutrition on the placenta, *Am J Obstet Gynecol* 123:191, 1975.
24. Luke B, Jonaitis MA, Petrie RH: A consideration of height as a function of prepregnancy nutritional background and its potential influence on birth weight, *J Am Diet Assoc* 84:176, 1984.

25. Mardones-Santander F, Rosso P, Stekel A et al: Effect of a milk-based food supplement on maternal nutritional status and fetal growth in underweight Chilean women, *Am J Clin Nutr* 47:413, 1988.

26. Mathematics Policy Research Inc: *The savings in Medicaid costs for newborns and their mothers from prenatal participation in the WIC Program,* Washington DC, 1990, U.S. Department of Agriculture, Food and Nutrition Services.

27. McDonald EC et al: Maternal nutritional supplementation and birth weight of offspring. *Am J Clin Nutr* 34:2133, 1981.

28. Naeye RL, Diener MM, Dellinger WS: Urban poverty: effects on prenatal nutrition, *Science* 166:1026, 1969.

29. Naeye RL: Nutritional/nonnutritional interactions that affect the outcome of pregnancy, *Am J Clin Nutr* 34:727, 1981.

30. Naeye RL: Causes of fetal and neonatal mortality by race in a selected U.S. population, *Am J Public Health* 69:857, 1979.

31. National Research Council, Food and Nutrition Board: *Committee on maternal nutrition: nutritional supplementation and the outcome of pregnancy,* Washington, DC, 1973, National Academy of Sciences.

32. Prentice AM, Cole TJ, Foord FA et al: Increased birthweight after prenatal supplementation of rural African women, *Am J Clin Nutr* 46:912, 1987.

33. Primose T, Higgins A: A study of human antepartum nutrition, *J Reprod Med* 7:257, 1971.

34. Report of Panel II-I: Pregnant and nursing women and young infants. In *White House Conference on Food, Nutrition, and Health, final report,* Washington, DC, 1970, Government Printing Office.

35. Rush D, Stein Z, Susser M: Controlled trial of prenatal nutrition supplementation defended, *Pediatrics* 66:656, 1980.

36. Rush D: *The national WIC evaluation: an evaluation of the special supplemental food program for women, infants, and children,* vol I and II, 1986, Research Triangle Institute and New York State Research Foundation for Mental Hygiene.

37. Schramm WF: WIC prenatal participation and its relation to newborn Medicaid costs in Missouri: a cost/benefit analysis, *Am J Public Health* 75:851, 1985.

38. Smith CA: Effects of maternal undernutrition upon the newborn infant in Holland, *J Pediatr* 30:229, 1947.

39. Splett PL: Federal food assistance programs. *Nutr Today* March/April 1994, p. 6-13.

40. Splett PL, Caldwell M, Holey ED et al: Prenatal nutrition services: a cost analysis, *J Am Diet Assoc* 87:204, 1987.

41. *Standards for obstetric-gynecologic services,* ed 5, Washington, DC, 1982, American College of Obstetricians and Gynecologists.

42. Stockbauer JW: WIC prenatal participation and its relationship to newborn Medicaid costs in Missouri: a second look, *Am J Public Health* 77:813, 1987.

42a. Susser M, Stein, I: Timing in prenatal nutrition: a reprise of the Dutch famine study, *Nutr Rev* 52:84, 1994.

43. Task Force on Nutrition: *Guidelines for assessment of maternal nutrition,* Chicago, 1978, American College of Obstetricians and Gynecologists.

44. Tompkins WT, Mitchell RM, Wiehl DG: Maternal and newborn nutrition studies at Philadelphia Lying-in Hospital. In *The promotion of maternal and newborn health,* New York, 1955, Milbank Memorial Fund.

45. Thomson AM, Bellewicz WZ, Hytten FE: The assessment of fetal growth, *J Obstet Gynaecol Br Commonw* 75:903, 1968.

46. Toverud KU, Stearns G, Macy IG: *Maternal nutrition and child health,* NRC Bull No 123, Washington, DC, 1950, National Academy of Science, National Research Council.

46a. Trouba PH, Okerke N, Splett PL: Summary document of nutrition intervention in prenatal care, *J Am Diet Assoc* (Suppl) S-21, 1991.

47. Villar J, Rivera J: Nutritional supplementation during two consecutive pregnancies and the interim lactation period: effect on birth weight, *Pediatrics* 81:51, 1988.

48. Winick M: Fetal malnutrition, *Clin Obstet Gynecol* 13:526, 1970.

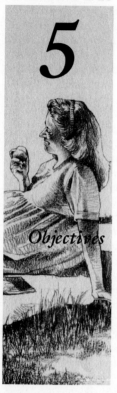

CHAPTER

5

Energy and Vitamin Needs During Pregnancy

Bonnie Worthington-Roberts

Objectives

✦✦✦

After completing this chapter, the student will be able to:

✓ *Describe known nutrient needs of the pregnant woman.*

✓ *Discuss the known effects of maternal nutrient deficiencies and excesses on pregnancy course and outcome.*

✓ *Define areas of research relevant to improving our understanding of nutrient deficiencies and excesses and human reproduction.*

Introduction

The low serum values of nutrients commonly seen during pregnancy and the tendency of the kidneys to excrete greater amounts have posed problems for setting nutrient requirements and making dietary recommendations. Some of the blood values typical in pregnancy would be viewed as borderline or deficient if they were seen in a nonpregnant woman. The picture is further complicated by the fact that most of the blood levels can be increased if oral supplements are given.

PROBLEMS IN DETERMINING NEEDS

If no physical symptoms of deficiency or consequences to the course or outcome of pregnancy are observed when serum values differ

from the norm, their clinical significance is difficult to determine. It is not presently known whether the total amounts of nutrients in the blood or their concentrations per 100 ml are more important for the mother and her growing child. Although the lower values may indicate increased needs, their nearly universal occurrence in pregnant women makes it hard to believe that they are all the result of dietary deficiencies.[70]

Most researchers who have made extensive studies on the physiology of pregnancy maintain that the profound changes that occur in maternal metabolism indicate that the pregnant woman cannot be judged by nonpregnant standards.[37] They assert that the alterations in nutrient levels that are so typical in pregnancy suggest a common purpose. They see no reason to assume that vitamins and minerals such as folic

128

acid, vitamin B_6, or iron require special attention, whereas other nutrients that are equally low (and usually less readily available as commercial supplements) are ignored.

Other clinicians have interpreted the lower serum values and altered rates of urinary excretion as indications of increased risk. They maintain that since intakes of nutrients necessary to achieve normal serum concentrations cannot be obtained without an inordinate increase in total calories, oral supplements should be used. Even though detrimental effects of the low serum values may not be apparent, these clinicians credit supplementation with the ability to prevent outright deficiencies that may be induced if women enter pregnancy with poor nutrient reserves.[11,12]

This controversy cannot be resolved without further research. Because pregnancy is a time of growth, the need for nutrients is increased. It stands to reason that women who enter pregnancy in poor nutritional status run a risk of having deficiencies develop that will have unfavorable effects on obstetrical performance. However, for healthy women who enter pregnancy in good nutritional status the picture is more obscure. Current standards used to monitor the nutrition of pregnant women cannot be viewed as absolute until more is known about maternal metabolism and its effects on nutrient requirements.

ENERGY

Supplying sufficient energy to maintain life is the principal task of the body's metabolism. All other metabolic processes are subservient to this aim. During pregnancy two factors that determine energy requirements are changes in the mother's usual physical activity and the increase in her basal metabolism to support the work required for growth of the fetus and the accessory tissues. The cumulative energy cost of this extra work has been estimated at about 85,000 kcal (Table 5-1).[36] This amount is derived from the caloric equivalents of protein and fat stored in the products of conception (~41,000 kcal) and from increased oxygen consumption of the mother (36,000 kcal). An additional 8,000 kcal are believed to be needed to convert dietary to metabolizable energy.

The energy demand is thought to be distributed fairly equally throughout the first three quarters of pregnancy. Deposition of about 3.5 kg of fat in the maternal compartment accounts for two thirds of the total energy need during the second and third quarters of pregnancy (Table 5-1). Fetal growth needs are greatest in the fourth quarter.

The total of 85,000 kcal for support of a pregnancy translates into about 300 extra kcal per day throughout pregnancy. A portion of the energy increment may be offset by the tendency of women to reduce their physical activity, especially

TABLE 5-1 *Cumulative Energy Cost of Pregnancy Computed from the Energy Equivalents of Protein and Fat Increments and the Energy Cost of Maintaining the Fetus and Added Maternal Tissues*

	Weeks of Pregnancy				Cumulative Total kcal*
	0-10	10-20	20-30	30-40	
	Equivalent, kcal per day				
Protein	3.6	10.3	26.7	34.2	5186
Fat	55.6	235.6	207.6	31.3	36329
Oxygen consumption	44.8	99.0	148.2	227.2	35717
Total net energy	104.0	344.9	382.5	292.7	77234
Metabolizable energy	114	379	421	322	84957

*Taken as 5.6 kcal/g for protein and 9.5 kcal/g for fat.
Based on data from Hytten FE, Chamberlain G: *Clinical physiology in obstetrics*, Oxford, 1980, Blackwell.

in the last trimester. Several investigators have clearly shown a reduction in work pace as weight gain proceeds.[6] Women who must continue a previous work pace or have chosen to do so will gradually build up their energy needs associated with movement of their larger body mass.[90,91]

The energy demand is not distributed equally through the course of pregnancy. Recent research assessing 24-hour energy expenditure in 12 healthy Dutch women demonstrated that energy expenditure gradually increased from pre-pregnant levels when measured at weeks 12, 23, and 34 of gestation.[24] No changes were recorded in digestibility or metabolizability of food. Virtually all of the change was directly related to the increasing resting metabolic rate. In this study, physical activity was held constant. Substantial differences in physical activity among pregnant women could further alter their total energy needs.

Actual energy intakes of pregnant women reveal several basic features in populations studied.[29a] First, intake is often less than recommended (Fig. 5-1),[59] this may be a result of omissions in recalls or records, extremely sedentary lifestyles, or purposeful restriction of weight gain. Second, pregnant women followed longitudinally over the course of a pregnancy often do not show a significant augmentation in kcalorie intake (Fig. 5-2). These observations have led researchers to reconsider the issue of kcalorie requirements during human pregnancy. In so doing, they have measured the two major components of energy expenditure: resting metabolism and activity energy expenditure.[43] These two aspects may account for 90% or more of the total energy expenditure.

The energy expenditure for basal or resting metabolism has been measured in several groups of pregnant women (Table 5-2). If the original estimates of resting energy needs are correct, a total of 36,000 kcal should be recorded during the course of a pregnancy.[8,37] In reality, much variability has been observed. The biggest net change was seen in Swedish women (46,500 kcal),[32] whereas the unsupplemented women in the Gambia had the lowest change—1000 kcal.[48] The longitudinal studies of Durnin et al[29] showed that resting metabolic rate dropped in early gestation and remained below pregravid levels until the 30th week (Fig. 5-3). If this phe-

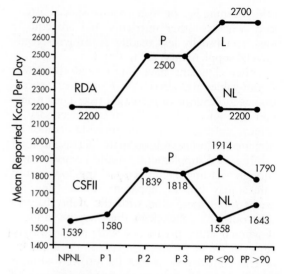

L = Lactating
NL = Not lactating
NPNL = Not pregnant not lactating
P = Pregnant
PP = Postpartum

FIG. 5-1   Longitudinal estimates of energy Intake in the Continuing Surveys of Food intakes by Individuals (CSFII), by reproductive state and comparison with 1989 Recommended Dietary Allowances (RDAs).

From Murphy SP, Abrams BF: Changes in energy intakes during pregnancy and lactation in a national sample of US women, *Am J Public Health* 83:1161, 1993.

nomenon is true, researchers assessing resting metabolic rate only in the later weeks of pregnancy may have grossly overestimated the total resting energy needs for pregnancy.

Observations made in the Gambia[48] suggest that maternal nutritional status influences the change in resting metabolism during gestation. The unsupplemented women who were consuming only 1,500 kcal per day had lower resting metabolic rates in the second and third trimesters than the women receiving supplements and consuming about 1,950 kcal per day. Calculations revealed that the supplemented women required 13,000 additional kcal for resting metabolism; only 1,000 was required by the

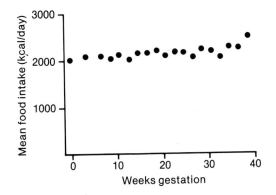

FIG. 5-2 Mean energy intakes of 67 Glasgow women at different stages of pregnancy.

From Durnin JVGA et al: Is nutritional status endangered by virtually no extra intake during pregnancy? *Lancet* 2:823, 1985.

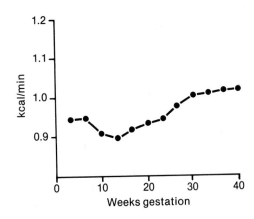

FIG. 5-3 Basal metabolic rates (BMR) during pregnancy—mean values of a longitudinal study of 67 Glasgow women.

From Durnin JVGA et al: Is nutritional status endangered by virtually no extra intake during pregnancy? *Lancet* 2:823, 1985.

TABLE 5-2 *Resting Metabolic Rate (RMR) of Pregnant Women*

| Population | Nonpregnant RMR (kcal/min) | Pregnant RMR | | | Total Increment in RMR (kcal) |
		1st Trimester	2nd Trimester	3rd Trimester	
Theoretical	1.07	+0.07 (10-20 wk)	+0.103 (20-30 wk)	+0.16 (30-40 wk)	36,000
Sweden	0.93	0.97	1.13	1.22	46,500
Glasgow	0.94	0.91	0.95	1.01	7,000
United States	0.86	—	1.01	1.15	—
United States	0.79	—	0.96	1.10	—
The Gambia*					
unsupplemented	0.97	0.94	0.94	1.05	1,000
supplemented	0.94	0.94	0.97	1.10	13,000

*Some women received dietary supplements; others did not.

unsupplemented women. It is logical that a smaller rise in resting metabolism may enable underfed pregnant women to sustain adequate fetal growth and development even with their limited energy stores.

In support of this idea is a report of altered **brown adipose tissue thermogenesis** during pregnancy in mice.[4] It was observed that in later pregnancy, there was a hypertrophy of brown fat, which reversed at parturition. However, food restriction prevented this hypertrophy such that the normal dietary stimulation of thermogenesis in response to **hyperphagia** was suppressed in the pregnant animal. The relevance of these observations to the pregnant human remains to be determined.

The Five-Country Studies

In light of the substantial controversy about the energy requirements of pregnancy and the degree to which these needs are met by extra food, a series of studies has been carried out in five countries around the world.[27,46,95,98] This integrated undertaking took place in two developed countries (Scotland and the Netherlands) and three developing countries (the Gambia, Thailand, and the Philippines). Methods of investigation were standardized in the five centers and in all cases women were recruited for participation early in pregnancy or in the preconception period. Throughout each pregnancy, an effort was made to evaluate body weight and body fat, energy intake, basal metabolic rate, and daily energy expenditure.

The characteristics of the study populations are defined in Table 5-3. It is clear that the populations are very diverse but the differences are much smaller when variables are expressed as a proportion of the initial body mass. The most startling observation is related to the Gambian women who seem to be the beneficiaries of a remarkable physiological adjustment; by becoming pregnant they save so much energy in basal metabolism that they end with a positive energy balance over the whole of pregnancy of about 11,000 kcal. Pregnancy, far from requiring extra energy, is a positive benefit to their state of energy balance.

After reviewing the results of this project, the following important observations should be emphasized[28]:

1. Although weight gain differed substantially among the populations, when expressed as a proportion of initial weight of the mother, more similarity is seen; the same applies to maternal fat (Table 5-4).

TABLE 5-3 *Initial Characteristics of the Subjects in the Five-Country Study (Mean)*

	Scotland	The Netherlands	The Gambia	Thailand	Philippines
Number	88	57	52	44	51
Age (year)	27.7	28.6	25.9	23.0	23.4
Parity	1.0	1.1	3.8	1.7	2.6
Height (m)	1.62	1.69	1.58	1.52	1.51
Weight (kg)*	57.3	62.5	51.4	47.6	44.4
Sum of 4 skin-fold measurements (mm)	49.3	55.3	31.3	41.1	46.5
Fat mass (kg)*	15.1	17.7	10.3	11.3	11.2
Fat mass as % body weight	26%	28%	20%	24%	25%
Fat-free mass (kg)*	41.9	44.7	41.0	36.4	33.2
Fat-free mass as % body weight	73%	72%	80%	76%	75%
Energy intake (kcal/day)*	2127	2127	—	1912	1745
BMR (kcal/day)	1338	1530	1315	1267	1195
BMR (kcal/kg weight/day)	23	25	26	27	27
BMR (kcal/kg fat-free mass/day)	32	34	32	35	36
Birth weight (gm)	3370	3458	2980	2980	2885
Placental weight (gm)	641	657	500	530	526

*Measured at or near 10 weeks' gestation. Fat mass and fat-free mass estimated from sum of four skin-fold measurements and body weight.

Based on data from Durnin JVGA: Energy requirements of pregnancy: an integration of the longitudinal data from the five-country study, *Lancet* 2:1131, 1987.

2. It is interesting that the Dutch women, who were bigger and slightly fatter than the Scottish women, deposited only about two-thirds the amount of fat, despite their higher energy intake and similar energy expenditure.

3. In none of the groups did fat gains come near the Hytten and Chamberlain[37] proposed value of 3.5 kg.

4. The total increase in basal metabolic rate (BMR) over the whole pregnancy differed by at least a factor of 10 between the Gambian women and those from the other centers. This enormous difference demonstrates a quite remarkable physiological adaptation, presumably not to pregnancy only, but to pregnancy in the face of severe nutritional stress.

5. The net energy cost of performing a given physical activity (calculated as energy per unit of body weight) fell slightly in most groups, but the change was small and never resulted in a reduced energy expenditure in absolute terms; even though a pregnant woman in the third trimester expends less energy doing a task per kilogram of her body weight than she did in her first trimester, she still expends more total energy.

6. There were apparent differences in the data on the energy cost of pregnancy from the different centers, but if they are standardized for body weight, total energy costs were about 59,750 kcal for all the groups except the Gambian women, and the small differences between the other groups were mostly the result of the variable amounts of maternal fat stored during pregnancy (Table 5-5).

7. With exception of the Thai groups, energy intakes did not conform, even remotely, to the theoretically expected quantities. There is no doubt that this result raises difficulties in relation to general recommendations of the energy requirements of pregnancy.

The overall conclusion from these studies is that the energy costs of pregnancy are about 59,750 kcal; this ought to imply that pregnant women, on the average, need an extra 59,750 kcal in their diet. These studies have also shown that this cost is not usually reflected in 59,750 extra kcalories being consumed in the diet. The usefulness of virtually all current guidelines for exogenous kcalorie requirements for pregnant women must therefore be questioned.

Further Observations on Energy Costs

Gambian women have provided an outstanding example of energy-sparing during pregnancy. This was illustrated in recent work using whole body calorimetry.[67] Components of daily energy expenditure were measured serially before pregnancy and at 6-, 12-, 18-, 24-, 30-, and

TABLE 5-4 *Weight and Fat Gain during Pregnancy*

Country	Mean Total Weight Gain (kg)*	Weight Gain as % of Initial Weight	Mean Fat Gain (kg)†	Fat Gain as % of Initial Weight
Scotland	11.7	20	2.3	4.0
The Netherlands	10.5	17	2.0	3.2
The Gambia	7.3	14	0.6	1.2
Thailand	8.9	19	1.4	2.9
Philippines	8.5	19	1.3	2.9

*From 10 weeks to term.
†Difference in maternal fat stores between 4 to 6 weeks postpartum and 10 weeks' gestation, calculated from sum of four skinfolds and body weight.
Based on data from Durnin JVGA: Energy requirements of pregnancy: an integration of the longitudinal data from the five-country study, *Lancet* 2:1131, 1987.

TABLE 5-5   *Energy Cost in Kcalories of Pregnancy in Different Centers*

	Scotland	The Netherlands	The Gambia	Thailand*	Philippines*
Fetus	8,126	8,222	7,146	7,146	6,907
Placenta	729	741	559	600	600
Expanded maternal tissues	2,891	2,940	2,486	2,486	2,414
Maternal fat	25,334	21,988	6,296	15,391	14,292
BMR	30,114	34,416	1,888	23,900†	18,881†
TOTAL	67,159	68,354	18,642	49,712	43,259

*Estimated from 10 weeks
†Estimated from 13 weeks
Based on data from Durnin JVGA: Energy requirements of pregnancy on integration of the longitudinal data from the five-country study, *Lancet* 2:1131, 1987.

36-weeks gestation. Weight gain was 15 lb (6.8 kg), fat deposition was 4.4 lb (2 kg) and lean tissue deposition was 11 lb (5 kg). Basal metabolic rate was depressed during the first 18 weeks of gestation. Individual responses to pregnancy correlated with changes in body mass. There was no significant increase in the cost of treadmill exercise, 24-hour energy expenditure, activity, or diet-induced thermogenesis during pregnancy in spite of body weight gain. Total energy costs over 36 weeks were markedly lower than reported for well-nourished Western populations. Fig. 5-4 through 5-7 illustrate some of these findings.

A cross-country analysis. In order to test whether energy-sensitive adjustments in gestational metabolism were apparent in women other than those studied in the Gambia and England, researchers from the United Kingdom conducted a retrospective analysis of data on basal metabolic rate and fat deposition in 360 pregnancies from 10 studies in a wide range of nutritional settings.[66] The energy costs of pregnancy varied widely between different communities: maintenance costs from −10,800 kcals to +50,400 kcals, fat deposition from −5520 kcals to +64,080 kcals, and total energy costs from −4800 kcals to 139,920 kcals. Total costs were correlated with prepregnancy fatness and pregnancy weight gain. Marginally nourished women conserved energy by suppressing metabolic rate and by gaining little fat. They also delivered smaller babies (Fig. 5-8).

Assessing the adequacy of energy intake. Comparing the estimated intake to a recommended intake is not desirable during pregnancy because energy needs differ from one woman to another. Requirements vary with prepregnancy weight and body composition, amount and composition of weight gain, and stage of pregnancy and activity level. It is therefore inappropriate to make a single energy recommendation for all pregnant women. Energy status may be estimated instead by evaluating the rate of weight gain. If the rate of weight gain is appropriate for the stage of pregnancy, it is assumed that the energy supply is adequate.

Sources of Energy

Theoretically the body can derive all of its energy from dietary or stored protein and fat. Carbohydrates are used preferentially by some cells and are required for intermediaries of the citric acid cycle, but they can be synthesized from protein. The exclusion of carbohydrate from the diet, however, has harmful effects. Since energy production is of primary importance, the body will use protein to manufacture citric acid cycle intermediaries and glucose if no preformed sources are available. This can impair growth. If the body must depend solely on dietary or stored fat for energy, metabolic products of fat oxidation accumulate in excess. These products, known as ketone bodies, cannot be metabolized when their concentrations reach high levels. Since they are acidic in nature, ketones disrupt

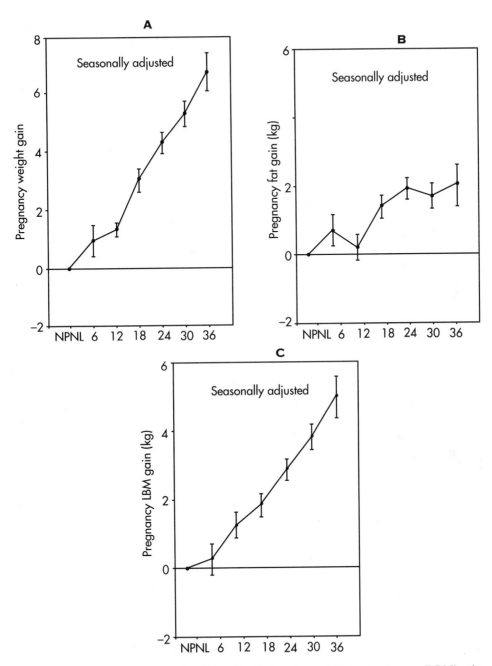

FIG. 5-4 **A,** Seasonally-adjusted weight gain, **B,** fat gain, and **C,** lean body mass (LBM) gain during pregnancy in 21 Gambian women. NPNL = nonpregnant, nonlactating. SEs represented by vertical bars.

From Poppitt SD et al: Evidence of energy-sparing in Gambian women during pregnancy: a longitudinal study using whole body calorimetry, *Am J Clin Nutr* 57:353, 1993.

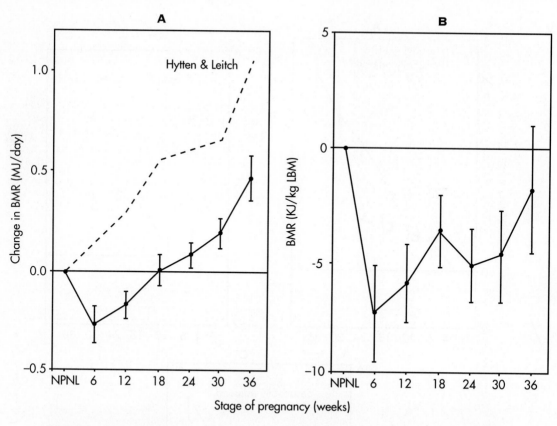

FIG. 5-5 The response of basal metabolic rate (BMR) to pregnancy in 20 Gambian women. **A,** Overall and the dotted line is the Hytten and Leitch predicted increase in BMR in well-nourished Western women. **B,** Mass-specific change in basal metabolic rate. NPNL = non-pregnant, nonlactating. SEs represented by vertical bars.

From Poppitt SD et al: Evidence of energy-sparing in Gambian women during pregnancy: a longitudinal study using whole body calorimetry, *Am J Clin Nutr* 57:353, 1993.

the body's acid-base balance and can eventually lead to coma and death.

Dieting, Fasting, and Food Restriction

The degree to which the mother is parasitized by the fetus has been the subject of much debate for many decades. Although it is known that the fetus can draw on maternal stores when maternal dietary input is limited, the extent and duration of this process is unknown. Several studies on the effect of food restriction on the body composition of pregnant and nonpregnant rats have provided new insights into the nature of maternal-fetal interactions during a reduced availability of nutrients. This work showed that at term, pregnant rats fed 50% of the food consumed by control animals had a similar body composition as pair-fed nonpregnant rats, whereas the mean body weight of the fetus was significantly reduced. These results support the idea that the pregnant, food-restricted rat is not extensively parasitized by the fetus. In addition, data suggest that important metabolic adjustments must occur to allow the mother to prevent fetal parasitism.

Human data are obviously limited, but the Dutch famine experience supports the idea that the malnourished mother is able to protect her

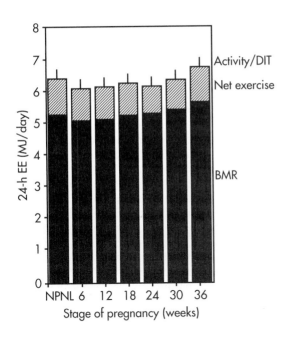

FIG. 5-6 The components of 24-hour energy's expenditure (24-hour EE), measured within a whole-body calorimeter in nine Gambian women during pregnancy. The components are basal metabolic rate (BMR), the net cost of a 1-hour period of treadmill exercise and the cost of other nonspecific activities including diet-induced thermogenesis (DIT). SEs represented by vertical bars. NPNL, nonpregnant, nonlactating.

From Poppitt SD et al: Evidence of energy-sparing in Gambian women during pregnancy: a longitudinal study using whole body calorimetry, *Am J Clin Nutr* 57:353, 1993.

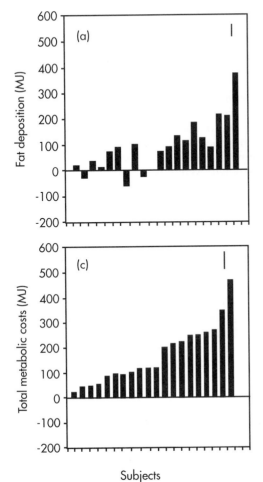

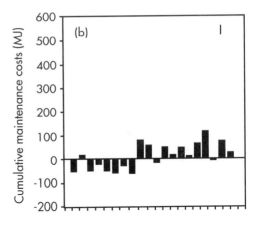

FIG. 5-7 The total metabolic costs of pregnancy are the sum of **A**), the energy deposited as fat, plus **B**), the cumulative maintenance costs, plus the cost of production of the fetus and associated structures (not shown on figure); **C**), represents total metabolic costs. Each column represents one Gambian woman during the weeks 6 to 36 of pregnancy.

From Poppitt SD et al: Evidence of energy-sparing in Gambian women during pregnancy: a longitudinal study using whole body calorimetry, *Am J Clin Nutr* 57:353, 1993.

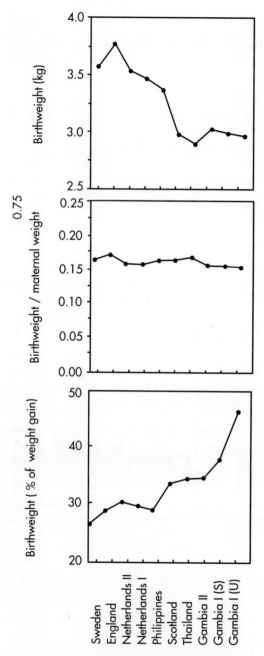

FIG. 5-8 Mean birth weight, ranked by country, in order of decreasing cost of pregnancy, plotted as absolute weight of the neonate (top), corrected for maternal body weight (middle), and as percentage of maternal pregnancy weight gain (bottom). S = supplemented; U = unsupplemented.

From Poppitt SD et al: Energy-sparing to protect human fetal growth, *Am J Obstet Gynecol* 171:118, 1994.

body stores of nutrients from fetal parasitism. Mean infant birth weight was reduced by 10%, but most mothers were estimated to lose less than 3% of their initial body weight during the stress of famine during pregnancy. The mothers appeared to be proportionately less affected than their infants, an observation consistent with that from animal data. Thus, optimal fetal growth occurs only when the mother is able to accumulate a critical amount of extra body stores during pregnancy. Evidence clearly contradicts the concept that the fetus is protected by the mother when nutritional status is less than optimal or that the fetus can protect itself by parasitizing the mother.

The fact that nature protects the mother more than the fetus seems reasonable from the point of view of survival of the species. During a famine caused by a serious crop failure, for example, a normal-sized newborn delivered by a nutritionally depleted mother would have little chance to survive if the mother could not initiate lactation, protect herself and her young, and cover enough ground during the day to secure food. A stronger or healthier mother who produces a small baby or few offspring probably has a better chance to survive and conceive again.

Although the food-restricted mother is known to adapt to her unfortunate predicament, the metabolic and physiologic mechanisms that allow for this adaptation are largely unknown. Major adaptations are known to occur in protein and amino acid metabolism, but these have not been defined. Food efficiency is known to increase, but the mechanism involved is still unknown. Many other factors are probably important, such as modified expansion in blood volume or deposition in maternal stores. It is possible that the normal sequence of physiologic adjustment to pregnancy is retarded in the face of nutritional deficit. The ultimate result might very well be suboptimal completion of the final stages of adjustment such that adequate growth of the conceptus is prevented.[71]

One recognized consequence of calorie restriction is the increased production of ketone bodies and their ultimate spillage into the urine. Although it is known that the fetus can metabolize ketone bodies to some degree, the consequences of maternal ketosis are not completely understood. Although severe ketoacidosis, as occurs in diabetics, is appreciated as harmful to the fetus, the short-term and long-term effects of maternal acetonuria are unclear. Churchill, Berendes, and Nemore[14,15] first reported that children whose diabetic and nondiabetic mothers had acetonuria during pregnancy had lower mental and motor scores at 8 months and lower IQ values at 4 years of age than children not so exposed. Stebhens, Baker, and Kitchell[84] later examined offspring of diabetic women and found a significant association of gestational acetonuria with lower IQ values at 5 years of age. Reports by Naeye and Chez,[13] however, have not confirmed these earlier reports; maternal acetonuria was not related to results of mental and motor tests administered to offspring at 4 to 7 years of age.

Data collected from both animals and humans indicate that ketone bodies are probably normally presented to the fetal brain at various times during pregnancy. After an overnight fast maternal ketone body concentrations are about threefold greater in pregnant than in nonpregnant women, and ketonuria will often be seen.[16,31,68] In one study Coetzee, Jackson, and Berman[16] found that urine concentrations of ketone bodies may abruptly increase in the presence of less than a twofold increase in blood concentrations; in addition, they found that blood levels generally fall within the upper limit of the normal range. These investigators tend to conclude that acetonuria in normal pregnancy "probably does not usually signify that any abnormality is present." More serious conditions of ketoacidosis should likely be viewed as more hazardous.

Another study in which acetonuria was assessed involved prenatal monitoring of pregnant adolescents.[60] Of the urine samples of 10- to 14-year-old mothers, 5% had 2+ or greater acetone versus only 2% of the older mothers. Mothers who had 2+ or greater acetone in one or more pregnancy urine samples had 56 fetal or neonatal deaths per 1,000 births versus 36 per 1,000 births when mothers had no acetonuria. Mothers whose acetonuria was no greater than 1+ during pregnancy had a perinatal mortality rate of 46 per 1,000 births. Naeye suggests that the young adolescent may very well exist in a circumstance of marked maternal-fetal competition for nutrients. He further points out that

high acetonuria may be a marker for maternal undernutrition and the associated increased risk of fetal or neonatal death.[60]

Also, the biochemical consequences of fasting during pregnancy may be associated with adverse consequences that are not yet understood. For example, Kaplan, Eidelman, and Aboulafia[39] reported that the number of deliveries among pregnant Jewish women in Jerusalem was significantly higher during the 24 hours after *Yom Kippur*. The number of deliveries was assessed in both 1981 and 1982, and in both cases the delivery rate increased after the total 24-hour fast engaged in during this annual holiday (Fig. 5-9). The clinical implications of this observation are by no means clear, but the researchers speculate that a special risk may exist for women with a tendency toward early delivery in that the biochemical changes associated with fasting may somehow precipitate labor.

PROTEIN

The promotion of optimal growth during pregnancy requires adequate supplies of energy and raw materials.[44] Protein is essential because it forms the structural basis for all new cells and tissues in the mother and fetus. Other key nutrients are vitamins and minerals, which participate in the biochemical reactions that build amino acids into new protein molecules and maintain the structural and functional properties of the cells.

Nitrogen is the key element in protein that makes it different from carbohydrate and fat. Protein requirements therefore are usually determined by measuring the amount of nitrogen retained in the body for metabolic use. One gram of nitrogen is equivalent to 6.25 gm of protein.

In the factorial method, protein needs are estimated by totaling all the ways that nitrogen can be lost from the body. This gives an indication of how much protein nitrogen must be replaced each day. Urinary excretion when subjects are consuming a protein-free diet is used to estimate basic endogenous needs. Loss in feces during protein restriction shows how much is sloughed from cells of the gastrointestinal tract. Integumental loss indicates replacement needs for nitrogen in sweat and desquamated cells of

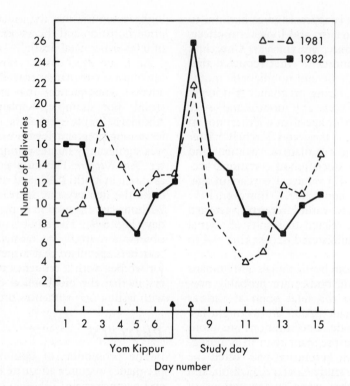

FIG. 5-9 Relationship of number of deliveries to day before, of, and after 24-hour fast.

From Kaplan M, Eidelman AI, Aboulafia Y: Fasting and the precipitation of labor; the Yom Kippur effect, *JAMA* 250:1317, 1983. Copyright 1983, American Medical Association.

the skin, hair, and nails. When these losses are calculated for the average woman used as a reference, requirements are 2.84 gm of nitrogen or 18 gm of protein per day.

Protein requirements during pregnancy are based on the needs of the nonpregnant woman used as a reference plus the extra amounts needed for growth. The easiest way to determine how much extra protein is needed daily to support the synthesis of new tissue is to divide the amounts contained in the products of conception by the average length of gestation. About 925 gm of protein are deposited in a normal-weight fetus and in the maternal accessory tissues. When this is divided by the 280 days of pregnancy, the average is 3.3 gm of protein that must be added to normal daily requirements. The rate at which new tissue is synthesized, however, is not constant throughout gestation.

Maternal and fetal growth do not accelerate until the second month, and the rate progressively increases until just before term. The need for protein follows this growth rate. Only about an extra 0.6 gm of protein is used each day for synthesis in the first month of pregnancy, but by 30 weeks' gestation protein is being used at the rate of 6.1 gm per day. If this is added to the normal maintenance needs of the reference woman, one finds that 18.6 to 24.1 gm per day of protein are required during pregnancy.

These calculations would equal dietary allowances if 100% of the protein eaten could be used in the body. In actuality the efficiency of protein utilization depends on its digestibility and amino acid composition. Proteins that do not contain all eight essential amino acids in amounts proportional to human requirements are utilized less efficiently, but the utilization of even a high-quality protein, such as that from eggs, is only about 70%. Utilization from a mixed diet or from one in which protein is supplied totally from vegetable sources is less efficient.

Protein utilization also depends on caloric intake. It has been shown that an extra 100 kcal during pregnancy will have the same effect on nitrogen retention as an additional 0.28 gm of nitrogen itself. This means that calories from nonprotein sources (i.e., carbohydrate and fat) have a sparing effect. If these calories are inadequate, protein requirements would increase.

Actual nitrogen retention has been measured in pregnant women by use of nitrogen balance methods. Observations in more than 150 women indicate that nitrogen retention is consistently greater than predicted levels. It has been suggested that pregnant humans, like pregnant rats, increase their lean body mass in early pregnancy in preparation for the demands of later pregnancy. Studies of nitrogen retention in nonpregnant women and those in the early and late stages of pregnancy, however, have not shown early deposition of nitrogen. It is therefore doubtful that a lean tissue store is gained by humans early in pregnancy. King[42] speculates that the difference between measured and predicted rates of nitrogen retention reflect errors in the methods.

Overall, the efficiency of protein utilization has not been quantitated in pregnant women. Assuming that only 70% of the dietary protein is retained in pregnancy, the National Research Council proposed that pregnant women consume an additional 10 to 12 gm of protein per day in order to retain 6 to 8 gm per day in the last half of pregnancy.[61]

Protein Deficiency

Adverse consequences of protein deficiency during pregnancy are difficult to separate from the effects of calorie deficiency in real-life situations. Almost all cases of limited protein intake are accompanied by limitation in availability of calories; under such circumstances decreased birth weight and greater incidence of preeclampsia have been reported. As previously mentioned in the Guatemala study,[34] provision of supplemental calories alone to patients with

deficient levels of protein intake was just as effective as provision of both protein and calories in influencing birth weight of babies. Zlatnik and Burmeister[98] also reported that birth weight and other anthropometric indexes of the newborn infant were not related to the level of dietary protein during pregnancy.

The notion that protein deficiency causes pregnancy-induced hypertension (PIH) is a highly controversial issue. Brewer[8] contends that consumption of adequate dietary protein will obliterate PIH. For several years he ran a prenatal clinic in northern California in which the value of a high-protein diet was stressed. In 1971, a scientific review group examined the records of patients from the clinic and from the Contra Costa Hospital for the frequency of PIH during the years 1965 to 1970. The frequency of PIH in the patients seen by Brewer was not significantly different than in those patients not seen by Brewer (9 of 548 vs. 12 of 367, respectively).[7] In his analysis of the data, Brewer removed six of the cases from his group, stating that he had not seen two, one was in the project for only 1 week, and three had no evidence of PIH in their records. He also removed three cases of preeclampsia from the hospital group. With these adjustments, there was a highly significant difference between the groups.

Osofsky[63] did a careful dietary survey on 118 low-income females attending the Temple University prenatal clinic. Their average protein intake was about 71 gm per day. He then gave 122 similar individuals a protein-mineral supplement. Their average protein intake was 80 gm per day. The latter group had a significantly lower incidence of blood pressure elevations.

Grieve[33] has advocated a high-protein/low-carbohydrate diet for his prenatal patients in Motherwell, Scotland. In a report in 1974, he had one case of PIH in 5,808 patients in the low-risk/good-diet group and 16 cases in 735 patients in the poor-diet group.

Although all of these studies support the role of protein deprivation in the etiologic factors of PIH, results from other studies cast doubt on this relationship.[50,96] In addition, other workers conducted a 12-day nitrogen balance study on 68 primigravidas who were between 30 and 35 weeks pregnant. These hospitalized patients were placed on a diet similar to the one they consumed at home. The diet was constructed after a careful diet history. Seven women developed preeclampsia. They had no significant difference in nitrogen intake or retention when compared with women in whom PIH did not develop.

The role of protein deficiency in the cause of preeclampsia has not been satisfactorily proved or disproved. Research in this area is lacking. Attempts to produce an animal model of PIH using a protein-deficient diet have proven unsuccessful. Given the body of evidence available to evaluate, one might suggest that encouraging sound dietary patterns among pregnant women is a justifiable practice but use of a protein supplement for prevention of PIH is not appropriate.

Protein Excess

Adverse effects of excessive protein during pregnancy are poorly understood at present. The New York supplementation study[74] has provoked much discussion of this issue, since use of the high-protein supplement was associated with an increased number of very prematurely born infants and excessive neonatal deaths. In light of these findings other data have been reviewed. Researchers reported in the 1970s that female monkeys reared on adequate diets showed an excessive number of very premature deliveries when provided with a high-protein diet during pregnancy. In addition, analysis of a number of past supplementation studies in human populations[75] has suggested that providing a supplement with more than 20% of the calories from protein is associated with retarded fetal growth, whereas supplements providing less than 20% of calories from protein yield increments in birth weight of offspring. Although these data suggest that too much protein (presented in an unbalanced nutritional package) may have negative effects on pregnancy course and outcome, data are limited, and the debate continues about the relevance of the observations that have been summarized.

ESSENTIAL FATTY ACIDS

Deficiency of essential fatty acids seems unlikely in a dietary environment rich in lipids.[18]

However, their importance in neural development suggests that a deficiency during the critical period of brain development may occur under adverse circumstances. The brain is 60% structural lipid; it universally uses arachidonic acid (AA) and docosahexanoic acid (DHA) for growth, function and integrity. Experimental evidence in animals has demonstrated that the effect of essential fatty acid deficiency during early brain development is deleterious and permanent. The risk of neurodevelopmental disorder is highest in very-low-birth-weight infants. Babies born of low birth weight or prematurely are more likely to have been born to mothers who were inadequately nourished and the babies tend to be born with AA and DHA deficits.

To test the hypothesis that maternal diet during pregnancy may impact fetal brain development, researchers in London studied 513 pregnancies in a population where the incidence of low birth weight is high.[27] They tracked 44 nutrients by use of a computerized nutrition database that provides a wide range of information on the nutritional quality of individual intakes. Results indicated that the diets of mothers who produced low-birth-weight babies were inferior to other mothers in many respects but among the dietary deficits was essential fatty acids. Also, reduced concentrations of arachidonic acid in maternal and cord blood phosphoglycerides were associated with low birth weight, head circumference and placental weight. This corresponds to a report by other researchers that a reduction in prostacyclin synthesis by the endothelium of the umbilical artery was correlated with low birth weight associated with lower maternal concentrations of arachidonic acid. Much remains to be learned about the importance of maternal dietary intake of essential fatty acids and the "quality" of the neonatal brain. This discussion applies equally to the importance of human milk fatty acid composition and postnatal brain development.

In recent years, interest has developed in the role essential fatty acids might play in the maintenance of normal vascular integrity and the prevention of preeclampsia.[1,2,51,93] Preeclampsia is a pregnancy-specific disorder complicating 5% to 7% of pregnancies and characterized by hypertension, proteinuria, edema and activation of the hemostatic system (see Chapter 8). It is one of the major causes of maternal and perinatal mortality and morbidity. The pathogenesis of preeclampsia remains obscure but dysfunction of the maternal vascular endothelial cells is considered to play a major role. It has been proposed that alterations in the circulating lipids may contribute to the induction of endothelial dysfunction in patients with preeclampsia. It has also been proposed that high intake of omega-3 fatty acids may improve birth weight and reduce the risk of intrauterine growth retardation. Thus far, evidence is insufficient to draw any conclusions. The door is open for further observation of the relevance of essential fatty acids in successful human reproduction.

VITAMINS
Thiamin, Riboflavin, and Niacin

The process of energy production involves several other nutrients in addition to those that yield calories. The oxidation of carbohydrate proceeds in a series of reactions that convert glucose to pyruvic acid and then to acetylcoenzyme A. This last step depends on a coenzyme, thiamin pyrophosphate (TPP). As its name implies, TPP contains the B vitamin thiamin, and its availability can limit the rate at which energy from glucose is produced.

Riboflavin and niacin are also concerned with energy production. These two B vitamins are parts of the coenzymes flavin adenine dinucleotide and niacin adenine dinucleotide, which assist in transferring hydrogen atoms through the respiratory chain in the cells. If protein must be used for energy, riboflavin is also needed as part of the coenzyme that helps to remove nitrogen from the amino acids.

Since thiamin, riboflavin, and niacin are all part of the reactions that produce energy in the body, requirements are related to caloric intake. The adult RDAs are 0.5, 0.6, and 6.6 mg per 1,000 kcal for thiamin, riboflavin, and niacin, respectively. Since caloric allowances increase during pregnancy, the allowances for thiamin, riboflavin, and niacin automatically increase too. In addition, evidence from urinary excretion studies indicates that pregnant women have higher requirements for thiamin and riboflavin

than nonpregnant women. The RDA for these two nutrients therefore contain additional adjustments.

Thiamin, riboflavin, and niacin are found in almost all foods, but only a few are exceptionally good sources. Whole grains, legumes, organ meats, and pork are high in thiamin, whereas riboflavin is more plentiful in milk, cheese, lean meats, and leafy green vegetables. Foods that are high in thiamin and riboflavin are also good sources of niacin. Niacin is not only found preformed in food but it can also be made in the body from the amino acid tryptophan. For every 60 mg of tryptophan in the diet, 1 mg of niacin will be formed. Foods that are sources of good-quality protein are therefore good sources of niacin as well. Foods that contain only fat or sugar have no thiamin, riboflavin, or niacin.

In animals, severe deficiencies of thiamin, riboflavin, or niacin during pregnancy have resulted in fetal death, reduced growth, and congenital malformation. The skeleton and organs that arise from the ectoderm appear to be especially susceptible to riboflavin deficiency. Lack of riboflavin in the mother's diet was once thought to be a cause of prematurity in humans, but studies have failed to find a correlation.

Researchers have also evaluated the thiamin status of pregnant women at various stages of gestation and have found that 25% to 30% have values that would be considered deficient by nonpregnant standards. Although there have been some reported cases of congenital beriberi from maternal thiamin deficiency, there is no evidence of functional impairment at the levels described.

The niacin status of pregnant women has been investigated; however, there are no cases that indicate that niacin deficiency in humans produces the malformations noted in animal experimentations.

Folic Acid

The central place that protein occupies in the synthesis of new tissue sometimes obscures the emphasis that should be given to other nutrients. Growth, however, is a complex process that requires more than an adequate supply of protein and energy. To make new cells, DNA must replicate and transmit its genetic information to RNA intermediaries. RNA acts as a template for every new protein synthesized in the body.

Both DNA and RNA are composed of purines and pyrimidines. These ringlike substances are synthesized in the body from one-carbon (methyl) fragments and nitrogen. Derivatives of the B vitamin folic acid accept the carbon fragments from their biochemical donors and transfer them to their sites in the purine and pyrimidine rings. Folic acid also acts as a coenzyme in the synthesis of a nonessential amino acid, glycine. Glycine, in its turn, is a carbon and nitrogen donor in the synthesis of purines. Thus, folic acid is involved in almost all aspects of DNA and RNA synthesis. If it is lacking, cell division cannot proceed normally. The effects are most detrimental in cells that have high turnover rates in the body.

One of the first signs of folic acid deficiency is megaloblastic anemia, which is caused by the production of abnormal red blood cells. These cells are arrested in their development so that bone marrow contains a large number of immature megaloblasts and hemoglobin levels are reduced.

The dietary availability of folic acid is somewhat limited and its content in specific foods is inherently variable. A large fraction of folate consumed each day comes from foods that are often ingested but are not particularly concentrated sources of the vitamin (Table 5-6).[65] Orange juice was found to be the largest contributor of folate in the American diet (9.7%). Those foods with the highest content of folate per serving are listed in Table 5-7.

Several factors are known to affect negatively the availability of dietary folate. These include

TABLE 5-6   *Major Contributors of Folate in the U.S. Diet (NHANES II Data, 1976-1980)*

Ranking	Description	Total % Folate in Daily Diet
1	Orange juice	9.70
2	White bread, rolls, crackers	8.61
3	Pinto, navy and other dried beans (cooked)	7.08
4	Green salad	6.85
5	Cold cereal, not bran or super-fortified	4.96
6	Eggs	4.63
7	Alcoholic beverages	3.85
8	Coffee, tea	3.40
9	Liver	3.07
10	Superfortified cereals	3.06
11	Whole milk, whole milk beverages	2.90
12	Bran and granola cereals	2.48
13	Whole-wheat, rye, and other dark breads	2.43
14	Corn	1.89
15	Spaghetti with tomato sauce	1.51

From Picciano MF, Green T, O'Connor DL: The folate status of women and health, *Nutr Today* 29(6):20, 1994.

TABLE 5-7   *Folate Content of Food Sources High in Folate*

Ranking	Description	Folate Per Usual Serving (ug)
1	Liver	383
2	Superfortified cereals	242
3	Cold cereals, not bran or superfortified	112
4	Pinto, navy and other dried beans (cooked)	84
5	Asparagus	82
6	Spinach	70
7	Instant breakfast, diet bars, supplements	65
8	Bran and granola cereals	58
9	Broccoli	53
10	Avocados	49
11	Okra	49
12	Brussels sprouts	47
13	Orange juice	43
14	Artichokes	43
15	Chili	36

From Picciano MF, Green T, and O'Connor DL: The folate status of women and health, *Nutr Today* 29(6):20, 1994.

overcooking, long-term thermal processing procedures and high-fiber diets. The forms of folate found in foods (polyglutamylated folates) are used less effectively than synthetic folic acid.

Low serum folate levels have been reported in as many as 60% of patients in some clinical studies, but only a few of these women exhibit signs of megaloblastic anemia. The low serum values of folic acid are believed to result from a number of factors. Problems with food selection, storage, and cooking losses, which place nonpregnant women in marginal status, are compounded in pregnancy by increased needs for folate to expand the maternal blood volume and for growth of the fetus. In addition, defects in the utilization of folic acid may be inherent in pregnancy because of the effects of steroid hormones. The folic acid absorbed from food is converted by a series of reduction reactions to its active coenzyme form in the liver. High steroid levels may interfere with this process, since the liver is also the site where progesterone and estrogen are deactivated before excretion. The reactions for both the activation of folic acid and the deactivation of steroids involve similar biochemical mechanisms. A relationship is suspected because sometimes folic acid deficiency develops in women taking oral steroid contraceptives.

Excitement in recent years has been centered on the recognition that folic acid deficiency may have a role to play in the cause of neural tube defect (NTD) (see box on p. 146). These congenital anomalies are among the most serious; they are usually seen as anencephaly and spina bifida (Fig. 5-10). Babies with anencephaly die

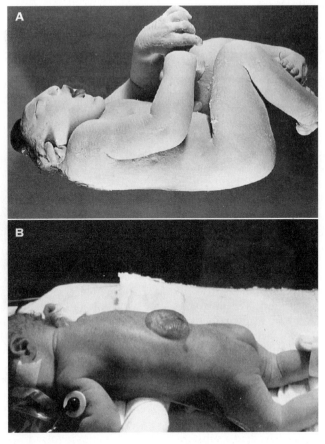

FIG. 5-10   Examples of neural tube defects. **A,** Anencephaly and **B,** spina bifida.

❖

FOLIC ACID FOR THE PREVENTIONOF NEURAL TUBE DEFECTS
COMMITTEE ON GENETICS, AMERICAN ACADEMY OF PEDIATRICS, 1993

Recommendations

1. *Prevention of Recurrence.* Patients with a history of a previous pregnancy resulting in a fetus with a NTD should be advised of the results of the MRC study. Unless contraindicated, they should be offered treatment with 4 mg of folic acid daily, starting 1 month before the time they plan to become pregnant and throughout the first 3 months of pregnancy. Patients should be advised not to attempt to achieve these doses of folic acid by taking over-the-counter or prescription multivitamins with folic acid because of the possibility of ingesting harmful levels of other vitamins, for example, vitamin A. It should be noted that 4 mg of folic acid did not prevent all NTDs in the MRC study. Therefore, high-risk patients should be cautioned that folic acid supplementation does not preclude the need for counseling or consideration of prenatal testing for NTDs.

2. *Prevention of First Occurrence.* The Academy endorses the PHS recommendation that all women of childbearing age who are capable of becoming pregnant should take 0.4 mg of folic acid daily.

3. *Implementation.* Because NTDs are among the most common and severe birth defects, it is important for women of childbearing age to receive folic acid as soon as possible. The Academy recommends that the Department of Health and Human Services expeditiously devise and implement a program, such as food fortification, that will prevent folate-related NTDs. The program should support surveillance with respect to effectiveness and/or adverse outcomes to further refine the effective folate dose and the mechanisms of its actions.

COMMITTEE ON GENETICS, 1993 TO 1994
Margretta R. Seashore, MD, Chairperson
Sechin Cho, MD
Franklin Desposito, MD
Judith G. Hall, MD
Jack Sherman, MD
Miriam G. Wilson, MD

Liaison Representatives
James W. Hanson, MD, American College of Medical Genetics
Michael Mennuti, MD, American College of Obstetricians & Gynecologists
Godfrey Oakley, MD, Centers for Disease Control & Prevention

AAP Section Liaison
Beth Pletcher, MD, Section on Genetics & Birth Defects

From Committee on Genetics: Folic acid for the prevention of neural tube defects, *Pediatrics* 93:408, 1993.

before or shortly after birth, whereas the majority of babies born with spina bifida grow to adulthood with paralysis of the lower limbs and varying degrees of bowel and bladder incontinence. This NTD may occur between postconceptional days 15 and 28 in humans. Thus NTD occurs so early that most women are unaware of their pregnancy.

In the 1980s, the introduction and efficacy of maternal alphafetoprotein and ultrasound screening, in addition to amniotic alphafetoprotein and other examinations have had a substantial effect. Nevertheless, selective abortion of a seriously malformed fetus should be considered a last resort rather than an optimal solution. Informed parents have to choose between terminating their pregnancy or having a malformed baby, with its long-term medical and social consequences. Many parents choose the first alternative and prevent the birth of the affected fetus. This scenario may be called secondary prevention but virtually everyone agrees that primary prevention is preferable. This is where folic acid becomes involved.

TABLE 5-8 *Controlled Trials of Folate Supplements and the Incidence of Neural Tube Defect*

Authors	Folate Dose	Incidence Rate/ 1,000 Births		Relative Risk	Recurrence or Occurrence
		Supplemented	Controls		
	mg/d				
Laurence et al[46]	4	33 [2]*	78 [4]	0.40	Recurrence
Smithells et al[82]	0.36	6.6 [3]	46 [24]	0.14	Recurrence
UK Vitamin Research Group[58]	4	10 [6]	35 [21]	0.36	Recurrence
Vergel et al[92]	5	0 [8]	35 [4]	0	Recurrence
Czeizel and Dudas[21]	0.8	0 [0]	3 [6]	0	Occurrence

*Number of cases in brackets.
From Rush, D: Periconceptional folate and neural tube defect, *Am J Clin Nutr* 59(suppl):511S, 1994

To date, it is known that neural tube defects appear to have some genetic base. That is, although they occur in about 0.1% of all pregnancies, the risk of occurrence is 0.3% to 1% if there is a close relative with NTD and recurrence risk is 3% to 4%. Chromosomal aberrations, gene mutations, and teratogenic factors (e.g., valproic acid) appear to account for a small fraction of the cases. The other 92% of cases may have multifactorial origins such as polygenic liability triggered by environmental factors.[20]

Among triggering environmental factors, undernutrition has been found to be a factor in the well-known association between NTD and poverty, seasonality, and rapid secular changes in the prevalence of NTD. In 1976, Smithells et al[81] reported lower concentrations of red cell folate and vitamin C during the first trimester of pregnancy in women who later delivered infants with NTD than in matched controls. The dietary study of Smithells et al[81] in which the 7-day food records of 195 mothers were studied in the first trimester of pregnancy, showed a social class gradient in intake of all nutrients. Laurence et al[47] retrospectively studied the interpregnancy diet of 415 mothers who had a child with NTD. A correlation was found between the mean serum and red blood cellolate concentrations and quality of the diet. Their subsequent prospective study showed that all five NTD recurrences (of 176 pregnancies) were from mothers with poor diets.[46]

From these early hints that some aspect of nu-

trition may alter a woman's risk of NTD pregnancy outcome, other evidence began to accumulate. Five sets of studies are available; these include the following:

1. From randomized and other controlled trials of folate or multivitamin supplementation and the prevention of NTD (Table 5-8)
2. Observational studies of the relationship between supplemental vitamin intake and rate of NTD (Table 5-9)
3. Studies of observed levels of dietary folate and incidence of NTD (Table 5-10)
4. One trial of dietary intervention to prevent NTD (Table 5-11)
5. The relationship of serum and red blood cell folate to the incidence of NTD (Table 5-12)

Smithells et al[82] and Laurence et al[46] organized the first intervention studies. Smithells et al[82] recruited women who had previously given birth to one or more infants with NTD into a trial of periconception multivitamins, specifically Pregnavite Forte F (a multivitamin-mineral product). Because two ethical committees refused to give permission for a randomized clinical trial, the control group was made up of women who had had one or more previous infants with NTD but were already pregnant when referred to the study centers or, in two cases, declined to take part in the trial. The time of supplementation was from at least 28 days before conception to the date of the second missed

TABLE 5-9 *Observational Studies of the Relationship Between Supplemental Vitamin Intake and Rate of NTD*

Author	Year	Impact of Periconceptional Supplementation
Khoury[a]	1982	Positive
Winship[b]	1984	Positive
Mulinare[c]	1988	Positive
Milunsky[d]	1989	Positive
Mills[55]	1989	Negative
Smithells[81]	1991	Positive
Werler[e]	1993	Positive
Shaw[f]	1995	Positive

a. Khoury MJ, Erickson JD, James LM: Etiologic heterogeneity of neural tube defects: clues from epidemiology, *Am J Epidemiol* 115:538, 1982.

b. Winship et al: Maternal drug histories and central nervous system anomalies, *Arch Dis Child* 59:1052, 1984.

c. Mulinare et al: Periconceptional use of multivitamins and the occurrence of neural tube defect, *JAMA* 260:3141, 1988.

d. Milunsky A et al: Multivitamin/folic acid supplementation in early pregnancy reduces the prevalence of neural tube defects, *JAMA* 262:2847, 1989.

e. Werler MM, Shapiro S, Mitchell AA: Periconceptional folic acid exposure and risk of occurent neural tube defects, *JAMA* 269:1257, 1993.

f. Shaw et al: Periconceptional vitamin use, dietary folate and the occurrence of neural tube defects, *Epidemiol* 6:219, 1995.

menstrual period. In the Yorkshire region of the United Kingdom, a 91% reduction in the recurrence rate was found and in Northern Ireland, an 83% reduction was found. However, Smithells was criticized for possible selection bias when it came to subject recruitment.

Laurence[46] organized a small, randomized double-blind trial in which women with a history of having a child with an NTD received either folic acid (4 mg daily) or placebo. This trial indicated a 58% risk reduction with folic acid; however, the difference was not significant.

In the early 1980s, the United Kingdom Medical Research Council (MRC) decided to organize a multicenter double-blind random-

ized trial;[58] 43% of the participants came from Hungary. (The United States did not participate.) Women who had already had an infant with an NTD were randomly divided into four supplementation groups:

• Folic acid (4 mg) only
• Folic acid and other vitamins
• Other vitamins
• Neither folic acid nor other vitamins.

A total of 1,195 pregnancies appeared to be sufficient to conclude that folic acid supplementation alone reduced NTD recurrences 71%. Other vitamins did not have a significant protective effect.

Research in Cuba provided similar results.[92] Folic acid at the level of 5 mg daily was provided to 81 women with a history of giving birth to babies with NTD. This product was taken before and throughout pregnancy; the control group of women did not follow this practice. The results indicated that there was no recurrence of NTD among the group of offspring whose mothers chose to use periconceptional folic acid supplementation. In the group of women who became pregnant without folic acid supplementation ($n = 114$), there were four recurrences of NTD.

A randomized trial with three treatments was initiated in Ireland in 1981 and ended in 1990 before the initial target number of study subjects was reached.

The goal of the Hungarian-controlled randomized trial of Czeizel and Dudas[21] was to determine efficacy of folic acid supplementation in the reduction in *first* occurrences of NTD. Women planning a pregnancy were randomly assigned to receive a single tablet of a multivitamin (including a physiological dose (0.8 mg) acid or a placebo-like trace element supplement daily for at least a month before conception and until at least the date of the second missed menstrual period. Overall, there were six children with NTDs, out of 2,391 offspring, in the trace element groups compared with none, out of 271 offspring, in the multivitamin group. The difference was significant.

Although these intervention trials provided valuable data, observational studies added fuel to the fire. In these studies, women were interviewed about their use of nutritional supple-

TABLE 5-10   *Dietary Intake of Folate and Neural Tube Defect: Observational Studies*

Authors

Milunsky et al[a]	Intake (µg/d)	<100	100+			
	RR*	1.00	0.42			
Bower and Stanley[b]	Intake (µg/d)	20–	175–	240–	350 – 1787	
	RR (vs other anomalies)	1.0	0.54	0.52	0.41	
	RR (vs community controls)	1.0	0.94	0.61	0.38	
Werler et al[c]	Intake (µg/d)	31–	197–	253–	311–	392 – 2195
	RR	1.0	1.0	0.7	0.6	0.6

*Relative risk.

a. Milunsky A et al: Multivitamin/folic acid supplementation in early pregnancy reduces the prevalence of neural tube defects, *JAMA* 262:2847, 1989.

b. Bower C, Stanley FJ: Dietary folate as a risk factor for neural tube defects: evidence from a case-control study in Western Australia, *Med J Austral* 150:613, 1989.

c. Werler MM, Shapiro S, Mitchell AA: Periconceptional folic acid exposure and risk of occurent neural tube defects, *JAMA* 269:1257, 1993.

From Rush D: Periconceptional folate and neural tube defect, *Am J Clin Nutr* 59(suppl):511S, 1994.

TABLE 5-11   *Dietary Counseling and Incidence of Recurrent Neural Tube Defect*

Treatment Group	Quality of Diet			Total
	Good	**Fair**	**Poor**	
Counseled	0/40	0/46	3/13	3/99 (28/1000)
Not counseled	0/13	0/39	5/17	5/69 (63/1000)

From Rush D: Periconceptional folate and neural tube defect, *Am J Clin Nutr* 59(suppl):511S, 1994.

ments before and during early pregnancy. Mothers of NTD offspring were compared with mothers of control infants. All but one of the studies showed fairly strong protective effects of using vitamin supplements around the time of conception. That is, mothers reporting that they had chosen to do so before and during early pregnancy had a significantly reduced risk of delivering a baby with NTD. In the case of the negative study by Mills,[55] it was well-executed and had a large sample size. However, it was conducted using a population from an area where NTD prevalence is low. Folate intervention may not apply in circumstances such as this.

Limited data are available on dietary folate intake and recurrence or occurrence of NTD. Not only were there technical shortcomings in data collection, but dietary information was also collected many months after neural tube closure. It is therefore amazing that any differences were seen between diets of NTD mothers and controls. In all three studies, the relative risk of NTD occurrence was significantly lowered by a dietary pattern rich in folic acid.

Laurence et al[47] performed the only reported trial of dietary education aimed at the prevention of NTD. When he compared the counseled with the noncounseled women (all of whom had a previous child with NTD), he found a fairly strong but not statistically significant association between higher levels of dietary folate and lower recurrence of NTD. This result was observed among women who were not taking nutritional supplements, so diet over supplements appears to make a difference.

Of considerable interest is the observation that in seven studies of serum and/or red blood cell concentration of folic acid, less than impressive differences were found between mothers of

TABLE 5-12 *Maternal Serum and Red Blood Cell Folate Concentrations and Neural Tube Defect*

Authors	Red Cell Folate		Serum Folate		When Specimens Collected
	Cases	Control Subjects	Cases	Control Subjects	
	nmol/L		*nmol/L*		
Emery, Timson, Watson-Williams[a]	—	—	11.1 [19]*	10.4 [37]	Presumably postpartum
Hall[b]	—	—	14.4 [11]	15.0 [2938] (Primigravida) 15.2 [2938] (Multigravida)	At booking
Smithells et al[82]	320† [6]	517 [959]	11.1† [5]	14.3 [953]	Early pregnancy
Molloy et al[c]			7.7 [32]	7.7 [384]	Early pregnancy
Yates et al[d]	403‡ [20]	607 [20]	6.3 [20]	7.5 [20]	After pregnancy
Holzgreve, Tercanli, Pietrzik[e]	—§ [17]	— [45]	—§ [17]	— [45]	
Mills et al[f]	—	—	9.36 [89]	9.70 [178]	Early pregnancy

*Numbers of subjects in brackets.
†‡§ Significantly different from control subjects: †$P < 0.001$, ‡$P < 0.01$.
§"No significant difference."
a. Emery AEH, Timson J, Watson-Williams EJ: Pathogenesis of spina bifida, *Lancet* 2:909, 1969.
b. Hall HM: Folates and the fetus, *Lancet* 1:648, 1977.
c. Molloy et al: Folate and vitamin B_{12} concentration in pregnancies associated with neural tube defects, *Arch Dis Child* 60:660, 1985.
d. Yates JRW et al: Is disordered folate metabolism the basis for the genetic predisposition to neural tube defects? *Clin Genet* 31:279, 1987.
e. Holzgreve W, Tercanli S, Pietrzik K: Vitamins to prevent neural tube defects, *Lancet* 338:639, 1991.
f. Mills et al: Maternal vitamin levels during pregnancies producing infants with neural tube defects, *J Pediatr* 120:863, 1992.
From Rush D: Periconceptional folate and neural tube defect, *Am J Clin Nutr* 59(suppl):511S, 1994

NTD offspring and mothers of normal infants. No standard time of blood collection was established throughout the studies. Two of three studies showed differences between cases and controls in red blood cell folate. Difference was found in only one of seven studies that measured serum folate. Hence, if folic acid status makes a difference in pregnancy outcome, why might it be that serum and red blood cell folate levels are not routinely low in mothers of NTD babies?

The underlying mechanisms of periconceptional multivitamin or folic acid supplementation in the prevention of NTD are still not understood. In general, women who have NTD-affected pregnancies have not been found to have lower serum or red blood cell folate values during pregnancy. However, Smithells et al[81] and Kirke et al[73] found a difference in red blood cell folate levels between women who had NTD pregnancies and controls. The risk of NTD is not dramatically altered by raising the red blood cell folate status from very low to a more normal value, whereas the risk is significantly reduced by attaining a red blood cell folate status of >300 or 400 μg/L. Thus a small change in folate status may profoundly reduce risk.

Recent epidemiological and biochemical evidence has suggested that the problem is not primarily a lack of sufficient folate in the diet. Instead, the problem appears to be rooted in changes in metabolism of folate in both maternal and fetal cells.[10,54] (Absorption of folate has been found to be normal in women with NTD pregnancies[23] and all pregnant women experience accelerated breakdown of folate during pregnancy.)[53] It is proposed that there is an interaction between a vitamin *dependency* (i.e., an inborn error of folate metabolism) and nutrition (e.g., a dietary vitamin deficiency) that may have a causal role in the origin of folic acid-related NTD. The effect on the embryo may be a localized folate deficiency. The supply of folate may be limited even in women with normal folate nutrition, resulting in impaired embryonic cell division at the crucial time of neural tube closure. Folate supplementation may cause an increase in folate concentrations in tissue fluids, and it may overcome this failure of local folate supply.

Although the pathogenesis of NTD is still unproven, three studies shed some light on the subject.[20] One found a possible role of methionine deficiency in the origin of NTD, based on cultures of whole rat embryos. Methionine is an essential amino acid, which is converted to S-adenosylmethionine; it is the ultimate methyl donor in humans:

Methionine ⟶ S–adenosylmethionine ⟶ CH–3
Methionine ⟵ S–adenosylmethionine ⟶ Homocysteine

Methionine deficiency may cause NTD at the period when the folds of the neural tube first become elevated and have started to appose opposite ridges. Other researchers reported that 31% of infants with NTD had methionine intolerance (with abnormally high serum homocysteine concentrations after an oral methionine load), whereas only 1% of people in the general population had such intolerance.[85] This finding may indicate a metabolic block of demethylation of homocysteine to methionine. Bunduki et al[10] reported a study of 14 NTD mothers and 14 controls. Mothers of NTD offspring had a significantly lower folate methylation rate than did mothers of normal infants.

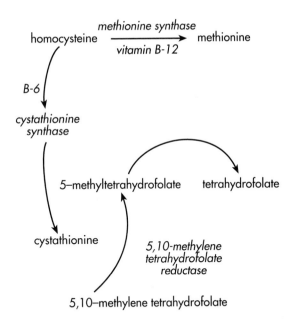

FIG. 5-11 Pathways of homocysteine metabolism.

A study showed that plasma vitamin B_{12} level is an independent risk factor for NTD offspring. Only one function in humans is independently influenced by both plasma folate and plasma vitamin B_{12}, and that is the action of the enzyme methionine synthase.[20]

Finally, Mills and colleagues[54] obtained blood during the pregnancies of 81 women who produced infants with NTD and 323 women who produced normal infants. Mothers of children with NTD had significantly higher homocysteine values than matched controls. The difference was significant in the 50% of women with the lowest plasma B_{12} concentrations. These researchers propose that an abnormality in homocysteine metabolism, apparently related to methionine synthase, is present in many women who give birth to children with NTD (Fig. 5-11). They also suggest that the most effective periconceptional prophylaxis to prevent NTD may require B_{12} as well as folic acid.

Although the mechanism of NTD prevention with folic acid is still poorly understood, important research is underway. At the very least, a marker may be found that could be used as a screening test for women at risk for NTD pregnancy (i.e., plasma homocysteine concentration). Such a marker could help identify, perhaps early in life or in prepregnancy counseling clinics, those who will require periconceptional supplementation.

In the United States, the current National Research Council (NRC)[61] Recommended Dietary Allowance (RDA) for women more than 14 years of age is 180 μg of folic acid, and the RDA during pregnancy is 400 μg (0.4 mg). Folic acid is available over-the-counter (OTC) in dosages of up to 0.8 mg and is also available by prescription in 1-mg tablets. Prenatal vitamins contain 0.8 or 1.0 mg of folic acid. Folic acid is water-soluble with no known toxicity; however, at high doses (more than 1.0 mg/day) the anemia of vitamin B_{12} deficiency (pernicious anemia) can be obscured, with progression of neurological sequelae. Because pernicious anemia is rare before the age of 50, this is likely to be a rare occurrence among women receiving folic acid during the reproductive years. Studies that definitively address the question of maternal and fetal safety of folic acid are not available. However, folic acid has been used extensively during later pregnancy without adverse effects.[97]

Based on the evidence available to date, the Public Health Service (PHS) has recommended that all women of childbearing age who are capable of becoming pregnant should take 0.4 mg of folic acid daily. Implementation of this recommendation is believed to have the potential of reducing the rate of NTD pregnancies by 50%. Regular and continuous ingestion of folic acid is necessary so that offspring of unplanned pregnancies benefit from this intervention. The PHS also points out that this recommendation should be followed by women who have previously had an affected pregnancy, even though they are not planning a pregnancy; by couples with a close relative with a NTD; women with insulin-dependent diabetes mellitus; and women with seizure disorders being treated with valproic acid or carbamazepine.

Can current recommendations for folate be met by diet alone? Is it practical to expect that women will be able to select foods to allow them to ingest 400 μg of folate daily? If the diet is meticulously designed according to the U.S.

Food Guide Pyramid or Canada's Food Guide to Healthy Eating, it is possible to provide the level of folate currently recommended to reduce the risk of an NTD-affected pregnancy (Table 5-13). However, women in the United States and Canada consistently select diets with less than 400 μg/day of folate. Nutrition education may help. The U.S. Food and Drug Administration recently authorized a health claim on food labels relating diets adequate in folate to reduction in risk of NTD pregnancies. They also proposed to require fortification of cereal grain products with folate at a level of 140 μg/100 grams and to allow fortification of breakfast cereals at 100 μg/serving.[65]

There has been much debate about the pros and cons of grain product fortification.[17,62]* Fortification can provide additional folate to women of childbearing age in a continuous and passive manner, whereas supplementation requires compliance for over 30 years. At the proposed level of fortification, some women still would not achieve the recommended level of 400 μg/day without changes in their food selections. Higher levels of fortification were not proposed because of potential risks to nontargeted populations of high intakes of folate (>1 mg/day) such as masking the hematological signs of vitamin B_{12} deficiency and delaying treatment while irreversible damage progresses.

As the debate about fortification continues, inputs continue to be published. Daly et al[22] used data from a recent case-control study, which related a woman's risk of having a pregnancy with NTD to her red cell folate level; a continuous dose-response relationship was found. These findings were used to calculate the reduction in NTD cases that would be expected under two different strategies to raise folate levels. Targeting high risk individuals has a small effect on the population prevalence but can substantially change an individual's risk. Targeting the population produces a small change in individual risk but has a large effect on the population prevalence. Supplementation of high-risk women was judged to be the most efficient method to implement the high-risk

---

*Grain product fortification was approved in 1996.

TABLE 5-13 *Sample Menus for a Woman of Child-Bearing Age Who Is Relatively Inactive*

	Folate (gm)
Menu 1	
Breakfast	
1 bowl cornflakes (30 g)	(18) (106)*
1 pumpernickel bagel with 5 mL margarine	14.9
250 mL 2% milk	12.9
1 medium banana	22.6
1 coffee	
125 mL orange juice (made from frozen concentrate)	57.9
Lunch	
Sandwich	
2 slices 60% whole-wheat bread	29.4
2 slices (50 g) chicken	2.5
5 mL margarine	Trace
1 large apple	4.6
1 medium carrot	7
250 mL milk	12.9
Supper	
250 mL baked beans (+tomatoes+onions+bacon)	61.9
Spinach salad	
250 mL leaves (raw)	112.5
2 slices tomato	4.5
1 green onion	2.3
25 mL oil and vinegar	Trace
1 slice whole wheat bread + 5 mL margarine	14.7
1 medium serving cantaloupe	23.1
Total	Total 402 μg or 490
Menu 2	
Breakfast	
1 slice 50% whole wheat bread	14.7
1 soft boiled egg	22
175 mL hot oatmeal cereal	7
250 mL 2% milk	13
1 medium apple	46.2
Lunch	
Macaroni and cheese	
250 mL cooked noodles 4.44	
5 mL margarine	
75 mL tomatoes 5.7	
25 g cheddar cheese 4.5	14.6
1 slice pumpernickel bread	7.5
5 mL margarine	Trace
125 mL raw broccoli	55.4
1 medium-sized wedge cantaloupe	23.1
250 mL orange juice (made from frozen concentrate)	115.8

*Cereals marketed in Canada are not fortified with folic acid whereas those in the U.S. can be. Sample menu no. 1 would provide 402 μg of folate/day to Canadian women and 490 μg/day to U.S. women.

Continued

TABLE 5-13 **Sample Menus for a Woman of Child-Bearing Age Who Is Relatively Inactive—cont'd**

	Folate (g)
Supper	
100 g roast chicken	5
250 mL cooked white rice	16.7
250 mL tossed garden salad	46.0
1 small whole-wheat bun	20.3
125 mL canned pears	2.7
125 mL 2% milk	6.5
15 mL Italian salad dressing	0
5 mL margarine	Trace
Total	417 µg

From Picciano MF, Green T, O'Connor DL: The folate status of women and health, *Nutr Today* 29(6):20, 1994.

strategy, whereas food fortification was considered preferable for the population approach. It was pointed out that the current guidelines for an increased intake of 0.4 mg per day would result in a 48% reduction in NTD, and that this may be optimal. These researchers emphasize that the two intervention strategies should be considered complementary in prevention of NTD.

Just what do women know about folic acid and birth defects? A Gallup poll was taken in early 1995 with the sponsorship of the March of Dimes Birth Defects Foundation.[56] This telephone survey (random digit-dialing) of 2,010 women age 18 to 45 asked questions about vitamins and birth defects. The response rate was 50%. Overall, 52% of women reported ever hearing of or reading about folic acid. Of these, 9% answered that folic acid helps to prevent birth defects and 6% that folic acid helps reduce the risk of spina bifida; 45% were unable to recall what they had heard or read. Fifteen percent of respondents reported having knowledge of the PHS recommendation regarding the use of folic acid; 4% reported that the recommendation was for prevention of birth defects and 1% for the prevention of spina bifida.

Another important and unexpected finding of the Hungarian NTD occurrence trial was a lower prevalence at birth of major congenital abnormalities other than NTD diagnosed during pregnancy and at birth after periconceptional multivitamin supplementation (9.0 per 1,000 vs. 16.6 in the trace element or placebo group). Some congenital abnormality groups such as congenital cardiovascular malformations, defects of the urinary tract, and congenital limb deficiencies, occurred less often in the multivitamin group than in the trace element group. Shaw reported in 1995[80] a reduced risk of orofacial clefts if a mother used multivitamins containing folic acid periconceptionally (overall risk reduction 25% to 50%). Also in 1995, Li et al[49] reported a case-control study using the Washington State Birth Defect Registry; their results indicated that early prenatal multivitamin use was associated with a reduced risk of congenital urinary tract defects. The bottom line is that folic acid (or some other vitamin) may play a role in the prevention of birth defects other than those related to neural tube closure.

Czeizel[20] points out in his recent discussion of this issue that the hour may have come for a more effective and primary prevention of birth defects (see box on p. 155). The recognition of this challenge led some experts to establish the World Alliance of Organizations for the Prevention of Birth Defects. Its manifesto declares: "We believe that children have the right to be free of preventable birth defects and that prevention must be accessible to all segments of the population."[19]

TESTING FOR GENETIC DISORDERS OR BIRTH DEFECTS

The following are relatively common screening tests:

MSAFP

MSAFP: This simple blood test can measure the amount of a substance called alpha-fetoprotein in the mother's system. Higher-than-normal levels are linked to a few major defects such as neural tube defects. Low levels are linked to certain chromosome disorders. In most cases, however, high or low levels are false alarms. The doctor may repeat the test, or discuss amniocentesis with the pregnant woman to rule out chromosomal abnormalities. For most women, this test provides reassurance that the fetus is not affected by the disorders in question.

Ultrasound

Ultrasound—the use of sound waves to show the physical outlines of the fetus on a screen—can detect many malformations such as spina bifida, heart or kidney problems and limb defects. It also can determine the age of the fetus and identify twins. The procedure involves moving an instrument over the mother's abdomen (or using one inside the vagina), which sends out sound waves to examine the shape, function and activity of the fetus, placenta and umbilical cord. Not all defects are detectable, and a normal ultrasound doesn't guarantee that the baby has no malformations. The procedure takes less than an hour, and can usually be done in the doctor's office.

The following diagnostic tests are done in some pregnancies when there are specific reasons, such as family history of inherited diseases or advanced maternal age:

Amniocentesis

Amniocentesis: This test detects all known chromosomal errors, and specific single-gene disorders through examination of fetal cells floating in the amniotic fluid surrounding the baby. The test is usually done between the 13th and 15th weeks of pregnancy. It entails using ultrasound imaging to "see" the fetus on a screen, and then withdrawing a small sample of amniotic fluid through a thin needle inserted through the mother's abdomen. Test results usually take two to four weeks, and can rule out abnormalities such as Down syndrome and other genetic conditions. Results are highly accurate, but many conditions cannot be detected by the test. There is a low risk (less than one in 200) of miscarriage or infection following the procedure.

Chorionic Villus Sampling

Chorionic Villus Sampling (CVS) is a newer diagnostic test that can be done earlier, during the 9th or later weeks of pregnancy. Either a needle is inserted through the abdomen or a slim tube is inserted through the vagina to take a tiny tissue sample from outside the sac where the fetus develops. The tissue is analyzed for chromosome disorders and certain gene conditions. Results of a CVS test may be ready in about 10 days. They are slightly less accurate than amniocentesis, and the risk of miscarriage appears to be higher—one in 50 to 100.

From Genetic Counseling. March of Dimes Birth Defects Foundation, 1994. National office-1275 Mamaroneck Ave White Plains, New York 10605

Vitamin B$_{12}$

Not only does folic acid deficiency cause megaloblastic anemia, but vitamin B$_{12}$ deficiency has the same result. However, it also causes irreparable damage to the nervous system. Nevertheless, a dietary deficiency of vitamin B$_{12}$ is rare, since it is present in all foods of animal origin. It is also manufactured in small amounts by microorganisms in the gastrointestinal tract. The most common cause of deficiency in humans comes from the inherited or acquired absence of intrinsic factor needed for the absorption of vitamin B_{12}. This occurs most often in older individuals, usually beyond reproductive age. In younger persons, a strict vegetarian diet may eventually be associated with vitamin B_{12} deficiency.

Vitamin B_{12} has recently been used in the prenatal treatment of a fetus with methymalonic acidemia. A fetus can be treated "nutritionally" by supplementing the mother with the appropriate nutrient for the special needs of the offspring. A good example is that of prenatal diagnosis of methylmalonic acidemia; this is achieved by measuring the levels of methylmalonic acid in amnionic fluid and maternal urine and by measuring the incorporation of propionate labeled with carbon-14 into protein or by assaying methylmalonyl-coenzyme A mutase activity in chorionic villi or amniocytes. Some of these babies are responsive in utero to large doses of vitamin B_{12}. That is, the early postnatal problems (lethargy, recurrent vomiting, dehydration, respiratory distress, and muscular hypotonia) may be prevented, and with institution of the appropriate low-protein diet and supplementation program, normal growth and development can be anticipated. Prenatal treatment with appropriate nutrient supplements may allow for much improvement in the prognosis of these infants with inborn defects.

Vitamin B_6

Vitamin B_6, or pyridoxine, is another important nutrient concerned with amino acid metabolism and protein synthesis. In its active form as pyridoxal phosphate, the vitamin is a cofactor in reactions involving a group of enzymes known as **transaminases.** These enzymes work in the body to transfer the nitrogen-containing portion of certain amino acids to keto acid intermediaries from the Krebs cycle to synthesize some of the nonessential amino acids. Vitamin B_6 also functions in the reactions that convert tryptophan to niacin. Niacin, in turn, works as nicotinamide adenine dinucleotide along with pyridoxal phosphate in some of the transamination reactions. This is another example of how interdependent the nutrients are in normal metabolism. Vitamin B_6 requirements increase in preg-

nancy not only because of the greater need for nonessential amino acids in growth but also because the body is making more niacin from tryptophan.

Urinary excretion of vitamin B_6 metabolites during pregnancy is 10 to 15 times higher than in nonpregnant women, whereas blood values are typically reduced. Investigators are not sure what the clinical significance of this is. For some time there have been efforts to link vitamin B_6 to preeclampsia because urinary excretion is even higher in patients with preeclampsia than it is in normal pregnant women. It is far more likely that the observed values are the result of preeclampsia rather than a cause of it.

There is evidence that the placenta concentrates vitamin B_6 and that levels in cord blood are much higher than in the maternal circulation. This could mean that the reduced maternal blood levels are simply the result of physiological adjustments. On the other hand, there is also evidence that the fetus takes up more vitamin B_6 and that maternal levels increase when oral supplements are given.

In neonatal animals and human infants, vitamin B_6 deficiency has been shown to produce neurologic impairment as manifested by marked irritability, ataxia, tremor, abnormal gait, and seizures. Even though much has been learned about the metabolic and neurochemical alterations associated with neonatal vitamin B_6 deficiency, the mechanism(s) underlying the neurologic abnormalities are not clearly known. New and sensitive analytical and behavioral methods are now being applied to determine, at the molecular level, how the lack or the excess intake of a dietary component such as vitamin B_6 can influence brain chemistry and ultimately brain function and behavior.

The dietary allowance of 2.2 mg per day recommended in pregnancy is less than the amounts used by clinical investigators to bring blood levels up to nonpregnant standards, but few clinically significant conditions can be attributed to the levels of vitamin B_6 that are commonly observed. Limited animal data suggest adverse pregnancy outcome in the presence of vitamin B_6 deficiency. In addition, Scandinavian workers[69] observed that the depth of pure pregnancy depression correlated negatively with serum vitamin B_6 concentration. American researchers observed significantly lower APGAR scores in newborns of mothers with evidence of vitamin B_6 deficiency when compared with offspring of controls.[77,78] The meaning of these observations remains to be determined, since lack of a relationship between vitamin B_6 status and maternal or fetal status has also been reported.

Although the precise cause of nausea and vomiting during pregnancy remains unknown, interest continues in the possibility that vitamin B_6 status may be important. Vitamin B_6 is known to catalyze a number of reactions involving neurotransmitter production, but a clear connection between vitamin B_6 status and pregnancy nausea remains to be observed.[77,78]

The first use of pyridoxine for severe nausea and vomiting of pregnancy was reported in 1942; individual injections ranged from 10 to 100 mg with total doses up to 1,500 mg being given. Satisfactory relief was obtained in most cases. Other clinicians subsequently reported successful treatment of nausea with injected or oral doses of this vitamin. None of these studies was controlled or double-blind.

Fifty-nine women completed a randomized, double-blind placebo-controlled study of vitamin B_6 supplementation for treatment of nausea and vomiting of pregnancy.[76] Thirty-one patients received vitamin B_6, 25-mg tablets orally every 8 hours for 72 hours, and 28 patients received placebo in the same regimen. The severity of nausea was scored using a numerical scale; vomiting episodes were also recorded. Results indicated that women with mild to moderate nausea did not benefit from B_6 supplementation. However, women with severe nausea and vomiting showed a substantial reduction in their symptoms. It appears, therefore, that some benefits may be derived from B_6 supplementation by women with the most problematic forms of nausea and vomiting during early pregnancy.

Vitamin A

Vitamin A is an essential nutrient for all animal species because of its critical role in reproduction, the immune system, and vision, as well as in the maintenance of cellular differentiation. Both vitamin A and carotene cross the placenta.

Most of our information regarding requirements for vitamin A during pregnancy are extrapolations from animal studies, studies of nonpregnant adult women or observational studies of women who report night blindness while consuming diets of a certain vitamin A content. Although the need in pregnancy is increased above the nonpregnant state, this additional amount is relatively small and confined mostly to the last trimester. Maternal reserves are generally adequate (at least in developed countries) to meet the need. Therefore the RDA during pregnancy is not different from that of the nonpregnant state. A chronically inadequate intake below the basal requirement must take place to critically deplete maternal body stores before detrimental effects occur in the mother.

Although vitamin A deficiency is associated with adverse pregnancy outcome in animals that have been studied, little information is available from human observations. Several recent reports, however, are worth noting. In Indonesia, the influence of vitamin A and iron supplementation was studied in anemic pregnant women in a randomized, double-blind, placebo-controlled field trial.[86] Subjects were randomly assigned to a supplement routine, which provided vitamin A, iron, or both; supplements were taken daily for 8 weeks. Maximum improvement in the anemic state was seen when both vitamin A and iron were provided. It was concluded that improvement in vitamin A status may contribute to the control of anemia in pregnant women.

A recent study in Malawi showed that vitamin A status is an important risk factor for the mother-to-child transmission of human immunodeficiency virus (HIV).[79] Among mothers with HIV infection, an association was observed between serum vitamin A and subsequent mother-to-child transmission rates. The relative risk of HIV transmission was four times greater in mothers with serum vitamin A less than 0.7-μmol/L compared with serum vitamin A greater than 1.40 μmol/L. This study suggests that vitamin A supplementation may be an economic and relatively simple intervention to reduce mother-to-child transmission of the virus.

Excessive consumption of vitamin A is known to be teratogenic in both animals and humans.[35] At least seven case reports of adverse pregnancy

TABLE 5-14   *Some Cases of Birth Defects Associated with High Maternal Intake of Vitamin A*

Maternal Intake	Duration	Symptoms	Other Conditions
Reports of individual cases			
~500 000 IU	Single dose, second month	Preauricular appendices, epibulbar dermatoid (eye malformations similar to Goldenhar's syndrome)	Dose caused acute toxicity in the pregnant woman
150 000 IU	Periconceptual −2 to +3 mo	Facial dysmorphism, pterygium colli, distended abdomen, absence of external genitalia and of anal and urethral openings, polycystic kidneys, dysmorphism of lumbar spine	Fetus aborted at 20 wk because of spinal abnormality and polycystic kidney
25 000 IU	0–13 wk	Unilateral ureteral duplication with one ureter ending in the vagina, hydronephrosis, hydroureters	
50 000 IU	14 wk to term		
Reports of multiple cases			
18 000–100 000 IU	Before and throughout pregnancy	Abnormalities of the head, face, ears, eyes, mouth, lips, jaws, heart, and urinary system; other defects	Cases reported by physicians to FDA; cases reported to NY State Birth Defect Registry

Data from Vallet H, et al: *Unpublished observations,* 1985.

outcome have been associated with a daily ingestion of 25,000 IU or more.[45] These data derive from 11 Adverse Drug Reaction Reports associated with the use of vitamin A during pregnancy that were filed with the Food and Drug Administration (FDA). Almost all of the FDA cases are brief retrospective reports of malformed infants or fetuses exposed to supplements of at least 25,000 IU per day of vitamin A during pregnancy (Table 5-14). In addition, epidemiologic evidence has accumulated that the drug isotretinoin (used for treatment of cystic acne) causes major malformations involving craniofacial, central nervous system, cardiac and thymic structures[5]; isotretinoin is a retinoid analog.

Since 1990, additional evidence has accumulated about the teratogenicity of vitamin A. Two epidemiological studies addressed the issue. Werler et al[95] examined 2,658 cases of birth defects (derived at least in part from neural crest cells), primarily craniofacial and cardiac malformations; these cases were compared with 2,609 infants with other malformations. Vitamin A supplementation was defined as daily use for at least 7 days of retinol alone or with vitamin D, or of fish oils. Information on vitamin A dose and nutrition was not available. Risk of neural crest-related birth defects was increased with reported vitamin A supplement use—2.5 times for lunar month 1, 2.3 times for lunar month 2, and 1.6 times for lunar month 3.

Martinez-Frias and Salvador[52] reported the results of an epidemiological study of prenatal exposure to high doses of vitamin A in Spain, using data from the Spanish hospital-based case-control registry. Results suggested that a teratogenic effect might exist for exposures of 40,000 IU or more.

Evans and Hickey-Dwyer[31] reported a case of hourglass cornea and iris with reduplicated lens in the left eye of an infant girl. An excess of vitamin A products had been taken by the mother during pregnancy. She had taken on average 10 capsules of royal jelly and six multivitamin tablets per week throughout the pregnancy. In addition, she had consumed three meals containing liver per week during the first trimester only, which she had been informed would be beneficial. Her estimated average daily dose of vitamin A was 25,000 IU in the first trimester.

Vitamin A is heavily involved in embryonic development. It has been referred to as a "morphogen;" it rapidly diffuses into susceptible tissues and changes cells' "positional information." In this capacity, it has the potential of altering developmental processes. Neural crest cells and their derivatives appear to be highly susceptible to this phenomenon. Recent evidence indicates that the teratogenic effect of retinoids may derive from an effect on the expression of a specific gene that regulates axial patterning in the embryo (see box at right).

The most impressive report to date on the teratogenicity of retinol derived from data collected by researchers at Boston University.[72] They interviewed 22,748 pregnant women when they underwent screening either by amniocentesis or by measurement of maternal serum alphafetoprotein. Information was obtained about the women's diet, medications, and illnesses during the first trimester, as well as information on their family and medical history and exposure to environmental agents. Information on the outcome of pregnancy was obtained largely from the obstetricians. Of the 22,748 women, 339 had babies with birth defects; 121 of these babies had defects occurring in sites that originated in the cranial neural crest. Results indicated that the higher the intake of vitamin A during the first trimester, the greater the risk of a birth defect associated with neural crest cells (e.g., craniofacial, cardiac, thymic, and central nervous system structures) (Table 5-15). The increased frequency of defects was concentrated among the babies whose mothers consumed high levels of vitamin A before the seventh week of gestation. Among the babies born to mothers who took more than 10,000 IU of preformed vitamin A per day in the form of sup-

❖

RETINOID THERAPY FOR SEVERE DERMATOLOGICAL DISORDERS

STATEMENT BY THE AMERICAN ACADEMY OF PEDIATRICS, COMMITTEE ON DRUGS

Recommendations

1. Isotretinoin should be prescribed only for patients with severe cystic acne who are unresponsive to standard therapies.
2. Isotretinoin should not be given to women of childbearing potential unless the following conditions are met: (a) the patient visits a health professional for contraceptive counseling, with which the patient must be able to comply, before beginning the drug; (b) results of serum pregnancy test are negative within 2 weeks of beginning the drug and every month during treatment; (c) the drug is started on the third day of a normal menstrual period; and (d) the patient has received oral and written warning of the reproductive hazards of isotretinoin and etretinate during pregnancy and has acknowledged in writing her understanding of those warnings. It must be emphasized that one third of the affected infants reported by Lammer et al[3] were born to mothers using contraception. The manufacturer recommends that two contraceptive measures be used simultaneously.
3. Etretinate should not be prescribed for women of childbearing potential.
4. Isotretinoin and etretinate should be prescribed only by those physicians with experience in the therapy (total and stepwise) of severe dermatological disorders.

From Committee on Drugs: Retinoid therapy for severe dermatological disorders, *Pediatrics* 90:119, 1992.

plements, it was estimated that about one infant in 57 would have a malformation attributable to the supplement (Fig. 5-12). The Teratology Society[87] urges that women in their reproductive years be informed that the excessive use of vitamin A shortly before and

TABLE 5-15 *Pregnancies Resulting in Neural Crest-Derived Birth Defects According to Daily Retinol Intake and Source of Retinol*

	# Defects	% Defects
Daily Retinol Intake (IU)		
0-5000	33	0.51
5001-10,000	59	0.47
10,001-15,000	20	0.63
>15,001	9	1.8
Retinol intake from food (IU)		
0-5000	114	0.52
5001-10,000	5	0.62
10,001-15,000	2	1.06
Retinol intake from supplements		
0-5000	51	0.46
5001-8,000	54	0.51
8001-10,000	9	1.18
>10,001	7	2.21

From Rothman KJ: Teratogenicity of high vitamin A intake, *New Engl J Med* 333:1369, 1995.

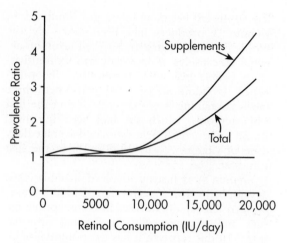

FIG. 5-12 Estimated prevalence ratio for birth defects related to the cranial neural crest, according to the retinol intake during the first trimester of pregnancy. The prevalence ratio is the ratio of the prevalence of defects among the babies born to women who consumed a given amount of vitamin A (from food and supplements—total—or from supplements alone) to the prevalence among the babies of women with a hypothetical intake of zero.

From Rothman KJ et al: Teratogenicity of high vitamin A intake, *New Engl J Med* 333:1369, 1995.

during pregnancy could be harmful to their babies. This group also suggests that manufacturers of vitamin A should lower the maximum amount of vitamin A per unit dosage to 5,000 to 8,000 IU and identify the source of vitamin A. They further support the practice of labeling of products containing vitamin A to indicate that consumption of excessive amounts of vitamin A may be hazardous to the embryo or fetus when taken during pregnancy, and that women of childbearing age should consult with their physicians before consuming these products.

Topical application of retinoids does not appear to pose a problem. Researchers in Seattle used information from the Group Health Cooperative of Puget Sound, Washington, USA, to evaluate the risk of birth defects in mothers exposed to topical tretinoin (a retinoid preparation used to treat acne) in the first trimester of pregnancy.[38] In the study, 215 women were identified who had delivered live or stillborn infants at

Group Health Cooperative hospitals and who were exposed to topical tretinoin early in pregnancy; 430 age-matched, nonexposed women who had delivered live or stillborn babies at the same hospitals comprised the control group. The prevalence of major anomalies among infants born to the exposed women was 1.9% and among babies born to the nonexposed women was 2.6%. It was concluded that topical tretinoin is not associated with an increased risk of major congenital disorders.

Vitamin C

Vitamin C functions in reactions that oxidize proline, a nonessential amino acid, to hydroxyproline. Hydroxyproline is used to form the collagen matrix in connective tissue, skin, tendons, and bones.

Vitamin C deficiency has not been shown to affect the course or outcome of pregnancy in humans. Questions have arisen, however, about its possible association with several specific conditions made known through isolated clinical observations; low plasma levels of vitamin C have been reported to be associated with premature rupture of the membranes and preeclampsia. An extra 15 mg of vitamin C is recommended daily for the pregnant woman; this total recommendation of 60 mg daily is easily met by the U.S. diet. Massive intake of vitamin C supplements may adversely influence fetal metabolism. Metabolic dependency on high doses may develop in the offspring such that scurvy may arise in the neonatal period.

Vitamin E

The most active form of vitamin E is alphatocopherol. Its principal function is to prevent the oxidation of unsaturated fatty acids, which make up the structure of cell membranes. Vitamin E also prevents the oxidation of vitamin A in the gastrointestinal tract so that more vitamin A in the diet can be absorbed.

Vitamin E needs are believed to increase somewhat during pregnancy, but deficiency in humans rarely occurs and has not been linked with either reproductive causality or reduced fertility. Since vitamin E deficiency in experimental animals has long been associated with spontaneous abortion, interest in the use of vitamin E for prevention of abortion has been a popular idea. In general, however, studies in humans have been negative in their support for this preventive measure. Several studies have shown, however, that the fetal vitamin E level is one-third to one-fourth the maternal concentration in both premature and term infants. Maternal levels of vitamin E rise during pregnancy such that by the third trimester these levels become 60% greater than in the nonpregnant controls. It has been found, however, that the maternal level must be from 150% to 500% of the value in the nonpregnant controls if the cord blood values are to reach the low-normal adult vitamin E concentrations.

Although the vitamin E level in the infant at birth is significantly less than in the mother, the infant's level has been shown to correlate directly with the maternal concentration. Attempts to raise the fetal level by supplementing the mother with vitamin E during the last trimester confirmed the direct correlation of fetal and maternal vitamin E concentrations but also indicated the great difficulty encountered by the administration of alphatocopherol to the mother. Thus it has been concluded that parenteral vitamin E administration to the mother before delivery is not enough to prevent an infant from having the hemolytic anemia of vitamin E deficiency. Since this problem develops within 6 weeks after birth, it can best be prevented by oral supplementation of the infant during the postnatal interval.

Vitamin D

Vitamin D has long been appreciated for its positive effects on calcium balance during pregnancy.[83] Evidence suggests that vitamin D may be involved in neonatal calcium homeostasis. Observations in Great Britain indicate that the peak season for neonatal hypocalcemia coincides with the time of least sunlight. In addition, serum vitamin D levels are often low in such infants, suggesting that some cases of neonatal hypocalcemia and/or **enamel hypoplasia** may relate to maternal vitamin D deficiency and subsequent limitation in placental transport of vitamin D to the fetus. One study of pregnant women and their offspring showed that vitamin D supplementation during the third trimester was associated with improved perinatal handling of calcium.[9,25]

Clinical osteomalacia is found in between 10% and 30% of the Asian immigrant population in northern Europe; between 25% and 53% have biochemical disease. Pregnancy is a serious risk factor following the increased requirements for calcium and vitamin D. Unfortunately, failure to recognize the clinical features of maternal osteomalacia still occurs. Problematic features include a small, deformed pelvis, which often precludes vaginal delivery; other musculoskeletal complications are also common, with bone pain and proximal myopathy both producing impairment in mobility. Routine biochemical screening for osteomalacia in this high-risk population is justified; other routine procedures might be vitamin D supplementation, placental function testing, predelivery pelvimetry and neonatal monitoring for hypocalcemia.[64]

Maternal ingestion of large amounts of vitamin D may be harmful to the developing fetus.[94] Data supporting the relationship between prenatal vitamin D excess and infantile hypercalcemia include the following:

1. Between 1953 and 1955 more than 200 cases were seen in Great Britain; at the same time fewer than 10 patients were reported in the United States. It was noticed that supplementation of vitamin D ensured that British subjects with a vitamin D intake approximately 5 to 6 times that of the U.S. average. When the British intake was reduced to 400 IU per day, infantile hypercalcemia promptly became a rarity.
2. Beuren et al (1964) noted similar facies and vascular lesions in German infants whose mothers had received several massive doses of vitamin D (500,000 IU) during pregnancy.
3. Friedman and Roberts (1966) showed a high incidence of arterial stenosis in rabbits whose mothers had been given large doses of vitamin D.

Vitamin K

Vitamin K is well-known to be essential for assisting in the normal process of blood clotting. Maternal dietary deficiency is almost unheard of, but transport of this vitamin across the placenta is slow. Newborns often have low body levels of vitamin K. This may be rectified by postnatal vitamin K supplementation of the baby, but concern is substantial for the infant who is born preterm. Risk of intraventricular (brain) hemorrhage is el-

❖ ❖ ❖

CASE STUDY

Folic Acid Supplementation

Marcia Nahikian-Nelms PhD, RD, Southwest Missouri State University

You are a nutritionist for a metropolitan clinic that serves a large multi-ethnic prenatal population. As part of the clinics health care team, you have been asked to evaluate the latest research and recommendations regarding the role of folic acid and neural tube defects (NTDs). From this data, you are to present to the staff your recommendations for supplementation and education to the clinic's prenatal population. Before you can make any recommendations, there is some basic information that you must clarify about folic acid.

1. What is the basic physiological role of folic acid?
   Why are those roles so critical in the prenatal period?
   What are the factors that increase the requirement during pregnancy?
2. What effects the availability of folic acid in the diet and why may that amount be so variable?
3. The deficiency of folic acid is megaloblastic anemia. Can someone have inadequate amounts of folic acid and not develop megaloblastic anemia?

Now that you are clear about the role of folic acid during pregnancy, you must tackle the latest research regarding the role of folic acid and NTDs.

3. At what point during the prenatal period do NTDs develop?
4. Do we understand the exact mechanism that folic acid supplementation may play in the prevention of NTDs?
   You have come to the conclusion that nutrition education and supplementation is warranted for your clinic populations.
5. What information can you use to justify and support your decision to provide supplementation and nutrition education to your clinic population?
   What clients would you target and why?
6. In a recent gallup poll, fewer than 50% of those surveyed had ever heard or read about folic acid. Design an outline for a nutrition class that would provide the necessary information about folic acid and nutrition recommendations that would meet the needs of your clinic population.

evated; this event still remains as the most devastating neurological happening in the perinatal period. Whether supplementing the mother before delivery with vitamin K will improve the condition of the newborn with regard to this vitamin remains to be determined. Evidence for[3,57] and against[26,40,41,88,89] this idea has been presented.

Summary   ~~Conclusion~~

Maintenance of health during the course of pregnancy obviously requires an adequate supply of calories and protein, as well as sufficient amounts of specific vitamins. Precise requirements for each of these nutrients have not been established, but recommendations for daily intake have been devised on the basis of available evidence. The consequences of specific nutrient deficiencies and excesses are only partially understood. Although a number of animal experiments have been completed during the past 30 years, data from humans largely represent only fortuitous observations of natural events in individual women.

Among the nutrients that have received special attention are folic acid, vitamin B_6, vitamin A, and vitamin D. Reports by European investigators suggest a relationship between folic acid deficiency and the incidence of neural-tube defects. Nausea and depression of pregnancy have been proposed to relate to vitamin B_6 deficiency; low APGAR scores have been reported among offspring of women whose diets and biochemical indicators of B_6 status suggest deficiency. Hypervitaminosis A in pregnant women has been anecdotally related to congenital malformations in their offspring. Poor enamel development and neonatal hypocalcemia have been associated with maternal vitamin D deficiency; excessive exposure to vitamin D prenatally is reportedly linked to neonatal hypercalcemia, calcification of soft tissues, and craniofacial abnormalities.

Although considerable controversy obviously exists about the etiologic relationships between nutrient status and pregnancy course and outcome, evidence supports some possible relationships that should be regarded as potentially significant.

REVIEW QUESTIONS

1. Explain why thinking about energy requirements during pregnancy is in the process of change.
2. Why has the issue of protein excess during pregnancy become a matter of concern?
3. What is known about the impact of specific vitamin deficiencies and excesses during pregnancy on pregnancy course and outcome?

LEARNING ACTIVITIES

1. Investigate the composition of available prenatal nutritional supplements.
2. Assess the nature of nutrition information provided to pregnant women in your area.
3. Determine the resources available in your community for nutrition information for pregnant women.

REFERENCES

1. Ackman RG: Birthweights in the Faroe Islands: possible role of isovaleric acid, *J Int Med* 255:73, 1989.
2. Al MD et al: The essential fatty acid status of mother and child in pregnancy-induced hypertension: a prospective longitudinal study, *Am J Obstet Gynecol* 172:1605, 1995.
3. Anai T et al: Can prenatal vitamin K-1 (phylloquinone) supplementation replace prophylaxis at birth? *Obstet Gynecol* 81:251, 1993.
4. Andrews JF et al: Brown adipose tissue thermogenesis during pregnancy in mice, *Ann Nutr Metab* 30:87, 1986.
5. Benke PJ: The isotretinoin teratogen syndrome, *JAMA* 251:3267, 1984.
6. Blackburn ML, Calloway DH: Energy expenditure of pregnant adolescents, *J Am Diet Assoc* 65:24, 1974.
7. Brewer TH: Metabolic toxemia of late pregnancy in a county prenatal nutrition education project: a preliminary report, *J Reprod Med* 13:175, 1974.
8. Brewer T: Role of malnutrition in pre-eclampsia and eclampsia, *Am J Obstet Gynecol* 125:281, 1977.
9. Brooke OG et al: Vitamin D supplements in pregnant Asian women; effects on calcium status and fetal growth, *BMJ* 1:751, 1980.

10. Bunduki, V., Dommergues, M., Zittoun, J., Marquet, J., Muller, F. and Dumez, Y. Maternal-fetal folate status and neural tube defects: a case-control study. Biol Neonate 67:154, 1995.

11. Burke BS: The influence of nutrition upon the condition of the infant at birth, *J Nutr* 26:569, 1943.

12. Burke BS, Harding VV, Stuart HC: Nutrition studies during pregnancy. IV. Relation of protein content of the mother's diet during pregnancy to birth length, birth weight, and condition of the infant at birth, *J Pediatr* 23:506, 1943.

13. Chez RA, Curcio FD: Ketonuria in normal pregnancy, *Obstet Gynecol* 69:272, 1987.

14. Churchill JA, Berendes HW: Intelligence of children whose mothers had acetonuria during pregnancy. In Perinatal factors affecting human development, Sci Rev, No. 185, Washington, DC, 1969, Pan American Health Organization.

15. Churchill JA, Berendes HW, Nemore J: Neuropsychological deficits in children of diabetic mothers, *Am J Obstet Gynecol* 105:257, 1969.

16. Coetzee EF, Jackson WPU, Berman PA: Ketonuria in pregnancy with special reference to caloric-restricted food intake in obese diabetics, *Diabetes* 29:177, 1980.

17. Crane NT et al: Evaluating food fortification options: general principles revisited with folic acid, *Am J Public Health* 85:660, 1995.

18. Crawford MA: The role of essential fatty acids in neural development: implications for perinatal nutrition, *Am J Clin Nutr* 57(suppl):703S, 1993.

19. Czeizel AE: Congenital abnormalities are preventable, *Epidemiol* 6:205, 1995.

20. Czeizel AE: Folic acid in the prevention of neural tube defects, *J Pediatr Gastroent Nutr* 20:4, 1995.

21. Czeizel AE, Dudas, I: Prevention of the first occurrence of neural-tube defects by periconceptional vitamin supplementation, *N Engl J Med* 327:1832, 1992.

22. Daly L et al: Folate levels and neural tube defects. Implications for prevention. *JAMA* 274:1698, 1995.

23. Davis BA et al: Folic acid absorption in women with a history of pregnancy with neural tube defect, *Am J Clin Nutr* 62:782, 1995.

24. de Groot L et al: Energy balances of healthy Dutch women before and during pregnancy: limited scope for metabolic adaptations in pregnancy, *Am J Clin Nutr* 59:827, 1994.

25. Delvin EE et al: Vitamin D supplementation during pregnancy: effect on calcium homeostasis, *J Pediatr* 109:328, 1986.

26. Dickson RC, Stubbs TN, Lazarchick J: Antenatal vitamin K therapy of the low-birth-weight infant, *Am J Obstet Gynecol* 170:85, 1994.

27. Doyle W et al: Maternal nutrient intake and birth weight, *J Hum Nutr Diet* 2:407, 1989.

28. Durnin JVGA: Energy requirements of pregnancy: an integration of the longitudinal data from the five-country study, *Lancet* 2:1131, 1987.

29. Durnin JVGA et al: Energy requirements of pregnancy in Scotland, *Lancet* 2:897, 1987.

29a. Durnin JVGA et al: Is nutritional status endangered by virtually no extra intake during pregnancy? *Lancet* 2:823, 1985.

30. Evans, K and Hickey-Dwyer, M.U. Cleft anterior segment with maternal hypervitaminosis A, *Br J Ophthamol* 75:691, 1991.

31. Felig P, Lynch V: Starvation in human pregnancy: hypoglycemia, hypoinsulinemia and hyperketonemia, *Science* 170:990, 1970.

32. Forsum E, Sadurskis A, Wager J: Energy maintenance cost during pregnancy in healthy Swedish women, *Lancet* 2:107, 1985.

33. Grieve JF: Prevention of gestational failure by high protein diet, *J Reprod Med* 13:170, 1974.

34. Habicht JP, Yarbrough C: Efficiency of selecting pregnant women for food supplementation during pregnancy. In Aebi, H, Whitehead, RG, editors: *Maternal nutrition during pregnancy and lactation*, Bern, 1980, Hans Huber.

35. Hathcock JN et al: Evaluation of vitamin A toxicity, *Am J Clin Nutr* 52:183, 1990.

36. Hurley LS: *Developmental nutrition*, Englewood Cliffs, NJ, 1980, Prentice-Hall.

37. Hytten FF and Chamberlain G: *Clinical physiology in obstetrics*, Oxford, 1980, Blackwell Scientific Publications.

38. Jick SS, Terris BZ, Jick H: First trimester topical tretinoin and congenital disorders, *Lancet* 341:1181, 1993.

39. Kaplan M, Eidelman AI, Aboulafia Y: Fasting and the precipitation of labor; the Yom Kippur effect, *JAMA* 250:1317, 1983.

40. Kazzi NJ et al: Maternal administration of vitamin K does not improve the coagulation profile of preterm infants, *Pediatrics* 84:1045, 1989.

41. Kazzi NJ, Iiagan NB, Liang K et al: Placental transfer of vitamin K_1 in preterm pregnancy, *Obstet Gynecol* 75:334, 1990.

42. King JC: Protein metabolism during pregnancy, *Clin Perinatol* 2:243, 1975.

43. Klebanoff MA, Shiono PH, Carey JC: The effect of physical activity during pregnancy on preterm delivery and birth weight, *Am J Obstet Gynecol* 163:1450, 1990.

44. Kramer MS: Effects of energy and protein intakes on pregnancy outcome: an overview of the research evidence from controlled clinical trials, *Am J Clin Nutr* 58:627, 1993.

45. Lammer EJ et al: Retinoic acid embryopathy, *N Engl J Med* 313:837, 1985.

46. Laurence KM et al: Double-blind randomised controlled trial of folate treatment before conception to prevent recurrence of neural-tube defects, *Br Med J* 282:1509, 1981.

47. Laurence KM et al: Increased risk of recurrence of pregnancies complicated by fetal neural tube defects in mothers receiving poor diets, and possible benefit of dietary counselling, *Br Med J* 281:1592, 1980.

48. Lawrence M et al: Energy requirements of pregnancy in the Gambia, *Lancet* 2:1072, 1987.

49. Li D et al: Periconceptional multivitamin use in relation to the risk of congenital urinary tract anomalies, *Epidemiol* 6:212, 1995.

50. Little RE, Sing CF: Association of father's drinking and infant's birth weight, *N Engl J Med* 314:1644, 1986.

51. Lorentzen B et al: Fatty acid pattern of esterified and free fatty acids in sera of women with normal and preeclamptic pregnancy, *Br J Obstet Gynecol* 102:530, 1995.

52. Martinez-Frias ML, Salvador J: Epidemiological aspects of prenatal exposure to high doses of vitamin A in Spain, *Eur J Epidemiol* 6:118, 1990.

53. McPartlin J et al: Accelerated folate breakdown in pregnancy, *Lancet* 341:148, 1993.

54. Mills JL et al: Homocysteine metabolism in pregnancies complicated by neural tube defects, *Lancet* 345:149, 1995.

55. Mills et al: and the National Inst Child Health Human Development Neural Tube Defects Study Group. The absence of a relation between the periconceptional use of vitamins and neural tube defects, *N Engl J Med* 321:430, 1989.

56. Morbidity and Mortality Weekly Report: Knowledge and use of folic acid by women of childbearing age-United States, 1995, *JAMA* 274:1190, 1995.

57. Morales WJ, Angel JL, O'Brien WF et al: The use of antenatal vitamin K in the prevention of early neonatal intraventricular hemorrhage, *Am J Obstet Gynecol* 159:774, 1988.

58. MRC Vitamin Study Research Group: Prevention of neural tube defects: results of the Medical Research Council Vitamin Study, *Lancet* 338:131, 1991.

59. Murphy, S.P. and Abrams, B.F. Changes in energy intakes during pregnancy and lactation in a national sample of US women, *Am J Public Health* 83:1161, 1993.

60. Naeye RL: Teenaged and pre-teenaged pregnancies: consequences of the fetal-maternal competition for nutrients, *Pediatrics* 67:146, 1981.

61. National Research Council, Food and Nutrition Board: *Recommended dietary allowances,* Washington, DC. 1989, National Academy Press.

62. Oakley G: Urgent need to increase folic acid consumption, *JAMA* 274:1717, 1995.

63. Osofsky HJ: Relationship between prenatal medical and nutritional measures, pregnancy outcome and early infant development in an urban poverty setting, *Am J Obstet Gynecol* 123:682, 1975.

64. Park W et al: Osteomalacia of the mother-rickets of the newborn, *Eur J Pediatr* 146:292, 1987.

65. Picciano, M.F., Green, T. and O'Connor, D.L. The folate status of women and health, *Nutr Today* 29(6):20, 1994.

66. Poppitt SD et al: Energy-sparing strategies to protect human fetal growth, *Am J Obstet Gynecol* 171:118, 1994.

67. Poppitt, S.D., Prentice, A.M., Jequier, E., Schutz, Y., and Whitehead, R.G. Evidence of energy sparing in Gambian women during pregnancy: a longitudinal study using whole body calorimetry. Am J Clin Nutr 57:353, 1993.

68. Prentice AM et al: Metabolic consequences of fasting during Ramadan in pregnant and lactating women, *Hum Nutr Clin Nutr* 37C:283, 1983.

69. Pulkkinen MO, Salminen J, Virtanen S: Serum vitamin B_6 in pure pregnancy depression, *Acta Obstet Gynecol Scand* 57:471, 1978.

70. Purdie DW, Aaron JE, Selby PL: Bone histology and mineral hemeostasis in human pregnancy, *Br J Obstet Gynecol* 95:849, 1988.

71. Rosso P: Nutrition and maternal-fetal exchange, *Am J Clin Nutr* 34:744, 1981.

72. Rothman KJ et al: Teratogenicity of high vitamin A intake, *N Engl J Med* 333:1369, 1995.

73. Rush D: Periconceptional folate and neural tube defect, *Am J Clin Nutr* 59(suppl):511S, 1994.

74. Rush D, Stein Z, Susser M: *Diet in pregnancy: a randomized controlled trial of nutritional supplements,* New York, 1980, Alan R. Liss.

75. Rush D, Stein Z, and Susser M. Controlled trial of prenatal supplementation defended, *Pediatrics* 66:656, 1980.

76. Sahakian V et al: Vitamin B_6 is effective therapy for nausea and vomiting of pregnancy: a randomized double-blind placebo-controlled study, *Obstet Gynecol* 78:33, 1991.

77. Schuster K et al: Morning sickness and vitamin B_6 status of pregnant women, *Hum Nutr Clin Nutr* 39C:75, 1985.

78. Schuster K, Bailey LB, Mahan CS: Effect of maternal pyridoxine HCl supplementation on the vitamin B_6 status of mother and infant and on pregnancy outcome, *J Nutr* 114, 977, 1984.

79. Semba RD et al: Maternal vitamin A deficiency and mother-to-child transmission of HIV-1, *Lancet* 343:1593, 1994.

80. Shaw GM et al: Risks of orofacial clefts in children born to women using multivitamins containing folic acid periconceptionally, *Lancet* 346:393, 1995.

81. Smithells RW, Schorah CJ: A possible role of periconceptional multivitamin supplementation in the prevention of the recurrence of neural tube defects. In Bendich A, Butterworth CE, Jr, editors: *Micronutrients in health and in disease prevention,* New York, Marcel Dekker, 1991.

82. Smithells RW et al: Apparent prevention of neural tube defects by periconceptional vitamin supplementation, *Arch Dis Child* 56:911, 1981.

83. Specker BL: Do North American women need supplemental vitamin D during pregnancy or lactation? *Am J Clin Nutr* 59(suppl):484S, 1994.

84. Stebhens JA, Baker GI, Kitchell, M: Outcome at ages 1, 3, and 5 years of children born to diabetic mothers, *Am J Obstet Gynecol* 127:408, 1977.

85. Steegers-Theunissen RP et al: Neural tube defects and elevated homocysteine levels in amniotic fluid, *Am J Obstet Gynecol* 172:1436, 1995.

86. Suharno D et al: Supplementation with vitamin A and iron for nutritional anemia in pregnant women in West Java, Indonesia, *Lancet* 342:1325, 1993.

87. Teratology Society: Teratology Society position paper: recommendations for vitamin A use during pregnancy, *Teratology* 35:269, 1987.

88. Thorp JA et al: combined antenatal vitamin K and phenobarbital therapy for preventing intracranial hemorrhage in newborns less than 34 weeks gestation, *Obstet Gynecol* 86:1, 1995.

89. Thorp JA et al: Antepartum vitamin K and phenobarbital for preventing intraventricular hemorrhage in the premature newborn: a randomized, double-blind, placebo-controlled trial, *Obstet Gynecol* 83:70, 1994.

90. van Raaij JMA et al: Energy cost of physical activity throughout pregnancy and the first year postpartum in Dutch women with sedentary lifestyles, *Am J Clin Nutr* 52:234, 1990.

91. van Raaij JMA et al: Energy cost of walking at a fixed pace and self-paced before, during and after pregnancy, *Am J Clin Nutr* 51:158, 1990.

92. Vergel, R.G., Sanchez, L.R., Heredero, B.L. et al: Primary prevention of neural tube defects with folic acid supplementation: Cuban experience, *Prenat Diagnos* 10:149, 1990.

93. Vilbergsson G, Samsioe G., Wennergren, M. and Karlsson, K: Essential fatty acids in pregnancies complicated by intrauterine growth retardation, *Int J Gynecol Obstet* 36:277, 1991.

94. Weisman Y, Harell A, Edelstein S: Infantile hypercalcemia: a defect in the esterification of 1,25-dihydroxyvitamin D? *Med Hypoth* 5:37 1979.

95. Werler MM et al: Maternal vitamin A supplementation in relation to selected birth defects, *Teratol* 42:497, 1990.

96. Williams C et al: Protein, amino acid and caloric intakes of selected pregnant women, *J Am Diet Assoc* 78:28, 1981.

97. Zimmerman MB, Shane B: Supplemental folic acid, *Am J Clin Nutr* 58:127, 1993.

98. Zlatnik FJ, Burmeister LF: Dietary protein in pregnancy: effect on anthrometric indices of the newborn infant, *Am J Obstet Gynecol* 146:199, 1983.

6

Mineral Needs During Pregnancy

Bonnie Worthington-Roberts

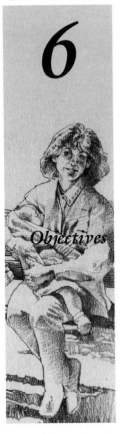

Objectives

✦✦✦

After completing this chapter, the student will be able to:

✓ *Discuss the pros and cons of iron supplementation during pregnancy*

✓ *Summarize the current research interests in the role that calcium might play in hypertensive disorders of pregnancy*

✓ *Define cretinism and indicate its role in the prevalence of mental retardation worldwide*

✓ *Outline what is known about other mineral deficiencies as far as human pregnancy and outcome is concerned*

Introduction

Minerals are inorganic compounds that are required for human survival. Needs for minerals during pregnancy increase; should diet not provide what is required, pregnant women will need to access their stores to assure the fetus of sufficient support. In the process, the mother may exit pregnancy with mineral depletion. At the same time, excess mineral intake may adversely affect mother and/or fetus. An appropriate balance is desirable.

MINERALS

Iron

The importance of folic acid and vitamin B_{12} in the production of red blood cells has been

discussed. These two nutrients must be accompanied by adequate amounts of protein and other vitamins and minerals for normal **erythropoiesis.** Adequacy of these supplies is indicated by the concentration of hemoglobin in the blood. Hemoglobin is responsible for carrying oxygen to the body's cells. One of its chief components is iron.

During pregnancy, iron is needed for the manufacture of hemoglobin in both maternal and fetal red blood cells.[6] The fetus accumulates most of its iron during the last trimester. At term a normal-weight infant has about 246 mg of iron in blood and body stores. An additional 134 mg is stored in the placenta, and about 290 mg is used to expand the volume of the mother's blood (Table 6-1).

TABLE 6-1   *Iron "Cost" of a Normal Pregnancy*

Iron contributed to the fetus	200-370 mg
Iron in placenta and cord	30-170 mg
Iron in blood lost at delivery	90-310 mg
TOTAL	310-850 mg*

*These figures are in addition to the normal excretory loss of 0.5 to 1.0 mg per day and ignore the demand during the second half of pregnancy for iron to support the expansion of red-cell mass. This latter amount (200 to 600 mg) is not included as an iron "cost" because it is largely conserved (and not lost from the body) when the red-cell mass returns to normal after delivery.

From Bothwell TH et al: *Iron metabolism in man,* Oxford, Blackwell, 1979.

Maintenance of erythropoiesis is one of the few instances during pregnancy when the fetus acts as a true parasite. It ensures its own production of hemoglobin by drawing iron from the mother. Maternal iron deficiency therefore does not usually result in an infant who is anemic at birth. The most common cause of iron deficiency anemia in the infant is prematurity. The infant who has a short gestation does not have time to accumulate sufficient iron during the last trimester.

Iron deficiency in the mother may have adverse effects on her obstetrical performance. As has been previously noted, a reduction in hemoglobin concentration means that the mother must increase her cardiac output to maintain adequate oxygen consumption by placental and fetal cells. This extra work fatigues the mother and makes her more susceptible to other sources of physiologic stress. A very low hemoglobin level places the mother at risk of cardiac arrest and leads to a poor prognosis for survival should she hemorrhage on delivery.

Setting requirements for iron during pregnancy is complicated by changes in the erythropoietic system. Even when women have adequate iron status at conception, the plasma volume increases faster than the number of red blood cells so that hemodilution occurs. However, erythropoiesis is stimulated in the last half of pregnancy, and the rate of hemoglobin production increases. If sufficient iron is available, hemoglobin levels should rise to at least 11.5 mg per 100 ml by term (Fig. 6-1).

It is generally conceded that the initial drop in hemoglobin is a normal physiological phenomenon, but there is concern that the usual iron intakes of pregnant women may not support increased erythropoiesis and fetal demands in the last half of pregnancy. Iron absorption from the gastrointestinal tract increases during pregnancy, possibly to as much as 50% compared with the usual 10% to 20% absorption from the diet.

French researchers provided evidence that the increased iron absorption during pregnancy may satisfy the iron needs of the pregnant women.[8] Twelve women were studied at intervals during gestation; eight of them were also evaluated in the postpartum period. The main absorption of iron at 24 weeks gestation was five times higher than at 12 weeks. It doubled once more, and by 36 weeks, it was 9.1 times the mean absorption at 12 weeks. The absorption of iron after delivery decreased to levels not significantly different from those found in early pregnancy. Calculations based on the available data indicated that the increase in iron absorption is sufficient to meet the increased requirements of pregnancy. Given the long evolution of the adaptations of human pregnancy, it would be surprising if iron absorption from dietary sources was not sufficient for most pregnancies. In other words, the findings in this study are precisely what should be expected.

It has been estimated that the pregnant woman probably needs 18 to 21 mg of iron in her diet each day. This could be supplied if large servings of iron-rich foods are eaten; unfortunately, such foods are limited in the U.S. diet. From an average mixed diet, approximately 6 mg of iron are obtained from each 1,000 kcal of food. At this rate a pregnant woman would have to eat 3,000 to 5,000 kcal per day to meet her iron needs. Furthermore, studies have shown that most women enter pregnancy with low iron stores so they have little to draw on to maintain normal hemoglobin concentrations in the later months. For these reasons the National Research Council recommends that pregnant

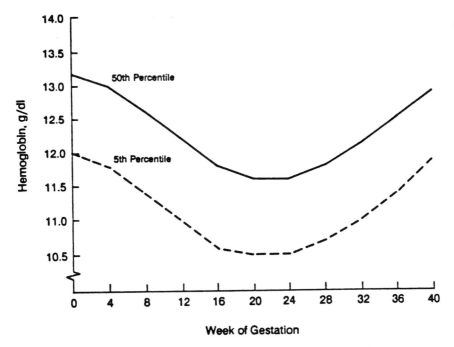

FIG. 6-1 Normal changes in hemoglobin concentration during course of pregnancy.

From Institute of Medicine: *Nutrition during pregnancy, part II: nutrient supplements,* Washington, DC, 1990, National Academy Press.

women receive an oral iron supplement of 30 mg per day.[28] This amount should maintain hemoglobin levels in normal pregnant women, but those who are anemic when they enter pregnancy will need a larger dose. Simple ferrous salts should be used. There are no advantages gained by using compounds purported to have unique properties that increase absorption or enhance erythropoiesis.

In a population of women who opt not to take iron supplements, evidence of iron deficiency without anemia has been reported.[32,51] Romslo et al.[51] evaluated 45 healthy pregnant women who were provided either oral iron or placebo. When the iron was not given, 15 of 23 women had exhausted iron stores and iron deficiency at term, as judged from low serum ferritin, low serum transferring saturation, and high erythrocyte protoporphyrin values (Fig. 6-2). In the iron-treated group none of the

women developed iron deficiency. The most significant known consequence of maternal iron deficiency is reduced fetal iron storage followed by increased risk of anemia during infancy. This may be prevented by maternal iron supplementation by about 20 to 24 weeks' gestation. In the absence of iron supplements, it appears to take up to 2 years after pregnancy before prepregnancy serum ferritin values are regained (Fig. 6-3).

However, the routine need for iron supplementation during pregnancy remains a controversial issue in obstetrics. In fact, one trial of routine iron prophylaxis during pregnancy showed that among well-nourished Finnish women, such prophylaxis is not crucial for the health of mothers or infants during pregnancy and through the first 8 weeks after delivery.[23] In a subsequent 7-year followup, a randomized trial was conducted comparing women who

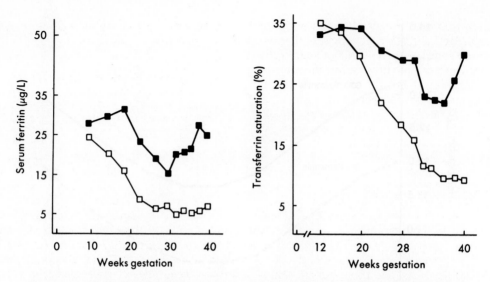

FIG. 6-2   Changes in serum ferritin and in transferrin saturation during pregnancy in women treated with (■) and without (□) oral iron supplementation. Results are given as means.

Modified from Romslo I et al: Iron requirement in normal pregnancy assessed by serum ferritin, serum transferrin saturation and erythrocyte protoporphyrin determinations, *Br J Obstet Gynaecol* 90:101, 1983.

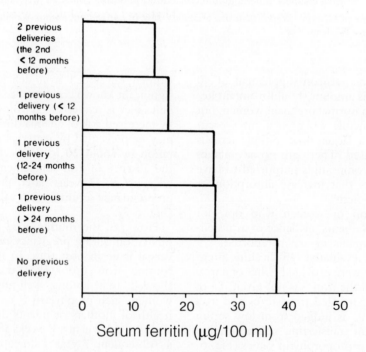

FIG. 6-3   Effect of childbearing and interval since last delivery on serum ferritin concentration.

were given iron only if needed and those given iron prophylactically. The outcomes of the two groups were similar—there were not statistically significant differences in deaths after birth, number of timing of infants' or mothers' hospitalization, reasons for mothers' first hospitalization, number or timing of subsequent miscarriages or births, or problems or outcomes in the next birth. (Interestingly, infants of the prophylactically supplemented group were more frequently hospitalized because of convulsions.) This study does not support routine iron prophylaxis for well-nourished pregnant women.

If iron supplements were completely innocuous, a rationale might be that so long as they are relatively inexpensive and the studies about effectiveness are equivocal, supplements might do some good. However, there are important questions about the safety of medicinal iron. A substantial number of prenatal patients develop diarrhea or more commonly constipation, which improves when they discontinue their iron supplements. Iron has been shown to depress the absorption of dietary zinc, and, the greatest danger of iron supplements for prenatal patients is that iron pills often resemble candy and are the leading cause of poisoning deaths in children under the age of 6. The Food and Drug Administration has proposed that packages of capsules and tablets containing iron be labeled with warnings not to leave the packages open or within the reach of children to prevent accidental and potentially fatal poisonings.

It seems practical, however, to monitor hemoglobin levels at the onset of pregnancy and at about 26 to 28 weeks gestation. If hemoglobin levels are less than 10 gm per 100 ml, a ferritin level should be drawn to determine whether there is iron deficiency. If the ferritin level is below normal, iron-rich foods or iron supplements should be added on a case-by-case basis. Response to therapy should be assessed with subsequent blood tests. All prenatal patients should be instructed about iron-rich foods, foods rich in vitamin C, and foods that inhibit bioavailability of iron.

Maternal anemia is the major clinical consequence of iron deficiency, but its effects on pregnancy outcome are poorly understood. Criteria recommended for the diagnosis of iron deficiency anemia are the following[28]:

1st and 3rd trimesters	
Hemoglobin (gm/100 ml)	<11.0
Hematocrit (%)	<33%
2nd trimester	
Hemoglobin (gm/100 ml)	<10.5
Hematocrit (%)	<32%

However, since both high altitude and smoking normally elevate hemoglobin and hematocrit levels, adjustments are necessary in these situations for diagnosis of anemia (see box on p.172).

An anemic woman is clearly less able to tolerate hemorrhage with delivery, and she is more prone to development of **puerperal infection.** Data suggest that the fetal effects of maternal iron deficiency are relatively mild, but several reports suggest that pregnancy outcome may be compromised. Observations in India in the early 1970s showed that moderate to severe anemia in pregnant women was associated with increased incidence of spontaneous abortion, premature delivery, low-birth-weight delivery, stillbirth, and perinatal death. It might be hypothesized that poor iron consumption leads to poor hemoglobin production, followed by compromised delivery of oxygen to the uterus, placenta, and developing fetus. If maternal cardiac output increased to accommodate the insufficiency in hemoglobin content per red cell, the added workload undertaken by the heart could unduly stress maternal systems.

Iron deficiency anemia. The pregnant woman with iron deficiency anemia should be treated for a finite period with iron supplements of appropriate dosage (100 mg or more per tablet). In a large proportion of anemic women treated in this fashion, an upward shift in the hematocrit level can be achieved easily. However, 15% or 20% of such women will not respond to typical iron therapy by obvious improvement in the hematocrit level; this group is suspected to represent women in whom expanded plasma volume is significantly greater than normal. This phenomenon is reportedly common in situations of multiple pregnancy. Supplementation with iron in excess of need has not been evaluated through critical research; one report, however, suggested that unneces-

❖

DOES ANEMIA OR IRON DEFICIENCY INCREASE RISK OF PRETERM DELIVERY?

Using criteria from the Centers for Disease Control, anemia and iron-deficiency anemia (anemia with serum ferritin concentrations (<12 µg/L) were assessed in more than 800 inner-city gravidas at entry to prenatal care. Iron deficiency anemia was associated with significantly lower energy and iron intakes early in pregnancy and a lower mean corpuscular volume. The odds of low birth weight were tripled and of preterm delivery, more than doubled with iron deficiency, but were not increased with anemia from other causes. When vaginal bleeding at or before entry to care accompanied anemia, the odds of a preterm delivery were increased fivefold for iron deficiency anemia and doubled for other anemias. Inadequate weight gain during pregnancy was more prevalent among those with iron deficiency anemia and in those with anemias of other etiologies. The prevalence of iron deficiency anemia (3.5%), however, was lower than anticipated for an inner-city, minority population in whom most anemias had been attributed clinically to iron deficiency.

From Scholl TO et al; Anemia vs iron deficiency: increased risk of preterm delivery, *Am J Clin Nutr* 55:985, 1992.

sary use of iron supplements led to macrocytosis in a small number of pregnant women.[61]

Efforts to reduce the prevalence of iron deficiency anemia may not work because of low compliance with an iron-supplementation program. This was shown in a study in Jakarta, Indonesia, where the prevalence of anemia was 42% among pregnant women.[53] After 2 months of supplementation with 300 mg ferrous sulphate per day, no decrease in the rate of anemia was observed. Questioning of the participants revealed that compliance was low. Such programs need reliable monitoring and evaluation systems.

Some patients with iron deficiency are found to exhibit a behavior called *pica*. Eating starch,

dirt, or clay has been implicated as a cause of iron deficiency in pregnancy; the opposite viewpoint has also been proposed—that is, iron deficiency is the etiologic factor behind pica. Coltman[13] has demonstrated the rapid remission of pagophagia (ice eating) with iron therapy; it is unlikely that ice would interfere with iron absorption from the gut. Crosby[14] suggests the following about pica:

1. The discovery of pica may be the first clue in establishing the existence of iron deficiency.
2. The abnormal craving is not always for a strange food or substance.
3. The patient's local (cultural) situation may influence the selection of the craving.
4. A sense of shame or guilt may interfere with eliciting a history of pica.

If either iron deficiency or pica is identified during pregnancy, a search should be initiated for the other problem.

High maternal hemoglobin levels. High maternal hemoglobin levels have been associated with increased risk of poor pregnancy outcome (Fig. 6-4).[25,41,52] Koller et al[34,35] found that out of 15 intrauterine deaths, 10 mothers had hemoglobin levels in late pregnancy than were more than two standard deviations above the mean. They also showed that 15 out of 24 mothers with small-for-gestational-age babies had high hemoglobin levels in the third trimester. Murphy et al.[41] reviewed data from 54,382 singleton pregnancies and found that both high (greater than 13.2 gm/100 ml) and low (less than 10.4 gm/100 ml) hemoglobin levels were associated with an adverse outcome. Significant differences emerged in perinatal mortality between those with high and those with intermediate hemoglobin values at 13 to 19 weeks' gestation. The frequencies of perinatal death, low birth weight, and preterm delivery were greater with high hemoglobin than with intermediate hemoglobin levels. There was a striking relation between initial hemoglobin value and subsequent frequency of hypertension ($p \leq 0.001$). In the primiparas, the frequency of subsequent hypertension ranged from 7% at hemoglobin levels under 10.5 gm/100 ml to 42% at hemoglobin concentrations over 14.5 gm/100 ml. Adverse findings among the high

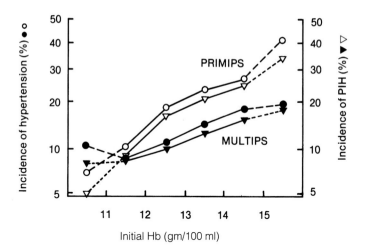

FIG. 6-4 Frequency of all hypertension in pregnancy and pregnancy-induced hypertension (PIH) among primiparous multiparas according to hemoglobin concentration at the initial prenatal visit. Points representing hemoglobin concentrations ≤10.5 gm/100 ml and ≥14.5 gm/100 ml have been joined to their neighbors by broken lines to indicate that these values may be inaccurate because of small sample sizes.

Modified from Murphy JF et al: Relation of haemoglobin levels in first and second trimesters to outcome of pregnancy, *Lancet* 1:992, 1986.

hemoglobin group reflect some failure in plasma volume expansion in these women. In addition, the high hemoglobin concentrations may have a deleterious effect on the uteroplacental circulation. If increased viscosity secondary to high hemoglobin concentration contributes to the formation of placental infarcts, as suggested by Naeye,[42] routine iron administration to these mothers may have a negative rather than a positive impact.

Calcium

Although ionic calcium and phosphorus both have important regulatory functions in the cells and blood, about 99% of the body's calcium and over 80% of its phosphorus are bound as hydroxyapatite, the primary structural component of bones and teeth. The importance of calcium and phosphorus during pregnancy is to promote adequate mineralization of the fetal skeleton and deciduous teeth.[48]

The fetus acquires most of its calcium in the last trimester, when skeletal growth is maximum and teeth are being formed. Widdowson[68] has calculated that the fetus draws 13 mg/hr of calcium from the maternal blood supply, or 250 to 300 mg per day. At birth the infant has accumulated approximately 25 gm. Additional calcium is believed to be stored in the maternal skeleton as a reserve for lactation.

Extensive adjustments in calcium metabolism are routinely observed in the pregnant woman.[12] Hormonal factors are largely responsible, with the following consequences known to occur:

1. Human chorionic somatomammotropin (from placenta)—Enhances the rate of bone turnover progressively through pregnancy.
2. Estrogen (largely from placenta)—Inhibits bone resorption and thus provokes a compensatory release of parathyroid hormone, which maintains the serum calcium level while enhancing intestinal calcium absorption and decreasing its urinary excretion.

The net effect is the promotion of progressive calcium retention. The prenatal changes begin well ahead of the time when fetal skeletal miner-

TABLE 6-2 *Selected Examples of Recommended Dietary Allowances for Calcium in Different Countries*

	Women	Pregnancy	Lactation
		mg/day	
Australia 1989	800	1100 (+300)	1200 (+400)
FAO/WHO 1974	450	1100 (+650)	1100 (+650)
France 1988	800	1000 (+200)	1200 (+400)
Indonesia 1980	500	600 (+100)	600 (+100)
Ireland 1984	800	1200 (+400)	1200 (+400)
Spain 1983†	600	1325 (+725)	1425 (+825)
United Kingdom 1991	700	700 (0)	1250 (+550)
United States 1989	800	1200 (+400)	1200 (+400)

alization ensues. It thus appears that anticipatory adjustments ready the maternal organism for the increased calcium demands later on. Mineralization of the fetal skeleton is ultimately stimulated, largely through active placental calcium transport leading to fetal hypercalcemia and subsequent endocrine adjustments. Vitamin D and its metabolites also cross the placenta and appear in fetal blood in the same concentration as found in the maternal circulation.

Recommendations for calcium intake. Organizations around the world differ in their recommendations for calcium intake during pregnancy (Table 6-2). In the United States, the current recommended dietary allowance (RDA) for calcium during pregnancy is 1,200 mg daily, a level 400 mg higher than recommended for the nonpregnant woman over age 24 years.[44] Some argue that this allowance is set too high, since apparently successful pregnancies occur in many other cultures with calcium intakes substantially below those recommended (Fig. 6-5). The explanation likely relates to the large calcium reservoir in the maternal skeleton, of which the total requirement of pregnancy (30 gm) amounts to about 2.5%.[58] It should also be noted that in many other cultures, diets are consumed that contain less phosphorus and protein; this factor might reduce the degree of calcium loss in the urine. Duggin et al.[16] have reported data from balance studies that suggest that if maternal intake of calcium is less than 2 gm per day, stores of calcium will be depleted to meet

the needs of the fetus. If this is the case, frequent pregnancies and consistently low calcium intakes throughout the childbearing years could contribute to osteoporosis in later life. Evidence of clinical manifestation of osteomalacia in multiparous women is available.[17] Neonatal bone density also may relate to adequacy of maternal calcium consumption during pregnancy.[49]

Milk and milk products constitute the most important sources of calcium in the diet, but additional amounts are supplied by legumes, nuts, and dried fruits. Dark leafy green vegetables such as kale, cabbage, collards, and turnip greens contain calcium in high amounts that can be well absorbed, but some of the calcium in spinach, chard, and beet greens is bound with oxalic acid, which makes it unavailable to the body.

The fairly common occurrence of dental caries during pregnancy has led to a widely held belief that calcium deficiency causes demineralization of the teeth. A number of chemical analyses have been performed on animal and human teeth during pregnancy, but none has confirmed that demineralization occurs. James[29] quotes an experiment in which a dog was maintained on a calcium-poor diet throughout pregnancy. The bones of the dog became so decalcified that they could hardly be seen on x-ray film, but its teeth showed no change. The dental caries that often accompanies pregnancy is more likely to be caused by a slight decrease in salivary pH. Proper oral hygiene and the avoidance of cariogenic foods can counter this effect.

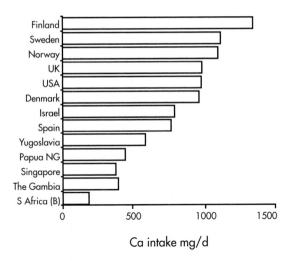

FIG. 6-5 Comparison of average calcium intakes in different countries.

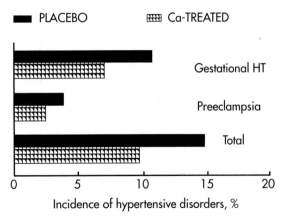

FIG. 6-6 Effect of calcium supplementation on the incidence of hypertensive disorders of pregnancy. Gestational hypertension was defined as a blood pressure greater than or equal to 140/90 mmHg. Preeclampsia was defined as the presence of both gestational hypertension and proteinuria. Calcium supplementation significantly reduced the risk of developing hypertensive disorders of pregnancy.

Data from Belizan JM et al: Calcium supplementation to prevent hypertensive disorders of pregnancy, *N Engl J Med* 325:1399, 1991.

In the early 1980s, an association was proposed between calcium deficiency and edema, proteinuria, and hypertension 183 183 (EPH gestosis) in pregnancy.[4,5,65,66,66a] Data are available indicating that in populations with low calcium intake the incidence of eclampsia is higher.[10] Calcium supplementation of pregnant women has also been associated with reduced blood pressure (Fig. 6-6).[10] It has also been noted that persons with high calcium intake have lower blood pressure, and rats with restricted calcium intake develop hypertension that is reversible with calcium administration. Furthermore, the eclampsia syndrome is similar to that of tetany caused by hypocalcemia (see box on p. 176).

Calcium intake and hypertensive disorders. In 1980, an inverse relationship was reported between calcium intake and hypertensive disorders of pregnancy.[37] It was proposed that satisfactory calcium intake may be protective against elevation in blood pressure during pregnancy. The hypothesis was based on the observation that Mayan Indians in Guatemala, who traditionally soak their corn in lime before cooking, had a high calcium intake and a low incidence of preeclampsia and eclampsia. Reports from other parts of the world have confirmed an inverse relationship between calcium intake and blood pressure during pregnancy (see box below). If calcium intake through food or supplements can significantly lower the risk of preeclampsia, strategies to achieve this goal are attractive interventions.[10]

In a recent report, available randomized trials in which the intervention included calcium supplementation during pregnancy were evaluated and summarized.[3,11] Twelve trials were located; three were excluded because true randomization to treatment or control groups was not carried out. This left 6 trials involving more than 1,700 women. Taken together, these trials suggest that calcium supplementation during pregnancy is associated with a substantial reduction in the risk of hypertension during pregnancy and of preeclampsia (Figs. 6-6 and 6-7). There was also evidence of moderate but promising reduction in preterm labor. The authors concluded that calcium supplementation during pregnancy appears to reduce the risk of preeclampsia and there is promising evidence of a reduction in the risk of preterm delivery. If these benefits lead to a reduction in the number of perinatal deaths or

❖

STUDY ON CALCIUM SUPPLEMENTATION TO PREVENT HYPERTENSIVE DISORDERS OF PREGNANCY

Background

Calcium supplementation has been reported to reduce blood pressure in pregnant and non-pregnant women. We undertook this prospective study to determine the effect of calcium supplementation on the incidence of hypertensive disorders of pregnancy (gestational hypertension and preeclampsia) and to determine the value of urinary calcium levels as a predictor of the response.

Methods

We studied 1194 nulliparous women who were in the 20th week of gestation at the beginning of the study. The women were randomly assigned to receive 2 g per day of elemental calcium in the form of calcium carbonate (593 women) or placebo (601 women). Urinary excretion of calcium and creatinine was measured before calcium supplementation was begun. The women were followed to the end of their pregnancies, and the incidence of hypertensive disorders of pregnancy was determined.

Results

The rates of hypertensive disorders of pregnancy were lower in the calcium group than in the placebo group (9.8% vs. 14.8%; odds ratio, 0.63; 95% confidence interval, 0.44 to 0.90). The risk of these disorders was lower at all times during gestation, particularly after the 28th week of gestation ($P = 0.01$ by life-table analysis), in the calcium group than in the placebo group, and the risk of both gestational hypertension and preeclampsia was also lower in the calcium group. Among the women who had low ratios of urinary calcium to urinary creatinine (≤ 0.62 mmol per millimole) during the 20th week of gestation, those in the calcium group had a lower risk of hypertensive disorders of pregnancy (odds ratio, 0.56; 95% confidence interval, 0.29 to 1.09) and less of an increase in diastolic and systolic blood pressure than the placebo group. The pattern of response was similar among the women who had a high ratio of urinary calcium to urinary creatinine during the 20th week of gestation, but the differences were smaller.

Conclusions

Pregnant women who receive calcium supplementation after the 20th week of pregnancy have a reduced risk of hypertensive disorders of pregnancy.

From Belizan JM et al: Calcium supplementation to prevent hypertensive disorders of pregnancy, *N Engl J Med* 325:1399, 1991.

diabled survivors, this would be a substantial advance in the care of women during pregnancy. However, since available evidence is still limited, calcium supplementation is not recommended for routine prenatal care at the present time.

Phosphorus

The RDA for phosphorus is the same as that for calcium—800 mg with an extra 400 mg during pregnancy. It is so widely available in foods that a dietary deficiency is rare. In fact, there is a possibility that the problem may be too much phosphorus rather than too little.

Calcium and phosphorus exist in a constant ratio in the blood. This ratio can be disturbed by the amounts of calcium and phosphorus in foods. If, for example, phosphorus is in excess, it will bind calcium in the gastrointestinal tract and limit the amount of calcium absorbed. A higher phosphorus:calcium ratio in the blood causes more calcium to be excreted in the urine.

The U.S. diet is high in phosphorus. In addition to the naturally high levels in most animal protein foods, even greater amounts are found in processed meats, snack foods, and carbonated beverages. With the exception of dairy products, foods that are high in phosphorus contain only small amounts of calcium.

Most adults can tolerate relatively wide variations in dietary calcium-to-phosphorus ratios

---

CALCIUM SUPPLEMENTATION DURING PREGNANCY

A randomized, controlled, double-blind trial of calcium supplementation was conducted with clinically healthy women of 17 years or less. These young women were followed at the Adolescent Pregnancy Clinic of The Johns Hopkins Hospital in Baltimore between 1985 and 1988. Patients were enrolled by the 23rd week of gestation and were provided either 2.0 g of elemental calcium per day or placebo. Dietary calcium was similar in both groups at about 1200 mg per day. The calcium group had

1. A lower incidence of preterm delivery—7.4% vs. 21%
2. A lower incidence of spontaneous labor and preterm delivery—6.4% vs. 17.9%
3. A lower incidence of low birth weight—9.6% vs. 21.1%

The researchers proposed that the observed effect could be mediated by a reduction in uterine smooth muscle contractility. If confirmed by future research, these results could represent an important preventive intervention for prematurity in high-risk populations.

From Villar J, Repke JT: Calcium supplementation during pregnancy may reduce preterm delivery in high-risk populations, *Am J Obstet Gynecol* 163:1124, 1990.

---

when vitamin D is adequate. However, pregnancy is a time when calcium reserves are severely stressed. Lowered serum calcium concentrations and the mild alkalosis from the mother's reduced PCO_2 tend to increase muscular irritability. When this is compounded by exceptionally high phosphorus intakes, a disturbance of the calcium-to-phosphorus ratio in the body could result.

Calcium-phosphorus balance is often discussed in relation to maintenance of neuromuscular normality. Many years ago, it was suggested that sudden clonic or tonic contractions (often at night) of the gastrocnemius muscle are caused by a decline in serum phosphate. Prevention or relief was proclaimed to be had through reduction in intake of milk (a high-phosphorus, high-calcium beverage). Supplementation with nonphosphate calcium salts was also recommended, along with regular ingestion of aluminum hydroxide to promote formation of insoluble aluminum phosphate salts in the gut. Several studies confirmed the benefit of these measures in the total serum calcium level in affected women. It is clear, however, that the clinical correlation of these observations is far from perfect, since some controlled and double-blind studies have failed to indicate a correlation between leg cramps and either intake of dairy products or the type of calcium supplement employed.

Magnesium

Magnesium is much like calcium and phosphorus in that most of it is stored in bones. The amounts that are biochemically active are concentrated in nerve and muscle cells. Deficiencies of magnesium produce neuromuscular dysfunctions characterized by tremors and convulsions. Magnesium-deficient pregnant rats show impaired abdominal contractions during parturition. However, there are no convincing data that magnesium supplementation of pregnant women improves pregnancy course or outcome.[50,54,59]

Studies of leg cramps have included both magnesium and calcium. Magnesium therapy as treatment for nightly leg cramps has been studied in several populations, including elderly men and women and people with Type 1 diabetes, with adequate results. Leg cramps have been reported in 5% to 30% of all pregnant women, most often during the latter months of pregnancy and without relationship to other complications or to unfavorable fetal outcome. Low serum magnesium levels have been reported in pregnant women with leg cramps. One uncontrolled therapeutic trial of magnesium supplementation indicated a positive effect.

Recently, Dahle et al[15] sought to determine whether low levels of serum magnesium occur in women with pregnancy-related leg cramps and

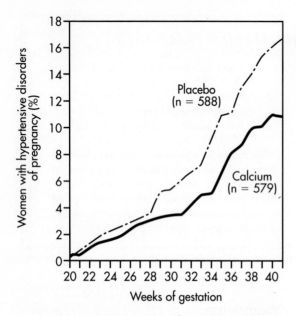

FIG. 6-7 Percentage of women in the calcium-treated and placebo groups in whom hypertensive disorders of pregnancy (gestational hypertension and preeclampsia) developed, according to the week of gestation.

Data from Belizan JM et al: Calcium supplementation to prevent hypertensive disorders of pregnancy, *N Engl J Med* 325:1399, 1991.

whether the symptoms can be alleviated by oral magnesium substitution. Seventy-three pregnant women with leg cramps participated in this controlled, prospective, and randomized double-blind trial. Inteviews and laboratory tests were performed before and after the 3-week intervention. Serum magnesium levels of these patients were at or below the lower reference limit, which is common for pregnant women. Oral magnesium substitution decreased leg cramp distress significantly but did not increase serum magnesium levels; excess magnesium was excreted as measured by an increase in urinary magnesium levels. The authors conclude that magnesium supplementation seems to be a valuable tool in the treatment of pregnancy-related leg cramps.

Not much is known about the need for magnesium during pregnancy. The RDA is based on estimates of the amounts accumulated by the mother and the fetus. Green vegetables are good sources of magnesium because the element is part of the green pigment chlorophyll, but the best sources are nuts, wheat bran, soybeans, and wheat germ. Animal products and fruits are relatively poor sources of magnesium.

Iodine

Iodine deficiency is by far the most common preventable cause of mental deficits in the world. The most severe form of endemic cretinism is characterized by a combination of mental deficiency, deaf-mutism, motor rigidity, and sometimes hypothyroidism. It occurs in parts of the world where iodine deficiency is sufficiently severe enough to cause goiter in 30% of the population. It is found in southern and eastern Europe and is common in Asia, Africa, and Latin America. Iodine injections in the form of iodized oil before but not during pregnancy will prevent cretinism. Studies in China showed that 2% of the infants of mothers who had injections in the second trimester of pregnancy compared with 9% of those whose mothers had injections in the second trimester had moderate or severe neurodevelopmental abnormalities. The importance of maternal thyroid hormone is supported by results of studies showing that maternal thyroxine is transported across the placenta to the fetus, and that iodine-replete but hypothyroid women have an increased frequency of stillbirths as well as cretinism and less severe neurological defects of motor and cognitive performance in live-born infants.

In 1990, the World Health Organization (WHO) estimated that 20 million people in the world had preventable brain damage resulting from the effects of iodine deficiency on fetal brain development.[24] They also set at 1 billion people the number at risk for iodine deficiency caused by low levels of iodine in the soil. Of these, 20% have goiter. Prevalence of neonatal hypothyroidism varies from 1 to 10% in these areas.

Other dietary compounds may affect iodine bioavailability. This is suspected to be the case in the Republic of Guinea where the overall prevalence of goiter is 70% among adults.[36] Thyroid swelling is sometimes present at birth and also affects 55% of schoolchildren. In this region, iodine deficiency is the primary causative factor but the diet also contains substantial amounts of thiocyanate anions which are likely to further depress iodine bioavailability. Other dietary components, notably flavonoids, are suspected to contribute.

It is also established that excessive exposure of a fetus to iodine during pregnancy can be problematic.[46] The major sources of iodine in excessive amounts were iodine solutions prescribed for maternal asthma, other respiratory problems, hyperthyroidism, hypothyroidism, or tachycardia. In one case the iodine source was a prenatal supplement. To date, there are no good data on the potential problem of excessive dietary iodine; the diet of a mother would have to be very unusual to achieve levels of iodine likely to be associated with fetal damage.

Zinc

Zinc has an active role in metabolism because it is a component of insulin. It also is part of the **carbonic anhydrase enzyme system** that helps to maintain acid-base balance in the tissues. The action of zinc in the synthesis of DNA and RNA makes it a highly important element in reproduction.

Zinc deficiency. Considerable interest has developed of late in the significance of zinc deficiency in adversely affecting pregnancy course and potential outcome. Zinc is a known constituent of a number of important metalloenzymes and a necessary cofactor for other enzymes. Zinc deficiency is highly teratogenic in rats and leads to the development of a variety of congenital malformations. Other adverse outcomes have also been reported (see the box above). Nonhuman primates also are affected, and abnormal brain development and behavior have been described in offspring of zinc-deficient monkeys. Unfortunately, it seems that a zinc-deficient diet does not effectively move zinc from maternal bones. This storage pool appears somewhat unavailable so that dietary deficiency can quickly have an impact on the mineral balance of the maternal organism.

Several studies involving laboratory rats relate to the consequences of prenatal zinc deficiency on offspring. In the first case, fetal and neonatal rats exposed to low levels of zinc through their pregnant or nursing mothers developed teeth with significantly reduced levels of zinc in both enamel (lower than 20%) and dentin (lower than

> ### ZINC DEFICIENCY AS A TERATOGENIC AGENT IN HUMANS
>
> **Observation**
> Neural-tube defects in regions of zinc deficiency
> Fetal death and malformation in acrodermatitis enteropathica
> Low maternal blood zinc and malformations in infants
> In Sweden
> In Turkey
> In Ireland
> Low maternal zinc and low birth weight

30%). When exposed to a cariogenic diet in early life, these offspring demonstrated a 42% greater buccal caries score than offspring of control dams.

In a second report, pregnant rats were provided either a low-zinc diet or a normal diet and then were given an intraperitoneal dose of a thalidomide analogue (EM_{12}). Offspring from mothers receiving adequate dietary zinc showed a 0% incidence of typical thalidomide malformations, whereas offspring born to zinc-deficient dams showed an incidence of 57.7% thalidomide malformations. This interaction between dietary deficiency and prenatal effect of a drug may very well be relevant to the human organism. Although no data exist to support this idea, additional research in rats suggests that various nutrient deficiency conditions might increase the harmful effects of noxious or foreign agents on the fetus.

Evidence from human populations suggests that the malformation rate and other poor pregnancy outcomes may be higher in populations in whom zinc deficiency has been recognized. In our discussion of preconceptional issues (Chapter 2), reference was made to the teratogenic effect of maternal zinc deficiency. Support for this proven phenomenon need not be repeated here. Suffice it to say, in cases of true maternal zinc deficiency, risk of congenital malformations in the offspring is probably elevated.

Other potential adverse pregnancy outcomes have been explored in human pregnancies with regard to their association with zinc deficiency. For example, the following reports are fascinating:

1. Maternal leukocyte zinc deficiency at start of third trimester as a predictor of fetal growth retardation—Leukocyte zinc levels were measured in 70 mothers at the beginning of the third trimester of pregnancy and compared with the weight centiles of their subsequently delivered babies. The median maternal leukocyte zinc concentrations rose progressively with the weight centile of the babies. A low maternal leukocyte zinc concentration strongly predicted a baby weighing less than the 10th centile. These findings suggest that maternal zinc status might have a role in antenatal screening for potential low birth weight.[67]

2. A positive association between maternal serum zinc concentration and birth weight—A study was conducted on a cohort of 476 women (mostly African American) who attended the Jefferson County Health Department clinic for their prenatal care. Serum zinc levels were measured in early pregnancy and related to the eventual birth weight of the babies. The data collected during the study indicated that there was a threshold for maternal zinc concentration below which the prevalence of low birth weight increases significantly. Pregnant women who had serum zinc concentrations in the lowest quartile had significantly higher prevalence of low birth weight than did those mothers who had serum zinc concentrations in the upper three quartiles during pregnancy. These findings suggest that maternal serum zinc concentration measured early in pregnancy could be used to identify those women at higher risk of giving birth to a low-birth-weight infant.[45]

3. Zinc status, pregnancy complications and labor abnormalities—Maternal zinc status was evaluated in 279 pregnant women at delivery and compared with the incidence of complications during the antenatal pe-

riod and major dysfunctional labor patterns. Patients were divided into "low zinc" and "high zinc" groups. Low plasma zinc was associated with more complications in the antenatal and intrapartum periods (Table 6-3). This specifically applied to pregnancy-induced hypertension, vaginitis, postdates, and with regard to labor, prolonged latent phase, protracted active phase, labor >20 hours, second stage >2.5 hours, and cervical and vaginal lacerations. The results suggest that plasma zinc screening might be a useful addition to a patient's antenatal workup.[38]

4. Zinc status in women with premature rupture of membranes at term—Zinc concentrations were measured in whole blood, scalp hair, pubic hair, and colostrum from patients at term with and without premature rupture of membranes (PROM). A maternal zinc index was established for each patient. The mean value of the maternal zinc index in patients with PROM was significantly lower than in patients without this complication. These results suggest that the subnormal tissue zinc content in pregnancy may play a role as a causative factor in PROM at term.[55]

5. Zinc nutriture of women living in a periurban Egyptian village was examined over the last 6 months of pregnancy and the first 6 months of lactation as one of several potential determinants of pregnancy outcome and infant development. Estimated bioavailable zinc intake was about 2 mg/day from diets high in phytate and fiber. Among numerous variables analyzed, early pregnancy weight (3 months) and plasma zinc concentrations in the second trimester formed the best predictor model of birth weight. Bioavailable zinc intake during pregnancy was also part of a profile of micronutrient intakes related to neonatal habituation behavior, a measure of early information processing. Performance on the Bayley motor test at 6 months of age was negatively related to maternal intakes of plant zinc, phytate, and fiber, suggesting that zinc bioavailability was involved.[33]

TABLE 6-3   *Relationship between Plasma Zinc and Antenatal and Intrapartum Complications*

| | Plasma Zinc | | |
	Low (*n* = 144) (%)	High (*n* = 135) (%)	*p* Value
Mild toxemia	5.6	0.7	0.02
Vaginitis	12.6	4.4	0.01
Postterm >42 wk	4.2	0	0.01
Prolonged latent phase	2.8	0	0.05
Protracted active phase	28.7	18.2	0.04
Labor >20 hr	6.3	1.5	0.03
Second stage >2.5 hr	6.3	0.7	0.01
Lacerations >3rd degree	7.0	1.5	0.02

From Lazebnik N, Kuhnert BR, Thompson KL: Zinc status, pregnancy complications and labor abnormalities, *Am J Obstet Gynecol* 158:161, 1988.

Zinc supplementation. Another approach to determining whether zinc status is related to the outcome of pregnancy is to supplement women suspected of having zinc inadequacy and look for improved pregnancy outcome.[26,30,31,39,43,57] Low-income Mexican-American women[26] supplemented with 20 mg of zinc daily had a lower incidence of PIH than did unsupplemented women; no difference in complications was associated with zinc supplementation. Supplementation of low-income women in India with a much larger amount of zinc, 300 mg $ZnSO_4$ daily, was stopped after three premature births and one stillbirth occurred consecutively.[39] Supplementation of a small number of presumably well-nourished women with a large amount of zinc (90 mg) had no deleterious effects, however.[30]

Since women with low serum concentrations of zinc are another group that may have inadequate zinc status, Jameson[30] investigated the effect of zinc supplementation on women in this category. Seven of the 20 women with low serum zinc concentrations and unsatisfactory hemoglobin concentrations in spite of oral iron and vitamin supplementation were supplemented with zinc, 90 mg daily, during a 10- to 12-day hospital stay. They presumably continued to take the supplements for the remainder of gestation (5 to 15 weeks). At delivery, these women had shorter labors and less blood loss than the 13 unsupplemented women, six of whom experienced "severe hemorrhage with uterine atony."

In a further study by Jameson, half the women with serum zinc concentrations less than the mean 65 μg/dl on week 14 of pregnancy were given 45 mg of zinc daily. Of 69 unsupplemented women, 33 had normal deliveries as compared with 40 of 64 supplemented women. Normal deliveries and infants resulted from only 26% of the pregnancies in which serum zinc at week 14 was less than the mean and declined thereafter.[31]

Zinc supplementation during pregnancy was recently evaluated in a a randomized, double-blind, placebo-controlled trial at the University of Alabama.[20] In the trial, 580 medically indigent, but otherwise healthy, African-American pregnant women with plasma zinc levels below the median at enrollment in prenatal care were randomized at 19 weeks gestation to receive either a daily dose of 25 mg of zinc or a placebo until delivery. (All women were taking a nonzinc-containing multivitamin-mineral tablet daily.) Daily zinc supplementation was associated with greater infant birth weights and head circumferences; the effect occurred predominantly in women who were not overweight.

However, Mahomed et al,[39] in a study in northern Europe involving zinc supplementation during much of the second and third trimesters, did not observe any impact on outcome. Mothers were randomly assigned to receive zinc supplementation or placebo in a double-blind trial. There was no difference between the groups given zinc and placebo in their social or medical backgrounds. Mothers in the active treatment group received one capsule of 20 mg of elemental zinc daily and those in the placebo group a capsule identical in appearance and taste with the active capsule but that contained inert substances. Various adverse outcomes were tested, including maternal bleeding, hypertension, complications of labor and delivery, gestational age, Apgar scores, and neonatal abnormalities. The main outcome measure was birth weight. *The result was there were no differences whatsoever between mothers given zinc supplement and those given placebo.* One must conclude that at least in this population, zinc supplementation did not seem to offer any benefits to the mother or her fetus.

Until more information is available about the potential value or lack of zinc supplementation during pregnancy, routine supplementation is not likely to be advocated by any of the established medical bodies. The Institute of Medicine indicated in their summary of recommendations about nutrient supplements during pregnancy that at this time, there is little justification for their use.[28] It is certainly reasonable, however, for prenatal nutrition counseling to include workable recommendations about food choices that maintain proper zinc status.

The RDA for zinc during pregnancy is 15 mg, about 30% to 40% higher than the estimated intake of most pregnant women. In 8 of 10 studies reviewed, zinc intake of pregnant women was remarkably similar, 9 to 11 mg, whether the women were Lebanese,[63] Mexican-American,[26] vegetarians,[2] middle-income Americans,[7,22,40] or Britons.[1] Other studies reported slightly higher intakes, 12 to 14 mg. and one reported 7 mg per day for Asian vegetarians.[1]

Observational data support the suspicion that prenatal iron supplementation may adversely affect maternal zinc status. Hambidge et al.[21] reported an inverse correlation between plasma zinc and the level of prenatal iron supplementation during the third trimester; Breskin et al.[7] confirmed these observations (Fig. 6-8), as did

Hambidge et al.[21] and Simmer, James, and Thompson.[56] Ideal levels of both iron and zinc have not yet been defined for prenatal vitamin and mineral supplements. However, attempting to counterbalance a large supplement of one trace element with a correspondingly large supplement of another may lead to unforeseen complications and should not be undertaken.

Other Minerals

One advance in nutrition research is the discovery that many other mineral elements are necessary for human reproduction, growth, and general health. Chromium, manganese, fluoride, cobalt, copper, selenium, molybdenum, vanadium, tin, nickel, and silicon have all been shown to be needed by the body. Like iodine, calcium, and phosphorus, these elements (and likely others as well) participate in reactions that control body processes. Studies in animals have revealed that deficiencies produce widespread and serious metabolic defects. Limited knowledge of requirements in humans makes it impossible to establish the RDA for the majority of these minerals. The 1989 edition of the RDA does, however, list estimated safe and adequate daily dietary intakes for copper, manganese, fluoride, chromium, selenium, molybdenum, sodium, potassium, and chloride. Because there is less information on which to base allowances for these nutrients, the levels are not presented in the main RDA table. They are given only as ranges of recommended intakes. No figures are available for pregnant women. Since toxic levels for many of the trace elements may not be much higher than usual intakes, pregnant women are advised not to take supplements that would greatly exceed the upper limits shown in Table 6-4.

Copper. Hurley et al[27] have been instrumental in defining the consequences of prenatal copper deficiency. In both experimental and field animals, copper deficiency has been found to be teratogenic. Lambs, rats, guinea pigs, and mice have been examined. Much of the reported work has related to observations of mouse mutants (quaking and crinkled) in which supplementation of the maternal diet with high amounts of copper has been found to markedly improve survival and reduce frequency of tremors in offspring. Preg-

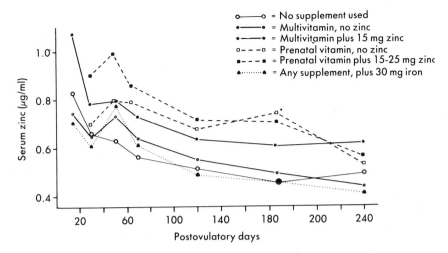

FIG. 6-8 Relationships between maternal zinc concentrations and use or nonuse of supplements by discrete time intervals. Supplement use is shown as none, multivitamins, multivitamins with 15 mg zinc, prenatal vitamins, prenatal vitamins with 15 to 25 mg zinc, and the use of any of the above supplements *plus* 30 mg or ore of iron. Multivitamins generally contain 18 mg of iron; prenatal vitamins contain 60 to 65 mg of iron; one of two women represented ate oysters regularly.

From Breskin MW et al: first trimester serum zinc concentrations in human pregnancy, *Am J Clin Nutr* 38:943, 1983.

nant rats provided D-penicillamine at dosages comparable to those provided to humans showed adverse pregnancy outcome when compared with controls not receiving the drug. Whereas control animals demonstrated a 2.3% rate of resorption and no offspring with malformations, dams exposed to D-penicillamine experienced a 4% resorption rate, and 40% of their live fetuses were malformed. Maternal plasma copper levels were 35% and liver copper concentrations 50% of control values; whole-body copper levels of experimental offspring were 30% those of controls. Teratogenic effects of D-penicillamine were reduced by copper supplementation of pregnant rats.

It is also possible that copper deficiency may compromise pregnancy outcome in humans. One case has been reported of a young woman treated with D-penicillamine during pregnancy who gave birth to an abnormal child.[27] The child had a connective-tissue defect including lax skin, hyperflexibility of the joints, fragility of the veins, varicosities, and impairment of wound healing; some of these features have been recognized previously as associated with copper deficiency. Since D-penicillamine is used clinically to remove copper from certain patients, copper deficiency may develop in such patients and subsequently harm the fetus.

It is presently unknown whether moderate dietary copper deficiency is of consequence to the developing human fetus. The only human situation of possible copper deficiency thus far observed has related to the use of D-penicillamine during pregnancy. Of interest, however, is a study in which copper and zinc balance was assessed in 20 pregnant women on self-selected diets.[60] In the case of copper, positive balance was achieved in these subjects only if a copper supplement was consumed. The authors suggest that the diets of many pregnant women may be marginal insofar as their copper content is concerned. Should these findings be confirmed and adverse consequences to the fetus suspected, copper supplementation may someday be advisable for selected women.

TABLE 6-4 *Estimated Safe and Adequate Daily Dietary Intakes of Additional Selected Vitamins and Minerals for Adolescents and Adults*

	Age Group	
	Adolescents	Adults
Age	11 +	
Vitamins		
Biotin (μg)	30-100	30-100
Pantothenic acid (mg)	4-7	4-7
Trace elements (mg)		
Copper	1.5-2.5	1.5-3.0
Manganese	2.0-5.0	2.0-5.0
Fluoride	1.5-2.5	1.5-4.0
Chromium	0.05-0.2	0.05-0.2
Molybdenum	0.075-0.250	0.075-0.250
Electrolytes (mg)		
Sodium	500	500
Potassium	2000	2000
Chloride	750	750

Modified from National Research Council, Food and Nutrition Board: *Recommended dietary allowances,* revised 1989, Washington, DC, 1989, Government Printing Office.

Fluoride. The role of fluoride in prenatal development is poorly understood at present. Some question has existed over the past 50 years as to the degree of fluoride transport across the placenta. Should it cross the placenta, questions still remain about its value in the development of caries-resistant permanent teeth. Development of the primary dentition begins at 10 to 12 weeks of pregnancy; from the sixth to ninth months of pregnancy the first four permanent molars and eight of the permanent incisors begin formation. Thus, 32 of the ultimate teeth are forming and developing during human pregnancy. Since there is no indication that color of the teeth is usually adversely affected and some evidence that caries resistance and morphological characteristics are improved, prenatal fluoride supplementation may be justified. *It should be recognized, however, that this issue is highly controversial, and to date, formal support for routine prenatal fluoride supplementation has not been voiced by any established medical or dental organization.*[20a,62]

This question is still the center of much debate, and the last word is not in. Researchers at Eastman Dental Center in Rochester, NY, are now testing the effectiveness of prenatal supplements for 1,100 children who live in nonfluoridated areas. Beginning in the fourth month of pregnancy, half of the mothers took 1 mg of fluoride daily—the standard dose—whereas the other half took a placebo. The goal is to determine whether prenatal treatment could reduce the incidence of tooth decay when the children reach 5 years of age.

Most of the children are still young; so far, results indicate that the treatment is safe—that is, miscarriages, premature deliveries, and other adverse outcomes are not more common in women who take prenatal fluoride. However, all of the children in the study have been found to exhibit good oral health—97% have no cavities. The true benefit of prenatal fluoride supplementation (if there is a benefit) has yet to be established.

Sodium. One final mineral to mention is sodium, which contributes significantly to fluid balance in the body. Sodium metabolism is altered during pregnancy under the stimulus of a modified hormonal milieu. Glomerular filtration increases markedly over time to "clean up" the increased maternal blood volume. An additional filtered sodium load of 5,000 to 10,000 mEq daily is typically seen during pregnancy. Compensatory mechanisms come into play to maintain fluid and electrolyte balance.

Restriction of dietary sodium has been common in the past among pregnant women suffering from edema, but moderate edema is normal during pregnancy and should not be combatted with diuretics or low-sodium diets. The increased fluid retained normally during pregnancy actually somewhat increases the body's demand for sodium. Rigorous sodium restriction in pregnant animals stresses the renin-angiotensin-aldosterone system to the point of breakdown; such animals show reduced weight gain and altered fluid consumption patterns,[9] and they tend to develop water intoxication along with renal and adrenal tissue degenera-

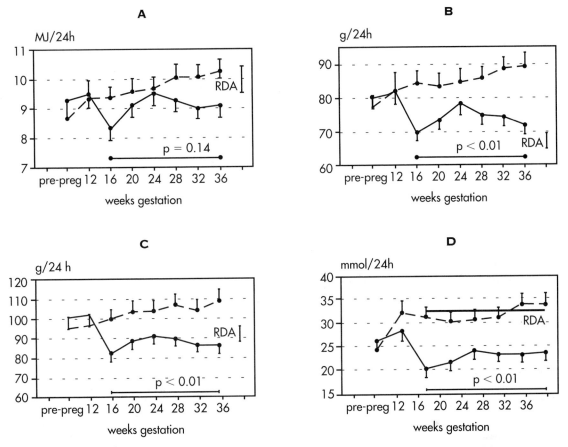

FIG. 6-9 Comparison of selected dietary components in women following a sodium re-stricted diet (———————) and women following a non-restricted diet (------------------------). **A**, energy, **B**, protein, **C**, fat, and **D**, calcium. Significance of difference (p) over the diet period is indicated by the horizontal line.

From: van Buul BJA et al: Dietary sodium restriction in the prophylaxis of hypertensive disorders of pregnancy: effects on the intake of other nutrients, *Am J Clin Nutr* 62:49, 1995.

tion.[47] Neonatal **hyponatremia** (low blood sodium) has been observed in offspring of women who unduly restricted their sodium intake before delivery. The potential for damage to the maternal renin-angiotensin-aldosterone system also exists.

Dietary sodium restriction is used in the Netherlands in the prophylaxis of preeclampsia. Researchers there studied the effects of long-term sodium restriction on the intake of other nutrients and the outcome of preg-

nancy.[64] In the study, 68 healthy pregnant women were randomly assigned to either a low-sodium diet or an unrestricted diet; the diet was consumed between 14 weeks gestation and delivery. Rigid dietary sodium restriction was associated with reduced intake of fat, protein and calcium; it tended to reduce energy intake and limit weight gain, as well as reduce maternal fat stores (Figs. 6-9 and 6-10). It had no major effect on birth weight. However, the undesirable impact that sodium restriction had on

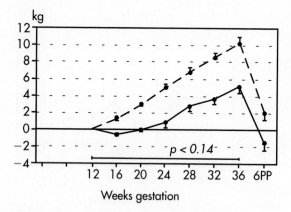

FIG. 6-10 Mean (±SEM) maternal weight gain compared with week 12 of gestation. 6PP, 6 wk after delivery. Broken line indicates the unrestricted group, solid line the low-sodium group. Significance of difference *(P)* over the diet period is indicated by the horizontal line.

From: van Buul BJA et al: Dietary sodium restriction in the prophylaxis of hypertensive disorders of pregnancy: effects on the intake of other nutrients, *Am J Clin Nutr* 62:49, 1995.

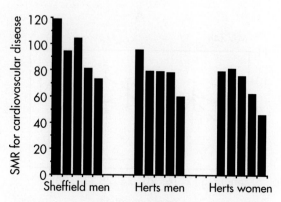

FIG. 6-11 Standardized mortality ratios (SMR) for cardiovascular disease according to birth weight. Categories of birth weight from left to right: <5.5 kg; 5.5–6.5 kg; 6.5–7.5 kg; 7.5–8.5 kg; >8.5 kg.

From Goldberg GR, Prentice AM: Maternal and fetal determinants of adult diseases, *Nutr Rev* 52:191, 1994.

dietary pattern may be of concern for those women who have poor nutritional status before pregnancy. Although moderation in the use of salt and other sodium-rich foods is appropriate for all people, aggressive restriction is unwarranted during pregnancy, when no less than 2 to 3 gm of sodium should be consumed on a daily basis.

MATERNAL AND FETAL DETERMINANTS OF ADULT DISEASES[18,19,8]

The notion that events occurring during the time of gestation might predispose an individual to chronic diseases later in life has recently been supported by epidemiological data. Observations made in the United Kingdom have led to the hypothesis that adverse nutritional experiences in utero have a powerful influence on the development of degenerative diseases in adult-

hood. Poor fetal growth appears to be a strong predictor of hypertension, diabetes, hyperlipidemia, alteration in clotting factors, Syndrome X (the combination of noninsulin-dependent diabetes, hypertension, and hyperlipidemia) and mortality from cardiovascular disease (Fig. 6-11) and chronic obstructive airway disease (COPD). The theory of fetal origins of adult disease proposes that early defects in the development, structure, and function of organs lead to programmed susceptibility, which interacts with later diet and environmental stresses to cause overt disease many decades after the original insult.

Barker has proposed that there are five testable hypotheses that deserve attention.[2a] These are that (1) undernutrition in early life has permanent effects; (2) undernutrition has different effects at different times in early life; (3) rapidly growing fetuses and neonates are more vulnerable to undernutrition than those growing more slowly; (4) undernutrition results from inadequate maternal intake, transport, or transfer of nutrients; and (5) the per-manent effects of undernutrition include reduced cell numbers, altered cell structure, and resetting of hormonal axes. Prospective studies in humans and animal models are underway in many labo-

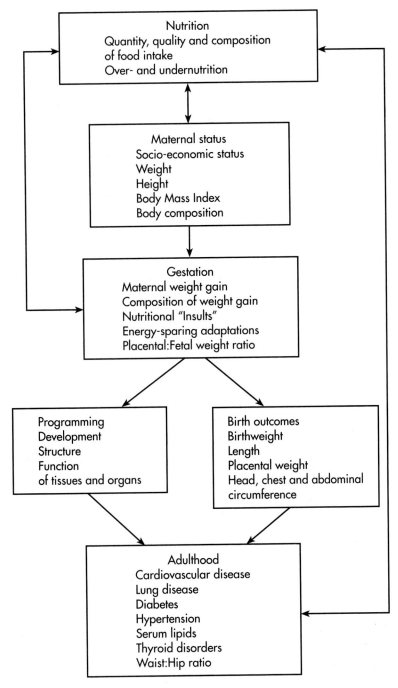

FIG. 6-12 The maternal and in utero nutritional influences on the fetus, and the subsequent effects of programming relevant to nutrition.

From Goldberg GR, Prentice AM: Maternal and fetal determinants of adult diseases, *Nutr Rev* 52:191, 1994.

❖

CRITERIA TO BE CONSIDERED BEFORE INSTITUTING A VITAMIN/MINERAL PREVENTION/INTERVENTION PROGRAM PRECONCEPTIONALLY OR PRENATALLY

1. The condition to be prevented is an important public health problem.
2. There is a safe and acceptable preventive method for women at high risk.
3. High-risk groups can be identified in a way that is acceptable to the population.
4. There is a known time period during which the treatment should be administered.
5. The natural history of the condition is understood.
6. The cost of identifying those at risk is economically feasible.
7. The cost of supplementation is insignificant as compared with the alternative, which is the possible cost of medical care.

From Murphy SP, Abrams BF: Changes in energy intakes during pregnancy and lactation in a national sample of U.S. women, *Am J Public Health* 83:1161, 1993.

raratories with a view to more clearly define the detailed mechanisms (Fig. 6-12).

RECOMMENDED DIETARY ALLOWANCES

The Food and Nutrition Board of the National Research Council is well aware of the problems of determining nutrient requirements during pregnancy and takes them into consideration when setting dietary allowances and making recommendations about the need for supplementation. Recommended Dietary Allowances (RDAs)[44] are based on the best available evidence from metabolic balance studies and from indirect estimates. Requirements for most nutrients are set at levels that prevent signs of deficiency and maintain intake in balance with urinary excretion. When making dietary recommendations, the requirements are adjusted upward to ensure that the amounts derived from experimental subjects will cover individual variations in digestion, absorption, and utilization in the general population. As new evidence concerning requirements becomes available, the allowances are revised (see box at left).

The 1989 edition of the RDA for pregnant and nonpregnant adult women is presented in Table 6-5. Women may need more or less of the amounts listed for calories and protein depending on body size, activity, and health status. The allowances for vitamins and minerals provide sufficient room for individual variation so that they can be applied to all healthy women. They may not be adequate for women who enter pregnancy in poor nutritional status or who have chronic diseases or other complicating conditions. They may not be appropriate for the primigravida who conceives for the first time after 35 years of age. The special needs of adolescent mothers will be discussed in Chapter 10.

RDAs have been set for only 18 of the 40 or so nutrients that are known to be needed to promote growth and maintain health. Strict attention to only those nutrients listed in Table 6-5 without regard for the general quality and variety of foods in the diet can lead to a false sense of security. Intakes can be inade-quate when highly fortified foods or vitamin pills are relied on as the primary source of nutrition, even though they contain 100% of the RDA. Daily consumption of foods from all of the food groups is recommended to make sure that nutrient needs, including those for which there is presently no RDA, are met.

Summary

Iron and calcium are key minerals required by mother and baby. They are also minerals that can be consumed in marginal amounts if the mother chooses to do so. Both maternal and fetal well-being is the obvious goal; providing satisfactory mineral support should be a goal of prenatal counseling. Avoiding excessive mineral supplementation is also necessary. In addition, undue sodium restriction should be avoided.

TABLE 6-5   Recommended Dietary Allowances for Women of Reproductive Age (1989)

Nutrient	Age 11-14	15-18	19-24	25-50	Pregnancy
Energy (kcal)	2200	2200	2200	2200	+300 (2nd and 3rd trimesters)
Protein (g)	46	48	46	50	60
Vitamin A (RE)*	800	800	800	800	800
Vitamin D (μg)	10	10	10	5	10
Vitamin E (mg)	8	8	8	8	10
Vitamin K (μg)	45	55	60	60	65
Vitamin C (mg)	50	60	60	60	70
Folic acid (μg)	150	180	180	180	400
Niacin (mg)	15	15	15	15	17
Riboflavin (mg)	1.3	1.3	1.3	1.3	1.6
Thiamin (mg)	1.1	1.1	1.1	1.1	1.5
Vitamin B_6 (mg)	1.4	1.5	1.6	1.6	2.2
Vitamin B_{12} (μg)	2.0	2.0	2.0	2.0	2.2
Calcium (mg)	1200	1200	1200	800	1200
Phosphorus (mg)	1200	1200	1200	800	1200
Iodine (μg)	150	150	150	150	175
Iron (mg)	15	15	15	15	30
Magnesium (mg)	280	300	280	280	320
Zinc (mg)	12	12	12	12	15
Selenium (μg)	45	50	55	55	65

*RE = retinal equivalent
From National Research Council, Food and Nutrition Board, *Recommended dietary allowances,* Washington, DC, 1989, National Academy Press.

REVIEW QUESTIONS

1. Provide a recommendation for a nonanemic pregnant woman.
2. Identify women at high risk for "mineral deficiency."
3. Evaluate the role that calcium may play in the prevention of PIH.

LEARNING ACTIVITIES

1. Determine the accepted policy in your community about iron supplementation during pregnancy.
2. Investigate mineral supplements available to pregnant women in local retail establishments and decide which ones might be appropriate for purchase by pregnant women.

REFERENCES

1. Abraham R: Trace element intake by Asians during pregnancy, *Proc Nutr Soc* 41:261, 1982.
2. Abu-Assal MJ, Craig WJ: The zinc status of pregnant vegetarian women, *Nutr Rep Intern* 29:485, 1984.
2a. Barker D et al: Growth in utero and serum cholesterol concentrations in adult life, *Br Med J* 307:1524, 1993.
3. Belizan JM et al: Calcium supplementation to prevent hypertensive disorders of pregnancy, *N Engl J Med* 325:1399, 1991.
4. Belizan JM et al: Calcium supplementation to prevent hypertensive disorders of pregnancy, *N Engl J Med* 325:1399, 1991.

❖ ❖ ❖

CASE STUDY

Calcium Needs During Pregnancy

Marcia Nahikian-Nelms PhD, RD, Southwest Missouri State University

Mrs. Romano is a 33-year-old woman who is pregnant with her third child. At 12 weeks gestation, she is referred to you for general nutrition counseling at her routine prenatal appointment. Mrs. Romano's previous pregnancies were complicated by both eclampsia and preterm labor. These pregnancies were eventual successful outcomes but both infants were born at about 35 weeks gestation with birth weights of 5 lbs 5 oz and 5 lbs 20 oz respectively. In addition, both pregnancies required that Mrs. Romano spend much of the last trimester at bedrest because she experienced preterm labor.

Mrs. Romano gives you the following food frequency:

- (AM) toast or bagel, fresh fruit, coffee and juice
  (mid-day) sandwich, soup and/or salad; fresh fruit; fruit juice or iced tea
- (PM) beef, chicken, or fish; pasta, rice, or potato; one or two fresh or frozen vegetables including broccoli, romaine lettuce, asparagus; fruit juice or iced tea
  (snacks) popcorn, fruit, frozen yogurt

When you ask her about her intake of milk and dairy products, she tells you that she has never really liked milk, and that her parents and other family members tend to avoid dairy products. She occasionally eats cheese but states that it is too high in fat. The only other dairy prod-

uct she consumes occasionally is frozen yogurt. She says, "I do take my prenatal vitamin everyday, and I know that it has calcium in it. I also eat lots of dark green vegetables, and I know there is lots of calcium there, too. And I use an antacid for heartburn that is advertised as containing calcium."

1. Compare Mrs. Romano's diet history with her recommended needs during pregnancy.
2. What is the physiological role of calcium in the body?
3. Mrs. Romano does appear to eat a variety of foods, but can she meet her calcium requirements without the consumption of dairy products? Using the food composition table, calculate the amount of calcium from her typical diet. Compare this with the requirements during pregnancy.
4. How may calcium intake be related to preeclampsia and the incidence of preterm labor?
5. How could you use this information to convince Mrs. Romano to increase her intake from dairy products? What strategies might you use to increase her calcium intake? At what point would you recommend additional calcium supplementation?
6. You also notice during your assessment that Mrs. Romano has multiple dental caries. Is this probably a result of low calcium intake during her previous pregnancy?

5. Belizan JM, Villar J: The relationship between calcium intake and edema-, proteinuria- and hypertension-gestosis; an hypothesis, *Am J Clin Nutr* 33:2202, 1980.
6. Bothwell TH et al: Iron metabolism in man, Oxford, Blackwell, 1979.
7. Breskin MW et al: First trimester serum zinc concentrations in human pregnancy, *Am J Clin Nutr* 38:943, 1983.
8. Bunin GR et al: Relation between maternal; diet and subsequent primitive neuroectodermal brain tumors in young children, *N Engl J Med* 329:536, 1993.

9. Bursey RG, Watson ML: The effect of sodium restriction during gestation on offspring brain development in rats, *Am J Clin Nutr* 37:43, 1983.
10. Bursey RG, Watson ML: Calcium supplementation prevents hypertensive disorders of pregnancy, *Nutr Rev* 50:233, 1992.
11. Carroli G et al: Calcium supplementation during pregnancy: a systematic review of randomised trials, *Br J Obstet Gynecol* 101:753, 1994.
12. Cole DE, Gundberg CM, Stirk LJ et al: Changing osteocalcin concentrations during pregnancy and lactation: implications for maternal mineral metabolism, *J Clin Endocrinol Metab* 65:290, 1987.

13. Coltman CA: Pagophagia and iron lack, *JAMA* 207:513, 1969.

14. Crosby WH: Food pica and iron deficiency, *Arch Intern Med* 127:960, 1971.

15. Dahle LO et al: The effect of oral magnesium substitution on pregnancy-induced leg cramps, *Am J Obstet Gynecol* 173:175, 1995.

16. Duggin GG et al: Calcium balance in pregnancy, *Lancet* 2:926, 1974.

17. Felton DJC, Stone WD: Osteomalacia in Asian immigrants during pregnancy, *BMJ* 1:1521, 1966.

18. Godfrey KM et al: Maternal nutritional status in pregnancy and blood pressure in childhood, *Br J Obstet Gynecol* 101:398, 1994.

19. Goldberg GR, Prentice AM: Maternal and fetal determinants of adult diseases, *Nutr Rev* 52:191, 1994.

20. Goldenberg RL et al: The effect of zinc supplementation on pregnancy outcome, *JAMA* 274:463, 1995.

20a. Groeneveld A et al: Fluoride in caries prevention: is the effect pre- or post-eruptive? *J Dent Res* 69(Spec. issue):751, 1990.

21. Hambidge KM et al: Acute effects of iron therapy on zinc status during pregnancy, *Obstet Gynecol* 70:593, 1987.

22. Hambidge KM et al: Zinc nutritional status during pregnancy: a longitudinal study, *Am J Clin Nutr* 37:429, 1983.

23. Hemminki E, Merilainen J: Long-term follow-up of mothers and their infants in a randomized trial on iron prophylaxis during pregnancy. *Am J Obstet Gynecol* 173:205, 1995.

24. Hetzel B: Iodine deficiency and fetal brain damage, *N Engl J Med* 331:1770, 1994.

25. Higgins AC et al: Maternal haemoglobin changes and their relationship to infant birth weight in mothers receiving a program of nutrition assessment and rehabilitation, *Nutr Res* 2:641, 1982.

26. Hunt IF et al: Zinc supplementation during pregnancy: effects on selected blood constituents and on progress and outcome of pregnancy in low-income women of Mexican descent, *Am J Clin Nutr* 40:508, 1984.

27. Hurley LS: *Developmental nutrition*, Englewood Cliffs, NJ, 1980, Prentice-Hall.

28. Institute of Medicine: *Nutrition during pregnancy: weight gain and nutrient supplements*, Washington DC, 1990, National Academy of Sciences.

29. James JD: Dental caries in pregnancy, *J Am Dent Assoc* 28:1857, 1941.

30. Jameson S: Effects of zinc deficiency in human reproduction, *Acta Med Scand Suppl* 593, 1976.

31. Jameson S: Zinc and pregnancy. In Nriagu JO, editor: *Zinc in the environment, part II: Health effects*, New York, 1978, Wiley & Sons.

32. Kaneshige E: Serum ferritin as an assessment of iron stores and other hematologic parameters during pregnancy, *Obstet Gynecol* 57:238, 1981.

33. Kirksey A et al: Relation of maternal zinc nutriture to pregnancy outcome and infant development in an Egyptian village, *Am J Clin Nutr* 60:782, 1994.

34. Koller O et al: Fetal growth retardation associated with inadequate haemodilution in otherwise uncomplicated pregnancy, *Acta Obstet Gynecol Scand* 58:9, 1979.

35. Koller O, Sandvei R, Sagen N: High haemoglobin levels during pregnancy and fetal risk, *Int J Gynaecol Obstet* 18:53, 1980.

36. Konde M et al: Goitrous endemic in Guinea, *Lancet* 344:1675, 1994.

37. Knight KB, Keith RE: Calcium supplementation on normotensive and hypertensive pregnant women, *Am J Clin Nutr* 55:891, 1992.

38. Lazebnik N, Kuhnert BR, Thompson KL: Zinc status, pregnancy complications and labor abnormalities, *Am J Obstet Gynecol* 158:161, 1988.

39. Mahomed K et al: Zinc supplementation during pregnancy: a double-blind randomised controlled trial, *BMJ* 299:826, 1989.

40. Moser PB, Reynolds RD: Dietary zinc intake and zinc concentrations of plasma, erythrocytes and breast milk in antepartum and postpartum lactating and nonlactating women: a longitudinal study, *Am J Clin Nutr* 38:101, 1983.

41. Murphy JF et al: Relation of haemoglobin levels in first and second trimesters to outcome of pregnancy, *Lancet* 1:992, 1986.

42. Naeye RL: Placental infarction leading to fetal or neonatal death, *Obstet Gynecol* 50:583, 1977.

43. National Institute of Nutrition: *Annual report*, Hyderabad, India, 1975.

44. National Research Council, Food and Nutrition Board: *Recommended dietary allowances,* Washington, DC, 1989, National Academy Press.

45. Neggers YH, Cutter GR, Acton RT et al: A positive association between maternal serum zinc concentration and birth weight, *Am J Clin Nutr* 51:678, 1990.

46. Pennington JA: A review of iodine toxicity reports, *J Am Diet Assoc* 90:1571, 1990.

47. Pike RL, Miles JE, Wardlaw JM: Juxtaglomerular degranulation and zona glomerulosa exhaustion in pregnant rats induced by low sodium intakes and reversed by sodium load, *Am J Obstet Gynecol* 95:604, 1966.

48. Purdie DW, Aaron JE, Selby PL: Bone histology and mineral hemeostasis in human pregnancy, *Br J Obstet Gynecol* 95:849, 1988.

49. Raman L et al: Effects of calcium supplementation to undernourished mothers during pregnancy on the bone density of the neonates, *Am J Clin Nutr* 31:466, 1978.

50. Raman L, Yasodhara P, Ramaraju LA: Calcium and magnesium in pregnancy, *Nutr Res* 11:1231, 1991.

51. Romslo I et al: Iron requirement in normal pregnancy assessed by serum ferritin, serum transferrin saturation and erythrocyte protoporphyrin determinations, *Br J Obstet Gynaecol* 90:101, 1983.

52. Sagen N et al: Maternal hemoglobin concentration is closely related to birth weight in normal pregnancies, *Acta Obstet Gynecol Scand* 63:245, 1984.

53. Schultink W et al: Low comliance with an iron-supplementation program: a study among pregnant women in Jakarta, Indonesia, *Am J Clin Nutr* 57:135, 1993.

54. Sibai BM, Villar MA, Bray E: Magnesium supplementation during pregnancy: a double-blind randomized controlled clinical trial, *Am J Obstet Gynecol* 161:115, 1989.

55. Sikorski R, Juszkiewicz T, Paszkowski T: Zinc status in women with premature rupture of membranes at term, *Obstet Gynecol* 76:675, 1990.

56. Simmer K, James C, Thompson RPH: Are iron-folate supplements harmful? *Am J Clin Nutr* 45:122, 1987.

57. Simmer K, Lort-Phillips L, James C et al: A double-blind trial of zinc supplementation in pregnancy, *Eur J Clin Nutr* 45:139, 1991.

58. Sowers M, Crutchfield M, Jannausch M et al: A prospective evaluation of bone mineral change in pregnancy, *Obstet Gynecol* 77:841, 1991.

59. Spatling L, Spatling G: Magnesium supplementation in pregnancy: a double-blind study, *Brit J Obstet Gynaecol* 95:120, 1988.

60. Taper LJ et al: Zinc and copper retention in pregnant women, *Fed Proc* 40:855, 1981.

61. Taylor DJ, Lind T: Haematological changes during normal pregnancy: iron-induced macrocytosis, *Br J Obstet Gynaecol* 83:760, 1976.

62. Thylstrup A: Clinical evidence of the role of pre-eruptive fluoride in caries prevention, *J Dent Res* 60:742, 1990.

63. Turnland JR et al: Zinc status and pregnancy outcome of pregnant Lebanese women, *Nutr Res* 3:309, 1983.

64. van Buul B et al: Dietary sodium restriction in the prophylaxis of hypertensive disorders of pregnancy: effects on the intake of other nutrients, *Am J Clin Nutr* 62:49, 1995.

65. Villar J, Belizan JM, Fischer PJ: Epidemiologic observations on the relationship between calcium intake and eclampsia, *Int J Gynaecol Obstet* 21:271, 1983.

66. Villar J et al: Calcium supplementation reduces blood pressure during pregnancy: results of a randomized controlled clinical trial, *Obstet Gynecol* 70:317, 1987.

66a. Villar J, Repke JT: Calcium supplementation during pregnancy may reduce preterm delivery in high-risk populations, *Am J Obstet Gynecol* 163:1124, 1990.

67. Wells JL, James DK, Luxton R, Pennock: Maternal leukocyte zinc deficiency at third trimester as a predictor of fetal growth retardation, *BMJ* 294:1054, 1987.

68. Widdowson EM: Growth and composition of the fetus and newborn. In Assali NS, editor: *Biology of gestation,* vol 2, New York, 1968, Academic Press.

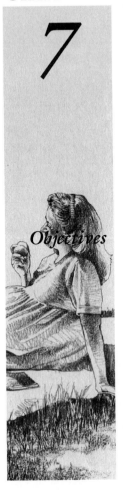

7

Lifestyle Concerns During Pregnancy

Bonnie S. Worthington-Roberts

Objectives

✦✦✦

After completing this chapter, the student will be able to:

✓ *Describe the typical food cravings and aversions of pregnant women and define the circumstance of pica.*

✓ *Summarize the characteristics of fetal alcohol syndrome and fetal alcohol effects.*

✓ *Discuss the current thinking about use of caffeine-containing products during pregnancy.*

✓ *Evaluate the potential adverse effects on pregnancy outcome of other foodborne compounds.*

✓ *Outline appropriate counseling recommendations to be made to pregnant women who wish to exercise during pregnancy.*

Introduction

Pregnancy outcome may be affected by factors other than nutrient deficiencies or excesses. Unusual eating behaviors are occasionally observed in this population, and the potential exists that such behaviors may adversely affect the mother or fetus. Alcohol, caffeine, drugs, tobacco smoke, and other such "chemicals" may also increase the risk of harm to the developing offspring. Rigorous exercise is rarely problematic but such a practice late in pregnancy may limit the growth of the fetus. This chapter deals with these agents and practices.

FOOD BELIEFS, CRAVINGS, AVOIDANCES, AND AVERSIONS[55]

Most women change their diets during the course of pregnancy. Some changes are based on medical advice, others on folk medical beliefs, and others on changes in preference and appetite that may be idiosyncratic or culturally patterned. Since those that are culturally sanctioned will affect a woman's willingness to follow prescribed dietary regimens, the health care provider should be sensitized to their existence.

193

Many beliefs have been recorded about prenatal diet, such as the idea that the mother can mark her child before birth by eating specific foods. Overuse of a craved food during pregnancy is thought to explain physical or behavioral peculiarities of the infant. More often, unsatiated cravings are thought to explain birthmarks that mimic the shape of the desired food (such as strawberry or drumstick-shaped marks). Behavioral markings have also been thought to derive from the prenatal diet; that is, the mother's consumption of certain foods has been said to cause the child to like such foods after birth.

Another important group of beliefs concerns dietary means by which the mother can ensure an easier delivery. Most important, from the biomedical viewpoint, are beliefs that lead a woman to avoid animal protein foods or to avoid "excessive" weight gain. Most lay people know very well that a smaller weight gain during pregnancy produces a smaller infant; since a smaller baby may be "easier to deliver," low weight gain has been proposed as desirable, especially since it is commonly believed that the baby can "catch up" after birth.

Food avoidances are those foods that the mother consciously chooses not to consume during her pregnancy, usually for a reason she can articulate and that seems reasonable to her. The four most commonly avoided foods are sources of animal protein: milk, lean meats, pork, and liver. Cravings and aversions are powerful urges toward or away from foods, including foods about which women experience no unusual attitudes outside of pregnancy. The most commonly reported craved foods are sweets and dairy products. The most common aversions are reported to be alcohol, caffeinated drinks, and meats. However, cravings and aversions are not limited to any particular foods or food groups.

The nutritional significance of these food-related behaviors is difficult to evaluate. Available information has often been collected in an anecdotal or one-sided manner. Thus, there is limited detailed information on dietary alterations that appear to be detrimental but little knowledge of total subcultural prenatal dietary intakes. As a result, it is difficult to quantify the nutritional effect of restrictive beliefs, avoidances, cravings, or aversions. The nutritional importance of such practices cannot be assessed without reference to the rest of the woman's diet. Overall, however, most cravings result in increased intakes of calcium and energy, whereas aversions often result in decreased intake of alcohol and caffeine but also decreased intake of animal protein. Cravings and aversions are not necessarily deleterious.

PICA[32]

Pica refers to the compulsion for persistent ingestion of unsuitable substances having little or no nutritional value. Pica of pregnancy most often involves consumption of dirt and/or clay (**geophagia**) or starch (**amylophagia**). However, compulsive ingestion of a variety of nonfood substances has been noted, such as ice, burnt matches, hair, stone or gravel, charcoal, soot, cigarette ashes, mothballs, antacid tablets, milk of magnesia, baking soda, coffee grounds, and tire inner tubes. The practice of pica is not new nor is it limited to any one geographical area, race, creed, culture, gender, or status within a culture.

Pica practices of pregnant women have been assessed through a systematic review of the literature for the period 1950 through 1990. Pica behavior was considered in terms of its prevalence, risk factors, clinical profile and effect on pregnancy outcome.[32] The prevalence of pica among pregnant women in high-risk groups declined between the 1950s and the 1970s but now remains steady; about one fifth of high-risk women are affected. Women at high risk for pica are more likely to be black, to live in rural areas and to have a positive childhood and family history of pica.

The medical implications of pica are not well understood, although several speculations have been put forward. The displacement effect of pica substances could result in reduced intake of nutritious foods, leading to inadequate dietary intakes of essential nutrients. Alternatively, substances that provide calories (e.g., starch) could lead to obesity if ingested in amounts above the usual dietary intakes. Some pica substances may contain toxic compounds or quantities of nutrients not tolerated in disease states. Some pica substances interfere with the absorption of certain mineral elements (such as iron). Other less commonly reported complications of pica are:

1. Congenital lead poisoning secondary to maternal pica for wall plaster
2. Tender, irritable uterus with dystocia associated with **fecal impaction** from clay ingestion
3. **Fetal hemolytic anemia** caused by maternal ingestion of mothballs and toilet air fresheners.
4. Parotid enlargement and gastric and small bowel obstruction from ingestion of excessive laundry starch
5. Parasitic infection from ingestion of contaminated soil or clay

The etiologic factors of pica are poorly understood, although several proposals have been put forth. One theory suggests that the ingestion of nontraditional substances relieves nausea and vomiting. The example of the dog who will eat dirt or grass during illness is often used to illustrate this theory. Some research indicates that pica is a normal behavioral response to gastrointestinal tract upset in rats. It has also been hypothesized that a deficiency of an essential nutrient such as calcium or iron results in the eating of nonfood substances that contain these nutrients. When prenatal patients were questioned concerning the practice of pica, a variety of answers were given:

1. A taste for clay
2. Clay kept the baby from being marked at birth
3. Nervous tension was relieved
4. Starch made the newborn lighter in color
5. Starch helped the baby to "slide out" more easily during delivery
6. Clay quieted hunger pains
7. Clay and starch were pleasant to chew
8. Social approval of pica

Many of these reasons are based on superstition, custom, and tradition, or practices that are passed from mother to daughter.

Health care professionals who counsel pregnant women need to be alert to the potential practice of pica in each client. Anemia and other poor pregnancy outcomes may occur as a result of excessive intakes of these nonfood items.

Consequently, all pregnant patients need to be asked about pica behavior; if present, they should be counseled about the possible effects and monitored for anemia and poor fetal development. Since our knowledge about adverse effects is limited, continued observation of patients with these interesting behaviors is warranted.

POTENTIALLY HARMFUL DIETARY COMPONENTS
Alcohol

During the past 20 years, health researchers have become aware of the adverse effect of excessive consumption of alcohol on fetal development.[7,26,35,46,64,78] In 1973 a University of Washington group[35] described a unique set of characteristics of infants born to women who were chronic alcoholics. These infants exhibited specific anomalies of the eyes, nose, heart, and central nervous system that were accompanied by growth retardation, small head circumference, and mental retardation. The investigators named the condition **fetal alcohol syndrome (FAS)** (Fig. 7-1; Table 7-1).

There is a high rate of prenatal mortality among infants with FAS. Infants who survive generally show signs of irritability and hyperactivity after birth. These symptoms are attributable to alcohol withdrawal. Physical and mental development is impaired. Infants with FAS exhibit poor rates of weight gain and failure to thrive despite concerted efforts at nutritional rehabilitation (see box on p. 196). The mental and growth deficits are generally seen at birth but follow-up of afflicted children later in life indicates that these deficits continue (Figs. 7-2 and 7-3).[17,70]

The impact of more moderate levels of alcohol consumption on fetal development has been the focus of much research during the past 20 years. It is now well-recognized that moderate drinkers may produce offspring with fetal alcohol effects (FAE); this term refers to the more subtle features of FAS. Diagnosis of FAE is by no means an easy task. For this reason the term possible fetal alcohol effects (PFAE) has been coined to describe individuals who have been prenatally exposed to alcohol and present with

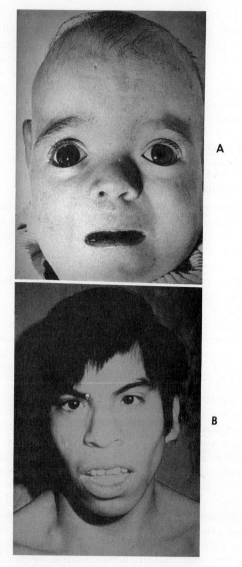

FIG. 7-1   **A,** A baby with FAS. **B,** A baby with FAS "grown up."

❖

MORE SUBTLE FEATURES OF FETAL ALCOHOL SYNDROME

Characteristics
Growth deficiency for height and weight
Distinct pattern of facial features and other physical abnormalities
Central nervous system dysfunction
Indicators of central nervous system dysfunction
Microcephaly (small head circumference)
Poor coordination
Lower average IQ
Hyperactivity
Attention problems
Learning difficulties
Developmental delays
Motor problems

cognitive and behavioral problems but do not have all of the facial characteristics of FAS. Simply put, PFAE is "FAS without a face." In the absence of the characteristic facial features, the cognitive/behavioral dysfunction in an individual cannot be directly and exclusively linked to the prenatal alcohol exposure. Therefore FAE is not a medical diagnosis at this time, and it is

more accurate to use the term *possible* fetal alcohol effects. PFAE is also not a mild form of FAS. In fact, individuals with PFAE can be just as severely affected cognitively and behaviorally as those with FAS. The needs of individuals with PFAE and their families may be just as acute as those with full FAS. However, it is often difficult for affected individuals to access services because they do not have a medical diagnosis.[70]

Animal studies are used to determine a median lethal dose (LD_{50}) of a toxic substance—the dose at which half of the fetuses will die. It is assumed that the individual differences in sensitivity to the exposure are distributed around the LD_{50}; some fetuses will die at a lower dose and others will survive at an even higher dose. If a large number of different doses are tested, with a large number of animals per dose, an S-shaped curve is observed (represented by the fetal death curve in Fig. 7-4). The threshold is the dose of alcohol at which all but the most vulnerable fetuses are affected. Certain outcomes are expected to have lower thresholds than others. Death would be expected to take place at the highest threshold, whereas milder forms of damage would occur at lower doses.[34]

TABLE 7-1 *Facial Characteristics in Fetal Alcohol Syndrome*[15]

	Features Necessary to Characteristic Face	Associated Features
Eyes	Short palpebral fissures	
Nose	Short and upturned in early child hood; hypoplastic philtrum	Flat nasal bridge; epicanthal folds
Maxilla	Flattened	
Mouth	Thinned upper vermilion	Prominent lateral palatine ridges; cleft lip with or without cleft palate; small teeth
Mandible		Retrognathia in infancy; micrognathia or relative prognathia in adolescents
Ears		Posterior rotation; abnormal concha

From Clarren SK: Recognition of fetal alcohol syndrome, *JAMA* 245:2436, 1981. © 1981, American Medical Association.

Mechanisms. At present, the mechanisms by which alcohol produces such widespread effects on the fetus are not completely understood.[47,61] Scientists have used experimental animals and in vitro methods (whole embryos or cells grown in a test tube or petri dish) to help them determine the molecular and cellular events affected by exposure of embryonic tissues to alcohol. Since alcohol can cross the placenta, the current hypothesis is that high levels build up in the fetus and produce direct toxic effects that are most adverse in the early phases of pregnancy during blastogenesis and cell differentiation. Another theory is that some of the effects of alcohol may be caused by maternal malnutrition. Women who derive a substantial portion of their daily caloric needs from alcohol may not have an appetite for more nutritious foods. Micronutrient deficiencies are often seen in alcoholics.

Besides the possible role of nutritional deficiencies in the manifestation of FAS, other theories have been introduced. Adverse changes have been proposed to occur in the following[47]:

- Hormonal factors
- Local growth factors
- Level and variety of prostaglandins
- Diminished oxygen delivery to fetal tissues
- Impaired cell migration and adhesion.

Many crucial biochemical and cellular events are affected by exposure of the fetus to alcohol during gestation. It is too early to speculate whether any one of alcohol's effects on molecular or cellular function is more significant than others.

In the developed world, FAS is the major cause of significant lifetime disabilities. Unlike many other birth defects, however, it is preventable. Prevention of FAS is a national health priority included in the *Healthy People 2000* objectives for health promotion and disease prevention. The specific health objective is to *reduce the rate of FAS to no more than 1.2 cases per 10,000 live births by the year 2000.* Surveillance programs allow for the tracking of the prevalence of a condition over time. Tracking the prevalence of FAS poses particular problems, however, since there is no "gold standard" of diagnosis. At the present time, the reported incidence rate of FAS is depressingly high (Fig. 7-5).[19,24]

The impact of binge drinking on the outcome of pregnancy has never been satisfactorily evaluated in human populations. Recently, however, use of a monkey model has allowed researchers to study the effects of one binge a week on pregnancy course and outcome.[16] Clarren, Bowden, and Astley exposed pigtailed macaques to various doses of ethanol once weekly. At doses of 2.5 gm/kg, pregnancy failure was seen in the early weeks of study; lower doses were associated with increased risk of spontaneous abortion. Viable offspring of the binge drinking mothers are currently under study. Preliminary data suggest permanent damage to the central nervous system manifested by abnormal behavior.

Need for intervention. It is imperative to identify alcohol and other drug use in pregnant

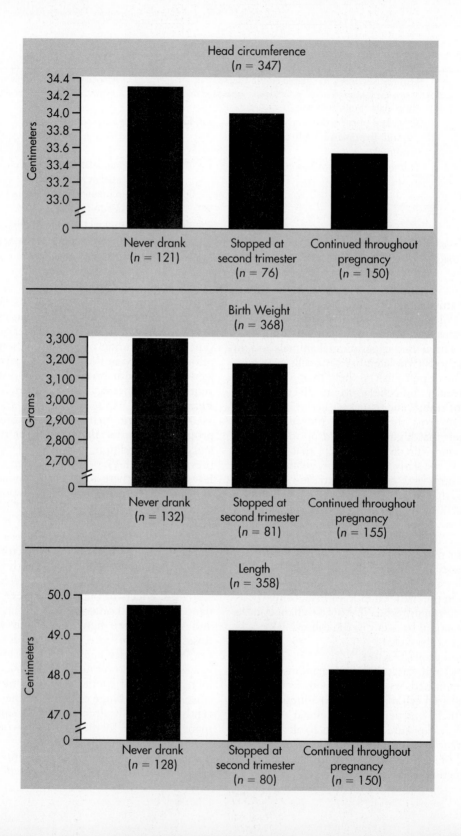

FIG. 7-2 Effects of alcohol exposure on growth. Growth was reduced the most in children whose mothers continued to drink throughout the pregnancy. Growth was not as affected in those whose mothers stopped drinking in the second trimester. These data suggest that exposure that continues throughout pregnancy produces fetal growth deficiencies that can be observed at birth.

From Coles, C. Critical periods for prenatal alcohol exposure. Evidence from animal and human studies, *Alcohol, Health Res World* 18:22, 1994.

women as early as possible during the course of prenatal care so that interventions may be applied.[65,66] However, many health professionals do not feel comfortable asking pregnant women about alcohol and other drug use. In addition, the time constraints of many busy prenatal clinics and private practices encourage health professionals to avoid adding time-consuming assessments to their already busy schedules[30] (see box at right).

Recent estimates, however, suggest that alcohol and drug use continues to escalate. Recent surveys indicate that 10% to 15% of women of childbearing age (15 to 44 years) are actively using alcohol or other drugs. Prospective studies in large metropolitan areas such as Boston have reported drug use in approximately 15% of the pregnant women evaluated. Another study in Florida found the same level of drug use and observed no substantial differences between clinic and private patients or between black and white patients.[30]

The Maternal Addiction Project (MAP) at St. Francis Medical Center in Pittsburgh has been treating pregnant women who use alcohol and other drugs since 1979. A major objective of this group is to improve identification of pregnant women using drugs in their geographic area. The following principles of identification have been put forward[30]:

1. All pregnant women should be asked about their use of alcohol and other drugs.
2. An identification method should not disrupt the flow of the prenatal clinic or office or be overly time consuming.
3. An interview style that incorporates respect and encourages trust will yield more truthful responses.

> ❖
> ### THE REAL WORLD—THE PREGNANT WOMAN WHO IS WORRIED
>
> Not uncommonly, a woman will find that she is pregnant well after the embryonic period. She remembers that she consumed a glass of champagne on her anniversary 6 to 8 weeks before. She is in a panic! One can generally be comfortable in explaining to the woman that chances are very good that the small level of alcohol consumed had no impact on the fetus. She should be encouraged to maintain a healthy lifestyle for the duration of the pregnancy without dwelling on this issue.

4. Specific questions about alcohol and other drug use can be readily incorporated into the usual history-taking process.
5. Drug and alcohol use during pregnancy has been associated with a number of risk factors in various studies. Determination of the presence of these risk factors can assist in identifying pregnant women who need further assessment.
6. Some women will need to be asked about alcohol and other drug use repeatedly for an honest answer to be obtained.
7. Some women who abuse alcohol and other drugs need to be confronted about their use to help them recognize that such use is a problem for them.
8. Identification can best be accomplished by combining a comprehensive interview

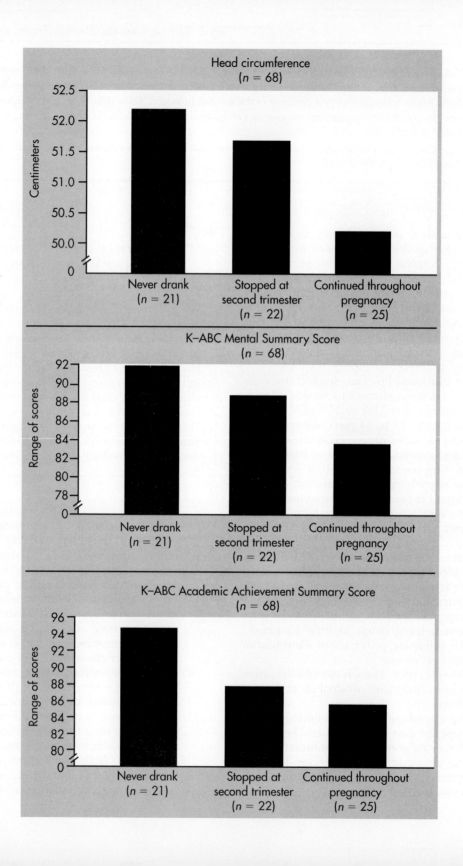

Head circumference
(*n* = 68)

Centimeters

52.5
52.0
51.5
51.0
50.5
50.0
0

Never drank
(*n* = 21)

Stopped at
second trimester
(*n* = 22)

Continued throughout
pregnancy
(*n* = 25)

K–ABC Mental Summary Score
(*n* = 68)

Range of scores

92
90
88
86
84
82
80
78
0

Never drank
(*n* = 21)

Stopped at
second trimester
(*n* = 22)

Continued throughout
pregnancy
(*n* = 25)

K–ABC Academic Achievement Summary Score
(*n* = 68)

Range of scores

96
94
92
90
88
86
84
82
80
0

Never drank
(*n* = 21)

Stopped at
second trimester
(*n* = 22)

Continued throughout
pregnancy
(*n* = 25)

FIG. 7-3 **A,** Reevaluation of growth in alcohol-exposed children at 5-7 years of age (head circumference). **B,** Effects on aptitude in alcohol-exposed children aged 2-12 years. **C,** Effects of academic achievement in alcohol-exposed children aged 2-12 years.

From Coles C: Critical periods for prenatal alcohol exposure. Evidence from animal and human studies, *Alcohol, Health Res World* 18:22, 1994.

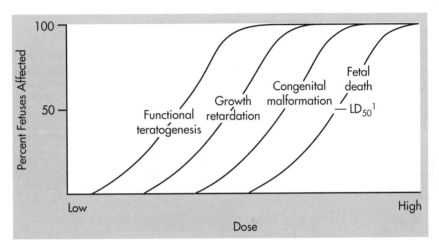

FIG. 7-4 Ideal dose-response curves for four domains affected by toxic exposure during fetal development. As dose of a toxic substance increases more fetuses are at risk of injury and effects become more severe ranging from functional teratogenesis which includes neurobehavioral outcomes to fetal death.

and urine drug screening. Although many pregnant women who use alcohol or other drugs can be identified through an interview method, some cannot. Urine screening for drugs should be used in combination with an interview, with the knowledge that some women who admit to use will have negative results on urine screening and some women who deny use will have positive results on urine screening. The presence of risk factors for alcohol and other drug use can be used to assist in determining which women should have their urine screened. Urine screening alone is inadequate for identifying alcohol and other drug use in pregnant women.

9. Risk factors associated with use of alcohol and other drugs may differ between pregnant teenagers and pregnant adult women. Although the approach to

recognition of alcohol and other drug use in teenagers may be similar to that in adult women, enough differences exist that we have designed a separate identification method for use with teenagers.

10. We recognize that many women who abuse alcohol and other drugs do not use prenatal care. Some of these women seek medical care only for a pregnancy-related problem (e.g., pain or bleeding) or at the time of delivery. These women also can be identified by using a risk assessment approach.

Paternal alcohol exposure. Paternal alcohol consumption may affect fetal development through a direct effect on the father's sperm or gonads. There are three possible mechanisms for the effect of paternal alcohol consumption on the offspring. First, alcohol may directly affect the characteristics and properties of sperm, per-

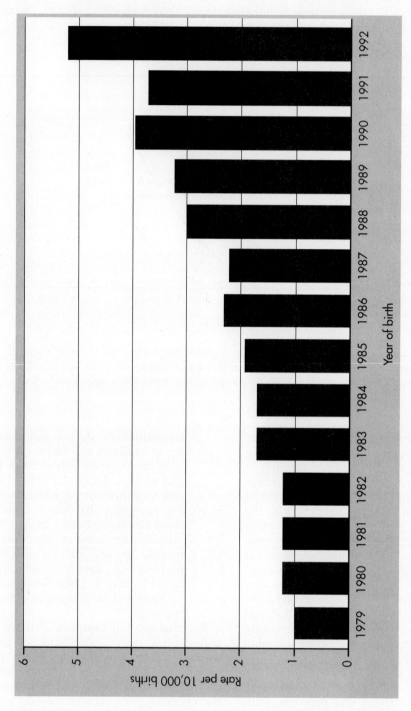

FIG. 7-5   Reported incidence rate of fetal alcohol syndrome by year of birth, from the Birth Defects Monitoring Program of the Centers for Disease Control and Prevention, 1979-1992.

From Cordero JF et al: Tracking the prevalence of FAS, *Alcohol, Health Res World* 18:82, 1994.

haps by causing mutations in the sperm's genetic material. Second, sperm may be "selected" in some way such that only a specific population is functionally intact following prolonged exposure to alcohol. Third, alcohol consumption might alter the chemical composition of semen so as to influence the activity of ejaculated sperm. Animal studies suggest that any of these possibilities holds true. Much more investigation of human males is required before useful light can be shed on this issue.[9]

Caffeine

In 1980 the Food and Drug Administration (FDA) warned pregnant women to restrict or even eliminate consumption of coffee based on studies showing teratogenic effects in rodents.[18] Although this advisory remains in effect, the implications of caffeine consumption during pregnancy remain controversial.

The results of studies in rodents indicate that caffeine, when administered in large single doses has teratogenic effects.[18] In addition to fetal resorptions, the most commonly seen malformations are those of the limbs and digits, as well as cleft lips and palates. Such malformations are observed, however, only in relatively high doses. Teratogenic effects usually appear only at doses high enough to cause toxicity in the mother and far higher than those consumed by humans, even those who drink large amounts of coffee. For example, a woman weighing 60 kg would have to drink about 10 to 14 cups of coffee in one sitting to achieve plasma caffeine concentrations comparable to those associated with teratogenic effects in the rat. Animal studies in which more moderate doses were administered over the course of a day (to mimic the typical pattern of human caffeine intake) have not shown teratogenic effects.

The available human evidence indicates that there is at most a very slight relationship between moderate caffeine consumption and the incidence of common congenital abnormalities.[56,60] Most epidemiological surveys have not shown an association between caffeine intake and the frequency of malformations. However, very little is known about the potential teratogenic effect of very large amounts of coffee (more than 8 cups per day).[33,49]

Animal studies suggest that maternal consumption of caffeine may have detectable effects on the behavior of the newborn.[22,48,58] Very few human studies have been performed on the neurobehavioral consequences of mothers' caffeine intake. A few studies have shown a positive association between maternal caffeine consumption and the incidence of neonatal apnea. However, no long-term consequence of prenatal caffeine exposure have been reported.[54]

Of significance is the reality that caffeine may have detrimental interactions with other substances that are harmful to the developing fetus. For example, most animal studies have reported that caffeine potentiates the teratogenic effect of alcohol. Interactions with other drugs are also possible; they may act in synergy with caffeine to induce constriction of blood vessels in the fetus. Other evidence suggests that caffeine may interact with tobacco to retard intrauterine growth.

A recent review of this issue by Nehlig and Debry provided the following conclusion:

> In the absence of more precise data and to avoid any fetotoxic risk, women should be advised to moderate their consumption of coffee during pregnancy and above all, to avoid tobacco and alcohol as well as other vasoconstricting medications such as anti-migraine drugs.

Herbal Teas

Herbal teas and herbal remedies have been part of folk medicine for centuries. There are currently more than 400 distinct herbs and spices commercially available to use either alone or in blended mixtures as tea. Many commercially prepared drugs originated from plants.[31,74] Consumers interested in "natural food" often turn to these products; other consumers looking for alternatives to caffeine-containing beverages often find herbal teas attractive[42] (see box on p. 204).

Pregnant women should be discouraged from unlimited consumption of herb teas. The major reason for this is that the composition and safety of most of them is unknown. Rather than seek FDA approval, most manufacturers of herbal tea preparations stopped marketing the mixtures as medicine and simply list the ingredients on the label.[25]

In 1983 the FDA officially designated 28 plants as unsafe to consume and wrote, "We

❖

> ### *MATERNAL USE OF GINSENG:*
> #### *AN INTERESTING CONSIDERATION*[3,40]
>
> There are some data suggesting that maternal use of ginseng may be associated with neonatal androgenization. The last word is not in.

Awang D: Maternal use of ginseng and neonatal androgenization, *JAMA* 265:1828, 1991

Koren G et al: Maternal ginseng use associated with neonatal androgenization, *JAMA* 264:2866, 1990

cannot conclude that all herbal teas are safe nor that it's safe to consume large amounts of any herbal tea over extended periods."[2] It is likely that many herbal teas are safe, but some (lobelia, sassafras, coltsfoot, comfrey, and pennyroyal) have been shown to have potentially harmful side effects; depressed breathing, convulsions and, in mice, malignancy have been reported.[2,41]

Because of the lack of safety testing, pregnant women should be cautious of herbal tea mixtures. They should be advised to choose only products in filtered tea bags, and in order to avoid displacing more nutritious beverages, to limit herbal tea consumption to two 8-oz servings per day.[42,75]

Food Additives

The teratogenicity of common food additives is largely unknown in human situations. Metabolites of **cyclamate** and red dye no. 2 reportedly damage developing rat embryos, but both of these additives have now been banned from use in the U.S. food supply. Artificial sweeteners have come under careful scrutiny in the past few years. Neither **saccharin** nor cyclamate has proven to be teratogenic in rodents. Kline et al[39] reported that the incidence of spontaneous abortion in a human population was not associated with ingestion of any sugar substitute. However, because saccharin has been shown to be weakly carcinogenic in rats, moderation in its use seems appropriate. This is especially true for the woman of reproductive age, since studies in rats indicate that saccharin is most effective as an initiator of bladder cancer when the mother is exposed to high doses before pregnancy and the offspring are exposed in utero and throughout their lives. Because saccharin can also markedly promote or enhance the potential of other carcinogens in rats, another basis for moderation in use is available.

Aspartame. Since the approval of **aspartame** for use in carbonated beverages, there has been much debate about the safety of the additive in the diets of pregnant women.[5] Major concern has been voiced about the added phenylalanine load since high circulating levels of phenylalanine (as are seen in women with poorly controlled phenylketonuria) are known to damage the fetal brain. However, individuals who do not have phenylketonuria have markedly lower serum phenylalanine levels, even those who are carriers for the phenylketonuria gene (heterozygotes). Phenylalanine-induced embryopathy is likely only if the phenylalanine values are continuously 1,200 μmol/L.

In normal persons fed 200 mg/kg aspartame, or the equivalent of 60 12-oz cans of diet soda at one time (or in heterozygotes fed 100 mg/kg), blood phenylalanine concentrations peak well below the sustained concentration level deemed harmful. To produce persistent phenylalanine concentrations of 600 μmol/L in pregnant heterozygotes, a woman would have to drink one can of diet soda every 8 minutes, 24 hours a day—a physical impossibility. In view of these practical considerations and the fact that no data exist to suggest that use of aspartame-containing products is associated with adverse pregnancy outcome, it seems unreasonable to direct pregnant women to avoid this artificial sweetener.[71]

Food Contaminants

Heavy metals. A number of "contaminants" are found in food, and some of these may adversely affect pregnancy course and outcome if consumed in sufficient amounts. Most heavy metals are embryotoxic, but only mercury, lead, cadmium, and possibly nickel and selenium have been implicated in this regard. Lead toxicity has long been known to be associated with abortion and menstrual disorders. Evidence as to whether lead is teratogenic is conflicting; whereas some authors report a correlation between atmospheric lead levels and congenital malformations, others deny these associations. In sheep, prenatal lead exposure has also been shown to affect the offspring's learning ability.

Probably the earliest instance of massive, unplanned exposure of a localized population to an environmental toxicant occurred in 1953, in and around Minamata, a town located on a bay in southern Japan. Unusual neurological problems (e.g., mental confusion, convulsions, and coma) began afflicting villagers. Over a third of the affected individuals died, and many infants and children suffered permanent brain damage from prenatal and neonatal exposure; mercury was transported across the placenta and also appeared in breast milk of mothers consuming contaminated fish. Eventually the source of the mercury was traced to the effluent discharged from a local plastics factory into Minamata Bay. A similar incident occurred in Niigata, Japan, in 1964.

Another massive methylmercury disaster occurred in Iraq during the winter of 1971 and 1972. In this case, barley and wheat grain treated with methylmercury as a fungicide had been purchased from Mexico. The grain sacks carried a written warning—but only in Spanish. Thirty-one pregnant women were hospitalized with methylmercury poisoning, and almost half of them died. Infants born to surviving mothers showed evidence of cerebral palsy, blindness and severe brain damage. Similar outbreaks have occurred in Russia, Sweden, and elsewhere.

Columbia University researchers have found that liquor kept in crystal decanters may contain undesirably high levels of lead; this metal is known to inflict irreversible damage on the brain, kidneys, and nervous system. The fact is that much of the fine crystal sold today is 22% to 30% lead by weight. Although lead may give crystal its brilliance, the bad news is that beverages stored in crystal absorb some of the heavy metal in a dissolved form. Columbia researchers advise pregnant women or women who think they might be (or become) pregnant not to use crystal decanters or glasses at all.

Several other heavy metals probably affect the fetus and infant. Cadmium, which is derived accidentally from tobacco smoke, the electroplat-

ing industry, and deterioration of rubber tires, is a known cause of developmental malformations in rodents. Nickel in low doses causes embryotoxicity in rats and eye malformations in the progeny. Selenium is also a suspect teratogen.

Chlorinated dioxin derivatives are among the most toxic substances known and may occur as contaminants in many substances such as herbicides and wood preservatives. The spraying of Agent Orange (a herbicide) in Vietnam has been suggested to be responsible for the increased incidence of abortion, stillbirth, and malformation among exposed persons, their spouses, or offspring. The spraying of 2,4,5-trichlorophenoxyacetic acid in parts of Oregon in the early 1970s to increase the productivity in commercial forests raised concern by the Environmental Protection Agency (EPA), whose officials were informed of the significant incidence of spontaneous abortion among women in an area exposed to the spray. A subsequent study reported in 1979 not only demonstrated the increased abortion rate throughout the spraying area but also showed that most of these miscarriages had occurred in the months of June and July, just after the peak spraying period of March and April. Breast milk of women from the same affected area also contained significant dioxin concentrations.

Dioxin derivatives are now well-known to act as potent teratogens in experimental animals, including primates. Rhesus monkeys exposed during pregnancy showed a marked increase in placental and fetal levels of dioxin derivatives and a marked increase in the rate of abortion and birth defects, particularly cleft palate and kidney abnormalities. Other studies have reported a significant concentration of these compounds in the fat of beef grazed on dioxin-sprayed rangelands. Unfortunately, almost nothing is known about the biochemical basis for the toxicity of these compounds, and safe or "threshold" levels of exposure have not been established.[67]

Polychlorinated biphenyls (PCBs), used as plasticizers and heat exchange fluids, comprise another group of chemicals that endanger health. In Kyushu, Japan, in 1968, ingestion of cooking oil contaminated with PCBs by pregnant and lactating women resulted in small-for-gestational-age infants with dark skin, eye defects, and other abnormalities. Although prenatal exposure was probably significant, evidence indicated that transfer of PCBs through breast milk was the most significant route of exposure. Polybromated biphenyl (PBB), produced commercially as a fire retardant, also provoked attention after its accidental entry into cattle feed in Michigan in 1973 and 1974. Over 30,000 cattle and many sheep, swine, and poultry died or had to be slaughtered. Contaminated meat, milk, and eggs were identified in local food supplies, and stillbirth among affected cattle increased. Adverse effects in human pregnancy have not yet been reported, but considerable concern still exists.

One report[6] suggests that consumption of **aflatoxin**-tainted foods by pregnant women significantly increases their risk of delivering mentally retarded children. Data supporting this relationship derive from observations of mothers and their children in two rural Georgia counties. The mothers of mentally retarded children had diets that differed from the average

in terms of foods but did not differ in terms of critical nutrients. The consumption of corn, rice, peanuts and milk (foods potentially high in aflatoxins) was significantly related to mental retardation of children; high levels of aflatoxin were found in the food supply. Although these findings are provocative, additional work is required to confirm the proposed relationship.

TOBACCO, MARIJUANA, AND COCAINE
Tobacco

Fetal growth retardation is often seen in offspring of cigarette smokers (Fig. 7-6). It has been postulated that this is a result of the reduced food intake of the mother, but observations have shown that this is not true[62,63]; women smokers often consume more kcalories per day than women who do not smoke (Fig. 7-7). The growth-retarding impact of smoking appears to be related to the effects of carbon

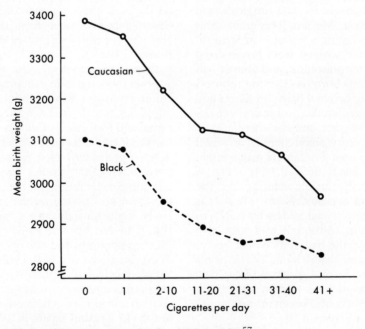

FIG. 7-6 Maternal cigarette use and infant birth weight.[57]

Modified from Niswander KR, Gordon M: *The women and their pregnancies*, Philadelphia, 1972, WB Saunders.

monoxide, nicotine, cyanides, and possibly other compounds on placental perfusion and oxygen transport to the fetus.[62,63] It is also likely that efficiency of kcalorie utilization is reduced in women who smoke.[62,63] Whether or not encouraging greater weight gain among smoking mothers will increase infant size is a question that has been inadequately addressed. However, several reports have suggested that greater prenatal weight gain is directly related to greater infant birth weight in this population.[45,59]

In 1992, 16.9% of U.S. mothers reported having smoked during pregnancy. Smoking was more common in white mothers than in blacks. In both groups, there has been a small reduction in the level of smoking since 1989. Smoking rates for Asian women are generally very low; this is also true of Hispanic mothers. In both cases, the level of smoking was observed to be less in foreign-born than U.S.-born mothers.[51]

With regard to pregnancy outcome, in 1992, babies born to smokers were at nearly twice the risk of low birth weight as babies born to non-smokers. The effect of smoking on infant birth weight becomes more severe with advancing maternal age. The percent of low birth weight for births to women who smoked the fewest cigarettes, less than 6 per day, was still 41% higher than for births to nonsmokers.[51]

So sizable is the number of babies affected by maternal smoking that the recommendation has been made to combine the key features into a case definition or a descriptive diagnostic term such as **fetal tobacco syndrome.** Providing such diagnostic criteria would serve to (1) facilitate identification, (2) allow a more precise epidemiologic assessment of population risks associated with cigarette smoking during pregnancy, (3) allow more precise evaluation of the effectiveness of smoking intervention programs, and (4) appropriately focus more public attention on this preventable cause of serious morbidity. The proposed definition of the fetal tobacco syndrome includes the following four conditions:

1. The mother smoked five or more cigarettes a day throughout the pregnancy.

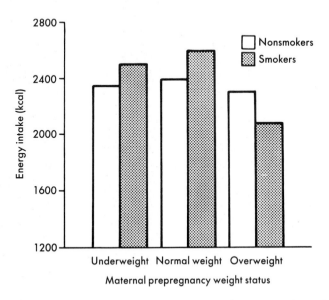

FIG. 7-7 Maternal energy intake of smokers and nonsmokers as seen in underweight (90% ideal), normal weight (90% to 110% ideal), and overweight (>110% ideal) women.

Data on public and private patients combined as reported by Haworth JC et al: Fetal growth retardation in cigarette smoking mothers is not due to decreased food intake, *Am J Obstet Gynecol* 137:719, 1980.

2. The mother had no evidence of hypertension during pregnancy, specifically no preeclampsia and documentation of normal blood pressure at least once after the first trimester.

3. The newborn has symmetrical growth retardation at term (≥37 weeks) defined as birth weight less than 2500 gm and a **ponderal index** greater than 2.32.

4. There is no other obvious cause of intrauterine growth retardation.

Adoption of this definition would help emphasize that cigarette smoking is the single most powerful determinant of poor fetal growth in the developed world.

The impact of smoking on fetal growth is well-established, whereas its impact on the production of congenital malformations is controversial. Although several studies[36,46,68] have reported positive associations between smoking and specific malformations, particularly oral clefts, others did not find such relationships. In one report, the association between cigarette smoking and oral clefts was examined using data from the Maryland Birth Defects Reporting and Information System. It was found that mothers of infants with oral clefts (cleft lip with and without cleft palate and cleft palate alone) smoked more during pregnancy than mothers or infants with other defects; there was also found to be a dose-response relation between the daily amount smoked and the risk of clefting. Adjustment for potentially confounding variables did not account for the association[36] (see box above).

Smoking is probably the most important modifiable cause of poor pregnancy outcome among women in the United States. Recent estimates suggest that the elimination of smoking during pregnancy could prevent about 5% of perinatal deaths, about 20% of low-birth-weight births and about 8% of preterm deliveries in the United States.

Maternal smoking is associated with several complications of pregnancy including abruptio placentae, placenta previa, bleeding during pregnancy, premature and prolonged rupture of the membranes and preterm delivery. Maternal smoking retards fetal growth, causes an average reduction in birth weight of 200 gm and dou-

---

PREGNANT WOMEN SHOULD NOT SMOKE![38]

It is estimated that if all pregnant women stopped smoking, the number of fetal and infant deaths would be reduced by approximately 10%.

From Kleinman JC, Pierre MB, Madans JH et al: The effects of maternal smoking on fetal and infant mortality, *Am J Epidemiol* 127:274, 1988.

bles the risk of having a low birth weight baby. Studies have shown a 25% to 50% higher rate of fetal and infant deaths among women who smoke during pregnancy, compared with those who do not. Women who stop smoking before becoming pregnant have infants of the same birth weight as those born to women who have never smoked.[72]

Effect of maternal age. A study was conducted in Alabama from January 1983 through January 1988; during this time, there were approximately 20,000 births in the two participating hospitals. The focus of the project was to determine if a relationship existed between smoking and maternal age and their combined effects on birth weight, intrauterine growth retardation, and preterm delivery. The effect of smoking on both fetal growth and gestational age was significantly greater as maternal age increased.

After adjusting for confounding variables, smoking was associated with a fivefold increased risk of growth retardation in women older than 35, but there was less than a twofold increased risk in women younger than 17. Smoking reduced birth weight by 134 gm in young women but 301 gm in women older than 35. Smoking in older women was also associated with more instances of preterm delivery and a lower mean gestational age when compared with women 25 or younger.[77]

Risk of sudden infant death. A population-based study was conducted in Sweden to assess risk factors for sudden infant death syndrome (SIDS). All infants surviving the first week of life were included (*n* = 279,938). The overall rate of SIDS was 0.7 per 1,000 first-week survivors; elevated relative risks were associated with low maternal age, multiparity, maternal smoking and male infants. *Maternal smoking doubled the risk; there was a clear dose-response rate.* Maternal smoking also seemed to influence the time of death; infants of smokers died at an earlier age. It would appear that in countries like Sweden, *smoking may be the single most important preventable risk factor for sudden infant death syndrome.*[28]

Smoking cessation programs are now available in many communities, and some of these are oriented specifically to pregnant women. The few studies that have examined their effectiveness indicate that if cessation or even marked reduction can be achieved, infant birth weight is increased.[68] Not all women will be able to respond successfully to this intervention, however, it makes sense that much effort should be made preconceptionally and prenatally to involve women who smoke in such programs.

Marijuana[21]

Although there have been reports of an association between prenatal marijuana exposure and smaller size at birth, these have been offset by reports that found no such effect. Growth deficits have not been found in studies with long-term follow-up. Similarly, recent data refute earlier reports of physical abnormalities resulting from prenatal marijuana exposure.

Studies of the effects of prenatal marijuana exposure on the brain and on intellectual and behavioral development have been provocative. Researchers studying the electrical activity of the brain during sleep in a subset of newborns found significant differences between marijuana-exposed and nonexposed subjects. Disturbed sleep patterns were still significantly associated with prenatal marijuana exposure in 3-year-old children.

Effects of marijuana exposure on the brain have been found in older children as well. Three-year-old children showed significant effects of first- and second-trimester exposure to marijuana on the composite score of the Stanford-Binet Intelligence Scale (4th edition) as well as on those portions of the scale that measure short-term memory, verbal reasoning,

and abstract/visual reasoning. These children showed the same effects at age 6. Other workers reported on the behavioral development of children who were part of the Ottawa Prenatal Prospective Study. At 4 years of age, prenatal marijuana exposure was significantly associated with lower scores on both the verbal and the memory domains of the McCarthy Scales of Children's Abilities. Six-year-old children prenatally exposed to marijuana performed poorly on tasks requiring attention and were described by their mothers as impulsive and hyperactive. In another project, behavior problems, including inattention and hyperactivity, also were significantly associated with prenatal exposure to marijuana among children ages 3 and 6.

Overall, the results suggest that prenatal exposure to marijuana has significant effects on sleep and, at older ages, on measures of intellectual development and behavior. There are few or no effects of prenatal exposure on growth or physical development.

Cocaine[21]

There are few consistent effects of prenatal cocaine exposure. When the offspring of cocaine-using women are compared with the offspring of women not using drugs, the exposed offspring display a broad variety of abnormalities. However, when the offspring of drug-using women are compared with one another, few defects emerge that can be ascribed uniquely to cocaine (see box on p. 210).

Some reports associate cocaine use with pregnancy complications. One group found increased rates of preterm labor, precipitous labor, and abruptio placentae (premature detachment of the placenta) in a cocaine-using group compared with women who were not exposed to any drugs. In other studies, however, there was no difference between cocaine users and nonusers in pregnancy, labor, or delivery complications. Other studies have reported that women who used cocaine and who received adequate prenatal care did not differ in the rate of abruptio placentae from non–cocaine-using controls.

Prenatal cocaine exposure also has been associated with decreased length of gestation and increased rate of prematurity. However, re-

❖

NUTRITIONAL EFFECTS OF MARIJUANA, HEROIN, COCAINE, AND NICOTINE[50]

A review by Mohs and colleagues summarizes nicely the impact of use of addictive drugs on food and liquid intake, taste preference, and body weight. Observations are also reported for changes in specific nutrient status and metabolism. For example, heroin addiction can cause hyperkalemia, and morphine use can result in calcium inhibition. Nutrition-related physiologic aspects, such as impaired gastrin release, hypercholesterolemia, hypothermia, and hyperthermia are also seen with morphine use. Diabetes decreases sensitivity to and dependence on morphine, protein deprivation produces preferential fat utilization with low cocaine use, and vitamin D deficiency decelerates morphine dependency. Data suggest that during use and/or withdrawal from nicotine, heroin, marijuana, and cocaine, major changes in food selection and intake occur; these may result in weight gain or weight loss. More human studies are needed to investigate the effects of drug use on the broad spectrum of nutrient deficiencies (or excesses).

From Mohs ME, Watson RR, Leonard-Green T: Nutritional effects of marijuana, heroin, cocaine, and nicotine, *J Am Diet Assoc* 90:1261, 1990.

searchers do not always control for the use of other drugs or for other factors associated with cocaine use and, therefore the effects cannot conclusively be attributed to cocaine. Data from one prospective study showed no effect of cocaine use on gestational age when the correlates of cocaine use were controlled.

Researchers have reported decreased weight, length, and head circumference in cocaine-exposed newborns, and others found that the duration of cocaine exposure during pregnancy was associated with decreased birth weight. However, other studies found no effects of prenatal cocaine exposure on growth.

Chasnoff and coworkers[8] compared the off-spring of three groups of women: cocaine, alcohol, and marijuana users; alcohol and marijuana users; and nonusers. The offspring were assessed at 3, 6, 12, 18, and 24 months. Infants in the two drug-exposed groups had smaller head circumferences than did the nonexposed infants at each follow-up point. However, the two drug-exposed groups did not differ from each other.

Most of the larger prospective studies have not found a relationship between prenatal cocaine exposure and physical defects.

Little is known about the effects of cocaine use on brain development because prospective studies have only begun recently. The Brazelton Neonatal Behavioral Assessment Scale (BNBAS) is used to measure the organization of the brain in the newborn and the infant's ability to interact socially. Cocaine-exposed newborns have been reported to perform differently than non-exposed newborns on the BNBAS.

Cocaine users may experience unpleasant withdrawal symptoms on terminating a period of heavy drug use. In adults, these symptoms may include decreased physical activity, lack of motivation, poor concentration, decreased libido, irritability, depression, and sleepiness. Withdrawal symptoms in newborns exposed prenatally may include jitteriness, poor muscle tone, and poor feeding.

In summary, negative effects of prenatal cocaine exposure have not been substantiated. Although some investigators have demonstrated significant effects of cocaine use during pregnancy, almost all of these relationships disappear when factors such as prenatal care, lifestyle, and multiple drug use are assessed. This pattern can be noted for the effects of prenatal cocaine exposure on length of pregnancy, growth, and physical characteristics. Thus, previous reports may have misattributed poor pregnancy outcomes to prenatal cocaine exposure because of the failure to control for associated factors. It is reasonable to conclude, that it is the lifestyle rather than the unique effect of cocaine exposure that leads to poorer outcomes in the offspring. However, there are few studies of the long-term effects of cocaine exposure, and judgment must be withheld until these data are available.

RIGOROUS PHYSICAL EXERCISE

The impact of exercise on the pregnant woman and the fetus has been the source of considerable debate resulting in conflicting recommendations. Physical fitness enthusiasts have championed maintenance of vigorous activity during pregnancy, whereas others, particularly those concerned with the effects of manual labor, have urged caution. Historically, traditional advice to women from the obstetric community has been to decrease activity and increase periods of rest during pregnancy, particularly in the third trimester (see box at right). Over the past decade, a number of studies have been conducted regarding this issue; unfortunately, most have been of weak scientific method and reflect the bias of the investigators.[37]

In 1982, the National Institutes of Health sponsored a planning workshop dealing with physical activity in pregnancy. This workshop identified dimensions of research needed, particularly prospective studies regarding both beneficial and adverse effects of exercise in pregnant women. Several extensive reviews of the physiology of exercise in pregnancy and its effects on the mother and fetus were published.[43,44] In addition, five other sets of authors reviewed the literature and made specific recommendations regarding exercise during pregnancy.[20,23,27,52,53]

To date the most sophisticated evaluation of rigorous exercise during pregnancy was completed by Clapp et al. Five reports were published between 1989 and 1995.[10-14] The results are intriguing. This research group evaluated the progress and outcome of pregnancy in women who were either very active or more sedentary. The results include the following:

1. Women who continued regular exercise during pregnancy gained less weight and less body fat than women who discontinued activity during this time. However, weight gain was within normal limits and all babies were healthy (Figs. 7-8 and 7-9).
2. Babies of very active women are not more likely to be aborted spontaneously than babies of more sedentary women.
3. Babies of very active women appear to present their mothers with fewer difficulties in the labor and delivery process.

❖

PHYSICAL ACTIVITY DURING PREGNANCY[76]

WHAT IS THE REAL CALORIC COST IF THE MOTHER IS SEDENTARY?

Basal metabolic rate, activity pattern and energy costs of some daily activities were measured in 25 Dutch women throughout pregnancy and in the first year postpartum. Typical women in this population demonstrated very low basal metabolic needs and very low levels of physical activity. The end result was that daily kcalorie needs were modest at best. Basal metabolic requirements at one year postpartum were 1,440 kcal per day; the costs of physical activity were modest. The conclusions of the researchers in this study were as follows:

For women with sedentary lifestyles, the energy saved during pregnancy and lactation because of decreased physical activity and decreased costs of activities will be limited.

From van Raaij IMA et al: *Am J Clin Nutr* 52:234, 1990.

---

4. Babies of very active women are smaller than those of sedentary women.
5. During pregnancy a wide range of exercise regimens appear to provide physiological benefit to both mother and fetus with little or no risk, but the lower limits, the upper limits and dose-response relationships of their beneficial effects remain to be established.

Much research remains to be done on the effects of specific exercise regimens during pregnancy, the effects on previously sedentary women, and the long-term health consequences to the offspring of women who perform vigorous exercise during pregnancy.[4,43,44]

Some high-risk women (i.e., those with diabetes, heart disease, history of spontaneous abortion, etc.) should be particularly cautious about the selection of exercise programs. The American College of Obstetricians and Gynecologists (ACOG) provides exercise guidelines for all pregnant women that go well beyond discouraging endurance training in the third trimester (see box on p. 212). Until more infor-

❖

AMERICAN COLLEGE OF OBSTETRICIANS AND GYNECOLOGISTS' GUIDELINES FOR EXERCISE DURING PREGNANCY AND POSTPARTUM[1]

Regular exercise (at least three times per week) is preferable to intermittent activity. Competitive activities should be discouraged.

Vigorous exercise should not be performed in hot, humid weather or during a period of febrile illness.

Ballistic movements (jerky, bouncy motions) should be avoided. Exercise should be done on a wooden floor or a tightly carpeted surface to reduce shock and provide a sure footing.

Deep flexion or extension of joints should be avoided because of connective-tissue laxity. Activities that require jumping, jarring motions, or rapid changes in direction should be avoided because of joint instability.

Vigorous exercise should be preceded by a five-minute period of muscle warmup. This can be accomplished by slow walking or stationary cycling with low resistance.

Vigorous exercise should be followed by a period of gradually declining activity that includes gentle stationary stretching. Because connective-tissue laxity increases the risk of joint injury, stretches should not be taken to the point of maximum resistance.

Heart rate should be measured at times of peak activity. Target heart rates and limits established in consultation with the physician should not be exceeded.

Care should be taken to rise from the floor gradually to avoid orthostatic hypotension. Some form of activity involving the legs should be continued for a brief period.

Liquids should be taken liberally before and after exercise to prevent dehydration. If necessary, activity should be interrupted to replenish fluids.

Women who have led sedentary lifestyles should begin with physical activity of very low intensity and advance activity levels very gradually.

Activity should be stopped and the physician consulted if any unusual symptoms appear.

Pregnancy only

Maternal heart rate should not exceed 140 beats/min.

Strenuous activities should not exceed 15 min in duration.

No exercise should be performed in the supine position after the fourth month of gestation is completed.

Exercises that employ the Valsalva maneuver should be avoided.

Calorie intake should be adequate to meet not only the extra energy needs of pregnancy, but also of the exercise performed.

Maternal core temperature should not exceed 38°C.

Reprinted with permission from the American College of Obstetricians and Gynecologists: *Exercise during pregnancy and the postnatal period (ACOG home exercise programs);* Washington, DC, 1985, American College of Obstetricians and Gynecologists.

mation is available to evaluate, common sense must be applied in the counseling of pregnant women about physical activity.

WEIGHT MANAGEMENT

Chapter 3 discussed the composition of weight gain during pregnancy. The tendency of some women to retain an excessive amount of weight in the postpartum period is of concern.

In this chapter, recent observations about weight gain patterns of pregnant women in the United States are summarized. Weight gain data have been available since 1989 when birth certificates were revised to include this and other information.

From 1990 to 1992 the proportion of mothers gaining 26 to 35 lb decreased from 35.6% to 34.8% with a concomitant rise in gains of more than 35 lb (28.4% to 19.9%). However, weight

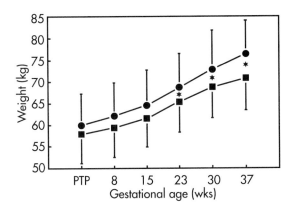

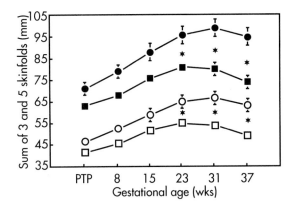

FIG. 7-8 The serial changes observed in maternal weight for the control (o) and continued exercise (n) groups throughout pregnancy. PTP = prior to pregnancy. The error bars indicate ± the standard error of the mean. The * indicates a significant between group difference in weight gain over the preceeding time interval.

From Clapp JF, Little KD: Effect of recreational exercise on pregnancy weight gain and subcutaneous fat deposition, *Med Sci Sports Exercise* 27:170, 1995.

FIG. 7-9 The serial changes observed in the sum of 3- and 5-site skinfold thicknesses on the control (●) and continued exercise (■) groups throughout pregnancy. The solid symbols represent the data for 5 skinfolds and the open symbols the data for 3 skinfolds. PTP = prior to pregnancy. The error bars represent ± the standard error of the mean, which, in many instances, was smaller than the size of the symbol. The * indicates a significant between group difference in the magnitude of the increase or decrease over the preceding time interval.

From Clapp JF, Little KD: Effect of recreational exercise on pregnancy weight gain and subcutaneous fat deposition, *Med Science Sports Exercise* 27:170, 1995.

gains of less than 16 lb—an amount associated with a greatly elevated risk of low birth weight—rose from 9.2% to 9.7%. Overall, median weight gain was almost unchanged, increasing from 30.4 to 30.5 lb.[51]

White mothers were more likely than black mothers to gain 26 to 35 lb and also more likely to gain 36 lb or more. Weight gains of less than 16 lb were nearly twice as common for black than for white mothers. Some of this racial disparity is explained by the generally shorter gestational age of black infants. A significantly higher proportion of black than white mothers reported weight gain advice that did not conform to the standards for maternal weight gain at that time.[51]

There were also substantial differences in weight gain among other racial groups. Only 7% of the Chinese mothers gained less than 16 lb in 1992 compared with 8% Filipinos, 8.9% Hawaiians, 9.3% Japanese, 11.5% Asian or Pacific Islander, and 14.0% of Native American mothers.[51]

Large differences in weight gain were also apparent among mothers of Hispanic origin.

Cuban and central and South American mothers were least likely and Mexican mothers the most likely to gain less than 16 lb; 11% of Puerto Ricans, "other," and unknown Hispanic origin mothers had this low same weight gain.[51]

Numerous studies have confirmed the positive relationship between weight gain and birth weight. The percent low birth weight declines dramatically for both white and black births with added weight gain, regardless of the period of gestation. However, for equivalent weight gain, the incidence of low birth weight is approximately twice as high for black births.[51]

IMPROVING THE OUTCOME OF PREGNANCY
Nutrition Relationships

There are sufficient parallels between animal and human research to conclude that maternal

TABLE 7-2 *Examples of Intensive Prenatal Nutrition Education Studies*[73]

Author (year)	Study Groups	Sample Size		Random Assignment	Birth Weight
		I	C		
Bruce and Tchabo (1989)	I = nutrition counseling C = no nutrition counseling	57	52	No	I = 3,157 gm C = 2,857 gm
Kafatos et al. (1989)	I = nutrition education C = no nutrition education	300	268	Yes By clinic	I = 3,391 gm C = 3,376 gm
Corbett and Burst (1983)	I = nutrition education using Higgins method C = no nutrition education	182	270	No	Birth weight distribution was significantly different ($p < 0.005$)
Ershoff et al. (1983)	I = nutrition counseling smoking cessation C = standard prenatal care	57	333	No	I = 3,447 gm C = 3,228 gm

I = intervention; C = control
Modified from Trouba PH, Okereke N, Splett PL: Summary document of nutrition intervention in prenatal care, *J Am Diet Assoc* (Suppl) S-21, 1991.

nutrition can influence reproductive performance, especially of women who have a high risk of giving birth to low-birth-weight infants. Birth weight, as a reflection of intrauterine growth, is a determinant of the child's potential for survival and future health (Fig. 7-10). This is true of both physical and mental performance.

There has been much discussion about the possible effects of prenatal nutrition on intelligence and learning ability. Whether an infant whose size and brain cells are reduced at birth from maternal malnutrition is going to have a permanent mental disability is not presently known. Given the understanding of growth and development, however, it is reasonable to suppose that the consequences will depend to some extent on the nutrition of the child in postnatal life, as well as the physical and social environment in which he or she is born. A follow-up study of children born during the World War II famine in Holland could find no evidence of lower-than-average intelligence or a higher incidence of mental retardation.[69] It is possible that acute dietary deprivation of previously well-nourished women during pregnancy can be compensated by adequate nutrition later on. However, the situation in Holland is not what typically occurs. Most women in good nutritional status before conception do not suddenly have poor diets during pregnancy and then try to make up for it by feeding their children well after they are born. The factors that place a pregnant woman at nutritional risk have operated over her lifetime and will continue to affect the nutritional status, growth, and development of her child. These include poverty, poor education, a deprived environment, and poor health. Surveys have shown clear associations between these factors and the nutritional status of infants, children, and women of childbearing age. Al-

Outcomes			
Weight Difference	LBW Rate	LBW Difference	Comments
+300 gm	I = 8.0% C = 17.0%	−9.0%	Birth weight was significantly different between smokers and nonsmokers 2 × higher LBW in control group Subjects from county health department and local hospital >75% WIC participation for both I and C
+15 gm	I = 3.9% C = 4.5%	−0.6%	Prematurity rate was 4.6% higher in C group I group had higher calorie and protein intake/day All subjects were from a rural area in Greece
	I = 9.1% C = 12.7%	−3.6%	Adolescent population
+219 gm	I = 7.0% C = 9.7%	−2.7%	No control for smoking 11.6% more quit smoking in I group 91% of I group made dietary changes vs. 68% of C group HMO with variety of SES and ethnicity

though all women need nutritional guidance during pregnancy, those who conceive in poor nutritional status and whose life circumstances impair their ability to secure adequate diets for themselves and their families require special care.

Nutritional Care for High-risk Mothers

Nutritional intervention to improve pregnancy outcomes must be both short and long term (Table 7-2). Nutritional status of the mother, as reflected by her height and prepregnancy weight, is a fixed variable not subject to manipulation once pregnancy occurs. Intervention must be directed at future generations of mothers to ensure that they receive adequate nutrition to reach their maximum growth potential and maintain optimal weight.

Special concern has been voiced for the current generation of adolescent females who appear to be entering the childbearing years with a less than optimal prognosis for successful pregnancy outcomes. These investigators point out that teenagers are frequently preoccupied with dieting in an attempt to maintain unrealistically low body weights. The problem of underweight females is compounded by the fact that according to current statistics, one third of females between 17 and 18 years of age smoke cigarettes. The number of teenagers who smoke more than one pack of cigarettes per day has tripled in recent years. Health education programs in the schools and in the community must work toward changing the behavior of this highly vulnerable group.

Diet after conception should also be made a focus of attention for women at high risk. Recent research on the effects of smoking and alcohol consumption should be used to discour-

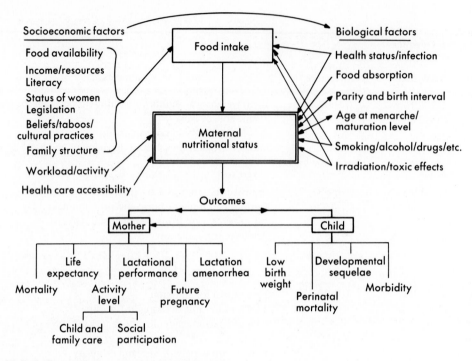

FIG. 7-10   Influences on and outcomes of maternal nutritional status.

Modified from Hofvander Y: *Maternal and young child nutrition,* Paris, 1983, United Nations Educational, Scientific and Cultural Organization.

age women from continuing these habits while they are pregnant. Often the motivation in pregnancy that is centered around the welfare of the unborn child can be a stimulus for women to modify their behavior permanently. Even a slight change is better than no change at all.

Summary

Issues related to weight gain and specific nutrients are areas of focus, whereas concerns about other food-related compounds, drug and alcohol use, and smoking deserve additional attention. Alcohol is clearly damaging to the fetus; caffeine may produce an impact on pregnancy course and fetal growth. Information about other dietary substances is less well understood but the dangers associated with drugs and smoking are clear. Exercise is generally healthful for pregnant women as long as common sense and moderation are kept in mind. Attention

should be given to all of these issues when counseling pregnant women.

REVIEW QUESTIONS

1. Describe the features of fetal alcohol syndrome.
2. Define the meaning of fetal alcohol effects.
3. Assess the impact of caffeine and other foodborne substances on pregnancy outcome.
4. Outline the recommendations of the American College of Obstetrics and Gynecology that relate to exercise during pregnancy.

LEARNING ACTIVITIES

1. Determine the policy in your state about dealing with alcohol sales and advertising for pregnant women.
2. Ask local clinicians about the degree to which pica is a problem and about what kinds of unusual cravings women report.

❖ ❖ ❖
CASE STUDY
Lifestyle Issues

Beth appears for prenatal care at 12 weeks gestation. She is concerned about the baby's well-being and seems to know much about what she should and should not do during pregnancy. She cries and tells you that she celebrated her anniversary about 8 weeks ago with a bottle of champagne; she did not know that she was pregnant and now she is afraid of what damage might have been done to the fetus.

This is not an uncommon scenario. what do you tell this woman?

It is very important that the rest of this pregnancy goes well. Outline your approach to counseling this woman the duration of this prenatal period

3. Explore the availability of treatment programs in your community for (a) pregnant women who smoke and (b) pregnant women who use dangerous drugs.

REFERENCES

1. American College of Obstetricians and Gynecologists: *Exercise during pregnancy and the postnatal period (ACOG home exercise programs),* Washington, DC, 1985, American College of Obstetricians and Gynecologists.
2. American Pharmacy: Herbs hazardous to your health, *Am Pharm* NS24:20, 1984.
3. Awang D: Maternal use of ginsengs and neonatal androgenization, *JAMA* 265:1828, 1991.
4. Bell R, O'Neill M: Exercise and pregnancy: a review, *Birth* 21:2, 1994.
5. Butchko HH, Kotsonis FN: Acceptable daily intake vs actual intake: the aspartame example, *J Am Coll Nutr* 10:258, 1991.
6. Caster WO: Dietary aflatoxin, intelligence and school performance in Southern Georgia, *Int J Vitam Nutr Res* 56:291, 1986.
7. Chasnoff IJ, Diggs G, Schnoll SH: Fetal alcohol effects and maternal cough syrup abuse, *Am J Dis Child* 135:968, 1981.
8. Chasnoff I et al: Cocaine polydrug use in pregnancy. Two-year followup, *Pediatrics* 89:284, 1992.
9. Cicero TJ: Effects of paternal exposure to alcohol on offspring development, *Alcohol Health & Res World* 18:37, 1994.
10. Clapp JF: The course of labor after endurance exercise during pregnancy, *Am J Obstet Gynecol* 163:1799, 1990.
11. Clapp JF: The effects of maternal exercise on early pregnancy outcome, *Am J Obstet Gynecol* 161:1453, 1989.
12. Clapp JF, Dickstein S: Endurance exercise and pregnancy outcome, *Med Sci Sports Exer* 16:556, 1984.
13. Clapp JF, Little KD: Effect of recreational exercise on pregnancy weight gain and subcutaneous fat deposition, *Med Sci Sports Exercise* 27:170, 1995.
14. Clapp JF, Little KD: The interaction between regular exercise and selected aspects of women's health, *Am J Obstet Gynecol* 173:2, 1995.
15. Clarren SK: Recognition of fetal alcohol syndrome, *JAMA* 245:2436, 1981.
16. Clarren SK, Bowden DM, Astley SJ: Pregnancy outcomes after weekly oral administration of ethanol during gestation in the pig-tailed macaque *(Macacca nemestrina), Teratology* 35:345, 1987.
17. Coles, C. Critical periods for prenatal alcohol exposure, *Alcohol Health & Res World* 18:22, 1994.
18. Collins TFN et al: *A comprehensive study of the teratogenic potential of caffeine in rats when given by oral intubation,* Washington, DC, 1980, Data Acquisition and Monitoring Division, Environmental Data and Information Services, National Oceanic and Atmospheric Administration.
19. Cordero JF, et al: Tracking the prevalence of FAS, *Alcohol Health & Res World* 18:82, 1994.
20. Dale E, Mullinax K, Bryan D: Exercise during pregnancy: effect on the fetus, *Can J Appl Sports Sci* 7:98, 1982.
21. Day NL, Richardson GA: Comparative teratogenicity of alcohol and other drugs, *Alcohol Health & Res World* 18:42, 1994.
22. Devoe LD et al: Maternal caffeine consumption and fetal behavior in normal third trimester pregnancy, *Am J Obstet Gynecol* 168:1105, 1993.
23. Diddle AW: Interrelationship of pregnancy and athletic performance, *J Tenn Med Assoc* May:265, 1984.

24. Dufour MC et al: Knowledge of FAS and the risks of heavy drinking during pregnancy, 1985 and 1990, *Alcohol Health & Res World* 18:86, 1994.

25. Dunlop M, Court JM: Effect of maternal caffeine ingestion on neonatal growth in rats, *Biol Neonate* 39:178, 1981.

26. Forrest F, Florey C, Taylor D et al: Reported social alcohol consumption during pregnancy and infants' development at 18 months, *BMJ* 303:22, 1991.

27. Goodlin RC, Buckley KK: Maternal exercise, *Clin Sports Med* 3:881, 1984.

28. Haglund B, Cnattingius S: Cigarette smoking as a risk factor for sudden infant death syndrome: a population-based study, *Am J Public Health* 80:29, 1990.

29. Haworth JC: Fetal growth retardation in cigarette smoking mothers is not due to reduced food intake, *Am J Obstet Gynecol* 137:719, 1980.

30. Hinderliter SA, Zelenak JP: A simple method to identify alcohol and other drug use in pregnant adults in a prenatal care setting, *J Perinatol* 13:93, 1993.

31. Hingson R et al: Effects of maternal drinking and marijuana use on fetal growth and development, *Pediatrics* 70:539, 1982.

32. Horner RD, Lackey CJ, Kolasa K et al: Pica practices of pregnant women, *J Am Diet Assoc* 91:34, 1991.

33. Infante-Rivard C et al: Fetal loss associated with caffeine intake before and during pregnancy, *JAMA* 270:2940, 1993.

34. Jacobson JL, Jacobson SW: Prenatal alcohol exposure and neurobehavioral development, *Alcohol Health & Res World* 18:30, 1994.

35. Jones KL et al: Pattern of malformation in offspring of chronic alcoholic mothers, *Lancet* 1:1267, 1973.

36. Khoury MJ et al: Maternal cigarette smoking and oral clefts: a population-based study, *Am J Public Health* 77:623, 1987.

37. Klebanoff MA, Shiono PH, Carey JC: The effect of physical activity during pregnancy on preterm delivery and birthweight, *Am J Obstet Gynecol* 163:1450, 1990.

38. Kleinman JC, Pierre MB, Madans JH et al: The effects of maternal smoking on fetal and infant mortality, *Am J Epidemiol* 127:274, 1988.

39. Kline J et al: Spontaneous abortion and the use of sugar substitutes, *Am J Obstet Gynecol* 130:708, 1978.

40. Koren G et al: Maternal ginseng use associated with neonatal androgenization, *JAMA* 264:2866, 1990.

41. Larkin T: *Herbs are often more toxic than magical.* In *FDA Consumer,* HHS Pub No 84-1112:1, Washington, DC, 1983, Government Printing Office.

42. Lesan SE: Potentially harmful beverages in pregnancy: recommendations and counseling strategies, *Topics Clin Nutr* 6:17, 1990.

43. Lotgering FK, Gilbert RD, Longo LD: The interactions of exercise and pregnancy: a review, *Am J Obstet Gynecol* 149:560, 1984.

44. Lotgering FK, Gilbert RD, Longo LD: Maternal and fetal responses to exercise during pregnancy, *Physiol Rev* 65:1, 1985.

45. Luke B, Hawkins MM, Petrie RH: Influence of smoking, weight gain and pregravid weight for height on intrauterine growth, *Am J Clin Nutr* 34:1410, 1981.

46. McDonald AD, Armstrong BG, Sloan M: Cigarette, alcohol and coffee consumption and congenital defects, *Am J Public Health* 82:91, 1992.

47. Michaelis EK, Michaelis ML: Cellular and molecular bases of alcohol's teratogenic effects, *Alcohol Health Res World* 18:17, 1994.

48. Miller RC et al: Acute maternal and fetal cardiovascular effects of caffeine ingestion, *Am J Perinatol* 11:132, 1994.

49. Mills JL et al: Moderate caffeine use and the risk of spontaneous abortion and intrauterine retardation. *JAMA* 269:593, 1993.

50. Mohs ME, Watson RR, Leonard-Green T: Nutritional effects of marijuana, heroin, cocaine, and nicotine, *J Am Diet Assoc* 90:1261, 1990.

51. *Monthly Vital Statistics Report* 43(#5 suppl), October 25, 1994 Advance Report of Final Natality Statistics, 1992.

52. Morton MJ, Paul MS, Metcalfe J: Exercise during pregnancy, *Med Clin North Am* 69:97, 1985.

53. Mullinax KM, Dale E: Some considerations of exercise during pregnancy, *Clin Sports Med* 5:559, 1986.

54. Narod SA, Sanjose S, Victoria C: Coffee during pregnancy: A reproductive hazard, *Am J Obstet Gynecol* 164:1109, 1991.

55. National Research Council, Food and Nutrition Board: *Alternative dietary practices and nutritional abuses in pregnancy,* Washington, DC, 1982, National Academy of Sciences.

56. Nehlig A, Debry G: Potential teratogenic and neurodevelopmental consequences of coffee and caffeine exposure: a review of human and animal data, *Neurotoxicol Teratol* 16:531, 1994.

57. Niswander KR: *The women and their pregnancies,* Philadelphia, 1972, WB Saunders.

58. Oei S, Vosters RPL, van der Hagen NLJ: Fetal arrhythmia caused by excessive intake of caffeine by pregnant women, *BMJ* 298:568, 1989.

59. Papoz L et al: Maternal smoking and birth weight in relation to dietary habits, *Am J Obstet Gynecol* 142:870, 1982.

60. Pastore LM Savitz DA: Case-control study of caffeinated beverages and preterm delivery, *Am J Epid* 141:61, 1995.

61. Phillips DK, Henderson GI, Schenker S: Pathogenesis of fetal alcohol syndrome, *Alcohol Health & Res World* 13:219, 1989.

62. Picone TA et al: Pregnancy outcome in North American women: I. Effects of diet, cigarette smoking and psychological stress on maternal weight gain, *Am J Clin Nutr* 36:1205, 1982.

63. Picone TA et al: Pregnancy outcome in North American women: II. Effects of diet, cigarette smoking, stress, and weight gain on placentas and on neonatal physical and behavioral characteristics, *Am J Clin Nutr* 36:1214, 1982.

64. Randall CL, Ekblad U, Anton RF: Perspectives on the pathophysiology of fetal alcohol syndrome, *Alcohol Clin Exp Res* 14:807, 1990.

65. Rosett HL et al: Patterns of alcohol consumption and fetal development, *Obstet Gynecol* 61:539, 1983.

66. Rosett HL, Weiner L, Edelin KC: Treatment experience with pregnant problem drinkers, *JAMA* 249:2029, 1983.

67. Rowland AS: Pesticides and birth defects, *Epidemiol* 6:6, 1995.

68. Sexton M, Hebel JR: A clinical trial of change in maternal smoking and its effect on birthweight, *JAMA* 251:911, 1984.

69. Stein Z et al: Nutrition and mental performance, *Science* 178:708, 1972.

70. Streissguth AP: A long-term perspective of FAS, *Alcohol Health & Res World* 18:74, 1994.

71. Sturtevant FM: Use of aspartame in pregnancy, *Int J Fertil* 30:85, 1985.

72. Surgeon General's 1990 report on the health benefits of smoking cessation, *MMWR Morb Mortal Wkly Rep* 39:RR-12, 1990.

73. Trouba PH, Okereke N, Splett PL: Summary document of nutrition intervention in prenatal care, *J Am Diet Assoc* (suppl)S-21, 1991.

74. Tyler VE: An expert answers questions on herbal teas, *Tufts Univ Diet Nutr Newslett* 4:4, 1986.

75. Tyler VE: *The honest herbal,* Philadelphia, 1982, George F. Stickney.

76. van Raaij IMA et al: Energy cost of physical activity throughout pregnancy and the first year postpartum in Dutch women with sedentary lifestyles, *Am J Clin Nutr* 52:234, 1990.

77. Wen SW, Goldenberg RL et al: Smoking, maternal age, fetal growth and gestational age, *Am J Obstet Gynecol* 162:53, 1990.

78. West JR, Goodlett CR, Brandt JP: New approaches to research on the long-term consequences of prenatal exposure to alcohol, *Alcohol Clin Exp Res* 14:684, 1990.

8

Nutrition Assessment and Guidance in Prenatal Care

Sue Rodwell Williams

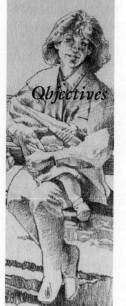

Objectives

✦✦

After completing this chapter, the student will be able to:

✓ *Promote healthy pregnancies and their successful outcomes by giving basic attention to the nutritional status of each individual mother.*

✓ *Identify each mother's prenatal nutritional care needs through a comprehensive nutrition assessment process, initial and ongoing, and use this information as a necessary base for developing practical personal food plans.*

✓ *Help avoid potential risk factors and ensure optimal nutritional support through continous personalized prenatal care based on background, living situation, and personal problems and needs.*

Introduction

The preceding chapters have discussed the unique physiologic changes in the pregnant woman's body that are specifically designed to support her pregnancy and its successful outcome. In the metabolic triad of maternal organism, fetus, and placenta is found a prime example of biologic **synergism** existing for the single purpose of bringing forth healthy new life. This enhanced metabolic work accounts for the increased nutrient and energy needs of pregnancy.

The process of comprehensive nutrition assessment is basic to all health care, but it has special importance in pregnancy. It provides the necessary foundation for planning personalized nutritional care, education, and guidance throughout the pregnancy, which is essential for healthy mothers and babies.

The necessity of this nutritional foundation during pregnancy and the urgency of its implementation in all health care practice and community program-planning has become increasingly evident. In the United States Department of Health and Human Services report, *Healthy People 2000,* setting national health objectives for the year 2000, a major priority area was assigned to Nutrition under Health Promotion and to Maternal and Infant Health under Preventive Services.[4,27] The Maternal and Child Health Bureau of the Department of Health and Human Services followed this report with a national workshop in which leaders in the field identified current issues and needs, set priorities, developed recommendations, and outlined action strategies.[23] Throughout these initial activities, the importance of early and ongoing nutrition assessment throughout the course of pregnancy for all women has been emphasized, with special attention to high-risk groups. In 1994, an interim report by the Healthy People 2000 Work Group indicated a mixed review of progress toward these objectives, with some falling short of their targets.[13] However, efforts are moving forward, based on the knowledge that positive nutritional support is fundamental to a healthy outcome in all pregnancies.

NUTRITION ASSESSMENT IN HEALTH CARE DURING PREGNANCY

Significance of Nutritional Status

Nutrition and the outcome of pregnancy. Evidence increasingly indicates that positive nutritional support of pregnancy promotes a positive outcome with increased health and vigor of mothers and infants alike. A healthy pregnancy in terms of each mother, infant, and family is the goal.

Perinatal concept. As nutrition knowledge and understanding have increased, health professionals realize that all of a woman's life experiences surrounding her pregnancy need to be considered. Her nutritional status and food patterns, which have developed over many years, and the degree to which she has established and maintained nutritional reserves, are important factors. In a real sense, a woman provides for the ongoing continuum of life throughout her own life by the food she eats. In this manner she pro-

vides direct nourishment for her unborn child during her pregnancy. She carries over her nutritional heritage, practices, and beliefs in the feeding and teaching of her growing child, who in turn passes on this heritage to the next generation. All of these factors surround and influence the total reproductive cycle.

Personal assessment and nutritional support. Each pregnancy presents a unique opportunity for positive nutritional guidance. Current perspectives on nutrition in pregnancy focus strongly on the preventive aspects of nutrition programs, identifying women at risk through careful assessment, recognizing special counseling needs, and planning optimum follow-up nutrition care. Nutritional demands of any pregnancy focus on nutrient needs basic to human growth and development, including increased protein, vitamins, and minerals to sustain the necessary building process, and sufficient energy input to do the work. However, a number of variables can combine to produce individual needs and problems that hinder obtaining an adequate diet. These needs may be physiologic, psychologic, situational, cultural, social, economic, or personal. Many disadvantaged women and adolescents receive little or no prenatal care, and sometimes those who have made the effort to engage in the prenatal care system receive prenatal care that is far from even minimally acceptable.[8]

Examples of personal risk factors affecting nutritional status that may be identified by sensitive counseling or medical/obstetric records include the following:[17]

- Low income and inadequate access to food
- Avoidance of certain types of food because of intolerance (e.g., milk, in cases of lactose intolerance), fad diets, or cultural taboos
- Use of strict vegetarian diet (vegan); lactoovovegetarianism adequate
- Substance abuse with alcohol, tobacco, or illicit drugs
- Diet restriction to lose weight
- Practice of pica, or eating of nonfood substances such as clay or laundry starch
- Lifestyle unlikely to support adequate purchase, preparation, or consumption of food (e.g., busy professional person or a poor woman living alone)

TABLE 8-1 *Nutritional Risk Factors in Pregnancy*

Risk Factors Present at the Onset of Pregnancy	Risk Factors Occurring During Pregnancy

Age
  15 years or younger
  35 years or older
Frequent pregnancies: three or more during a 2-year period
Poor obstetric history or poor fetal performance
Poverty
Bizarre or faddist food habits
Abuse of nicotine, alcohol, or drugs
Therapeutic diet required for a chronic disorder
Inappropriate weight
  Less than 85% of standard weight
  More than 120% of standard weight
	Low hemoglobin and/or hematocrit
	  Hemoglobin less than 12.0 gm
	  Hematocrit less than 35.0 mg/100 ml
	Inadequate weight gain
	  Any weight loss
	  Weight gain of less than 2 lb per month after the first trimester
	Excessive weight gain: greater than kg (2 lb) per week after the first trimester

- Fear, unhappiness, or depression because of the pregnancy
- Substantially underweight or overweight
- Early teenage pregnancy
- Multiple pregnancy (e.g., twins or triplets)
- Anemia

Such risk factors, summarized in Table 8-1, present special nutritional needs and require personal attention. Dietary intervention and improvement provides the best answer to such problems, but in the real world of 20th century America and elsewhere such patterns may be unlikely, or impossible, to change and nutrient supplementation is needed. Whatever the problem, if the vital component of nutrition in prenatal health care is to be fulfilled, it must meet such human needs, both physically and personally.

Influences on the Process of Health Care During Pregnancy

Nutrition is essential to health on two levels. On a physiologic level, nutrients and energy from food build and maintain body tissues, and the healthy functioning of the body depends on the fundamental integrity of these tissues. On a personal level, food has many meanings and ful-

fills social and cultural needs. Both of these roles of nutrition in health care are present throughout the life cycle, but they take on special meaning for the pregnant woman and must be considered in assessing her needs and goals.

Changing community, family, and personal needs. Far-reaching social changes mean that many young adults are not conforming to previous patterns of American life. They are marrying later, divorcing more often, postponing childbirth (if electing to have children at all), and setting up smaller households. An increasing number are burdened by economic stresses of unemployment, low wages, a changing workplace, and high-priced housing. Faced with increasing health care costs, many lack even minimal health insurance. In such situations, when pregnancy does occur, planned or unplanned, it poses problems for many.

At best, pregnancy is a period of normal physiologic stress. However, in poor circumstances this normal stress is compounded by inadequate nutrition, increasing the risks to both mother and child. Ongoing nutrition assessment can identify specific needs, help prevent problems or complications, and promote a healthy pregnancy for mothers and babies.

METHODS OF NUTRITION ASSESSMENT

Phases of the Person-Centered Maternity Care Process

Optimum nutrition, vigorously supported with initial and ongoing preventive nutrition services, is an integral part of sound maternity care. Ideally, preconception nutrition assessment and education, with correction of any deficits and promotion of fertility for a planned pregnancy, provides the best possible foundation. To ensure that this fundamental requirement for successful pregnancy is met, an initial individual assessment of nutritional status and needs must be made. Records of plans, procedures, and progress guide actions and instructions for continuing self-care.

The methods used in any nutrition assessment may be grouped into four types of activities that provide data necessary to determine needs: (1) clinical observations and physical examination, (2) anthropometry, (3) laboratory data, and (4) history. The procedures briefly outlined here provide a good base in general practice for assessing and monitoring nutritional status, planning care, and promoting health. Here these methods focus on the pregnant woman.

Clinical Observations

Valid clinical observations require trained observers. Careful observations of physical signs of possible malnutrition provide important individual data for evaluation. However, in assessing possible nutritional relationships from clinical observations, two problem areas exist. First, observers' interpretation of physical signs may vary for several reasons: (1) differences in expertise and experience, (2) problems in standardization of definition of a particular sign, or (3) the low general prevalence and nonspecificity of clinical evidence of malnutrition in developed areas except in high-risk groups. Second, there is sometimes confusion in specific interpretation of signs during pregnancy. For example, *gingival hypertrophy* may sometimes occur normally in pregnancy and is not necessarily a sign of ascorbic acid deficiency. Some general *edema* of the feet and hands usually reflects the normal increase in total body water during pregnancy and is not necessarily a sign of protein deficiency. Nonetheless, together with more definitive data from laboratory studies of hemotologic and biochemical analyses and from careful evaluation of medical, obstetrical, social, and nutritional histories, much valuable information may be gained from good clinical observations by trained observers.

General examination of skin, mucous membranes, gums, teeth, tongue, eyes, and hair provide useful information for assessing nutritional status during pregnancy. These signs must, of course, be evaluated in relation to other data from laboratory procedures and histories, recognizing that various signs have different degrees of reliability. However, they present useful clues for further investigation or monitoring. Table 8-2 summarizes clinical signs of nutritional status.

Anthropometric Data

Anthropometry is the process of measuring various dimensions of the human body. A number of these measures provide valid estimates of fat and muscle components of body composition.[20] The results of such measurements help to assess preconception nutritional status or to initiate prenatal care in early pregnancy. The measures commonly used in practice include weight-height assessments and various body skinfold and circumference determinations. These accurate individual baseline values are important in follow-up monitoring during pregnancy.

Weight. Typical beam balance scales with nondetachable weights give the most accurate measurement. After carefully reading and recording the woman's weight, check the measurement against standard weight-height tables. However, do not apply such tables to individuals as "ideals." Experienced clinicians recognize that using "ideal" weight-height tables developed for medium-frame adults ignores the wide normal variations in healthy bodies. Also, self-reported usual prepregnant weight of overweight and underweight pregnant adolescents and adult women may be inaccurate. Those who are overweight tend to underestimate their

TABLE 8-2   *Clinical Signs of Nutritional Status*

Body Area	Signs of Good Nutrition	Signs of Poor Nutrition
General appearance	Alert, responsive	Listless, apathetic, cachectic
Weight	Normal for height, age, body build	Overweight or underweight (special concern for underweight)
Posture	Erect, arms and legs straight	Sagging shoulders, sunken chest, humped back
Muscles	Well developed, firm, good tone, some fat under skin	Flaccid, poor tone, undeveloped, tender, "wasted" appearance, cannot walk properly
Nervous control	Good attention span, not irritable or restless, normal reflexes, psychological stability	Inattentive, irritable, confused, burning and tingling of hands and feet (paresthesia), loss of position and vibratory sense, weakness and tenderness of muscles (may result in inability to walk), decrease or loss of ankle and knee reflexes
Gastrointestinal-tract function	Good appetite and digestion, normal regular elimination, no palpable organs or masses	Anorexia, indigestion, constipation or diarrhea, liver or spleen enlargement
Cardiovascular function	Normal heart rate and rhythm, no murmurs, normal blood pressure for age	Rapid heart rate (above 100 beats/min tachycardia), enlarged heart, abnormal rhythm, elevated blood pressure
General vitality	Endurance, energetic, sleeps well, vigorous	Easily fatigued, no energy, falls asleep easily, looks tired, apathetic
Hair	Shiny, lustrous, firm, not easily plucked, healthy scalp	Stringy, dull, brittle, dry, thin and sparse, depigmented, can be easily plucked
Skin (general)	Smooth, slightly moist, good color	Rough, dry, scaly, pale, pigmented, irritated, bruises, petechiae
Face and neck	Skin color uniform, smooth, healthy appearance, not swollen	Greasy, discolored, scaly, swollen, skin dark over cheeks and under eyes, lumpiness or flakiness of skin around nose and mouth
Lips	Smooth, good color, moist, not chapped or swollen	Dry, scaly, swollen, redness and swelling (cheilosis), or angular lesions at corners of the mouth or fissures or scars (stomatitis)
Mouth, oral membranes	Reddish pink mucous membranes in oral cavity	Swollen, boggy oral mucous membranes
Gums	Good pink color, healthy, red, no swelling or bleeding	Spongy, bleed easily, marginal redness, inflamed, gums receding
Tongue	Good pink color or deep reddish in appearance, not swollen or smooth, surface papillae present, no lesions	Swelling, scarlet and raw, magenta color, beefy (glossitis), hyperemic and hypertrophic papillae, atrophic papillae
Teeth	No cavities, no pain, bright, straight, no crowding, well-shaped jaw, clean, no discoloration	Unfilled caries, absent teeth, worn surfaces, mottled (fluorosis), malpositioned

TABLE 8-2 *Clinical Signs of Nutritional Status—cont'd*

Body Area	Signs of Good Nutrition	Signs of Poor Nutrition
Eyes	Bright, clear, shiny, no sores at corner of eyelids, membranes moist and healthy pink color, no prominent blood vessels or mound of tissue or sclera, no fatigue circles beneath	Eye membranes pale (pale conjunctivae), redness of membrane (conjunctival infection), dryness, signs of infection, Bitot's spots, redness and fissuring of eyelid corners (angular palpebritis), dryness of eye membrane (conjunctival xerosis), dull appearance of cornea (corneal xerosis), soft cornea (keratomalacia)
Neck (glands)	No enlargement	Thyroid enlarged
Nails	Firm, pink	Spoon shape (koilonychia), brittle, ridged
Legs, feet	Good color, no tenderness, weakness, or swelling	Edema, tender calf, tingling, weakness
Skeleton	No malformations	Bowlegs, knock-knees, chest deformity at diaphragm, beaded ribs, prominent scapulas

usual weight and those who are underweight tend to overestimate it.[25] Nonetheless, the mother's preconception or early pregnancy weight should be interpreted in terms of percentage of her usual body weight, with general reference to standard tables. Recent significant weight loss, either from dieting or some other cause, should be investigated.

Height. Accurate height is best measured by a stationary rod securely fastened to the wall, but may be obtained for practical purposes with the movable measuring rod on the platform clinic scale, using a consistent method. The woman stands as straight as possible, without shoes or cap, heels together, and looking straight ahead; the heels, buttocks, shoulders, and head should touch the surface of the measuring rod.

Mid-upper-arm circumference (MAC). Using a nonstretchable centimeter tape, measure the upper arm at its midpoint. The measure should be accurately read, recorded to the nearest tenth of a centimeter, and compared with standard tables as well as with any previous individual measures to note possible changes.

Triceps skinfold thickness (TSF). TSF provides an estimate of the subcutaneous fat. Together with the MAC at the same spot, the mid-

arm muscle circumference can be calculated to give a good estimate of the skeletal muscle mass. Use a standard millimeter skinfold caliper, such as the Lange caliper. Have the woman stand with her previously measured arm hanging loosely to her side. Then with the thumb and forefinger at the back of her arm, about 1 to 2 cm from the previously measured mid-point of the upper arm, gently pull a vertical pinch of the skin and subcutaneous fat away from the underlying muscle. Place the caliper jaws over the lifted skinfold mid-point while the skinfold is held. Release the caliper extender within 2 or 3 seconds and read the measure of the compressed skinfold to the nearest full or fraction of a millimeter. Avoid excessive pressure or delayed reading. For increased accuracy, take three measures and use the mean for calculations. Record results and compare with standard tables and with previous individual measures to note any changes.

Mid-upper-arm muscle circumference. As indicated, this derived value gives a good indirect measure of the body's skeletal muscle mass, a major indicator of the tissue protein integrity. First, convert the TSF mean value (millimeters) to centimeters to match the other two measuring units involved (divide millimeter value by

10). Then calculate the mid-upper-arm muscle circumference (MAMC) by the following formula:

$$MAMC(cm) = MAC(cm) - [3.14 \times TSF(cm)]$$

Alternately, the TSF can be left in millimeters as measured and the value of the factor (pi) in the formula changed to the value of 0.314. Compare the results with standard percentiles for women given in reference tables.

Weight evaluation in maternity care. Of all the initial anthropometric data for assessing nutritional status before pregnancy or at its beginning, maternal body weight is most significant. It is the baseline by which the mother's increasing weight during pregnancy can be monitored carefully, and is an indicator of adequate nutritional support for a healthy course and outcome.

Prepregnant weight. The mother's prepregnant weight and her pattern of gain or loss during her pregnancy are important clinical parameters predictive of the birth weight of the child. Prepregnancy weight is the result of the mother's genetic pattern, her previous nutritional history, and her environment, given no other coexisting serious illnesses. Extremes of being underweight and overweight should be investigated for underlying problems such as poor eating habits, environmental or social factors, or illness.

Weight Gain During Pregnancy

A number of factors must be considered in counseling women concerning weight gain during pregnancy: the nutritional quality of the gain, range of individual needs, energy requirement to support adequate gain, importance of weight gain to the pregnancy course and outcome, and the general amount and rate of gain for a healthy pregnancy.

Quality of weight gain. Although the amount of gain is important, the central concern is with the nutritional quality of the gain. The woman should be encouraged to consume foods high in nutrient density to achieve this crucial quality of weight gain. The critical role of sufficient energy intake (kcalories) to meet the in-

creased metabolic needs must be stressed. Clearly, severe caloric restriction is an unphysiologic and potentially harmful practice for both the developing fetus and the mother. Usually it is accompanied by restriction of vitally needed nutrients essential to the growth process during pregnancy, the most rapid period of human growth throughout the life cycle.

Individual needs. As indicated above, weight gain alone gives a partial, though important, indication of the health status during pregnancy. It must be interpreted on an individual basis in terms of weight history, nutritional-medical-obstetric histories, current nutritional status and reserves, and overall weight pattern during the pregnancy. Each pregnant woman must be carefully assessed in terms of her own particular health status and life situation; then person-centered care and guidance can be provided accordingly.

Energy requirement. As indicated in previous chapters, a total of about 60,000 to 80,000 additional kcalories, or 200 to 300 kcal/day above nonpregnant needs, is required to develop a healthy fetus and necessary maternal tissues. An energy intake at this level will usually result in a weight gain of about 26 to 35 lb (10 to 12 kg) by term. However, energy intakes and weight gains that support healthy pregnancies vary widely. Weight gains and energy needs during pregnancy are influenced by many factors, including prepregnancy weight, energy expenditure (Fig. 8-1), preparation during pregnancy for lactation, and multiple gestation.

Importance of weight gain to pregnancy outcome. A woman's weight before pregnancy and her weight gain during pregnancy directly affect infant birth weight and incidence of infant morbidity and mortality. Over four decades (1947-1987), infant mortality in the United States declined from a rate of 32.2 per 1,000 live births to a rate of 10.1.[31] However, significant declines occurred at only two points over these decades: (1) in the 1940s, a 37.9 percent decline with the advent of antibiotics and its effect primarily on postneonatal mortality, and (2) in the 1970s, a 37.0 percent decline with the spread of neonatal technology and intensive care units and its effect mainly on neonatal mortality. Furthermore, between these two decades of the 1940s

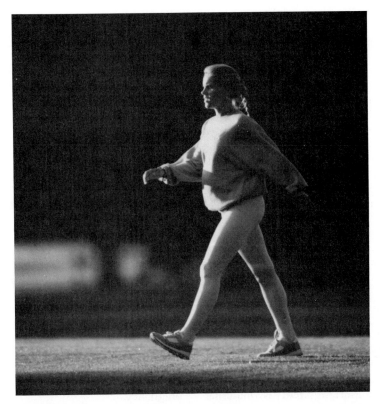

FIG. 8-1 Regular, moderate exercise such as walking is an important component of good health during pregnancy.

and the 1970s and since 1980, declines have been only minimal, holding the United States at comparatively high infant mortality rates, ranking twenty-second among the developed industrialized nations of the world. Also particularly alarming through these recent years are the increasing black/white infant mortality ratios (see Chapter 1), perhaps reflect the invasion of illicit drugs into already hazardous and impoverished neighborhoods together with a neglect of human services.[12,25,31]

Women who are poorly nourished and underweight at the beginning of pregnancy are at a higher risk of delivering vulnerable, low-birth-weight infants and of experiencing preterm labor and delivering small, underdeveloped premature babies. Inadequate weight gain during pregnancy—less than 1 kg/month during the last two trimesters—is associated with the deliv-ery of of low-birth-weight infants. The use of additional energy foods of high nutrient quality in the mother's diet will ensure optimal weight gains and increased infant birth weights. The importance of adequate weight gains during pregnancy must be emphasized to the underweight woman.

Women who are overweight at the beginning of pregnancy should be given individualized attention.[30] Overweight women do not necessarily have adequate nutrient stores, since the quality of the diet may not have been adequate. However, weight reduction during pregnancy is not recommended under any circumstances, although controlled weight gain at the lower end of the recommended range for overweight women may be indicated. Inappropriate reduced energy intake during pregnancy can result in ketosis, which can be harmful to fetal neurologic development. In any event the energy intake required for optimum protein utilization should not fall below 36 kcal/kg current maternal body weight; 45 kcal/kg meets average energy intake needs though some women may require more.

General amount of weight gain. Healthy women produce healthy babies over a wide range of total weight gains, but the quality of the diet is paramount. Optimum maternal weight gain from a quality diet throughout pregnancy makes an important contribution to successful course and outcome. An average weight gain during pregnancy is about 25 to 30 lb (11 to 14 kg). Many individual variations occur around this average. There is no specific rigid norm or restriction to which all women must be held regardless of individual needs. Such an approach is obviously unwise and unscientific. Current recommendations, therefore, are usually stated in terms of ranges to accommodate variances in needs. An initial basis for evaluation, however, may be the average weight of the products of conception as shown in Table 8-3. In addition to the components of growth and development usually attributed to a pregnancy, another important item is maternal stores. This laying down of extra adipose fat tissue is necessary to provide maternal energy reserves to sustain rapid fetal growth during the latter part of pregnancy and energy for labor and delivery and maintaining lactation after birth. About 4 to 8 lb (1.8 to 3.6 kg) of adipose tissue are commonly deposited for these needs.

Although a relatively wide range of weight gains can support healthy pregnancies and healthy babies, some approximate ranges based on prepregnant weight-for-height may be recommended and can serve as general guidelines. A National Academy of Sciences report, *Nutrition During Pregnancy,* recommends setting weight gain goals together with the pregnant woman according to her prepregnant nutritional status and weight-for-height category using the measure of body mass index (BMI) as a more specific indicator (BMI = weight = weight/height^2).[17] These recommended gains according to individual BMI are given in ranges: normal weight, 25 to 35 lb (11.5 to 18 kg); underweight 28 to 40 lb (12.5 to 18 kg); over-

TABLE 8-3   *Average Weight of the Products of Pregnancy*

Products	Weight (lb)
Fetus	7.5
Placenta	1.0
Amniotic fluid	2.0
Uterus (weight increase)	2.5
Breast tissue (weight increase)	3.0
Blood volume (weight increase)	4.0 (1,500 ml)
Maternal stores	4.0-8.0
TOTAL	24-28 lb

weight, 15 to 25 lb (7 to 11.5 kg). Adolescent mothers should strive for the upper end of the recommended range, and mothers carrying twins should gain 35 to 45 lb (16 to 20.5 kg). In any case, the important consideration is not only the quantity of weight gained but also the quality of the gain and the foods consumed to bring it about. There is a definite connection between high-risk, low-birth-weight babies, and inadequate maternal weight gain during the pregnancy.[17]

Rate of weight gain. A useful overall index is the rate of weight gain during pregnancy. On the whole, about 2 to 5 lb (1 to 2.3 kg) comprise an average gain during the first trimester. Thereafter about 1 lb (2.2 kg) per week, more or less, during the remainder of the pregnancy is usual. There is no scientific justification for routinely limiting weight gain to lesser amounts. Unusual patterns of gain, such as a sharp sudden increase in weight at about the twentieth week of pregnancy, may indicate abnormal fluid retention that should be monitored closely, especially if it occurs in conjunction with blood pressure elevation and proteinuria.

Despite efforts of practitioners over the past few years to dispel former myths and practices, many women still have misconceptions about how much weight they should gain during pregnancy, some of which stem from inappropriate advice about weight gain given to them by their physicians, or a course of prenatal care that does not include the fundamental dietary assessment and nutrition counseling recommended by the

TABLE 8-4 *Normal Adjustments in Vitamin and Mineral Serum Levels During Pregnancy*

Decreased	Variable	Increased
Plasma	**Serum**	**Serum**
Inorganic iodine	Folacin	Copper
Pyridoxal phosphate	25-Hydroxycholecalciferol	Vitamin A
	Iron	Vitamin E
Serum		
Ascorbic acid		
Vitamin B_{12}		
Calcium		
Inorganic phosphate		
Magnesium		
Selenium		
Zinc		

Modified from Beal VA: *Nutrition in the life span,* New York, 1980, John Wiley & Sons; King JC: Dietary risk patterns during pregnancy. In Weiniger J, Briggs G, eds: *Nutr Update* 1:206, 1983.

National Academy of Sciences (NAS) report.[17] Worse still, an increasing number of high-risk adolescent and adult poor women receive little or no prenatal care or sound advice at all.[8] Implementation of the NAS recommendations in *Nutrition During Pregnancy,* which identifies a primary need for routine nutritional assessment and guidance for all pregnant women in the United States, calls for major changes in a number of health care policy areas.[17]

Laboratory Data

More objective and precise data concerning nutritional status may be obtained by laboratory methods. However, for assessment during pregnancy, some problems in interpretation exist here also. These problems include (1) a lack of established norms for pregnant women for some of the tests and (2) a need for more knowledge about the relation of certain nutrients to prepregnant and pregnant states. For example, the use of steroid contraceptives has been implicated in changes in serum folate, vitamin B_6, vitamin B_{12}, and vitamin C, which may be important in developing chronic depletion of maternal stores. Also, more knowledge is needed about the effects of maternal distribution of plasma proteins, serum cholesterol, and triglycerides on the future health of the infant.

Despite these limitations, however, laboratory data provide vital baseline information for nutritional assessment at the beginning of pregnancy, as well as ongoing monitoring of its course throughout gestation. In general, laboratory tests can help determine deficiencies, needs, or effects on pregnancy in several nutrient areas. Table 8-4 shows specific physiologic diseases and increases in blood levels of various vitamins and minerals during pregnancy.

Blood-forming nutrients. Measures of the blood-forming nutrients—iron, folate, pyridoxine (B_6), and cobalamin (B_{12})—are important guides for use in preventing and treating the anemias often associated with pregnancy or with depletion of prepregnant stores of these hematologic agents. Along with protein, these agents are necessary to combat nutritional anemia, a common complication of pregnancy and the interconceptual period, by providing materials for the synthesis of red blood cells and their essential component, hemoglobin. Five biochemical tests serve as early mirrors of nutritional deficiency and provide serum markers for determining needs. The first two (hemoglobin and hematocrit) are routine in prenatal care; the others (transferrin, ferritin, and total iron-binding capacity) may be added as indicated.

Hemoglobin. Hemoglobin is a conjugated protein in red blood cells made up of two essential parts: (1) *globin*, the protein part, structured from four large polypeptide chains, each made up of 141 to 146 specifically sequenced amino acids, and (2) *heme*, the nonprotein part, a red pigment compound. Each globin peptide chain binds a heme group, and each heme group carries a molecule of iron attached at its center. Together these parts form a convoluted sphere with the heme held in crevices or "pockets" on the surface of the large completed structure of folded peptide chains. Normal hemoglobin (HbA) is a unique structure that can form a stable oxygen complex, **oxyhemoglobin,** in which the iron remains in its ferrous form (Fe+++). Thus hemoglobin provides a stable carrier to deliver vital oxygen to the cells for cell metabolism, work that is increased during pregnancy. The increase in circulating blood volume during pregnancy is a normal adaptation to support the increased metabolic load. This fluid increase contributes to a normal physiologic dilution anemia, for which increased intake of blood-forming nutrients is necessary to restore normal levels. A hemoglobin level less than 11 gm/100 ml late in pregnancy is suspect for unreplenished nutritional anemia, and hemoglobin less than 10 gm/100 ml is a certainty for it.

Hematocrit. **Hematocrit** is a measure of packed volume of red blood cells, the cells that carry the hemoglobin. Together with hemoglobin values, this measure can reflect impending or frank anemia. Hematocrit levels less than 32% late in pregnancy indicate such a deficient state.

Transferrin and ferritin. **Transferrin** is the plasma protein beta-globulin that binds absorbed iron and carries it to its tissue storage sites in the bone marrow, spleen, and liver, where the iron is then transferred to its storage protein ferritin. Serum transferrin levels determine the amount of carrier protein available to supply iron to tissue sites that synthesize red blood cells. A measure of serum **ferritin** indicates the extent of iron reserves, an important consideration in high parity women.

Total iron-binding capacity. **Total iron-binding capacity** values indicate how much iron the available transferrin is carrying. Nor-mally, only about 20% to 35% of the iron-binding capacity of transferrin is filled, leaving an unsaturated latent reserve in the plasma for handling variances in iron intake. If the transferrin level falls, as in protein-energy malnutrition or unreplenished plasma dilution in pregnancy, there is less total transport capacity and the cells' source of iron diminishes, contributing further to the anemia. Further examination of a stained **erythrocyte** smear will help determine the specific cause of the anemia. Measures of serum iron, free red blood cell **protoporphyrin,** and red blood cell count help to evaluate iron deficiency more specifically.

Serum protein. Of special interest during pregnancy is the serum level of **albumin,** the major blood protein controlling the capillary fluid shift mechanism and hence water balance throughout the body. This basic homeostatic mechanism maintains the normal flow of tissue fluids from the circulating blood into and through the tissues for nourishment of cells and back into the blood circulation. The operation of this important mechanism depends on a normal balance between two pressures: the blood pressure pushing fluids and their nutrients across capillary membranes into the tissues, and the colloidal osmotic pressure of serum albumin drawing tissue fluids and their metabolites back across capillary membranes and into circulation for constant renal control of fluids and metabolites. The increased total body water during pregnancy requires increased serum albumin to sustain levels necessary to support normal tissue circulation. Thus a protein deficit would contribute to a lower plasma albumin level and in turn to an imbalance in the fluid shift mechanism with resulting edema. An acceptable level of serum albumin during pregnancy is 3.5 gm/100 ml or above.

Other measures of protein metabolism. In high-risk populations, women may enter pregnancy in a more serious condition of borderline nutritional status or frank malnutrition. The increased metabolic demands of the pregnancy may then compromise their tenuous nutritional status even further. In such cases additional measures of protein balance may be used to assess needs. These measures include tests for urinary creatinine and urinary urea nitrogen.

Urinary creatinine is a metabolic product of tissue protein breakdown. The amount excreted indicates the extent of the tissue catabolism. The 24-hour excretion is interpreted in terms of ideal creatinine for height, with height used as a basic indicator of body protein mass. Standard ideal creatinine values in relation to height and weight (the creatinine-height index) are found in nutrition texts.[30]

Urea is the chief end product of dietary protein metabolism, so its urinary excretion rate in relation to dietary protein intake is a basic measure of the body's protein balance. This balance is expressed in terms of nitrogen balance, the unique constituent element in protein. A 24-hour urinary urea nitrogen excretion is used with the calculated dietary nitrogen intake over the same period of time to determine the woman's nitrogen balance. Since every 6.25 gm of dietary protein digested and metabolized results in 1 gm of nitrogen urinary excretion, the following formula is used to derive the overall nitrogen balance:

$$\text{Nitrogen balance} = [\text{protein intake} \div 6.25]$$
$$- [\text{urinary urea nitrogen} + 4]$$

The formula factor of 4 represents additional nitrogen loss through feces and skin.

Other vitamins and minerals. According to individual indication, tests of other vitamin and mineral levels may be used to measure nutritional status. These tests may include determinations of the water-soluble vitamins thiamin, riboflavin, niacin, and vitamin C. Tests for levels of fat-soluble vitamins A, D, E, and K may be indicated, as well as for zinc and other trace elements.

Blood lipids, glucose, and enzymes. Routine testing for blood glucose levels, as well as urine sugar and ketones, is used to screen for and monitor latent diabetes mellitus or gestational glucosuria. More extensive monitoring and care can then be provided for those mothers indicated. Other tests may be indicated in other preexisting chronic conditions such as cardiovascular disease or maternal phenylketonuria (PKU). Such complicating conditions during pregnancy require special care and are discussed in Chapter 9.

Historical Data

The most important method of nutritional assessment in pregnancy is that of history taking. These data must include baseline and continuing information from careful medical, obstetrical, nutritional, family, social, and personal histories, all of which influence nutritional status (Fig. 8-2). Historical data that should be included are age, previous obstetrical history, background medical conditions and their course and treatment, socioeconomic and cultural background, personal needs, and nutritional history and diet evaluation.

Age. Pregnancy at either end of the general reproductive cycle carries added risk of potential problems. Pregnancy in an adolescent involves not only physiologic demands added to the young teenager's own growth needs, but also emotional, social, educational, and other personal and family problems.

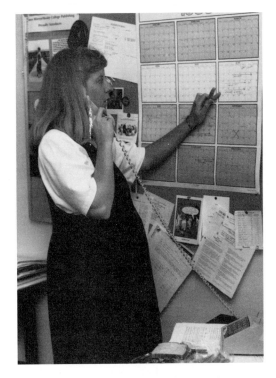

FIG. 8-2 Careful history taking in prenatal care includes gathering data on all related areas of a client's life.

In older women, especially in the "elderly" primigravida, pregnancy poses other problems associated with more mature ovulation and physiologic changes in the latter stages of the reproductive cycle. Women 35 years of age or older who are pregnant for the first time carry added risks and need close monitoring throughout pregnancy to avoid complications. The problem needing the most nutritional intervention in the older primigravada is the tendency toward elevated blood pressure. Though monitoring is needed, dietary recommendations for the hypertensive pregnant woman are the same as for the normotensive pregnant woman. However, resting metabolism and activity tend to decline with age so the older pregnant woman may have total energy needs about 4% lower than that of a younger pregnant woman of comparable size. Since protein, vitamin, and mineral needs would not be lowered correspondingly, a diet of higher nutrient density should be recommended.

Obstetrical history. Poor reproductive history may indicate nutritional deficiencies. Data should be gathered about previous pregnancies:

- *Parity and outcome.* Sequential listing, noting time intervals, of all previous pregnancies and their results, including stillbirths, premature infants, and abortions (spontaneous and therapeutic).
- *Infant birth weights.* Low birth weights, which may suggest nutritional problems, or higher birth weights, which may be associated with latent diabetes.
- *Maternal weight changes in previous pregnancies.* Amount and pattern of weight gain as a potential indicator of possible high-risk mothers.
- *Interconceptual period.* Repeated pregnancies or lactation within 1-year intervals with depletion of nutritional reserves; use of steroid contraceptives, which affect nutritional status through inhibition of folate absorption; intercurrent illnesses or conditions of a metabolic nature such as diabetes mellitus, which pregnancy intensifies; or infections or neoplastic disease.
- *Lactation experience.* Breast-feeding experience with previous infants; awareness of lactation preparation during pregnancy.

Medical history. In addition to the incidence of intercurrent illnesses, chronic conditions such as insulin-dependent diabetes mellitus (IDDM), renal disease or heart disease, metabolic genetic disease such as PKU, galactosemia or fructose intolerance and the course of its management and control, as well as any overt signs or family history of diabetes, should be noted and will require special attention during the pregnancy. Any prior incidence of hypertension, venereal disease, tuberculosis, or other infections must be reported. Previous nutritional deficiencies should be described fully.

Social history. Living situation, family, housing, economic status (and family income available for food), and the need, accessibility, and use of family assistance programs are prime factors of concern in nutrition assessment in pregnancy. The occupation and physical activity of the mother are also important. Food habits are closely related to ethnic patterns, so data concerning cultural background and food beliefs and values are especially significant.

Personal history. Personal data should include habits related to smoking and use of drugs and alcohol, all of which should be avoided during pregnancy, and the degree of physical activity. All medications used should be reviewed, exploring possible nutrient-drug interactions. During pregnancy, all drugs that are not specifically prescribed and administered under medical supervision should be avoided.

Nutrition history. In addition to data concerning food habits, many additional items such as allergies, food intolerances, dieting experiences, and other problems related to food will need to be explored in detail. This information is basic to nutrition assessment in pregnancy and planning of realistic food patterns. The following section discusses needs and approaches in this fundamental area of dietary evaluation.

INDIVIDUAL NUTRITION ASSESSMENT

In all health care and education, but especially in maternity care, the guiding principle is to begin where the client is, to focus on her concerns, her thinking, her situation, her needs. Thus, in nutrition assessment in pregnancy, a time in the human life cycle when nutrition is of special importance, it is particularly necessary to learn who the mother is, how mature she is in her own values and thinking, and how her individual needs can best be met. Only in this context of personal life situations and needs can realistic guidance be provided. Nutrition assessment in pregnancy, therefore, involves three basic areas: (1) background data, (2) diet history, and (3) diet analysis.

Personal Background Data

The life situation and values, as well as physical and emotional factors, are closely related to food habits and attitudes. Information about the following items will provide important background data with which the nutritionist can help the mother develop her own personalized food plan.

Living situation. Details of the mother's living situation help nutrition counselor and client work together to plan a food guide that will meet the mother's individual needs during her pregnancy. This information will include any contingencies or influences on food use and eating behavior, such as home setting, housing, lifestyle, family members, occupation, general socioeconomic status, food assistance needs, and family roles and attitudes about food, especially food practices in pregnancy.

Cultural-ethnic food practices. Any culturally related food patterns will be explored, including types of food, ethnic dishes, food sources, methods of food storage, preparation, and cooking, and any taboos associated with pregnancy. The pregnant woman receives much culturally based advice about what she should eat from many sources in her community and family.

Special diet practices. Any personal diet beliefs, values, practices, and experiences will also be explored. Areas that may bring out special nutritional needs include any recent dieting that may have reduced her nutritional reserves and any faddist or unusual food patterns that may be nutritionally unsound. Pica patterns, such as eating laundry starch or clay, can be damaging.[10] Highly restrictive vegetarian regimens, such as a macrobiotic diet, fruitarianism, or any other arbitrarily adopted food pattern can be harmful to her pregnancy.

Food allergies or intolerances. Any food allergies, milk or lactose intolerance, or other indications for omission of certain foods need to be explored. The problem may be a true allergy requiring elimination of certain foods, or an intolerance requiring modification of the food. For example, in cases of lactose intolerance resulting from a lack of the enzyme lactase, the missing enzyme in the form of products such as Lactaid can be added to milk, allowing the use of milk with no problem. In other cases the problem may be one of simple dislike or unpleasant association with the food, and discussion about the cause or alternate ways of using that food or nutritionally similar foods may be the solution.

Medications or supplements. The use of all medications or supplements needs to be explored. Drugs should be avoided during pregnancy, and if needed, used only under medical supervision. Nutrient supplements should be discussed in terms of individual needs and situations in which inadequate diets are unlikely to improve. In clinics where nutritional services for dietary assessment and counseling do not exist, a multivitamin-mineral supplement may well be the only practical means of improving nutrient intake.[17] In general practice, some form of vitamin-mineral supplementation is used in most prenatal clinics, and specific attention is given to iron and folate supplements. Counseling should include making the individual aware that excessive intake of any nutrient may be toxic. Excesses of iodine and vitamins A, D, C, and B_6, especially should be discouraged.

Alcohol, cigarettes, and drugs. The use of alcohol, cigarettes, and drugs should be strictly avoided during pregnancy. Studies indicate that intrauterine growth retardation has been consistently observed with such habits, especially the dramatic effect of fetal alcohol exposure.[14]

1. *Alcohol.* Extensive and habitual alcohol use during pregnancy, especially during the early weeks of cell differentiation and fetal tissue development, leads to the irreversible tragedy of fetal alcohol syndrome (FAS).[24] FAS has become a leading cause of preventable birth defects and developmental disabilities in the United States.[2,26] It is characterized by a specific set of alco-

hol-related birth defects including facial deformities, impaired nervous system, a stunted brain, and mental retardation.[14] Even small amounts of alcohol may be injurious in some cases, so abstinence is the best policy during pregnancy.

2. *Cigarettes.* Cigarette smoking during pregnancy poses special high-risk problems resulting in placental abnormalities and fetal damage including prematurity and low birth weight.[1,7] Moreover, a long-term study of air pollution and lung hazards indicates that maternal smoking can affect the child's lung function into adulthood.[18] These investigators also found that long-term smoking by both parents creates health dangers for children, and those who grow up breathing passive smoke in smoking households have diminished air volume exchange in breathing and increased risk of many lower respiratory problems, such as shortness of breath, chronic cough and wheezing, bronchitis.[29] Smoking has also been found to deplete vitamin C from the mother and fetus.[3]

3. *Drugs.* Cocaine, highly addictive in all its various forms, is a major illicit drug used in the United States. Reported use crested in 1985 at 5.8 million users and dropped to 1.3 million users in 1993, with peak ages of use being 18 to 34 years (60% of users).[28] These years are also the prime child-bearing years. Cocaine exposure alters normal fetal growth. It crosses the placenta, causing fetal hypertension, ischemia, and hypoxia. Fetal growth is also affected by maternal drug-associated prepregnancy malnutrition, caused by being underweight, lack of funds for food, or drug-induced anorexia, as well as lack of prenatal care. Other related behaviors common among drug-users that affect fetal growth include tobacco and alcohol abuse and unprotected sex, leading to increased risk from multiple unplanned pregnancies and sexually transmitted diseases.[9]

4. *Caffeine.* The daily intake of caffeine in the United States, in caffeinated beverages such as coffee, tea, and soft drinks averages about 200 mg, with little change in use during pregnancy.[16] Study of such maternal caffeine use has indicated acute cardiovascular effects in the mother and fetus affecting maternal blood pressure and fetal heart rate. Though these changes are small and do not appear to have adverse effects, they may have important clinical implications. Investigators have found that caffeine is also related to miscarriage.[11]

Physical activity. The extent of physical exercise in either recreation or work should be explored. Strenuous "fitness" programs may result in low-birth-weight infants with insufficient body fat development. The American College of Obstetricians and Gynecologists (ACOG) has produced a helpful guide for appropriate exercise during pregnancy. Also, adverse or heavy working situations can contribute to prematurity.[15,21]

Diet History

Food intake. Measures of nutrition assessment center mainly on dietary intake surveys and nutrient analyses. Together with comparative data from biochemical tests, anthropometry, and clinical observations, these measures provide an appraisal of the individual's nutritional status, as well as practical information about response to individual food plans or nutrition intervention programs. Methods for assessing dietary intake may take many forms, depending on such factors as the resources of the health care center and the background and nature of the individual clients. At best, however, the methodology is imperfect. Americans are a multiethnic and multiracial population with great diversity in cultural food patterns that are influenced further by economic, psychologic, and physiologic factors. Dietary surveys or histories can only attempt to describe food behavior, and that behavior is constantly changing. Nonetheless, the traditional dietary assessment methods briefly described here have been used alone or in various combinations to indicate nutrition and health needs.

Usually nutritionists use several basic tools to obtain needed information about food intake of different individuals.

24-hour recall. Individuals are asked to recall the specific food items they ate during the previous day, describing the nature and amount of each. This method is simpler and less costly than some of the others, but has the disadvantages of memory limitations and measurement problems in determining actual amounts of food eaten.

Food records. Individuals are asked to record their food intake for a brief period of time, from 1 to 3 or 7 days, or on certain days periodically. Obtaining accurate information about actual food intake is difficult at best. Thus discussion about the purpose and method of recording is essential, with clear directions for describing food items used singly or in combination and for simple ways of measuring amounts eaten. Studies indicate that a 1-day record gives a rather meaningless estimate of a person's usual eating habits, but may provide a reasonable estimate for a group of individuals. A 3-day record provides more accurate information to help account for daily variation. A combination of methods may be used with a follow-up 3-day food record. Table 8-5 gives an example of a general form that may be used for recording food intake.

Food frequency questionnaire. A food frequency questionnaire (FFQ) is helpful in combination with actual food records or diet history. Its purpose is to help determine food intake over an extended period of time, such as the course of the pregnancy, especially where risk factors are involved and need closer monitoring. This method provides useful data for investigating the relation of individual diets to these risks. The FFQ has two basic parts: a list of foods and a scale for checking frequency of use over a given period of time. The food list may be comprehensive to assess overall food habits, or specific, to focus on use of particular food sources related to the condition being monitored. The FFQ may also include a means of measuring amounts of the foods used. Diet diversity indexes have been developed on the basis of food frequency studies; they give further descriptive information to help measure cultural aspects of the diet.

Diet history interview. The classic in-depth diet history technique requires a highly trained nutritionist who determines a full picture of the usual total diet and interprets its nutritional significance. Such an in-depth method may be unrealistic in general practice, but can be highly valuable with high-risk cases. However, nutri-

TABLE 8-5 **Food Record: Diet History**

Name _____

Medical record no. _____

Date _____

	Total Food Intake					Comments
Meals and Snacks	Description of Food Items					
Time	Place	Food	Amount	Type or Preparation	With Whom Eaten?	Any Related Factors? (Associated Activity, Place, Persons, Money, Feelings, Hunger, etc.)

tionists have developed and used successfully modified diet history methods in a variety of situations. For example, an activity-associated approach or a carefully constructed questionnaire can easily be adapted for use in prenatal care.

1. *Activity-associated general day's food intake pattern.* For most people, eating is related to a usual activity pattern. An activity-associated food intake history uses a series of memory hints about food habits as the interviewer leads the person through a typical day, first a weekday and then a weekend day, attaching questions about food intake to the typical day's routine (i.e., where they are, what they are doing, and with whom). This structured process brings out many details about habits and schedules that will aid in constructive food planning with the individual. Fig. 8-3 is an example of a form that may be used for developing such an activity-associated food intake pattern.

2. *Diet history questionnaire.* A carefully developed and pretested diet history form combining FFQ techniques with family living situation, a day's typical food pattern, and methods of accurately measuring food portions can be used by the nutritionist as a basis for follow-up food planning with the mother. This approach uses adapted diet history methods to obtain valid information with the assistance of trained support-level staff or lay interviewers, in the clinic or in the home, with personal follow-up nutrition assessment and care planning. It is especially effective with persons from multiethnic backgrounds, incorporating a variety of representative ethnic foods in the questionnaire's food lists and portion-sized illustrations, and using trained community workers in the homes.

Diet Analysis

Once food habit information has been obtained by any of the described methods, the findings must be analyzed and the results used as a basis for nutrition counseling in terms of the increased demands of pregnancy. Two methods used for analysis are nutrient calculations and general check by food groups.

Nutrient calculation. Most nutrient calculations of food intake data are done today using a number of available programs and data bases. The largest computer data bank is maintained by the U.S. Department of Agriculture, and individual software programs draw from these data and other resources for particular food items. Constant revision and additions of items as new food composition data are developed improve the usefulness of these evaluation resources.

General nutrient check by food groups. Lacking computer access or knowledge, however, a basic evaluation and education tool that can be used with the mother is the basic grouping of these foods according to major nutrient contributions. Various ethnic foods contributing the major nutrients can also be added for use with particular food patterns. An effort is made to determine amounts of food from each group outlined to meet the increased needs for key nutrients during pregnancy. The nutritional analysis form in Table 8-6 provides such a guide. Using this guide, the counselor helps the mother become familiar with the basis of the groupings according to the major nutrients each contains, having her add other equivalent items from her own ethnic food as desired. This review offers initial and ongoing opportunity to check diet adequacy, discuss basic nutrients needed during pregnancy, why they are necessary, major food sources of these nutrients, and ways they can be included in her diet.

NUTRITION EDUCATION AND GUIDANCE

What can be done at this point with the findings from diet surveys in the prenatal clinic? What kind of educational program and continuing guidance is needed to build and strengthen healthy food practices? Fundamental answers involve recognition of a varity of food practices and how people learn.

As the personal diet history of each mother is analyzed, a variety of individual food practices will be found. Some of these will be beneficial and will only need encouragement and positive reinforcement. Some may be harmless and can generally be ignored. However, some practices may be harmful because they produce deficien-

Name _____ Date _____

Age _____ Height _____ Prepregnancy weight _____

Gravida _____ EDB* _____ Present weight _____

Activity-Associated General Day's Food Intake Pattern

Living Situation

Housing _____

Members of household _____

Culture _____

Occupation: Husband _____

Self _____

Recreation, physical activity _____

Present Food Habits	Place	Time	Checklist
Morning			Protein foods

Present Food Habits   **Place**   **Time**

Morning

_____

_____

_____

Noon

_____

_____

_____

Evening

_____

_____

_____

Snacks

_____

_____

Comments

_____

_____

_____

Checklist

Protein foods
  - Milk   Fish
  - Cheese   Poultry
  - Meat   Eggs

Breads, cereals, legumes
  - Breads (whole-grain, enriched)
  - Cereals
  - Pastas
  - Dried beans, peas, lentils

Vegetables
  - Dark yellow   Potato
  - Deep greens   Others

Fruits   Fats and oils
  - Citrus   Butter
  - Others   Margarine
  -      Others

Desserts, sweets
Soft drinks, candy
Alcohol
Vitamin, mineral supplements
Medications, drugs

*Expected date of birth.

FIG. 8-3   Nutrition interview: diet history.

TABLE 8-6   Nutritional Analysis Sheet

Food Groups	Major Nutrient Contributions	Recommended Daily Intake (Number of Servings)	My Intake	Analysis of Food Needs
Protein-rich foods				
Milk, cheese	Protein (complete, high biologic value); calcium, phosphorus, magnesium; vitamin D; riboflavin	1 qt milk 2 oz cheese or ½ cup cottage cheese		
Egg, meat	Protein (complete, high biological value); B complex vitamins; folic acid (liver); vitamin A (liver); iron	2 eggs (unless contraindicated) 2 servings meat (3-4 oz each)		
Vitamin- and mineral-rich foods				
Grains, whole or enriched, breads or cereals, legumes	Protein (incomplete, supplementary); B complex vitamins; iron, calcium, phosphorus, magnesium; energy (protein sparing)	4 or more servings		
Green and yellow vegetables	Vitamin A; folic acid	1-2 servings		
Citrus fruits and other vitamin C-rich fruits and vegetables	Vitamin C	2 servings		
Potatoes and other vegetables and fruits	Energy (protein sparing); added vitamins and minerals	1 serving or as needed for calories		
Fats—margarine, butter, and oils	Vitamin A (butter, fortified margarine); vitamin E (vegetable oils); energy (protein sparing)	1-2 tbsp as needed for calories		
Iodized salt	Iodine	Use with food to taste		

cies in specific nutrients or directly affect fetal development. These practices need to be corrected. All of these situations present educational and counseling challenges. Because the successful outcome of each pregnancy is of particular personal and social concern and nutrition plays such a primary role in determining that outcome, meeting these challenges is becoming increasingly important. This is especially true, considering the dramatic increases in the number of low-birth-weight babies being born today in major American cities. In addition to the unmeasurable human costs of a poor outcome, the incremental monetary cost alone of these poor outcomes in intensive neonatal services and long-term disability care is far greater than the cost of good prenatal care for all pregnant women. Thus nutrition education and guidance become major responsibilities of policymakers administering prenatal care programs, to supply sufficient personnel qualified to provide essential preconceptual and prenatal nutrition services.

Learning New Ideas and Food Behaviors

The learning process is not a simple matter. Essentially, learning means change and when this applies to food habits, very personal behaviors are involved. Often this process involves deeply rooted habits, values, and beliefs, and such change is seldom easy. The counselor will need to remember and apply three basic principles of learning:

1. *Learning is very personal and individual.* It cannot be imposed from the outside. Rather, it takes place inside a person in response to personally felt needs and through interaction with the environment. Therefore valid learning must meet personal needs and involve the learner directly.

2. *Learning is associative or developmental.* It builds on prior learning, experience, and knowledge. Thus valid learning must start where the person is and blend the new with the familiar.

3. *Learning results in changed behavior.* It brings new attitudes and values and actions. Therefore valid learning must be measured in terms of changed behavior.

Learning Framework: Concept of Building

The familiar concept of building provides a useful framework for prenatal education. The idea is a concrete one with numerous illustrative associations from prior learning and experience. Applied to pregnancy, it gives a dynamic notion to the profound reality of building a new human life. Using this concept, nutrition principles can be presented, interpreted, and learned in relation to the basic idea of growth and development, with each nutrient providing a necessary part for the successful outcome of the building process. In this manner, for example, protein may be viewed as the essential building material, kcalories as the necessary energy for the building work, and vitamins and minerals as required structural elements as well as vital control agents for regulating the building process.

Positive Approach to Build Motivation for Learning

Perhaps at no other time in the human life cycle is a person more open to nutrition education or more motivated by a sense of responsibility for another human life than during the period of pregnancy. A positive personalized approach can build on this feeling of responsibility and anticipation of parenthood to develop motivation for learning. Moreover, nutrition education during this period will go far in carrying over to the parents' attitudes toward feeding their children as they continue to grow through infancy, childhood, to maturity and in turn contribute to the health habits of another generation.

Personal motivation, then, is a prime requisite for learning. Without it, an educational program is not put into action. With such motivation, learning becomes a very human adventure. The whole business of motivation is tied up with sending learners away from instruction anxious to use what the counselor has taught them—and eager to learn more. A positive personalized approach in individual prenatal counseling can help to accomplish this goal.

Yet how will the counselor begin? In general, two types of food behavior will be discovered in prenatal clinic work with mothers: (1) good food intake that meets all the recommended nutrient needs and ensures optimum nutritional intake for pregnancy and (2) inadequate food intake that does not meet needs and creates deficiencies that contribute to complications. In each case an analysis of individual food habits and positive reinforcement of good habits and positive teaching to correct deficiencies will be useful. Then, on this basis, a personal food plan may be developed.

Positive reinforcement of good food habits. To strengthen good food habits, the clinician can give positive feedback immediately for behaviors that help fulfill recommended choices and amounts for pregnancy. A clinician may provide positive reinforcement for this desired behavior in several ways:

1. Relate the mother's food behavior to her pregnancy. The clinician should guide her to identify for herself how her particular food practices are meeting the nutritional needs of her pregnancy. Table 8-7 relates

TABLE 8-7 *Nutrient Needs of Pregnancy*

Nutrient	Amount (RDA 1989)		Reasons for Increased Nutrient Need in Pregnancy	Food Sources
	Nonpregnant Adult Need	Pregnancy Need		

Protein	46-50 gm	60 gm	Rapid fetal tissue growth
			Amniotic fluid
			Placenta growth and development
			Maternal tissue growth: uterus, breasts
			Increased maternal circulating blood volume:
			  a. Hemoglobin increase
			  b. Plasma protein increase
			Maternal storage reserves for labor, delivery, and lactation
				Milk
				Cheese
				Egg
				Meat
				Grains
				Legumes
				Nuts

Calories	2200	2500	Increased basal metabolic rate, energy needs Protein sparing	See individual foods
Minerals Calcium	800 mg	1200 mg	Fetal skeleton formation Fetal tooth bud formation Increased maternal calcium metabolism	Milk Cheese Whole grains Leafy vegetables Egg yolk
Phosphorus	800 mg	1200 mg	Fetal skeleton formation Fetal tooth bud formation Increased maternal phosphorus metabolism	Milk Cheese Lean meats
Iron	15 mg	30 mg	Increased maternal circulating blood volume, increased hemoglobin Fetal liver iron storage High iron cost of pregnancy	Liver Meats Egg Whole or enriched grain Leafy vegetables Nuts Legumes Dried fruits
Iodine	150 μg	175 μg	Increased basal metabolic rate—increased thyroxine production	Iodized salt
Magnesium	280 mg	320 mg	Coenzyme in energy and protein metabolism Enzyme activator Tissue growth, cell metabolism Muscle action	Nuts Soybeans Cocoa Seafood Whole grains Dried beans and peas

TABLE 8-7   *Nutrient Needs of Pregnancy—cont'd*

Nutrient	Amount (RDA 1989)		Reasons for Increased Nutrient Need in Pregnancy	Food Sources
	Nonpregnant Adult Need	Pregnancy Need		
Vitamins				
Thiamin	1.1 mg	1.5 mg	Coenzyme for energy metabolism	Pork, beef Liver Whole or enriched grains Legumes
B_6 (pyridoxine)	1.6 mg	2.2 mg	Coenzyme in protein metabolism Increased fetal growth requirement	Wheat, corn Liver Meat
B_{12}	2.0 μg	2.2 μg	Coenzyme in protein metabolism, especially vital cell proteins such as nucleic acid Formation of red blood cells	Milk Egg Meat Liver Cheese

some specific key foods a mother uses to the nutrients needed.

2. Review the reasons for these increased needs. The mother's good habits should be further reinforced her by guiding her to see *why* it is important that she get these increased nutrients during her pregnancy. The clinician should relate the functions of the key nutrients to the changes taking place in her body and to the rapid growth of her baby and its protection. The reasons for increased need given in Table 8-7 may be useful here.

3. Recognize her efforts. The clinician should commend her openly and warmly for her good food habits. Everyone needs to hear simple phrases such as "Good work!" or "You're doing a good job."

Positive teaching to correct nutritional deficiencies. To correct inadequate food practices, the clinician should provide positive teaching rather than dire pronouncements to encourage the mother to change those food habits that need improving. The clinician may provide positive thinking and concern for habit change through the following actions:

1. Help the mother relate her food habits to unmet nutrient needs of her pregnancy. The clinician can guide her to identify for herself ways in which her particular food intake fails to meet the nutritional demands of her pregnancy. Table 8-7 includes the key nutrients she needs more of and some specific foods that supply them.

2. Review the reasons for these increased nutrient needs of pregnancy. Again, this is the previous approach, but here the clinician is trying to build motivation for making the desired behavior change by helping the mother to see *why* it is important for her to do so. Point to the positive results for her baby's health, as well as for her own health. Here, also, Table 8-7 may be a useful guide for discussion.

3. Identify reasons for the deficiencies. What are her problems in obtaining needed foods? What limiting factors exist in her personal living situation? A variety of factors may be involved, often interrelated. Some may be simple reasons of which the mother is aware and can readily change.

Others, however, may be larger problems requiring team help from the nutritionist, the social worker, the nurse, and the physician. In any event, possible problem areas should be considered in an analysis of the mother's needs:

A. *The food supply.* There may be a lack of food available because of insufficient funds, poor shopping resources, inadequate storage facilities with spoilage and waste, or lack of skills in general food management and preparation.

B. *The person herself.* Physical problems may be present, such as underlying disease, food intolerances or aversions, poor appetite, low energy level, and low nutritional reserves or frank signs of malnutrition. Personal problems may include ignorance of food needs or food values, special beliefs concerning food, lack of education, illiteracy, language barrier, carelessness, lack of concern or general apathy, and underlying psychologic or emotional needs.

C. *The environment.* Too often, problems attributed to personal factors, as just listed, are in reality the result of environmental factors that have overwhelmed the mother's coping resources, and she needs assistance in dealing with them. She may not be living in her own home and may have little control over food selection and preparation. Also, there may be cultural or family food customs, especially during pregnancy, that limit food choices. There may be added socioeconomic problems from low income, unemployment, or poverty. Moreover, in some communities there may be attitudes or political influences that limit the availability of food assistance programs for pregnant women.

4. Explore possible solutions to problems or alternative practices available. Whatever the situation discovered, the clinician should identify any problems, needs, or limitations on the mother's ability to make the desired changes and explore with her possible solutions:

A. *Low income.* Depending on degree of need, two areas of assistance may be discussed: (1) economical buying suggestions to help her spend her limited funds wisely and (2) food assistance programs available to her in the community through agencies such as Women, Infants, and Children (WIC), church or lodge groups, or other local food programs or food banks. Consultation with the team social worker will provide guidance.

B. *Food aversions or intolerances.* The basis for the food rejection should be reviewed as a means of securing acceptance of foods in question, or determining another form of the particular foods or other foods supplying similar nutrients.

C. *Cultural food patterns.* Nutrition needs should be related to a variety of acceptable food forms and preparations within the personal cultural food pattern. However, within a general cultural group, individual food habits may vary widely so that careful exploration of individual needs and desires is necessary.

D. *Vegetarian food patterns.* The type of vegetarian food pattern the mother is following must be determined. Many vegetarian food plans exclude only meat, some even allowing fish or poultry. In these cases, ample complete protein with essential amino acids may be obtained from dairy foods and eggs. However, if a strict vegetarian diet is followed, as with vegans, careful planning is necessary to obtain sufficient complete protein from mixtures of complementary plant protein food sources. A general vegetarian food guide is given in Table 8-8, and because well-planned vegetarian food patterns have become more widely used now, many expanded references are available. However, among strict vegans, low prepregnancy weight and optimum weight gains during pregnancy may be a problem. Added energy-dense foods will be helpful for ensuring increased energy intake so that

TABLE 8-8   *Vegetarian Food Guide*

General guidelines

1. Follow nutrition guide for regular food plan during pregnancy as outlined in Table 6-10.
2. Eat a wide variety of foods, including milk and milk products and eggs.
3. If no milk is allowed, use a supplement of 4 μg of vitamin B_{12} daily. If goat and soymilk are used, partial supplementation may be needed.
4. If no milk is taken, also use supplements of 1,200 mg of calcium and 10 μg of vitamin D daily. Partial supplementation will be necessary if less than four servings of milk and milk products are consumed.
5. Select a variety of plant foods (especially grains, legumes, nuts, and seeds) to obtain "complete" proteins by complementary combinations, as indicated in the list below.
6. Use iodized salt.

Complementary plant protein combinations

Food	Amino Acid Deficiencies	Complementary Protein Food Combinations
Grains	Isoleucine Lysine	Rice + legumes Corn + legumes Wheat + legumes Wheat + peanut + milk Wheat + sesame + soybean Rice + brewer's yeast
Legumes	Tryptophan Methionine	Legumes + rice Beans + wheat Beans + corn Soybeans + rice + wheat Soybeans + corn + milk Soybeans + wheat + sesame Soybeans + peanuts + sesame Soybeans + peanuts + wheat + rice Soybeans + sesame + wheat
Nuts and seeds	Isoleucine Lysine	Peanuts + sesame + soybeans Sesame + beans Sesame + soybeans + wheat Peanuts + sunflower seeds
Vegetables	Isoleucine Methionine	Lima beans Green beans Brussels sprouts } + Sesame seeds or Brazil nuts or mushrooms Cauliflower Broccoli Greens plus millet or rice

protein utilization will not be compromised. The absence of vitamin B_{12} (from lack of its source—animal protein foods), as well as the high-fiber and phytate consumption from vegan diets, which may bind and reduce calcium availability, requires alternative sources of these nutrients, such as calcium-fortified soy milk, vitamin B_{12}-fortified soy products, nutritional yeasts, or vitamin-mineral supplements.

Common Functional Problems

As the pregnancy progresses, general nutritional guidance may also be needed for common functional gastrointestinal difficulties encountered. These complaints are highly individual in form and extent. The mothers will need individual counseling and assurances for control. Usually these difficulties are relatively minor. However, if they persist or become extreme, they will need medical care. In most cases, general investigation of food practices will reveal some areas where diet adjustments may help to relieve them. Some of the more common difficulties include nausea, constipation, hemorrhoids, and heartburn.

Nausea and vomiting. Difficulty with nausea and vomiting is usually mild and limited to early pregnancy. It is commonly called "morning sickness" because it occurs more often on arising than later in the day. A number of factors may contribute to this condition. Some are physiologic, based on hormonal changes that occur early in pregnancy, for example, a placental rise of human chorionic gonadotropin (HCG). Other factors may be psychologic, such as situational tensions or anxieties concerning the pregnancy itself, or dietary, such as poor food habits. Simple treatment generally improves food toleration. Small frequent meals, fairly dry and consisting chiefly of easily digested energy foods such as carbohydrates, are more readily tolerated. Cooking odors should be avoided as much as possible. Liquids are best taken between meals instead of with meals. However, if the condition persists and develops into *hyperemesis gravidarum*—severe, prolonged, persistent vomiting—a more creative approach to food selection provides helpful suggestions for patients who are able to consume food orally.[5] However, if the condition persists, a medical/nutrition team administers intravenous (IV) fluid and electrolyte replacement to prevent complications of dehydration, followed as necessary by an enteral tube feeding of appropriate formula.[6,22] However, such an increase in symptoms is usually rare. Most conditions respond to simple diet adjustments.

Constipation. This condition is seldom more than minor. Hormonal changes in pregnancy tend to increase relaxation of the gastrointestinal muscles. Also, increasing pressure of the enlarging uterus on the lower portion of the intestine, especially during the latter part of pregnancy, may make elimination somewhat difficult. Increased fluid intake, use of natural laxatives such as whole grains, fibrous fruits and vegetables, dried fruits (especially prunes and figs), and other fruits and juices generally induce regularity. Laxatives should not be used, except in special situations under medical supervision.

Hemorrhoids. A fairly common complaint during the latter part of pregnancy is that of hemorrhoids. These are enlarged veins in the anus, often protruding through the anal sphincter, caused by the increased weight of the fetus and its downward pressure. Hemorrhoids may cause considerable discomfort, burning, and itching. Occasionally they may rupture and bleed under pressure of a bowel movement, causing still more anxiety for the mother. The difficulty is usually controlled by the dietary suggestions given above for constipation. Sufficient rest during the latter part of the day may help relieve the pressure of the uterus on the lower intestine.

Heartburn or gastric pressure. Pregnant women sometimes experience the related complaints of "heartburn" or a "full feeling." These discomforts may occur especially after meals, usually caused by the pressure of the enlarging uterus crowding the adjacent digestive organ, the stomach. Gastric reflux of some of the food mixture, now a semiliquid chyme, may occur in the lower esophagus, causing a "burning" sensation from the gastric acid mixed with the food mass. This burning sensation is commonly called heartburn because of the close proximity of the lower esophagus to the heart. Obviously, however, it has nothing to do with the heart and its action. A full feeling comes from general gastric pressure, caused by a lack of normal space in the area, and is accentuated by a large meal or gas formation. These complaints are usually remedied by dividing the day's food intake into a series of small meals, avoiding eating large meals at any time. Attention may be given to relaxation, adequate chewing, eating slowly, and avoiding tensions during meals. Loose-fitting clothing provides comfort. The physician may occasionally prescribe an appropriate antacid, but home remedies such as baking soda should not be used.

Effects of iron supplements. During pregnancy an iron supplement in the form of ferrous sulfate is usually given to maintain maternal iron stores. However, further supplementation beyond the iron in routine prenatal vitamin-mineral tablets may not be necessary unless hemoglobin falls to 10.5 gm/100 ml or below. Effects of iron medication include gray or black stools, and occasional symptoms of nausea, constipation, or diarrhea. To help avoid food-related effects, the iron supplement should be taken 1 hour before or 2 hours after meals with liquid such as water or orange juice.

PLANNING AND IMPLEMENTING PERSONAL NUTRITION PROGRAMS
A Personal Food Plan

On the basis of individual findings the nutritionist and the mother can plan together a personal food guide that the mother can enjoy, one that provides for variety, a realistic pattern, and follow-up support.

Food variety. A diet consisting of a variety of foods can supply needed nutrients and make eating a pleasure. A core plan, such as that in Table 8-9, may be used initially. Additional foods may be added or changed according to individual needs, cultural patterns, or personal lifestyles. An expanded daily food guide for women, such as the plan outlined in Table 8-10, may be useful for long-term counseling and nutrition education.[19]

Realistic pattern. In each case the food plan must be practical and realistic to be useful. Many women have broad food habits and few if any limitations exist. For these women basic guidance and encouragement will suffice to meet needs. However, for some women with real problems that carry risks for a successful pregnancy, careful planning is necessary and may well determine the outcome of their pregnancies. In any case, resource materials are available for use in early pregnancy guidance to help with practical nutritional needs, food choices, marketing, and preparation.

Follow-up support. Some form of follow-up support and evaluation should be built into the continuing plan of care throughout the pregnancy. Ongoing nutrition awareness and concern should be made an integral part of every clinic visit, with the nutritionist, the nurse, and the physician showing positive interest for continuance of the food plan. They should continue to look for any problems that may require adjustment of the plan, and the nutritionist may use occasional food records for continuing evaluation of nutritional needs. It is encouraging to the mother to see ways in which her food habit changes are indeed making actual increases in her nutrient intake and hence providing the necessary nutritional support for her pregnancy.

Community Nutrition Services

Changing health care needs and systems. An increasing variety of health services in prenatal care are developing in communities as people become more aware of health needs. In our changing society and health care system in the United States, public and professional groups increasingly see relationships between social issues and health/disease problems, and are seeking ways of reaching high-risk populations and involving people more in their own health care. More community programs are developing around these principles of positive health maintenance and identification of risk factors. As a result of these trends, health-centered care of the mother, where she is a major member of the prenatal care team, is an increasing pattern. Such team prenatal care is supported by a group of professionals working in a variety of community health care settings and drawing on other community resources as needed. However, too often among disadvantaged women, this ideal care is still not the typical experience, especially with the young and uneducated who lack power with an intimidating bureaucratic establishment.[8]

Private settings. Women with sufficient financial resources may seek out and employ the services of a private medical specialist, an obstetrician-gynecologist, receive care at his or her private office, and be delivered at a private hospital used by the physician. This has been the traditional medical model. However, with rising costs of such care, this model is being diffused to involve more childbirth education for par-

TABLE 8-9   Daily Food Plan for Pregnancy: Protein, Minerals, Vitamins, and Energy

Foods	Daily Amount	Suggested Uses
Protein-rich foods		
Primary protein		
Dairy products	1 qt milk	Beverage, in cooking, or milk-based desserts such
Milk, cheese	2+ oz brick cheese or ½ cup+ cottage cheese	as ice milk, custards, puddings, cream soups; cheese in cooked dishes, salads, or snacks throughout the day
Eggs	2	Breakfast use, chopped or sliced hard eggs, in salads, custards, whole boiled eggs, deviled eggs, plain or in sandwiches
Meat	2 servings (total of 6 oz), liver frequently, 1-2 times per week	Main dish, sandwich, salad, snack
Supplementary protein		
Grains	4 to 5 slices or servings	Bread, plain or toast, sandwiches, with meals,
Enriched or whole grains, breads, cereals, crackers	whole grain or enriched	snacks, cereal (breakfast or snack), cooked grain as meal accompaniment (corn, rice, pasta, grits, hominy, hot breads such as corn bread, biscuits, etc.)
Legumes, seeds, nuts	Occasional servings as	Cooked and served alone or in combination with
Dried beans and peas	meat or grain substitute or in combination with meat or grains	grains, cheese, or meat; soups, salads; nuts as snacks or in salads; peanut butter sandwich
Lentils		
Mineral-rich foods		
Calcium-rich dairy products	1 qt milk (as above)	As above
Grains, whole or enriched	4-5 slices or servings (as above)	As above
Green leafy vegetables	1 serving	Cooked or raw in salads
Iron-rich		
Organ meats, especially liver	1-2 servings per week	
Grains, enriched	4-5 slices or servings	Breakfast cereals, main dish, or in combination with meats, cheese, egg, cooked grain foods, enriched breads
Egg yolk	2	As above
Green, leafy vegetables or dried fruits	1-2 servings	Cooked or stewed, raw in salads, snacks
Iodine-rich		
Iodized salt	Daily in cooking and on foods	On salads, in cooked food dishes, according to taste
Seafood	1-2 servings per week	Main dish, salad, sandwiches

TABLE 8-9 *Daily Food Plan for Pregnancy: Protein, Minerals, Vitamins, and Energy—cont'd*

Foods	Daily Amount	Suggested Uses
Vitamin-rich foods		
Vitamin A		
Animal sources		
Butterfat (whole milk, cream, butter)	2 tbsp butter (or fortified margarine)	In cooking or on foods
Liver	1-2 servings per week	Main dish
Egg yolk	2 (as above)	As above
Plant sources		
Dark green or deep yellow vegetables or fruits	1-2 servings	Cooked dishes, salads, snacks
Fortified margarine	2 tbsp	In cooking and on foods
Vitamin C		
Fruits		
Citrus	1 or 2 servings	Snacks, salads, juices
Other fruits—papayas, strawberries, melons	Occasional serving to substitute for one citrus portion	Salads, snacks
Vegetables		
Broccoli, potatoes, tomato, cabbage, green or chili peppers	1 serving as a substitute for 1 citrus occasionally	Cooked, snacks, salads, juices
Folic acid		
Liver, dark green vegetables, dried beans, lentils, nuts (peanuts, walnuts, filberts)	1 serving	Cooked as main dish or soups, snacks, in salads
Additional energy foods (as needed)		
Carbohydrates		
Grains, breads, legumes, vegetables, fruits	Added portions (as above)	
Fats		
Butter, margarine, oil, mayonnaise, salad dressing, etc.	Moderate additions (as above), in cooking or on foods	

TABLE 8-10 *Daily Food Guide for Women*[1]

Food Group	One Serving Equals	Recommended Minimum Servings		
		Nonpregnant		Pregnant/ Lactating
		11-24 yrs.	25+ yrs.	
Protein foods Provide protein, iron, zinc, and B-vitamins for growth of muscles, bone, blood, and nerves. Vegetable protein provides fiber to prevent constipation.	**Animal protein** 1 oz cooked chicken or turkey; 1 oz cooked lean beef, lamb, or pork; 1 oz or ¼ cup fish or other seafood; 1 egg; 2 fish sticks or hot dogs; 2 slices luncheon meat **Vegetable protein** ½ cup cooked dry beans, lentils, or split peas; 3 oz tofu; 1 oz or ¼ cup peanuts, pumpkin, or sunflower seeds; 1½ oz or ⅓ cup other nuts; 2 tbsp peanut butter	5 A half serving of vegetable protein daily	5	7 One serving of vegetable protein daily
Milk products Provide protein and calcium to build strong bones, teeth, healthy nerves and muscles, and to promote normal blood clotting.	8 oz milk; 8 oz yogurt; 1 cup milk shake; 1½ cups cream soup (made with milk); 1½ oz or ⅓ cup grated cheese (like cheddar, monterey, mozzarella, or Swiss); 1½-2 slices presliced American cheese; 4 tbsp parmesan cheese; 2 cups cottage cheese; 1 cup pudding; 1 cup custard or flan; 1½ cups ice milk, ice cream, or frozen yogurt	3	2	3
Breads, cereals, grains Provide carbohydrates and B-vitamins for energy and healthy nerves. Also provide iron for healthy blood. Whole grains provide fiber to prevent constipation.	1 slice bread; 1 dinner roll; ½ bun or bagel; ½ English muffin or pita; 1 small tortilla; ¾ cup dry cereal; ½ cup granola; ½ cup cooked cereal; ½ cup rice; ½ cup noodles or spaghetti; ¼ cup wheat germ; 1 4-inch pancake or waffle; 1 small muffin; 8 medium crackers; 4 graham cracker squares; 3 cups popcorn	7 Four servings of whole-grain products daily	6	7

Food group	Foods		Servings
Vitamin C–rich fruits and vegetables. Provide vitamin C to prevent infection and to promote healing and iron absorption. Also provide fiber to prevent constipation.	6 oz apricot nectar or vegetable juice cocktail; 3 raw or ¼ cup dried apricots; ¼ cantaloupe or mango; 1 small or ½ cup sliced carrots; 2 tomatoes	½ cup cooked or 1 cup raw spinach; ½ cup cooked greens (beet, chard, collards, dandelion, kale, mustard); ½ cup pumpkin, sweet potato, winter squash, or yams	1 1 1
Other fruits and vegetables. Provide carbohydrates for energy and fiber to prevent constipation.	6 oz fruit juice (if not listed above); 1 medium or ½ cup sliced fruit (apple, banana, peach, pear); ½ cup berries (other than strawberries); ½ cup cherries or grapes; ½ cup pineapple; ½ cup watermelon	¼ dried fruit; ½ cup sliced vegetable (asparagus, beets, green beans, celery, corn, eggplant, mushrooms, onion, peas, potato, summer squash, zucchini); ½ artichoke; 1 cup lettuce	3 3 3
Unsaturated fats. Provide vitamin E to protect tissue.	⅛ medium avocado; 1 tsp margarine; 1 tsp mayonnaise; 1 tsp vegetable oil	2 tsp salad dressing (mayonnaise-based); 1 tbsp salad dressing (oil-based)	3 3 3

Modified from California Department of Health Services, Maternal and Child Health Branch and WIC Supplemental Foods Branch: *Dietary guidelines and daily food guide*. In *Nutrition during pregnancy and postpartum period; a manual for health care professionals*, Sacramento, Calif, June 1990, Department of Health Services.

Single, photo-ready copies of this food guide in English and Spanish are available from Maternal and Child Health Branch, Department of Health Services, 714 "P" Street, Room 760, Sacramento, CA 95814, (916) 327-8176.

NOTE: The Daily Food Guide for Women may not provide all the calories you require. The best way to increase your intake is to include more than the minimum servings recommended.

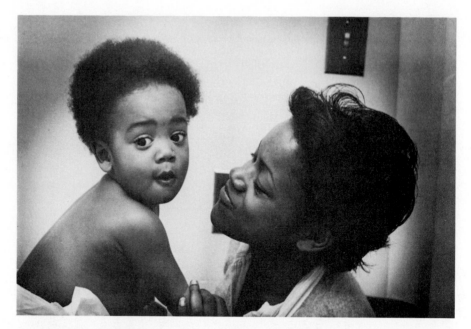

FIG. 8-4   Healthy child and mother—happy participants in the WIC program.
From Williams SR: *Nutrition and diet therapy,* ed 7, St. Louis, 1993, Mosby.

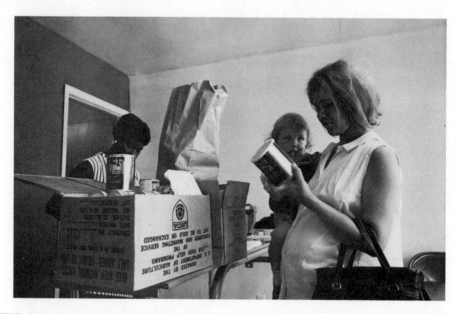

FIG. 8-5   Pregnant mother and her child participating in Supplemental Commodities Distribution Program.
From Williams SR: *Nutrition and diet therapy,* ed 6, St. Louis, Mosby.

✦ ✦ ✦

CASE STUDY

A Personal History of Maria's Pregnancy

You are working as a public health nutritionist in a large city health department. One day when you are on your usual weekly assignment in a busy district prenatal center, the clinic nurse brings in a thin, anxious teenage girl, apparently unwell, to see you for nutritional care. The physician at the clinic has just confirmed her pregnancy and referred her to you, with a note attached to the chart: "This is Maria. She needs our help. After you see her today, we can review her situation at team conference. Thanks."

Using the chapter material presented here, put yourself in the role of this public health nutritionist, and write your history of Maria's pregnancy. How would you start your assessment of Maria's situation? What is her living situation? What problems does she face? How would you follow-up with her on-going care?

What is the course and outcome of her pregnancy?

Write your story of Maria's pregnancy and its outcome as if you were recording her personal history in her clinic chart. Describe your actions, your findings, and Maria's concerns. Outline the assessment procedures you used and the results, giving a picture of her life situation, her problems, and her needs. Describe her food habits from her diet history and the food plan you worked out together. What were the results? Was she able to make the necessary nutritional improvements to support her pregnancy and her own health? What resources or referrals did you use? Complete your history with the condition of her baby at delivery and your conclusions about the role of nutrition in prenatal care.

---

ents, alternative birth centers with a more "homelike" atmosphere, and a family-centered maternity care program.

Community settings and programs. Various health maintenance organizations (HMOs) provide maternity care through community health centers and clinics. Other special government-funded programs, such as the Special Supplemental Food Program for Women, Infants, and Children (WIC), reach underserved or economically depressed areas to provide additional outreach services. These programs have proved to be effective in supporting a healthy pregnancy course and outcome for many high-risk mothers and infants, as shown in Fig. 8-4. Another source of nutrition support for low-income pregnant women and their families is the supplemental Commodities Distribution Program, administered by the United States Department of Agriculture (Fig. 8-5). These surplus foods include agricultural products such as meat and poultry, fruits and vegetables, eggs, dried beans and peas, dairy products, fats and oils, peanuts, wheat, rice, and other grains. Other programs stem from var-

ious community action groups. Innovative health projects and food advocacy programs have resulted, often reaching out to meet needs beyond the mainstream of medical care.

Community resources. In any setting of prenatal care a number of possible community resources for nutritional needs may exist. These should be explored, constantly updated, and used for consultation, referral, and sources of materials or services. Some of these resources include public health nutritionists in public health departments, nutritionists with the Agricultural Extension Service at state universities, registered dietitians on the staff of local community hospitals and clinics, nutritionists with advanced training and skill working in practice in the community, and nutritionists associated with community professional groups or volunteer health organizations. In the area of prenatal care, as well as infant and early childhood care, these nutritionists and dietitians, working together with physicians, nurses, and social workers, provide sound professional support for parents. Such persons bring particular skills and personal strengths to help ensure healthy pregnancies in family-centered maternity care programs.

Summary

A positive course and outcome of pregnancy is built on positive nutritional support throughout prenatal care. This sound approach is based on scientific knowledge and demonstrated nutritional needs of both mother and child. It is best provided by a skilled and sensitive nutritionist and health care team, working closely with the mother.

To assure that these increased nutritional needs are met, the process of nutrition assessment, initial and ongoing, is fundamental in all prenatal care. This general process includes clinical observations, body measures with attention to a good quality weight gain, biochemical tests for monitoring nutritional status, and obtaining significant social, medical, and family histories as background for nutrition education and guidance. A personal food plan incorporates both physiologic requirements and personal needs and uses community resources as indicated.

REVIEW QUESTIONS

1. After studying this chapter, what is your own definition of a "healthy pregnancy?" If you were developing a maternity care program to achieve a healthy pregnancy for each mother, describe what your primary goal would be and some ways in which you might reach that goal.
2. Describe some general changes occurring in prenatal health care and account for them in terms of human needs.
3. What is the function of nutrition assessment in prenatal care? Describe methods used to achieve this assessment.
4. Identify phases of the health care process and relate nutrition assessment activities to each phase.
5. Select and describe a particular pregnant woman, in terms of all the data you would need to collect about her and her needs. Outline the nutrition education and counseling approach you would use to help meet her needs, indicating any materials, resources, consultations, or referrals you might use in your planned follow-up.

LEARNING ACTIVITIES

1. Develop a reasonable daily menu for a pregnant vegetarian woman.
2. Evaluate the materials related to diet during pregnancy that are distributed to local health facilities.
3. Produce a list of dietary recommendations for a pregnant woman who chooses to use no dairy products.

REFERENCES

1. Armstrong BG et al: Cigarette, alcohol, and coffee consumption and spontaneous abortion, *Am J Pub Health* 82(1):85, 1992.
2. Centers for Disease Control and Prevention: Trends in fetal alcohol syndrome—United States, *MMWR* 44(13):249, 1995.
3. Cunningham J et al: Maternal smoking during pregnancy as a predictor of lung function in children, *Am J Epidemiology* 139(12):1139, 1994.
4. Danford DE, Stephenson MG: *Healthy People 2000:* development of nutrition objectives, *J Am Diet Assoc* 91(12):1517, 1991.
5. Erick M: No more morning sickness: A survival guide for pregnant women, New York City, 1993, Penguin/Plume Books.
6. Erick M, Hahn NI: Battling morning (and noon and night) sickness, *J Amer Diet Assoc* 94(2):147, 1994.
7. Eskenazi B et al: Passive and active maternal smoking as measured by serum cotinine: the effect on birthweight, *Am J Public Health* 85(3): 395, 1995.
8. Hansell MJ: Sociodemographic factors and the quality of prenatal care, *Am J Pub Health* 81(8): 1023, 1991.
9. Harsham J et al: Growth patterns of infants exposed to cocaine and other drugs in utero, *J Am Diet Assoc* 94(9):999, 1994.
10. Horner RD et al: Pica practices of pregnant women, *J Am Diet Assoc* 91(3):34, 1991.
11. Infante-Rivard C et al: Infante-Rivard C et al: Fetal loss associated with caffeine intake before and during pregnancy, *JAMA* 270 (24):2940, 1993.
12. Joyce T: The dramatic increase in the rate of low birthweight in New York City: An aggregate time-series analysis, *Am J Pub Health* 80(6):682, 1990.

13. Lewis CJ et al: *Healthy People 2000:* report on the 1994 Nutrition Progress Review, *Nutr Today* 29(6):6, 1994.

14. Lewis DD, Woods SE: Fetal alcohol syndrome, *Am Family Physician* 50:1025, 1994.

15. Marbury MC: Adverse working condition and premature delivery, *Am J Public Health* 81(2):973, 1991.

16. Miller RC et al: Acute maternal and fetal cardiovascular effects of caffeine ingestion, *Am J Perinatology* 11(2):132, 1994.

17. National Research Council, Food and Nutrition Board, Committee on Nutrition status during pregnancy and lactation, Institute of Medicine, National Academy of Sciences: *Nutrition during pregnancy,* Washington DC.

18. Neus L et al: Concentration of indoor particulate matter as a determinant of respiratory health in children, *Am J Epidemiol* 139, 139(11):1088, 1994.

19. Newman V, Lee D: Developing a daily food guide for women, *J Nutr Educ* 23(2):76, 1991.

20. Orphanidou C et al: Accuracy of subcutaneous fat measurement: comparison of skinfold calipers, ultrasound, and computed tomography, *J Am Diet Assoc* 94(8):855, 1994.

21. Peoples-Sheps MD et al: Characteristics of maternal employment during pregnancy: effects on low birthweight, *Am J Public Health* 81(8):1007, 1991.

22. Sanders SL, Greenspoon JS: New protocol to manage hyperemesis gravidarum (letter), *J Amer Diet Assoc* 94(12):1367, 1994.

23. Sharbaugh CO, ed: *Call to action: better nutrition for mothers, children, and families,* Washington DC, 1991, National Center for Education in Maternal and Child Health.

24. Steinmetz G: Fetal alcohol syndrome, the preventable tragedy, *Nat Geograph* 181(2):37, 1992.

25. Stevens-Simon C et al: Relationship of self-reported prepregnant weight gain during pregnancy to maternal body habitus and age, *J Am Diet Assoc* 92(1):85, 1992.

26. Streissguth AP: A long-term perspective of FAS, *Alcohol Health Res World* 18:74, 1994.

27. US Department of Health and Human Services, Public Healic Service: *Healthy People 2000: national health promotion and disease prevention objectives* (PHS Pub No 79-55071), Washington DC, 1990, Government Printing Office.

28. US Department of Health and Human Services, Public Health Service, Substance Abuse and Mental Health Services Administration: *Preliminary estimates from the 1993 National Household Survey on Drug Abuse,* Rockville, MD, 1994, Government Printing Office.

29. Wang X et al: A longitudinal study of the effects of parental smoking on pulmonary function in children 6-18 years, *Am J Respiration, and Crit Care Med,* 149(6):1420, 1994.

30. Williams SR: *Nutrition and diet therapy,* ed 8, St Louis, 1996, Mosby.

31. Yankauer A: What infant mortality tells us, *Am J Pub Health* 80(6):653, 1990.

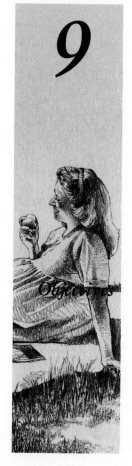

9

Management of Pregnancy Complications and Special Maternal Disease Conditions

Sue Rodwell Williams
Cristine M. Trahms

Objectives

+++

After completion of this chapter, the student will be able to:

✓ *Identify risk factors that complicate pregnancy and determine appropriate intervention therapy.*

✓ *Prevent problems during pregnancy from preexisting maternal conditions through collaborative health team care for each mother.*

✓ *Provide personalized care for each mother, especially high-risk ones, to reduce risks and achieve a healthy pregnancy course and outcome.*

Introduction

In Chapter 8, ways of helping pregnant women have healthy pregnancies through comprehensive assessment of personal and nutritional needs were considered. In this important assessment process, various risk factors for health problems during pregnancy can be identified and personal care plans formulated to promote healthy pregnancies.

In this chapter specific conditions that contribute to high-risk pregnancies will be considered. On the basis of time of onset, two types of conditions complicate pregnancy: conditions that are induced by the pregnancy itself and pre-

existing disease conditions of the mother. Methods of screening and managing these health problems are discussed, focusing on the nutritional aspects of care.

MANAGEMENT OF HIGH-RISK PREGNANCIES
Current Focus in General Health Care

For the past few years, general health care in America has begun to move from the traditional medical model of disease intervention with a curative approach to a more comprehensive personal model of health promotion with a preventive approach. Americans in general and their health care officials in particular have increasing concerns about chronic disease, which often has its roots in family history and changing lifestyles. These concerns are evident in reports from national health agencies, such as the U.S. Surgeon General's health objectives for the nation, the Public Health Service of the U.S. Department of Health and Human Services publication *Healthy People 2000,* setting defined goals; the Maternal and Child Health Bureau's call for strategic actions to achieve better nutrition for mothers, children, and families; and the American Public Health Association's report *Healthy Communities 2000.*[4,6,69,70] Many of these national goals to reduce health risks have integral nutritional components, involving care by a professional team, and a number of them specifically target improvements in maternal and infant care.

These changes in general health care practices emphasize risk reduction for underlying disease through personal health maintenance and fitness. They have had two major effects on maternity care: (1) a more active role of the mother in her own care and (2) a more coordinated team of professionals working closely with the mother to provide this care. This is especially true in the management of high-risk pregnancies. Risk factors that may complicate pregnancy are summarized in Table 9-1, grouped according to personal characteristics that cannot be changed, lifestyle behaviors that can be changed, and background obstetrical and medical conditions that can be screened and either prevented or controlled. Basically, pregnancy problems stem from two types of conditions: (1) complications induced by the pregnancy itself and (2) preexisting chronic disease in the mother.

Problems such as anemia, hyperemesis gravidarum, or pregnancy-induced hypertension (PIH) are directly related to the pregnancy itself. In some cases, the normal physiologic stress of the pregnancy imposes demands on a relatively poor maternal nutritional status or on reserves that are inadequate to meet the new needs. Preexisting disease in the mother, such as insulin-dependent diabetes mellitus (IDDM), phenylketonuria (PKU), or chronic hypertension, brings risk to the pregnancy. The mother's background condition places special additional metabolic and physiologic demands on her body.

TABLE 9-1 *High-Risk Pregnancies: Risk Factors in Pregnancy-Induced Complications and Preexisting Chronic Conditions in the Mother*

Personal Characteristics (Cannot Change)	Personal Habits, Living Situation (Seek to Change)	Chronic Preexisting Maternal Medical Problems (Screen, Treat)	Obstetric History (Screen, Prevent)	Current/Potential Pregnancy-Induced Problems (Screen, Prevent, Treat)
Gender	Smoking	Hypertension	Low birth weight	Anemia
Age	Alcohol/drug use	Insulin-dependent diabetes mellitus	Macrosomia	Iron deficiency
Adolescent	Poor diet	Non-insulin-dependent diabetes mellitus	Stillbirth	Folic acid deficiency
Older woman	Malnutrition	Heart disease	Abortion	Pregnancy-induced hypertension
Family history	Obesity	Pulmonary disease	Fetal anomalies	Gestational diabetes
Diabetes	Underweight	Renal disease	High parity	
Heart disease	Sedentary lifestyle	Maternal phenylketonuria	Multipara	
Hypertension				
Phenylketonuria				

Other preexisting maternal conditions have developed more over the past decade from social problems such as drug addiction and the epidemic of **acquired immunodeficiency syndrome (AIDS).** Other problems may arise with extremes of eating disorders, from chronic obesity to the life-threatening starvation of anorexia nervosa or pain of bulimia. In all of these cases, sensitive team care by specialists is required. With some mothers an alternate mode of enteral or parenteral feeding may be indicated.

TYPES OF ANEMIAS IN PREGNANCY

Anemia is by far the most common complication of pregnancy. The term *anemia* refers to a lack of sufficient red blood cells and thus a significant reduction in hemoglobin, the carrier of vital oxygen to the body cells for cell metabolism. During pregnancy, the woman's metabolic rate increases about 15% and her need for oxygen increases accordingly. Anemia is often compounded by lowered socioeconomic status. However, its incidence is not confined to poorer living situations with more apparent malnutrition. Clinical experience indicates that neither the absence of poverty nor regular use of prescribed nutrient supplements guarantees optimum dietary intakes during pregnancy. The majority of anemia cases in any population are nutritional in origin, with iron deficiency being the main cause. A related cause is acute blood loss from hemorrhage. A less common nutritional anemia is caused by a deficiency of folate. The causes of anemias of pregnancy in the United States, as reported by the National Research Council in order of incidence, are given in Table 9-2.

Iron Deficiency Anemia

A characteristic **microcytic hypochromic anemia** is produced by a deficiency of iron, the major mineral element required for the synthesis of hemoglobin. Because of the widespread incidence of iron deficiency among adolescents and young women during their reproductive years of menstruation, they become highly vulnerable to iron deficiency anemia when pregnancy places a greater physiologic demand on their already

TABLE 9-2 *Acquired and Hereditary Causes of Anemias in Pregnancy in the United States in Order of Incidence*

Acquired	Hereditary
Iron deficiency anemia	Thalassemia
Hemorrhagic anemia	Sickle cell anemia
Folate deficiency anemia (megaloblastic)	Sickle cell disease
Anemia caused by infection	Other hemoglobinopathies
Acquired hemolytic anemia	Hereditary hemolytic anemia without hemoglobinopathy
Aplastic or hypoplastic anemia	

Based on data from the National Research Council.

tenuous iron balance. As indicated in Table 9-3, the iron cost of a pregnancy is high, and negative balances can easily occur. Iron deficiency anemia accounts for about 75% or more of the nonphysiologic anemias in pregnancy.

The typical pregnant woman may not have adequate iron stores or dietary iron intake sufficient to meet the increased need for iron during the second half of the pregnancy. This increased amount is needed not only for hemoglobin synthesis but also for fetal liver storage to meet iron needs of the infant during the first 6 months of life. In addition, up to 2 years of normal diet are required to replace the iron lost during pregnancy and delivery. Hence if there is a shorter time interval between pregnancies, an even greater drain is placed on the mother's depleted iron stores. To counteract this tendency toward iron deficiency anemia in pregnancy, the current recommended dietary allowance (RDA) of the National Research Council for iron intake during pregnancy is 30 mg/day, double the amount needed by nonpregnant women. In addition to dietary intake, a routine iron supplement is prescribed in most prenatal clinics. Commonly used iron compounds are ferrous sulfate or ferrous fumarate, both of which contain about 33% elemental iron. However, there are problems with routine iron supplements for

TABLE 9-3   *Maternal and Fetal Iron Balances*

Input		Output	
Stores		**Increased requirement**	
Normal adult female iron stores (total)	2 gm	Maternal red blood cell mass	450 mg
		Fetus (single), placenta, cord	360 mg
Red blood cells (60%-70%)	1.2-1.4 gm	TOTAL	810 mg
Liver, spleen, and bone marrow (10%-30%)	0.3 gm	Lactation (daily)	0.5-1.0 mg
Other cell compounds (remainder)		**Losses**	
		Gastrointestinal, renal, sweat (280 days)	0.5-1.0 mg/day
Diet			
Average absorption (280 days)	1.3-2.6 mg/day*	Birth† (including placenta and lochia)	200-250 mg
Supplementation			
Daily iron supplement	30-60 mg		
12%-25% absorption: ferrous sulfate, ferrous fumarate, 33% iron; ferrous gluconate, 11% iron			

*Some investigators estimate that a pregnant woman requires more than 4 mg of iron per day, an amount that exceeds that absorbed from a normal diet, even if the woman is iron deficient.
†Cesarean section or birth of twins results in an additional loss of approximately 140 mg of iron.

all pregnant women, such as unpleasant gastrointestinal side effects and less motivation to maintain a good diet, or imbalances with other trace elements such as zinc. Also, excess iron intake when not needed may potentially mask inadequate pregnancy-induced hemodilution, a normal pregnancy adaptation that puts less strain on the maternal heart; may minimize hemoglobin loss with blood loss at delivery; and may increase nutrient flow to the fetus. Some prenatal clinics follow revised protocols that prescribe prenatal vitamins with iron at the first clinic visit with additional iron supplementation only if hemoglobin falls to 10.5 gm/100 ml or less at any time during the pregnancy.

The diagnosis of iron deficiency anemia is made on the basis of a hemoglobin concentration value of 10 gm/100 ml of blood or less, a hematocrit value of 30% or less, and the appearance of characteristic red blood cells on a stained erythrocyte smear. The cells are smaller than usual (microcytic), with a fading red color (hypochromic). As the anemia develops, the first changes that occur are the depletion of iron stores in the liver, spleen, and bone marrow, followed by a decrease in serum iron and an increase in serum total iron-binding capacity (TIBC). Finally, the anemic state develops as hematocrit levels drop below normal, and the change in red blood cell maturation follows. Usually the microcytosis precedes the hypochromia. A serum iron level below 50 to 60 µg/100 ml and less than 15% to 16% saturation of transferrin usually indicate iron deficiency anemia, if other causes of decreased serum iron have been ruled out.

Treatment of iron deficiency anemia centers on the correction of the low hemoglobin concentration with iron, usually a therapeutic dose up to 200 mg/day, depending on the severity of the anemia. Moreover, it can be prevented by appropriate iron supplementation and emphasis on food sources of iron in the daily diet. Simple teaching tools, such as an iron checklist to guide food choices, help increase dietary intake through greater awareness of iron food values and comparative bioavailability. A prenatal diet such as that outlined in Chapter 8 will help to prevent such a nutritional anemia.

Folate Deficiency Anemia

A deficiency of the B vitamin folate during pregnancy produces a characteristic **megaloblastic anemia.** This condition can exist as a single deficiency state but is more commonly found in association with iron deficiency. Folates have widespread physiologic functions, participating as they do in biosynthesis of methionine, purine, and thymine. They not only assist in hemoglobin synthesis, but also are necessary for synthesis of DNA. Thus a deficiency has far-reaching consequences for fetal development.

The nonpregnant adult woman requires about 50 to 100 µg/day of folate. To ensure the absorption of this quantity, the RDA standard for women is 180 µg/day. In pregnancy the RDA rises to 400 µg/day. This increased demand for folate in pregnancy results from increased maternal and fetal tissue synthesis needs. In folate deficiency anemia the characteristic red

blood cell is larger than normal and immature, a hematologic condition called **megaloblastosis.**

Food sources of folate, such as leafy vegetables, liver, nuts, cheese, eggs, and milk, should be emphasized in the diet. A food plan such as that described in Chapter 8 provides helpful guidelines. Such a diet emphasis along with supplementation as needed will help prevent the incidence of serum folate depletion found among pregnant women in the United States.

Table 9-4 presents a summary of guidelines for laboratory evaluation of anemia in pregnancy.

HYPEREMESIS GRAVIDARUM
Incidence and Etiologic Factors

In the early months of pregnancy, many women experience mild nausea and vomiting, especially in the morning, thus giving this condition the common name "morning sickness."[16,17,41] At least 50% of all pregnant women, most of them primiparas, have this sign of pregnancy, beginning during the fifth or sixth week of pregnancy and usually lasting only until the fifteenth or sixteenth week. However, usually in early pregnancy, in a small number of women (approximately 3.5 pregnant women per 1,000 pregnant women), the more serious condition of **hyperemesis gravidarum** develops.[15] This condition is associated with alterations in

---

TABLE 9-4   Guidelines for Laboratory Evaluation of Anemia in Pregnancy

	Hemoglobin (gm/100 ml)	Hematocrit (Packed Cell Volume %)	Serum Iron (µg/ 100 ml)	Transferrin Saturation (%)	Serum Folacin (ng/ml)*	Serum B_{12} (pg/ml)†
Pregnant woman						
Deficient	<9.5	<30	<40	<15	<2.0	<100
Marginal	9.5-10.9	30-32	40	15	2.1-5.9	100
Acceptable	>11.0	>33	>40	>15	>6.0	>100
Nonpregnant woman						
Normal values	>12.0	36-50	>50	>15	6.0-25.0	>100

*Nanograms per milliliter.
†Picograms per milliliter.
Modified from U.S. Department of Health, Education, and Welfare: *Ten state nutrition survey, 1968-1970,* DHEW Pub No (HSM) 72-8130, Atlanta, 1972, Centers for Disease Control.

fluid and electrolyte balance, weight loss, nutritional deficits, and dehydration. The severe and prolonged vomiting may continue throughout the pregnancy and become life-threatening if not controlled. If the condition continues unchecked, clinical effects of dehydration, acidosis, weight loss, avitaminosis, and jaundice increase. The severe vomiting causes hemoconcentration, a decrease in serum protein and buffering alkali reserves, and elevation of serum sodium and chloride, serum potassium, and blood urea nitrogen. Ketones appear in the concentrated urine, and there is proteinuria. Enteral feeding of appropriate formula by nasogastric (NG) tube may be offered if oral intake problems persist, but to prevent dangerous dehydration and malnutrition in intractable cases, total parenteral nutrition (TPN) may be necessary.[64] (See section on TPN during pregnancy, p. 284.)

The precise cause of vomiting during pregnancy is unknown, but various pregnancy-associated physiologic mechanisms, as well as psychogenic factors, have been suggested. *Hyperolfaction*, acute sensitivity to various odors, not merely foods but the total environment, appears to be a strong factor.[15] Since the condition occurs to its greatest extent during the same time human chorionic gonadotropin (HCG) is secreted in large quantities by the placenta, there has been speculation that this placental hormone is somehow responsible. Despite this association of timing, however, a direct causal relationship has never been proved.

Another physiologic event occurring early in pregnancy is the rapid invasion of the trophoblast into the endometrium lining the uterus. Because the cells of the trophoblast digest portions of the endometrium as they invade, it has been suggested that degenerative products resulting from this invasion are responsible for the nausea and vomiting. This may be possible since similar results do occur in other parts of the body from degenerative tissue effects of such clinical events as radiation therapy and burns. Another possible theory is that such vomiting during pregnancy is related to the large quantities of *estrogen* secreted by the placenta. This theory is supported by the fact that large doses of estrogen injected daily over many weeks in persons with other clinical conditions often cause the same nausea and vomiting response.

In addition, there may be emotional disturbances associated with acceptance or denial of the pregnancy, or a distorted body image, particularly if there is a history of bulimia or anorexia nervosa. Such psychogenic factors may enhance the physiologic nausea and vomiting.

Nutritional Management

Hospitalization is usually required for women in whom hyperemesis gravidarum develops. Initial intravenous (IV) fluid and electrolyte replacement is essential to correct dehydration, followed by more extensive enteral or parenteral feeding if the woman still cannot retain food. As soon as possible, when the mother can eat regularly, she may tolerate a fairly dry diet in small feedings during the day, with liquids between these snacks. Actually, food tolerances and desires are highly individual, so best results come from a close association with the mother as the nutrition counselor probes, observes, and tests reactions to a variety of foods.[15-17] Usually fats are avoided at first, as well as foods with strong odors, spiced dishes, or any items that do not appeal to the mother. Continued personal support and reassurance are important.

HYPERTENSIVE DISORDERS

Hypertension in pregnancy may be defined basically according to its relation to the pregnancy: (1) PIH caused by the pregnancy itself, or (2) preexisting chronic hypertension in the mother before the pregnancy, adding a risk factor to her current pregnancy. A late transient hypertension may occur briefly during labor or early postpartum, but returns to normal in a few days. The basic characteristics of these hypertensive disorders of pregnancy are summarized in Table 9-5 for comparison. Because PIH presents a serious complication to a woman's pregnancy, and because it has significant nutritional relationships, this condition is the focus of our discussion here.

Incidence and Etiologic Factors of Pregnancy-Induced Hypertension

Approximately 4% to 5% of all pregnant women in North America experience a rapid rise in arterial blood pressure during the latter few

TABLE 9-5   *Hypertensive Disorders of Pregnancy*

Disorder	Characteristics
Pregnancy-induced hypertension	
Preeclampsia	Hypertension with proteinuria and/or edema developing after the twentieth week of pregnancy: almost exclusive incidence in primigravidas and affects women at reproductive age extremes (under 20 or over 35)
	Hypertension: 140/90 or increase of 30 mm Hg systolic or 15 mm Hg diastolic above woman's usual base line; at least two observations 6 or more hours apart
	Proteinuria: 500 mg or more in 24-hour urine collection or random 2+ protein; develops late in course of PIH
	Edema: significant; usually in face and hands
Severe preeclampsia	One or more of following symptoms: systolic pressure 160 mm Hg or diastolic 110 mm Hg on two observations 6 or more hours apart at bed rest; proteinuria at least 5 gm/24 hours or random 3 to 4+; blurred vision, headache, altered consciousness; pulmonary edema
	Advancing disease: epigastric or upper quadrant pain, impaired liver function, thrombocytopenia
Eclampsia	Extension of preeclampsia with grand mal seizure, occurring near time of labor
Chronic hypertension	Blood pressure 140/90 mm Hg before pregnancy
	Blood pressure 140/90 mm Hg before twentieth week of pregnancy or persisting indefinitely after delivery
	Plasma urea nitrogen 20 mg/100 ml; plasma creatinine 1 mg/100 ml
Chronic hypertension with preeclampsia	Often a quick progression to eclampsia, developing before the thirtieth week of pregnancy
	Documented record of chronic hypertension
	Evidence of a superimposed process: elevation of systolic pressure 30 mm Hg or of diastolic pressure 15 to 20 mm Hg above base line on two observations at least 6 hours apart; development of proteinuria; edema as observed in preeclampsia
Late transient hypertension	Transient blood pressure elevations observed during labor or early postpartum, returning to normal within 10 days postpartum

Modified from Willis SE: Hypertension in pregnancy: pathophysiology, *Am J Nurs* 82:792, 1982; in Gant NF and Worley RJ: *Hypertension in pregnancy: concepts and management*, New York, 1980, Appleton-Century-Crofts.

months of pregnancy, associated with loss of large amounts of protein in the urine, and accompanied by generalized edema and rapid weight gain.[25] Arterial spasm occurs in vital body organs, most significantly in the liver, kidneys, and brain. The precise underlying pathogenesis of this syndrome remains unclear, but several theories have been put forth as detailed below.

Excessive weight gain or prior obesity. Although this has been a popular theory in the past, current studies provide no supporting evidence.[58] To the contrary, most women who develop PIH have total weight gains that are below average, thus low early gains may be a marker, or even a determinant, of subsequent gestational hypertensive disorders.

Hormonal basis. Despite past attempts to prove that excessive secretion of placental or adrenal hormones cause PIH, proof is still lacking.[25]

Autoimmunity. Because the acute symptoms disappear with the birth of the infant and release of the placenta, it has been speculated that some autoimmune process related to the presence of the fetus, and perhaps the placenta, underlies the thickening of glomerular basement membranes that causes the renal effects.[25] Both the renal blood flow and the glomerular filtration rate are decreased, which is exactly opposite to the changes that occur normally in the pregnant woman.

Genetic basis. Speculation has also centered on the possibility that a genetic mechanism is involved, but as yet, no definitive proof exists.

Whatever may develop with further research, it is evident from studies of the incidence of PIH in the United States, together with associated concerns about infant mortality rates, that lack of prenatal care and poor nutritional status contribute in large measure to pregnancy-induced complications.[76] In summary, the following conditions are associated with the incidence of PIH:

1. *Inadequate diet, nutritional deficiencies.* Poor nutritional status with varying degrees of malnutrition, including deficits in energy, protein, vitamins and minerals, contributes to pregnancy risks such as PIH and poor nutritional outcome.
2. *Primigravidity and age.* About 65% of the cases of PIH occur with first pregnancies, especially if the first-time mother is under age 17 or over age 35.
3. *Multiple pregnancies.* Progressive incidence occurs with number of fetuses involved (twins, triplets).
4. *Vascular disease.* Incidence is more common in women with preexisting vascular disease such as essential hypertension, hypertensive renal disease, and insulin-dependent diabetes mellitus (IDDM), all

of which carry a genetic factor in their development.
5. *Familial predisposition.* The family history may reveal relatives who have had PIH.

Clinical Nature of Pregnancy-Induced Hypertension

Sometimes when a clinical condition is not clearly understood, many confusing clinical names are given to it. This is the case with PIH. Historically, the term **toxemia** was used, but it is a misnomer here because its actual meaning—*blood toxins*—does not apply. The term **eclampsia,** which means a "sudden development," has been retained because its meaning does apply to sudden development of PIH in the latter part of pregnancy with varying degrees of severity. The terms *preeclampsia* and *eclampsia* are used to refer to the nature and degree of the symptoms involved in PIH. The current term *pregnancy-induced hypertension* more accurately describes this hypertensive disorder unique to pregnancy and "cured" only by the termination of the pregnancy. PIH may be better understood by a review of its cardinal symptoms: **hypertension, proteinuria,** and **edema,** usually occurring after week 20 of gestation.

Hypertension. Usually PIH is defined as a systolic blood pressure of 140 mm Hg or a diastolic pressure of 90 mm Hg, or both. These blood pressure levels must be observed on two or more occasions at least 6 hours or more apart. However, there are problems with this diagnostic level. Many younger women and adolescents have normal blood pressures at lower levels of about 120/80 mm Hg, and the usual minimum diagnostic values of 140/90 mm Hg may thus miss hypertensive conditions in younger mothers displaying these lower values. For example, young teenagers have blood pressures of about 90/60 mm Hg, and it is in this group of young primiparas that the risk factor is greatest. Thus a more significant level for determining hypertension would be based on *individual blood pressure:* a rise of 20 to 30 mm Hg in systolic pressure and/or of 10 to 15 mm Hg in diastolic pressure observed on two or more occasions at least 6 hours apart. Further confusion lies in the common problem of distinguishing between preexisting chronic hypertension in the mother, complicated now by her pregnancy, and true PIH. In any event, the use of blood pressure values of 140/90 mm Hg as the upper limits of normal appears to have little real meaning in pregnancy. Blood pressures above 125/75 mm Hg before 32 weeks' gestation are usually associated with significant increases in fetal risk, as are pressures above 125/85 mm Hg at term.

Proteinuria. Although the degree of proteinuria varies with the degree of PIH involved, it rarely exceeds 5 gm/day. Often it is fluctuating or transient and may be minimal even in severe cases. These observations of proteinuria must be made on clean voided specimens, two or more taken at least 6 hours apart.

Edema. The normal physiologic edema of pregnancy, manifested mainly in the extremities, is not to be confused with the pathologic generalized edema associated with PIH. Thus the accumulation of fluid in the legs alone is not significant in the diagnosis of the preeclampsia stage of PIH. In the majority of pregnant women, some degree of edema develops in the third trimester. In the preeclampsia stage additional common complaints include dizziness, headache, visual disturbances, upper abdominal pain, facial edema, anorexia, nausea, and vomiting. Sometimes further probing may disclose a history of poor food intake as a result of gastrointestinal problems, superimposed on an underlying chronic state of poor nutrition, often related to socioeconomic, personal, and psychologic problems. The more severe stage of eclampsia is distinguished by characteristic convulsions.

Incidence of Pregnancy-Induced Hypertension

As indicated, the incidence of PIH in the United States and related concerns about infant mortality rates generally indicate a close association with low income, poverty, and a relative lack of prenatal care. The United States' poor ratings in pregnancy outcomes among the industrialized nations of the world reflect these problems, and the mortality rate for nonwhite infants, especially blacks, remains nearly twice as high as that for whites.[76] Historically, mortality rates from acute PIH have striking relationships

to economic factors, and this association persists. This correlation supports a long-held view that living standards, hence quality of prenatal care and nutritional status, are significant factors in the incidence of PIH. The greater incidence in nonwhite minority groups, especially blacks, is not related to race, per se, but to deeply rooted social issues, including medical care and nutrition, associated with the home and community and political environment. Official awareness and concern is evident in revisions of the U.S. certificates of fetal deaths and livebirths, in which specific checkboxes for pregnancy risk factors have replaced an open-ended medical statement. The checklist of risk items includes PIH and eclampsia, chronic hypertension, anemia, diabetes mellitus, cardiac disease, acute and chronic lung disease, renal disease, obstetrical history, and personal habits of tobacco, alcohol, and other drug use.

Nutritional Factors in Pregnancy-Induced Hypertension

As discussed here and in previous chapters, pregnancy presents the human maternal organism with a profound physiologic and metabolic challenge. It is not surprising that the integrity of all body tissues, especially highly metabolic organs such as the liver, depend on optimum nutritional intake of varied nutrient materials and their myriad metabolites. Nutritional factors in PIH include directly or indirectly all the nutrients and their metabolites, with particular emphasis on certain members of each group.

Protein. Since protein provides the basic structural units for all human tissue—the amino acids, it holds a primary position in human metabolism in close interrelationships with other nutrients. Such is true of the fundamental growth process that characterizes pregnancy. Especially, however, in relation to PIH, three functional roles of protein are important.

Fluid and electrolyte balance. The major homeostatic mechanism maintaining the vascular volume and tissue fluid circulation is the **capillary fluid-shift mechanism.** This mechanism operates on a balance between two major fluid pressures: (1) the hydrostatic pressure of regular heart and blood vessel contractions (blood pressure), and (2) the colloidal osmotic pressure of circulating plasma protein, mainly albumin. This normal tissue fluid circulation nourishes cells, maintains blood volume, and prevents edema. Any situation in which serum albumin decreases alters this balance of fluid pressures and fosters edema. Thus albumin is the major plasma protein responsible for maintaining serum osmotic balance and in turn overall tissue fluid balance. Each gram of albumin per 100 ml serum exerts an osmotic pressure of 5.54 mm Hg, whereas the same quantity of serum globulin, for example, exerts a pressure of only 1.43 mm Hg. One gram of albumin will hold 18 ml of fluid in the blood. Albumin infusions of 25 gm in 100 ml of fluid base are equivalent in osmotic effect to 500 ml of citrated blood plasma.[54] Such albumin infusion would benefit any clinical situation, such as PIH, where the objective is to remove excess fluid from the tissues, returning it to the blood circulation and increasing the blood volume.

The liver is the sole source of albumin synthesis, using amino acids derived largely from dietary protein. The most effective food proteins that supply materials for regeneration of plasma proteins are lactalbumin (a milk protein), egg white, beef muscle, liver, and casein (the major milk protein). Thus the two factors necessary for the synthesis of plasma albumin for normal circulation of tissue fluids through the body and prevention of edema are a constant optimum dietary source of adequate protein to supply the essential amino acids and a healthy liver to do the metabolic work.

Lipid transport. Protein functions also as the major means of transporting lipids in a water medium—the blood stream. These transport vehicles, the lipoproteins, are formed mainly in the absorbing intestinal wall and in the liver. To the degree that there is inadequate dietary protein supply or diseased liver tissue, this metabolic work of packaging fat with water-soluble protein coverings for transport as lipoproteins cannot take place and fats accumulate abnormally in the liver. Fatty infiltration of liver tissue is a pathologic state that can ultimately prevent normal cell functions in this vital metabolic tissue.

Tissue synthesis. Protein, through its constituent amino acids, is the basic necessity for

building and maintaining all tissue protein. Especially here in these metabolic relationships described, a healthy functioning liver, as well as other vital organs, depends on optimum protein supply and utilization.

All of these basic protein functions relate to overall body metabolism, especially to metabolic functions of the liver, and in turn to PIH. Characteristic clinical findings in PIH, preeclampsia and eclampsia, are **hypoalbuminemia** and **hypovolemia,** with subsequent **hemoconcentration** often masking anemia and lowered total serum albumin. Blood volume in some cases may be reduced 35% to 50%, and serum albumin may be as low as 2 gm/100 ml (it should be 3.5 gm/100 ml to be acceptable).

Energy. Always associated with protein functions in tissue synthesis is a sufficient supply of nonprotein kcalories to ensure the crucial increased energy needs of pregnancy and prevent protein breakdown to supply energy. This is especially true in pregnancy. The former practices of restricting dietary energy (kcalories) to control weight to reduce risk of PIH complications are unwarranted, unscientific, and dangerous. On the contrary, there is a greater incidence of PIH among underweight women who fail to gain weight normally during pregnancy.[58] The overwhelming evidence indicates that an optimum individual range of weight gain to support the pregnancy is vital, and that the nutritional quality of the weight gain determined by the positive nutritional value of the diet as well as the regular pattern of that gain throughout pregnancy are significant contributing factors.

Minerals. The full spectrum of major minerals and trace elements is required to support the enhanced metabolic and structural functions during pregnancy, as discussed in previous chapters. This need includes the long-demonstrated essential role of sodium (Na+) in fluid balance, and the more recently studied possible role of calcium (Ca++) in reducing the incidence of PIH.

Sodium. In its ionized form (Na+), sodium is a major mineral specifically required for control of the body's extracellular fluid compartment. In prior obstetrical practices, especially in PIH, sodium was erroneously restricted by low sodium diets to 500 to 1,000 mg sodium/day.

Current practice usually follows a regular diet with moderate sodium intake to taste, about 2 to 3 gm/day. Measures of ad libitum sodium intake by pregnant women during their second and third trimesters have found their daily sodium intake in the two trimesters to be about those moderate amounts. When the total extracellular fluid is increased as it is in pregnancy, the total amount of its major cation sodium must be present in adequate amounts to maintain a normal ionic concentration. In pregnant women with PIH, the increased sodium retention is in direct relation to increased edema. Decreased edema, along with decreased retention of sodium, follows the restoring of normal circulating blood volume through correction of the hypoalbuminemia and its related hypovolemia, and hence better operation of the failing capillary fluid shift mechanism. Thus the correct treatment is increased albumin through diet or infusion if needed, not undue sodium restriction.

Calcium. Extensive study of nonpregnant adults has found an inverse relationship between calcium intake and blood pressure, a finding further extended to pregnant women in clinical trials in the United States (Maryland) and in South America (Argentina and Ecuador).[5] Daily calcium supplementation of 1,500 to 2,000 mg reduced the incidence of PIH in the two South American countries but not in Maryland. Pathophysiologic basis for these associations is still unclear, as is the effect of calcium supplementation on pregnancy outcome, necessitating more extensive clinical trials to explore the relationship further.[58]

Vitamins. The full spectrum of vitamins is also required during pregnancy. Their need and metabolic rationale have been discussed in previous chapters. Basic to the full use of needed protein and other nutrients to reduce PIH risks are those vitamins especially related to protein and energy metabolism. Vitamins A, C, D, and E have particular structural functions, and the B vitamins are closely related as coenzyme factors in protein and energy metabolism.

Nutritional Management

Pregnancy-induced hypertension. Certainly the best approach to clinical management of PIH is its prevention, and significant among the factors related to its prevention is good prenatal care based on sound nutrition. It is evident from accumulating research that vigorous nutritional support is basic to a healthy pregnancy and the avoidance of complications. If PIH should develop, the same high quality diet should be followed with attention to sufficient protein (60 to 80 gm), kcalories (2,500 kcal), and sodium (2 to 3 gm) to control its symptoms and to maintain nutritional support of the pregnancy. Maintenance of good nutritional status can be achieved through sound knowledge of nutrition applied in a culturally acceptable manner to meet individual personal and socioeconomic needs.

Preexisting hypertension. Medical therapy for preexisting hypertension in the mother will continue to be guided by individual needs for its control. Effort is made, however, to minimize or remove drug use during the pregnancy. Instead, emphasis is given to nondrug approaches such as sound prenatal diet as outlined, avoiding excessive weight gain, and using a moderate sodium intake as described above. Bed rest may be used as needed.

DIABETES MELLITUS

During their pregnancies women with preexisting chronic disease require special care. This is especially true of diabetes. Today, however, improved expectations for the diabetic mother's pregnancy is one of the success stories of modern medicine. This "sweet success" marks the experience of highly motivated diabetic women enrolled in a growing number of education and support groups across the United States affiliated with the American Diabetes Association. These programs seek to enroll diabetic women before they become pregnant so that good blood glucose control can be established before conception and maintained throughout pregnancy. Using a team approach, studies have demonstrated that education and intensive management for glycemic control, especially before and during early pregnancy, enable women with diabetes to have healthy pregnancies that produce healthy babies, reducing risk of complications to the same level as that found in nondiabetic pregnant women.[31,36]

A number of factors have helped to achieve these improved expectations for the course and outcome of the diabetic mother's pregnancy. Current advances in obstetric technology in monitoring fetal development, increased knowledge of nutrition and diabetes, and especially management refinements in "tight" self blood glucose monitoring and control have all played a part. The provision of care by a team of specialists including internist, obstetrician, diabetes nurse educator, clinical nutritionist, and social worker has helped most of all to apply this increased knowledge of diabetes in pregnancy and self-care skills, all in a manner that is tailored to meet individual needs.

Care of the diabetic mother during her pregnancy requires a full knowledge not only of the normal physiologic changes of pregnancy but also of the altered metabolism of diabetes and the interrelationships of both states. Maternal metabolic control has a direct influence especially on early embryo development, making normalization of blood glucose levels in the immediate preconception period and early pregnancy important for normal organ development and avoidance of diabetes-related defects.[19] Essentially the metabolic processes involved in energy and growth systems provide the physiologic environment that both supports the pregnancy and controls the diabetes. Here, then, we can better understand and meet these objectives of care by looking first at the energy adaptations in pregnancy in terms of the maternal-fetal-placental fuel and hormone relationships, comparing them with changes taking place in the diabetic state, and then basing plans for care on these principles.

Energy Metabolism

In pregnancy, energy needs are increased, and thus the fuel requirements to meet these needs are also increased. In the human energy system glucose and fatty acids provide the main fuel sources, with some additional supply if needed from deaminated amino acids. However, glucose is the primary fuel. This is especially true in the developing fetus, who depends heavily on glucose to meet growing energy demands. To meet this energy demand the rate of fetal uptake of glucose is approximately twice that of the adult. Since the fetus preferentially uses glucose to meet energy needs, at term the fetal energy need is approximately 30 gm of glucose daily.

Fetal-maternal fuel-insulin relationships. The relatively large glucose requirement of the fetus to meet its energy needs is facilitated by the rapid transfer of glucose from the mother to the fetus in two ways. First, since fetal blood glucose levels are usually only 0.55 to 1.1 mmol/L (10 to 20 mg/100 ml) lower than those of the maternal circulation, simple diffusion would account for movement of glucose across the placental membranes. Second, since glucose is the only significant fuel used by the fetus and vital to its survival, additional rapid absorption is ensured by carrier-mediated diffusion or active transport. However, maternal insulin does not cross the placental membrane, although it is the ultimate mediator of the whole system of fuels available for transfer across the placenta. The fetus depends on its own supply of insulin for development. Fetal insulin is already present at 12 weeks' gestation, stimulated by increased glucose available from maternal circulation, as well as by increased amino acids present. Amino acids are actively transported by the placenta from maternal to fetal circulation to meet fetal tissue synthesis needs. Amino acids not only serve these vital synthesis needs in the fetus but also provide energy support. Thus fetal demands for glucose and key glucose precursor amino acids, notably alanine, pose a constant pull on the maternal metabolic supply.

Maternal fasting blood glucose levels. As a result of rapid fetal uptake of glucose and glucose precursor amino acids, there is a fall in the maternal fasting levels of blood glucose. At 15 weeks' gestation, for example, maternal glucose levels after an overnight fast during sleep are 0.8 to 1.1 mmol/L (15 to 20 mg/100 ml) lower than levels in the nonpregnant woman. If breakfast is skipped and fasting extends beyond 12 hours, the maternal blood glucose level may drop as low as the dangerous level of 2.2 to 2.5 mmol/L (40 to 45 mg/100 ml). In turn, this increased incidence, varying from 3% to 12%, and its association with significant pregnancy complications such as **macrosomia,** perinatal mortality, and prematurity, even with only moderately elevated blood glucose levels of approximately 6.6 to 9.0 mmol/L (120 to 165 mg/100ml). However, California researchers Jovanovic-Peterson and Peterson[31] have recently shown in their elegant study of women with gestational diabetes that dietary intervention in a strict **euglycemia** regimen can prevent macrosomia.[31] Their euglycemic diet is based on body weight—30 kcal/kg for ideal weight women, 24 kcal/kg for overweight ones—with total day's kcalories divided 40% carbohydrate, 20% protein, 40% fat, distributed in a 113131/10 meal-snack pattern: 10% of the kcalories at breakfast, 10% at midmorning snack, 30% at lunch, 10% at mid-afternoon snack, 30% at dinner, and 10% at evening snack. Tight surveillance based on four daily self-tests of blood glucose—a fasting test each morning before eating and 1 hour after each meal—guided food adjustments and any insulin addition. Results indicated that of the 30 women in the diet trial group, by 32 weeks gestation only 8 (26%) required insulin, and all 30 of the infants in this group had healthy weights in the 50th to 60th percentile for gestational age. Furthermore, in past years of their practice of prescribing the "euglycemic diet" to over 300 pregnant women at risk with gestational diabetes, none of the infants have had growth retardation or macrosomia, a zero rate in sharp contrast to the general reported macrosomic rates in gestational diabetes—20% to 40%!

The National Institutes of Health (NIH) classifications of diabetes in pregnancy are summarized in Table 9-6.

TABLE 9-6 *Classification of Diabetes Mellitus during Pregnancy**

New Classifications	Former Names	Clinical Characteristics
Type I insulin-dependent diabetes mellitus (IDDM)	Juvenile diabetes Juvenile-onset diabetes Brittle diabetes Ketosis-prone diabetes	Ketosis prone: insulin deficient because of loss of islet cells; often associated with human leukocyte antigen types, with predisposition to viral insulitis or autoimmune (islet-cell antibody) phenomena; can occur at any age, but more common in youth
Type II non-insulin-dependent diabetes mellitus (NIDDM) Nonobese Obese	Adult diabetes Adult-onset diabetes Maturity-onset diabetes Stable diabetes Ketosis-resistant diabetes Maturity-onset diabetes of youth	Ketosis resistant: occurs at any age but more frequent in adults; majority are overweight; may be seen in families as an autosomal dominant genetic trait; may require insulin in times of stress; usually requires insulin during pregnancy
Gestational diabetes	Gestational diabetes	Classification retained for women whose diabetes begins (or is recognized) during pregnancy; carries above risk of perinatal complications; transitory glucose intolerance, which frequently recurs; diagnosis: at least two abnormal values on a 3-hour oral glucose tolerance test (100 g glucose) Fasting plasma glucose 105 mg/100 ml 1 hour 190 mg/100 ml 2 hour 160 mg/100 ml 3 hour 145 mg/100 ml

*This classification replaces the White classification for pregnancy, which was based on age at onset, duration of the disease, and complications.

Diagnosis of diabetes in pregnancy. Universal screening for gestational diabetes is important for all pregnant women, especially because of the increased knowledge about its significant incidence and relation to pregnancy complications.[31,36] It is especially important for women over the age of 30 who are overweight and not physically fit and those who have a history of (1) family diabetes, (2) previous unexplained stillbirths, (3) giving birth to babies weighing 4 kg (9 lb) or more, (4) habitual abortion, (5) birth of infants with multiple congenital anomalies, and (6) excessive obesity.

Screening should be done at 24 to 28 weeks of gestation with a blood sugar test 1 hour after the ingestion of 50 gm of oral glucose. If the test result is greater than 7.8 mmol/L (140 mg/100 ml), a complete 100-gm, 3-hour glucose tolerance test (GTT) should follow with the woman in a fasting state. A 3-hour test is sufficient for diagnosis, with venous blood samples taken at 1-, 2-, and 3-hour intervals after the oral glucose dose. Criteria for diagnosis of gestational diabetes include a fasting plasma glucose above 5.8 mmol/L (105 mg/100 ml) and two or more remaining test values elevated: 1-hour value above 10.6 mmol/L (190 mg/100 ml), 2-hour value above 9.2 mmol/L (165 mg/100 ml), 3-hour value above 8.0 mmol/L (145 mg/100 ml).[30] Since the renal threshold for glucose is normally lower in pregnancy, transient glycosuria is not uncommon in the presence of normal glucose levels. Continued monitoring of pregnant women, especially those with suspect histories, is part of good preventive prenatal care.

Course of diabetes in pregnancy. Usually the course of diabetes in pregnancy follows a varying pattern from the first stages of the pregnancy, through the second half, and into the postpartum period. The early stages of pregnancy are characterized by an increasing transfer of maternal glucose to the fetus to meet fetal energy demands. This "siphoning" of glucose by the fetus, plus a lowered food intake resulting from nausea and vomiting of early pregnancy, usually reduces insulin requirements. This reduced insulin need is not the result of changed tissue sensitivity or altered diabetes status but, rather, of less available circulating blood glucose.

In the second half of pregnancy the increased diabetogenic effects of the placental hormones outweigh the continuous drainage of glucose by the fetus, and insulin requirements are increased some 65% to 70%. At the same time that insulin effectiveness is diminished, the tendency toward ketoacidosis is increased in the face of blood glucose levels that are markedly increased. Some confusion may occur because the ketonuria may reflect a starvation ketosis rather than diabetic ketosis, indicating the need for glucose rather than insulin. Thus close monitoring of all parameters is imperative.

After childbirth, maternal levels of the gestational hormones HCS, estrogen, and progesterone fall rapidly. Continued suppression of the growth hormone release is also seen. These hormonal changes cause a reduction in maternal insulin requirements, usually to levels below the prepregnant dose.

Management of Diabetes in Pregnancy

It is essential to a successful outcome of a diabetic woman's pregnancy that care be planned on the following: (1) sound principles of both pregnancy and diabetes management; (2) close attention to the basic components of diet, insulin, and exercise; (3) a schedule of care to meet changes throughout gestation; and (4) adjustments for birth and postpartum needs. This close management should involve frequent evaluation, team care, and personalized individual therapy.

Clinicians agree from experience that there is no substitute for frequent contacts with the mother and close observation of the changing course of metabolism and its effects during the pregnancy. In most prenatal clinics all diabetic mothers are seen every 2 weeks until the twenty-sixth week and every week, or more often if needed, thereafter.

Because of the variable aspects of diabetes and its course during pregnancy, as well as the altered course of pregnancy in the presence of diabetes, an interdisciplinary team of specialists can best meet the changing needs of the mother. This team includes the internist, obstetrician, nurse, nutritionist, and pediatrician at the baby's birth. Since nutritional management is fundamental to sound and safe care in both diabetes and pregnancy, the clinical nutritionist becomes a highly significant member of the care team. With this team approach the mother plays a central role. Ideally, with preexisting diabetes, the pregnancy is planned and good diabetes control is established before conception, through diabetes and pregnancy education and refined skills in self-monitoring of blood glucose levels, as well as management of diet, insulin, and exercise balances. Throughout the pregnancy, progress is continually assessed and self-care modified according to clinical symptoms.

Because diabetes, pregnancy, and people in general vary in their natures and needs, it is imperative that close, supportive individual therapy be followed. A primary medical concern is good control of the diabetes, with optimum nutritional support and insulin coverage to prevent fetal damage. Obstetrical concern centers on constant surveillance to maintain maternal and fetal health throughout the pregnancy and minimize risk to mother and infant.

Principles of nutritional therapy. Careful constant management of the basic components of diet and insulin, together with appropriate exercise, help to ensure an optimum outcome of the pregnancy. The fundamental cornerstone of diabetes management at any time is dietary management and control. This factor becomes even more important during pregnancy, in both preexisting chronic diabetes and gestational diabetes.

Since the onset of insulin-dependent diabetes mellitus (IDDM) occurs during childhood or adolescence, the prepregnant woman with IDDM has been exposed to prior nutritional counseling about her disease management. Sometimes a liberal diet has been permitted, or she has not formed habits of good blood glucose control. During pregnancy, however, she is usually more motivated and realizes that to achieve a successful pregnancy and outcome she must learn about her special nutritional needs and the importance of rigid blood glucose control. Dietary changes will be needed, and this is usually a good time for fine tuning her self-management skills.

Special attention must be given to distribution of both kcalorie and carbohydrate intake at frequent times during the day to minimize blood glucose fluctuations. A consistent daily schedule of self-monitoring of blood glucose levels is recommended to enable the diabetic mother to maintain close control of her glucose levels throughout the day. However, there must be sufficient energy intake in food to support appropriate weight gain during the pregnancy.

Tight control of maternal blood glucose levels is necessary for the management of gestational diabetes as well as IDDM. Nutritional care for the pregnant women with diabetes of any type must be individualized because the nutritional needs differ depending on prepregnancy weight and overall health, prepregnancy dietary habits and food plan, nutrition knowledge, and insulin therapy.

In the care of diabetes, especially during pregnancy, principles of diet management are based on the concept of *balance:*

1. *Total energy balance.* Energy intake as measured in kcalories is balanced with energy output needs, both basal metabolic and physical activity, to achieve and maintain ideal weight gain. In pregnancy, total energy requirements are governed by the demands of maternal-fetal growth and overall heightened metabolic needs. Energy needs are usually calculated on the basis of about 30 to 35 kcal/kg ideal body weight. The RDA of 300 kcal added to the average allowance for adult women gives a recommendation of about 2,200 to 2,400 kcal, which for a 55 kg woman translates to about 40 kcal/kg.

2. *Nutrient balance.* The ratio of energy nutrients—carbohydrate, protein, and fat—is important in diabetes to meet metabolic needs. During pregnancy, moderate total carbohydrates spaced through the day is important for diabetes control, as well as fetal needs for glucose. In current therapy, this need translates to approximately 40% of the total kcalories as carbohydrate. The greater proportion of carbohydrate kcalories should come from complex carbohydrate foods such as starch to provide more sustained glucose release, with lesser amounts from simple sugar food forms.

    Protein needs are increased in pregnancy as described in previous chapters. Optimal protein intake is also important in diabetes control. Thus the diet of a pregnant woman with diabetes should contain approximately 20% of total kcalories as protein.

Fat intake should be moderate for both diabetes and pregnancy needs. Thus the remainder of the kcalories, or approximately 40% of the total energy, comes from fat. In general, the use of more highly saturated fats should be controlled.

3. *Distribution balance.* In diabetes, the regular distribution of the total diet throughout the day to balance with insulin activity is necessary to avoid hypoglycemia and provide a sustained release of glucose. This is especially true in pregnancy to avoid both "starvation ketosis" as well as diabetic ketoacidosis. A consistent daily schedule of frequent smaller meals and snacks is a usual pattern. Each meal and snack should contain both protein and complex carbohydrate to smooth out the resulting glucose release. Meals, especially breakfast, and snacks through the day and at bedtime should not be missed and should follow a regular pattern each day, accompanied by regular self-monitoring of blood glucose levels.

In planning the diabetic mother's diet during her pregnancy, the regular food exchange system, developed jointly by the American Diabetes Association and the American Dietetic Association, may be used for calculating the diet and making a variety of food choices. The current 1995 food exchange revisions have incorporated desired changes in nutrient values, food portions, and fat modifications.[68,73] For example, a diet prescription and food exchange pattern applying the current principles of diet management of diabetes in pregnancy for an ideal weight woman weighing 140 lb (64 kg) would follow this approximate energy and nutrient balance:

Energy	2,240 kcal	(35 kcal/kg)
Carbohydrate	224 gm	(40% of total kcal)
Protein	112 gm	(20% of total kcal)
Fat	99 gm	(40% of total kcal)

Excellent resources are available from the American Dietetic Association to add variety, flexibility, and interest to food plans based on the exchange system,[3] and to provide guidelines for meeting cultural needs, such as Jewish dietary laws.[59]

Management of insulin balance. During pregnancy, changes in insulin therapy must occur to meet the changing metabolism of the pregnancy and balance with the food intake and exercise pattern. As with all aspects of care, insulin therapy must be individualized. However, usually in early pregnancy, injections twice daily of mixed doses of intermediate and regular insulin provide good control. By the twenty-fourth to twenty-eighth week of pregnancy, when the activity of hormonal insulin antagonists peak, more frequent use of regular insulin with additional intermediate insulin as needed is required. For example, for tight control at this time, regular insulin may be used three times a day before meals and additional smaller amounts of NPH intermediate insulin at breakfast and at supper or bedtime. With other women, a combination of NPH and regular insulins at breakfast, regular at dinner, and NPH later in the evening at about 11:30 PM will suffice.

As indicated, insulin requirements usually fall during the first half of pregnancy because of continuous fetal use of glucose, and the mother may need no more than two thirds of her prepregnant amount. In the second half of pregnancy, however, the progressive rise of the placental hormones HCS and progesterone and of maternal cortisol creates the need for more insulin. Dosage requirements increase approximately 70% to 100% above prepregnancy needs.

Tight metabolic regulation is current practice in management of diabetes in pregnancy. A reasonable goal of insulin therapy for the diabetic mother during pregnancy is to maintain blood glucose at approximately normal levels of 3.3 to 6.6 μmol/L (60 to 120 mg/100 ml), with postprandial rise to no more than 7.8 μmol/L (140 mg/100 ml). In comparison, most women with gestational diabetes have a threshold glucose value of 7.8 μmol/L (140 mg/100 ml).[19] With good management this can generally be achieved without risking hypoglycemia. In any event, starvation ketosis must be distinguished from diabetic ketoacidosis and both should be avoided.

Starvation ketosis. Starvation ketosis may occur more readily in pregnancy because of the accelerated fetal uptake of glucose and is accentuated by early nausea and vomiting or by self- or physician-directed restriction of kcalories. In such cases, after overnight or extended fasts, blood ketone levels may rise to two or three times the normal nonpregnant level, but hyperglycemia is *not* present. This lack of hyperglycemia, characteristic of diabetic ketoacidosis, is the distinguishing feature. The treatment consists of glucose solutions and foods rather than supplemental insulin. Since ketonuria during pregnancy is undesirable, the practice of skipping the morning meal either by personal desire or for medical testing should be avoided during both normal pregnancy and pregnancy complicated by diabetes. Declining maternal blood glucose may be one of the factors leading to ketonemia. Therefore it is wise not to restrict carbohydrates during pregnancy, and the bedtime snacks needed to carry over through the night are desirable.

Diabetic ketoacidosis. Diabetic ketoacidosis occurs in the face of elevated blood glucose levels. Treatment is directed toward correcting the metabolic acidosis and discovering the underlying cause of the ketoacidosis. Usually regular insulin is given, along with hypotonic fluids (4.5% saline) and potassium supplements. Bicarbonate therapy is given only in more severe cases. Continued monitoring of blood glucose, blood ketones, and arterial pH provides a basis for determining additional insulin needs.

Schedule for prenatal care. Ideally, the diabetic woman planning a pregnancy would have been working closely with the maternal diabetes team, especially the nutritionist, to achieve good control before conception. If this has not occurred, then at earliest pregnancy confirmation a special prenatal clinic visit with the care team should include an extensive medical-obstetrical workup, complete with the nutritionist's personalized assessment process described in Chapter 8. An initial problem-oriented plan of care, including refinement of self-management skills with blood glucose monitoring and individually adapted diet prescription, calculation, and food plan developed by the clinical nutrition specialist working with the care team.

At each subsequent clinic visit (every 1 or 2 weeks until the twenty-sixth week and every week thereafter), the diabetic mother is evaluated by the medical-obstetrical-nutritional team of specialists. The mother's own record of self-monitoring blood glucose is reviewed carefully, as well as intermittent food records. Weight, blood pressure, and signs of edema are checked regularly. The ocular fundus is examined often.

Control of **perinatal risk** is essential. Some important goals for the treatment team include control of maternal glycemia, elimination of any trauma complications, prevention of iatrogenic prematurity, and detection of intrauterine distress before fetal damage can occur. In combination with increased sophistication in fetal monitoring and fetal intensive care, frequent clinic visits, and a liberal attitude about hospitalization when optimum control cannot be maintained on an outpatient basis, the current practice of tightened control of maternal diabetes throughout pregnancy as described has reduced problems in pregnancies complicated by diabetes.

Birth and Postpartum Care

The goals of modern obstetrical management of diabetes at most care centers are to permit pregnancy to be carried to term and to accomplish vaginal delivery, whenever possible, without compromising the fetus. These goals have largely been met through use of **ultrasonography** as a primary tool, enabling most diabetic mothers in good metabolic control to be hospitalized only at term. This primary obstetrical surveillance tool helps to maintain fetal health to term by (1) monitoring fetal growth throughout pregnancy, (2) evaluating early development, especially when **glycosylated hemoglobin** is increased in early pregnancy, (3) confirming gestational age, (4) detecting macrosomia, particularly in the third trimester, and (5) assisting in detection of central nervous system, cardiac, or skeletal malformations.

The objectives of diabetes management during labor are to maintain normal blood glucose levels and prevent ketosis. To achieve these goals, clinicians usually give IV glucose with limited regular insulin as needed according to frequent monitoring of blood glucose levels throughout labor. With this monitoring, many diabetic mothers are found to require little if any insulin during labor, despite their large insulin requirements during pregnancy.

After birth, because of the rapid clearing of placental hormones and continued suppression of maternal growth hormone, there is a dramatic decline, often 50% or more, in maternal insulin requirements. Resumption of the mother's full diet is encouraged as soon as possible to restore nutrition reserves and support lactation. Breastfeeding presents no problem in control of maternal diabetes but does require additional energy intake, usually about 35 to 45 kcal/kg. During the postpartum period and continuing, the insulin need varies, and women are encouraged to continue their good diabetes management skills with frequent self-monitoring of blood glucose levels.

MATERNAL PHENYLKETONURIA

Phenylketonuria (PKU) is a recessively inherited metabolic disorder which, if left untreated, is a major cause of mental retardation. In PKU the liver fails to synthesize phenylalanine, an essential amino acid, into tyrosine because of the lack of the enzyme **phenylalanine hydroxylase.** The result is a toxic buildup of phenylalanine in the blood, which interferes with brain development and function. Newborn screening, resulting in early diagnosis for **phenylketonuria,** has had a remarkable effect. Infants who begin treatment in the early neonatal period and continue intensive long-term treatment achieve their genetic potential for intellectual development. By 1988 the first group of early and continuously treated individuals were of college age and were bearing out this observation.

Although early and aggressive treatment of PKU leads to successful outcomes, that is, normal intelligence and motor function, the well-managed individual with PKU still has an elevated blood phenylalanine level. Effective treatment of women with PKU has led to a new public health concern. Maternal PKU causes congenital abnormalities in infants of women with PKU. It is well known that young women with PKU are at risk for bearing children with lowered IQs, microcephaly, heart defects, and low birth weight. Paternal PKU does not seem to cause mental or physical defects in offspring (see box above).

PATERNAL PKU

Although there is an inverse relationship between sperm count and semen volume and serum phenylalanine levels, men with PKU are able to father children. Children whose fathers have PKU do not appear to be at greater risk for physical or mental disabilities that are other children. However, all of these children are carriers for the gene for PKU.

From Fisch RO et al: Children of fathers with phenylketonuria and international survey, *J Pediatr* 118:739, 1991; and Levy H et al: Paternal phenylketonuria, *J Pediatr* 118:741, 1991.

The Problem

It has been estimated that there are 2,000 to 4,000 women in the United States who have PKU and are of childbearing age. Furthermore, it has been estimated that in North America, 1 in 30,000 females of childbearing age has hyperphenylalaninemia that is undetected because of normal or near normal intelligence. The offspring of these women are at significant risk for abnormal in utero development and at slightly increased risk for phenylketonuria.

It is feared that given average rates of reproduction (two children per woman) the number of children with PKU-related mental retardation, that is, children who are damaged because of untreated maternal PKU, will be equal to or greater than the mental retardation caused by untreated phenylketonuria.[35,51] The birth of numbers of severely damaged infants to women with PKU would soon eliminate the advantages gained by newborn screening, that is, the prevention of mental retardation caused by phenylketonuria.

Spontaneous abortion, microcephaly, congenital heart disease, low birth weight, and mental retardation have become the recognized problems associated with maternal phenylketonuria.[38,47,52]

As shown in Table 9-7, retrospective surveys have indicated that the probability for women with phenylketonuria to bear children with ma-

TABLE 9-7   Frequency (%) of Abnormalities in Offspring of Women with Untreated PKU,
According to Maternal Blood Phenylalanine Level

Complication	20 mg/ 100 ml	16-19 mg/ 100 ml	11-15 mg/ 100 ml	3-10 mg/ 100 ml	Normal Frequency (%)
Mental retardation	92	73	22	21	5.0
Microcephaly	73	68	35	24	4.8
Congenital heart disease	12	15	6	0	0.8
Low birth weight	40	52	56	13	9.6

From Lenke RR and Levy HL: Maternal phenylketonuria and hyperphenylalaninemia: an international survey of the outcome of untreated and treated pregnancies, *N Engl J Med* 303:1202, 1980.

jor problems is much greater than that expected in the general population. These problems are independent of the infant's having phenylketonuria.[47] Thus women who have blood phenylalanine concentrations >1200 μmol/L (>20 mg/100 ml) have the greatest risk of having an affected child.

The normal physiology of pregnancy mandates a preconceptual and rigorous decrease in blood phenylalanine concentrations. The fetal-maternal plasma ratio is higher in early pregnancy. This ratio is estimated to be 1.5:1.[22] The heart is most vulnerable to maldevelopment in the first 8 weeks of pregnancy. A significant increase in cardiac malformation is demonstrated when maternal blood phenylalanine concentrations are >900 μmol/L (>15 mg/100 ml).[43] The 1993 status report of the Maternal PKU Collaborative Study showed that of 318 pregnancies there were 207 live births. Fifteen infants (7.2%) born to women without biochemical control by 10 weeks of gestation had cardiac anomalies. The rate in the general population is about 0.5—1.0%.[39]

Facial dysmorphology is correlated with high maternal blood phenylalanine concentrations. When blood phenylalanine concentrations are consistently <360 μmol/L (<6 mg/100 ml) facial dysmorphology diminishes.[63]

Status of Treatment

Reported outcomes following dietary treatment during pregnancy vary from normal to severely affected infants. However, most of these children are young, less than 5 years of age, and their eventual intellectual development has not been documented and reported.

There appears to be an inverse relationship between the maternal levels of phenylalanine and the effect on the fetus. Drogari et al[13] noted that on average, for each 200 μmol/L (3.3 mg/100 ml) rise in phenylalanine values at conception, birth weight fell by 110 gm and head circumference by 0.5 cm.

Outcomes have been described as: (1) an unaffected infant was born to a mother after treatment was begun in the last third of the first trimester,[12] (2) early intervention provided no protection at all,[66] (3) extremely variable fetal outcomes are common.[61] These variable outcomes can, in part, be explained by the timing of the reduction of the maternal blood phenylalanine level to the low levels of 120 to 360 μmol/L (2 to 6 mg/100 ml) that are hypothesized to prevent fetal damage. However, blood phenylalanine levels probably do not explain all problems demonstrated by the infants. Other factors that may play a significant role in fetal outcome are genetic makeup and enzyme activity of the mother, willingness or ability of the pregnant woman to comply with the restricted phenylalanine food pattern, and nutritional status before and during pregnancy.

Even though the maternal blood phenylalanine concentration at conception appears to be a predictor of fetal status at birth, less than 20% of the women enrolled in the Maternal PKU Collaborative Study started therapy before conception. Only a small percentage of these women had brought their blood phenylalanine concen-

TABLE 9-8   *Preliminary Results from the National Maternal PKU Collaborative Study*

Group	Number of Pregnancies	Birth Length (cm)	Birth Weight (kg)	Head Circumference (cm)
Non-PKU control	52	52	3480	35.5
PKU group				
Blood level <600 μmol/L achieved by				
Prepregnancy	14	50.8	3423	33.7
0-10 weeks	24	50.8	3210	33.8
11-20 weeks	51	49.5	3022	33.0
>20 weeks	77	47.8	2794	31.5

Adapted from Koch R et al: *Acta Paediatr Suppl*, 1994.

trations into the desired range of control before conception, even though they had made efforts to do so. More than half the women in the study did not start management of blood phenylalanine concentrations until the first trimester of pregnancy.[40]

Outcome of Treatment

It is hoped that these risks of maldevelopment can be reduced to an acceptable degree if the woman is to maintain a very low blood phenylalanine concentration before conception and throughout pregnancy. At this time, no safe maternal blood phenylalanine level has been demonstrated. Until a safe level has been established, it is recommended that blood phenylalanine levels be reduced to and maintained at 120-360 μmol/L (2-6 mg/100 ml) both before conception and during the entire pregnancy. Several programs have recommended more-stringent guidelines. For example, guidelines from the United Kingdom suggest 60-180 μmol/L (1-3 mg/100 ml) and 120-300 μmol/L (2-5 mg/100 ml). These goals of management still provide a blood phenylalanine level significantly greater than normal [30-60 μmol/L (0.5-1.0 mg/100 ml)].

The Maternal PKU Collaborative Study (MP-KUCS) was organized in 1984 as a prospective study to evaluate the effectiveness of dietary treatment in reducing the damage to offspring associated with maternal PKU.[38] It included, as controls, peers without PKU. The study attempted to answer a series of questions related to dietary treatment during pregnancy and condition of the infant at birth and to ascertain at what blood levels the risks were diminished.

The United Kingdom research group proposed that fetal damage is to a large extent determined by the level of blood phenylalanine around conception and there is still some risk when maternal phenylalanine concentrations are no more than 2 to 3 times normal.[67] It is also believed that it is not possible to define an absolute threshold value below which there is no risk to the fetus.[43]

Table 9-8 summarizes the birth size of MP-KUCS infants by time of metabolic control of the women with PKU. Birth outcomes (length, weight, head circumference) were progressively diminished and directly related to increased maternal phenylalanine level. All infants born to mothers with PKU were smaller than infants born to mothers without PKU. Although the results are not definitive the trend is encouraging; the best chance of a good pregnancy outcome in women with PKU results from initiation of biochemical control (preconception low blood phenylalanine levels and diet therapy) and strict control of maternal phenylalanine levels throughout pregnancy.[39,40] Unfortunately, in this study, small numbers of women with PKU achieved biochemical control before pregnancy and had a planned, well-controlled pregnancy experience. The optimal conditions for treatment are yet to be established. The results suggest an "effect on the fetus from even mildly elevated phenylalanine levels in the mother."[50,55] Results of MPKUCS indicate that the time at which phenylalanine restricted diet is initiated (e.g., gestational age) has effect on outcome. Median head circumference percentiles of infants of women initiating treatment before conception and that of women in the first trimester differed; the preconception infants had increased head circumferences. The infant head circumferences of women whose plasma phenylalanine was <360 μmol/L (<6 mg/100 ml) by 10 weeks gestation were greater than offspring of women whose plasma phenylalanine was 360-600 μmol/L (6-10 mg/100 ml).[39-40,58]

The children were all too young to report definitive cognitive progress and status. Children whose mothers achieved biochemical control before conception or very early in pregnancy and maintained it during the pregnancy had higher general Cognitive Index Scores on the McCarthy Scales of Children's Abilities.[40]

Identifying Women at Risk

Identification is one of the single impediments to treatment of women in their reproductive years who have phenylketonuria. Many women born before 1968, when newborn screening began, have either not been identified or have been lost to follow-up. Many women born before 1975 were identified by newborn screening but were discontinued from diet during the school years and then lost to follow-up. Also, many women with elevated blood phenylalanine concentrations—(240-600 μmol/L [4-10 mg/100ml]) on an unrestricted diet—were not treated with diet therapy but are nonetheless at risk for producing affected infants.[50] Many of these women are unknown to health care professionals and may not realize themselves that they have PKU (see box at right).

Canada has developed a maternal PKU registry in an effort to track and educate all women of childbearing age with elevated blood phenylalanine levels.[10] The Canadian program[26] recommends that all women be screened by

❖

> ### *RECOMMENDATIONS FROM THE COMMITTEE ON GENETICS FOR THE AMERICAN ACADEMY OF PEDIATRICS*
>
> #### *Maternal Phenylketonuria*
> 1. To optimize pregnancy outcome for women with PKU, the pediatrician should refer all young women with hyperphenylalaninemia to appropriate treatment centers, where careful monitoring by the physician and nutritionist will allow for adequate maternal and fetal nutrition. This referral should antedate pregnancy.
> 2. Women who give birth to children with microcephaly and retardation, without a known cause, should have a blood screening test for hyperphenylalaninemia.
> 3. In cooperation with newborn screening programs and physicians caring for children with PKU, state health departments should develop a plan to establish and/or maintain contact with women identified as having elevated blood phenylalanine concentrations so that these women may be kept informed about the implications of their condition and available treatment.

Guthrie bacterial inhibition assay during preconceptual counseling if their history reveals any of the following situations:
- A mentally retarded child, especially if that child has microcephaly or congenital heart disease.
- A miscarriage
- A family history of phenylketonuria

In the United States, the American Academy of Pediatrics[11] and the American Public Health Association[4] advocate the development of a system to maintain or reestablish contact with all women who are at risk because of elevated plasma phenylalanine concentrations.

Reproductive Counseling for Women with PKU

The discussion of pregnancy and childbearing and childrearing alternatives should be initiated well before a woman with PKU reaches her childbearing years. The woman with phenylketonuria should be well aware of the significant risks to the fetus as well as the need to have very low blood phenylalanine levels before conception. She needs to know that even careful and controlled management of blood phenylalanine levels before conception and during pregnancy do not insure the delivery of a normal infant. No safe range of maternal phenylalanine levels during pregnancy have been established.

Since more abnormal than normal births have been reported and attempts at dietary management are often unsuccessful, a discussion of pregnancy alternatives is warranted. Alternatives for women with PKU and their partners to consider, given the risks to the fetus, are: (1) adoption, (2) in vitro fertilization using parental gametes, and (3) avoiding pregnancy.[21] Another option is to delay pregnancy until more information on an intervention program that reduces the risks to the fetus to a more acceptable level is available.

Barriers to effective pregnancy planning for women with PKU have been assessed.[71] Personal beliefs about contraception, sexual activity and childbearing, as well as presence or lack of social support for family planning, were among the many factors regarding pregnancy planning. Compared with the other groups of women, the young woman with PKU has little knowledge of family planning. The risks to the fetus and the need to evaluate other options for achieving parenthood are not clearly understood by these young women. Nor do they seem to understand the mandate for prepregnancy planning to increase the possibility of a good outcome. A greater emphasis on reproductive decision making is clearly needed.[72]

Nutritional Management in Maternal PKU

There appears to be a mitigating effect on fetal damage by the reduction of maternal blood phenylalanine levels to very low concentrations before conception and throughout the pregnancy. The low-phenylalanine diet for preconception and pregnancy is more rigorous than the usual prescription for children and adolescents with PKU. The goals for management

of maternal phenylketonuria as stated by both the American Academy of Pediatrics[11] and the Maternal PKU Collaborative Project[51] are to maintain blood phenylalanine levels between 120-360 μmoi/L (2-6 mg/100 ml) before and during pregnancy and at the same time to meet all the nutritional needs of pregnancy. This rigorous goal cannot be attempted without the use of medical foods to provide a significant percentage (80% to 90%) of protein and energy intake during pregnancy. Nutritional inadequacies are possible if adequate medical food is not ingested.[2] There are several medical foods available that theoretically meet the protein needs of the pregnant woman while restricting phenylalanine and supplementing tyrosine (Table 9-9). These products are free of phenylalanine and supplemented with tyrosine. The necessity for additional tyrosine supplementation during pregnancy is an unsettled issue. However, L-tyrosine should be supplemented if the maternal plasma concentration is below normal.

During pregnancy, the recommendation for protein is 75 gm/day and 2,200 to 2,400 kcal (Table 9-10). Assuming 80% of the protein is from medical foods, meeting this recommendation would require 300 gm of Phenyl-Free, 88 gm of PKU, 3,250 gm of Phenex 2, or 154 gm of MAXAMUM-XP per day. Since both PKU-3 and MAXAMUM-XP are essentially free of fat and carbohydrate, they require the addition of a major source of these components to the formulation. Usually oil, corn syrup, and **Polycose** are used for this purpose. The medical foods must be supplemented with a source of phenylalanine from foods. Phenylalanine-free nonprotein foods such as low-protein specialty products are needed to meet energy needs.

Meeting phenylalanine requirements and energy needs from foods is also problematic. A typical intake of 300 to 500 mg of phenylalanine per day is easily met and exceeded from traditional protein foods such as milk, eggs, meat, and cheese. For example, 1 oz of cheddar cheese, 1 cup of milk, and 1 oz of cooked beef each contain 345 to 360 mg of phenylalanine. Grain products such as bread, cereals, pasta, and rice, as well as starchy vegetables such as potatoes, peas, and corn, all contain relatively high percentages of phenylalanine (160 to 290

TABLE 9-9 **Medical Foods for the Treatment of Women with PKU**

	Phenyl-Free*	PKU-3*	Phenex 2†	Maxamum-XP**
Composition				
Protein	Amino acids	Amino acids	Amino acids	Amino acids
Carbohydrates	Sucrose, corn syrup solids, tapioca starch	Sucrose	Corn starch	Sucrose, corn starch
Fat	Corn oil, coconut oil	0	Palm oil, coconut oil	0
Nutrients (per 100 gm powder)				
Protein (gm)	20	68	30	39
Fat (gm)	6.8	0	15.5	<1
Carbohydrate (gm)	66	1.7	30	45
Energy (kcal)	405	280	410	340
Tyrosine (mg)	930	600	2440	403
Phenylalanine (mg)	0	0	0	0
Iron (mg)	12.2	21	13	23.5
Calcium (mg)	510	1310	880	670
Zinc (mg)	7.1	24	13	13.6
Vitamin A (IU)	1220	4000	μgRE 660	2350 (RE 705)
Vitamin D (IU)	152	480	μg 9.9	320
Vitamin E (IU)	10.2	12	mg α-TE 12.1	7.8
Ascorbic acid (mg)	53	100	60	90
Thiamin (μg)	610	1800	4000	1400
Riboflavin (μg)	1020	1800	1800	1400
Niacin (μg)	8100	18000	equiv mg 31700	13600
Vitamin B_6 (μg)	910	3200	1300	1200
Vitamin B_{12} (μg)	2.5	5	9.5	4
Folacin (μg)	127	950	430	500
Pantothenic acid (μg)	3000	8300	14000	5000
Biotin (μg)	30	179	130	140

*Dietary management of metabolic disorders, Mead Johnson Nutritionals, Evansville, IN, 1991.
†Metabolic checklist, Scientific Hospital Supplies, Gaithersburg, MD, 1993.
**Nutrition support protocols, The Ross Metabolic Formula System, Ross Laboratories, Columbus, OH, 1993.

TABLE 9-10 **Guidelines for Nutrient Intakes**

Nutrient	Recommendation
Protein	75 gm
Energy	2,200 to 2,400 kcal
Phenylalanine	200 mg as base-line minimum, adjusted to calibrate blood phenylalanine concentrations at acceptable levels
Vitamins and minerals	1989 RDA for pregnancy
Tyrosine	As needed to maintain normal plasma concentrations
Weight gain	Usual recommendations based on age, height, pregnancy weight

From Maternal PKU Collaborative Study: *Maternal PKU Collaborative Study protocol*, 1992.

phenylalanine/1 cup serving) and must be carefully measured and restricted. Fruits and vegetables contain lower percentages of protein as phenylalanine and can be included more liberally. Low-protein wheat-starch products such as bread, pasta, and baked products must be included to meet energy needs and to satisfy appetite while maintaining a very restricted phenylalanine intake. Nutritional guidelines for management of the pregnant woman with PKU are shown in the box below).

The physiologic changes of pregnancy pose difficulties for rigorous dietary management. The gradient of amino acids across the placenta changes with the stage of the pregnancy, and thus a maternal blood phenylalanine level of 240 μmol/L (4 mg/100 ml) would be amplified depending on the stage of pregnancy. Not only is the technology required for monitoring this important variable unavailable, but the maternal responses to fluctuating and changing hormones also may make it difficult for the pregnant woman to sustain a stable appetite and consequent ingestion of the medical foods.

The semisynthetic nature of the medical foods and supplement foods required for the management of pregnancy mandate the careful management of other aspects of pregnancy, which include the biochemical and nutritional parameters of weight gain, energy, phenylalanine and protein intake, blood levels for amino acids, ferritin, hematocrit, hemoglobin, cholesterol, and folate. Nutrient intake from prescription and actual food records should be monitored weekly. A daily food intake record provides the woman with supportive information for her treatment. Table 9-11 indicates the schedule of assessments necessary for monitoring the pregnancies of women with PKU. Frequent changes in individualized diet prescription as pregnancy pro-

---

GUIDELINES FOR NUTRITIONAL MANAGEMENT FOR THE PREGNANT WOMAN WITH PKU

Goals of Nutritional Management

1. Maintain serum phenylalanine levels as low as possible. The U.S. Maternal Collaborationtive Study recommends concentrations between 120-360 μmol/L (2-6 mg/100 ml).
2. Maintain adequate and consistent weight gain.
3. Maintain serum tyrosine in the normal range.
4. Meet pregnancy nutrient requirements for protein, energy, vitamins and minerals using the current RDA.

Tasks of Nutritional Management

1. Stress the special nutritional needs during pregnancy.
2. Stress the importance of strictly following the phenylalanine prescription to achieve the necessary rigid control of blood phenylalanine levels.
3. Calculate a food pattern to provide adequate energy, protein, phenylalanine, vitamins, and minerals.

4. Provide a food pattern for the individual that is based on a phenylalanine-free protein source (formula/medical food).
5. Provide a meal guide and serving lists that indicate protein, energy, and phenylalanine content of foods.
6. Provide education on foods: selection, purchasing, preparation using low phenylalanine recipes, and recording intake as needed.
7. Review and calculate diet records for accuracy.
8. Compare recorded and calculated food intake with blood phenylalanine levels and weight gain.
9. Adjust food pattern and meal guide as necessary to meet individual needs.
10. Monitor plasma amino acid levels.
11. Monitor indices of nutritional status for pregnancy.

gresses are based on: (1) plasma concentrations of phenylalanine, tyrosine, and other amino acids; and (2) weight gain.[2] Birth measures of infants of women with PKU are negatively correlated with plasma concentrations and positive correlation with maternal energy and protein intake and weight gain.[55] The pregnancies of these women should be considered very high risk and monitored rigorously. All other obvious risks such as smoking, alcohol consumption, medications, and substance abuse are clearly contraindicated.

The difficulties of compliance with this rigorous treatment protocol are obvious. Satisfactory compliance is often unattainable even with intensive patient instruction and extensive support. Thus the frequent nausea and vomiting components of pregnancy can greatly interfere with management of plasma phenylalanine concentrations. Women often require hospitalization to bring blood phenylalanine levels into the acceptable range and then are able to maintain them only with difficulty. Management of these high-risk pregnancies requires extensive commitment of the clinic staff, including the physi-

cian, nutritionist, nurse, social worker, and public health nurse, as well as the expertise of an obstetrical team with experience in high-risk pregnancy management. Programs such as Medicaid, WIC, Home Health Aides, and other community resources are needed to provide support for the pregnancy as well as intervention with the handicapped children that result.

The time commitments required of health care providers and the financial impact of pregnancies of women with PKU and their children have not been fully appreciated. A cost accounting of the time resources and commitment from all health care providers and resources such as medical food and laboratory analyses indicated that management of the pregnancy of an intellectually normal and compliant woman, including preconceptual management, was about $30,000. Much of the time, resources were donated to the family.

It appears that some infants of mothers with PKU are less damaged than others. Currently, there is no basis for differentiating these women and their infants from those who will be severely damaged without rigorous treatment. Treatment during pregnancy can mediate the in utero risks to the fetus but no guarantees can be made that even with rigorous maternal therapy the fetus will be unaffected. The infants of mothers who endeavour to follow the rigorous therapy during pregnancy will need to be closely monitored as they grow and develop (central nervous system functioning is of particular concern). Only then can the long-term effect of the therapy during pregnancy be evaluated objectively.

There are indications that intellectual deficits can be lessened and that the risk for physical deformities can be reduced but not eliminated. The data currently available indicate that the severity of damage to the fetus appears to be directly related to maternal blood phenylalanine levels, that introduction of the diet before conception and at various points during pregnancy may be helpful but with inconsistent results, and that the only risk-free choice for women with PKU is to avoid pregnancy.[51] The summary of the MPKUCS states that preliminary findings have indicated that phenylalanine restriction should begin before conception for

TABLE 9-11 *PKU-Specific Parameters to Monitor during Pregnancy*

Assessment	Frequency
Blood phenylalanine level	Weekly
Clinical evaluation	Monthly
3-day diet record	Weekly*
Calculated nutrient intake	Monthly
Ultrasound	20, 28, 34 weeks
Plasma amino acids	Monthly
Serum ferritin	Monthly
Hemoglobin, hematocrit	Each trimester
Serum total protein	Each trimester
Serum total albumin	Each trimester
Serum total cholesterol	Each trimester
Whole-blood red-cell folate	Each trimester
Vitamin B$_{12}$	Each trimester

*Daily records are necessary to support reasonable monitoring of nutrient intakes.
From Maternal PKU Collaborative Study: *Maternal PKU Collaborative Study Protocol,* 1992.

females with PKU planning a pregnancy. Dietary control should maintain maternal blood phenylalanine levels between 120 and 360 μmol/L (2-6 mg/100 ml) and should provide adequate energy, protein, vitamin and mineral intake.[40]

It is hoped that women who have remained on treatment and have continued to monitor their blood phenylalanine levels since infancy and who have normal intelligence will evaluate the risks and make informed decisions about childbearing.[62]

SPECIAL WEIGHT PROBLEMS IN PREGNANCY

Adolescent girls and young adult women enter pregnancy with wide variances in prepregnancy weights. Although a majority are of an appropriate medium or standard weight-for-height, a number of them are at either end of the weight spectrum, being overweight or obese on the one hand or underweight on the other. Both extremes carry pregnancy risks and need initial assessment and ongoing monitoring to help ensure a successful outcome.

Assessing Prepregnancy Weight-for-Height

An accurate determination of maternal preconception body size, especially for underweight and overweight clients, is especially critical in prenatal care but is difficult to obtain. The initial prenatal clinic visit usually follows pregnancy confirmation at about 8 to 12 weeks, or in the case of late registrants may be much later, and weight recall by overweight and underweight mothers may be biased, making gestational evaluation more difficult. Studies of pregnant adolescents and adults indicate that overweight individuals tend to underestimate their prepregnancy weights and those who are underweight tend to overestimate their weights.[70] Accurate measures of weight and height can be taken at first clinic visit and weight related to gestational week based on last menstrual period. Then as accurate a weight history as possible can be obtained along with the general nutrition interview or questionnaire.

Body Mass Index

Weight-for-height measure. The most widely used indicator of maternal nutritional status, not only in the United States but in other developed countries, is the calculated value for the **body-mass index.** It is a better nutritional indicator than weight alone because it factors in the height, an important consideration in prenatal assessment, especially in short women. This weight-for-height value is easily calculated by the following formula:

$$BMI = [weight(kg)] \div [height(cm)]$$

Metric units of weight in kilograms and height in centimeters are generally used, but may be converted easily to pounds and inches equivalents.

$$BMI = [weight(lb) \times 0.4536] \div [height(in) \times 0.0254]$$

Prepregnancy weight-for-height categories. In their recent report the subcommittee on Nutritional Status and Weight Gain During Pregnancy of the Institute of Medicine, U.S. National Academy of Sciences, has recommended the following prepregnancy weight-for-height categories, based on derived BMI values, to serve as guidelines for planning sufficient weight gain during pregnancy.[58] These BMI values correspond to percentages of the usual standard weight-for-height reference tables in general use as indicated here:

Under-weight	Normal Weight	Overweight	Obese
BMI <19.8	BMI 19.8-26.0	BMI 26.0-29.0	BMI >29.0
<90% of normal weight	90% to 120% of normal weight	120% to 135% of normal weight	>135% of normal weight

On the average, overweight women gain less weight during their pregnancies than do thinner women, but there is wide variation in weight gain by women with normal pregnancies within each prepregnancy weight-for-height category. The highest variation occurs among obese women.[58]

Obesity in Pregnancy

Prevalence. U.S. population trends in women's weights indicates that during the past two decades women have become heavier and taller. In fact, recent statistics derived from current U.S. studies of health and nutrition, the third National Health and Nutrition Examination Survey (NHANES III), revealed what many have already observed—Americans of all ages, genders, and ethnic groups are gaining weight.[44] Previous surveys from 1960 to 1980 showed small progressive increases of 24% and 25% overweight, but the current NHANES III reported that 33.4% of Americans are overweight. This current NHANES study defined overweight of women as a body mass index (BMI) of 27.3 or more (120% of desirable). The relative rates of overweight reported for women according to ethnic group were:

- Black women—48.6%
- Mexican-American women—46.7%
- White women—32.9%

A recently reported long-term study of women's health, *The Nurses' Health Study,* showed similar relations of overweight and health problems. Reported problems of diabetes and hypertension, conditions complicating pregnancies, were two to six times more prevalent among women in the heavier groups.[53]

Other factors in obesity prevalence among American women also relate to socioeconomic status, age, and marital status. Kahn's study of race and weight changes in U.S. women indicates that greater obesity risk is associated with education below college level, entering marriage, and very low family income.[33]

Pregnancy risks. The increased prevalence of overweight among U.S. women of reproductive age has brought concerns about the influence of these changes on pregnancy outcomes. During the past two decades, the incidence of **macrosomia,** large infants weighing 4,000 gm (4 kg, or 8.8 lb) or more at birth, among white women has increased by 31% and among black women, 17%.[58] The prevalence of maternal obesity may contribute to this incidence of high-birthweight babies, who at birth have a rounded cushingoid face and a body bloated with enlarged viscera and increased fat, and who are often in respiratory distress. Maternal obesity and overnutrition sets up the cascading events of increased blood glucose that stimulates increased fetal insulin, resulting in abnormally increased li-pogenesis and excessive adipose tissue deposits—an overly fat baby at risk. Obese mothers as much as 150% overweight are at risk themselves for developing gestational diabetes, elevated blood pressure, and increased blood lipids.

Neonatal mortality occurs at both extremes of birth weight. Among low-birth-weight infants the death rate decreases sharply with increasing birth weight toward a normal developmental plane at weights of about 3,000 gm (3 kg, or 6.6 lb) to 4,000 gm (4 kg, or 8.8 lb). Then, as the birth weight rises, the neonatal mortality rate also rises again, increasing sharply when the weight reaches 4,250 gm (4.25 kg, or 9.35 lb) and above.[26,27]

Individual assessment. Assessing individual prepregnancy weight-for-height and monitoring amount and pattern of weight gain during the pregnancy are important health care procedures for obese pregnant women. As indicated in the National Academy of Science report *Nutrition During Pregnancy,*[58] in the BMI weight-for-height categories the central normal weight category is designated as a prepregnancy BMI of 19.8 to 26.0 (90% to 120% ideal body weight), with a recommended weight gain of 11.5 to 16.0 kg (25 to 35 lb). The overweight category is a pregnancy BMI of 26.0 to 29.0 (120% to 135% overweight), with a recommended weight gain of 7.0 to 11.5 kg (15 to 25 lb).

The obese category is a prepregnancy BMI above 29.0 (135% to 150% or more over ideal weight-for-height), with a recommended weight gain of at least 15 lb. However, the target for obese women should be determined on an individual basis since many obese women with good pregnancy outcomes do gain somewhat more or less than the stated goal. Nonetheless, an obese woman's pregnancy should be monitored carefully throughout to ensure that her nutritional needs are met and her weight gain is sufficient to support ideal fetal growth and development.

Nutritional care. Since the obese pregnant woman is at high risk for developing gestational diabetes, she is often found on screening to have elevated blood sugars. Thus, using the regular exchange system for a dietary calculation and management tool, her basic nutritional therapy is usually developed on the pattern of that used for control of gestational diabetes[21]:

1. *Energy.* Basal energy expenditure (BEE) may be calculated by the usual formula for women, using her prepregnancy weight:

$$BEE = 655 + [9.6 \times wt\ (kg)]$$
$$+[1.7 \times ht\ (cm)] - (4.7 \times age)$$

   Add physical activity factor, usually a fairly sedentary estimate of 30% of basal needs (BEE), plus the pregnancy factor of 300 kcal. Sometimes the additional pregnancy kcal factor is waived as a result of the obesity. As an alternate process, the RDA guide for kcalories according to age may be used as an energy base with the added 300 kcal pregnancy allowance. The resulting energy need will usually range about 2,000 to 2,500 kcal, depending on body size. In the past, obese pregnant women were sometimes put on low-energy 1,200-kcal diets, which they either did not follow, eating to appetite to the body's advantage, or strictly followed the order with disastrous results. Recent study has shown the metabolic danger of such restricted diets in obese pregnant women at risk for gestational diabetes.[31]

2. *Carbohydrate.* This is the key energy nutrient to be monitored carefully by continuing blood sugar tests to avoid both hyperglycemia and hypoglycemia, as well as dipstick urine tests for ketonuria. To achieve this glucose control, the carbohydrate allowance needs to be lowered somewhat to 40% of the day's total kcalories, distributed for general purposes in a 23131/10 pattern for meals and snacks: breakfast 2/10, lunch 3/10, mid-afternoon snack 1/10, dinner 3/10, and evening snack 1/10.[21] Foods carrying high simple sugar loads, such as fruit juices or dried fruit and sometimes milk (lactose), are curtailed or avoided, depending on the difficulty of controlling maternal blood sugars.

3. *Protein.* This important growth nutrient is held at the usual 20% of total day's kcalories level. Complete protein foods of animal origin are used to achieve a balance of required essential amino acids, or if the mother is a vegetarian, a lactoovovegetarian pattern to omit only meat. If the mother is a strict vegan, the diet will need to be carefully planned to achieve a complimentary balance of the remaining nonessential amino acids to supply her essential needs.

4. *Fat.* This energy nutrient is increased somewhat to 40% of the day's total kcalories to supply the basic energy deficit to balance with the tighter carbohydrate control. Food sources should be mainly monounsaturated or polyunsaturated in nature.

Each obese pregnant woman should receive individual dietary assessment and nutrition counseling, both initially at the beginning of the pregnancy and continuing throughout its course.[58] The mainstay of management for these women at risk is dietary, with adjustments in energy intake and distribution according to follow-up monitoring, with the goal of maintaining normal blood sugars to help ensure a healthy course and outcome for both mother and baby. A carefully supervised exercise program involving daily walking, as well as upperarm conditioning exercises using medium resistance or weights, may be a helpful adjunct for both cardiovascular fitness and a sense of well-being, as well as for maintaining normal blood sugar levels.[32]

General Underweight

The problem of underweight. Although general underweight is a less common problem in the American population than is overweight, it does occur in a small percentage, estimated at somewhat less than 10%, who have trouble gaining and maintaining weight. The underweight condition may be associated with poverty, poor living conditions, and inadequate food intake. It may result from malabsorption of nutrients as a result of gastrointestinal disease or abuse of laxatives. In some cases it may relate to energy imbalance from greatly increased physical activity without a corresponding increase in food. Maternal factors relating to an underweight prepregnancy state may also be associated with an increased risk of low weight gain during the pregnancy itself, for example, low family income, unmarried status, young age, and low educational level.[58]

Individual assessment. As indicated for the obese woman, the underweight pregnant adolescent or young woman presents special weight-related problems and needs, especially of inadequate total weight gain during the pregnancy and the pattern of the gain. Gestational weight gain, particularly during the second and third trimesters, is an important determinant of adequate fetal growth. Thus in any case, following the procedures outlined in Chapter 8, a comprehensive nutrition assessment of the underweight adolescent or adult mother is necessary. It should include a sensitive personal history of weight background and living situation, to determine her needs and plan care to help meet the increased physiologic demands of her pregnancy.

The underweight category is a prepregnancy BMI under 19.8, or under 90% of the ideal weight-for-height standard. For example, for a maternal height of 158 cm (62.2 in) this underweight category would include maternal weights under 49 kg (108 lb) ranging downward to about 40 kg (88 lb). The recommended weight gain during pregnancy for these underweight mothers is 12.5 to 18.0 kg (28 to 40 lb). For women who were underweight before pregnancy, the greater the gain during pregnancy, the lower the neonatal mortality rate.[58]

Nutritional care. A main goal of nutritional care for underweight mothers is to supply sufficient increased energy intake to ensure the needed weight gain for a successful course and outcome of the pregnancy. Following the RDA standard for age, an initial goal of 2,500 kcal/day is reasonable, with adjustments as needed according to ongoing individual monitoring and counseling throughout the pregnancy. The general food plan in Chapter 4 may serve as a guide, with multiple snacks through the day to accommodate the increased intake of nutrient dense food selections. Supplementation is needed for these at-risk underweight mothers with limited nutritional body reserves.

Eating Disorders

Prevalence. The incidence of the eating disorders *anorexia nervosa* and *bulimia nervosa*, as well as *bingeing disorder*, which mainly affect adolescent girls and young women in their early reproductive years, has been dramatically increasing over the past decade. Anorexia nervosa now affects about 1 of every 100 in a vulnerable population such as female high school or college students.[42] Bulimia is even more prevalent, reported to affect from 3% to 19% of young women.[46] Workers in this field express concern about this growing number and indicate that this is a true increase, not merely a factor of increased reporting. The food behaviors and malnutrition involved in these psychophysiologic eating disorders seriously complicate a pregnancy that may occur. Such situations require the sensitive and skilled care of a team of specialists including internist, obstetrician, psychiatrist, nurse, and clinical nutritionist.

Anorexia nervosa. The more extreme form of disorder, anorexia nervosa, has a long history. It was first described and named over a hundred years ago by the British physician Sir William Gull in his original classic papers of 1858 and 1874.[24] As originally described by Dr. Gull, these patients are usually of high intelligence, introverted, perfectionistic, compulsive, and overly sensitive. Their response to food is one of revulsion and disgust with vomiting usually following any forced feeding. Sometimes there is a preceding history of the opposite reaction to food, overeating and obesity, followed with shame at being fat. Usually there is hostility in parental relations at home, especially with the mother, or in sibling rivalry and jealousy. Occasionally a pregnancy fantasy may have triggered the desire to "diet," with complete refusal of food.

The pioneering clinical work of American psychiatrist Hilda Bruch laid the foundation for our current understanding of this psychophysiologic disorder, deeply rooted in a distorted body image, inability to eat, and an extreme fear of fatness in the midst of a culture that reveres and rewards thinness in women.[8] Bruch called this distorted body image and its self-induced starvation the "golden cage" that virtually imprisons the young patient.[9] This personal prison often develops through childhood in a controlling mother-daughter relationship that prevents the emerging adolescent girl from realizing her own true self-identity, filling her with such psychic pain from her distorted self-image that she can only escape by not eating. Current studies reinforce these relationships of poor family communication and self-concept to abnormal eating patterns in disturbed adolescents and young women.[46,77]

Pregnancies are not common among adolescents and young women with anorexia nervosa. Psychologically, the body image distortion affects sex-role identification and often there is little or no interest in sex. Also, physiologically, the monthly female reproductive cycle is usually not functioning normally and the fertility rate is low.[7,68] The severe long-term malnutrition in anorexic adolescents and young women contributes to a number of problems including menstrual abnormalities such as amenorrhea, irregular cycles, and anovulatory cycles, effectively preventing conception. This condition is especially true in female ballet dancers, for example, in whom high levels of exercise and exceptionally thin bodies are requisites for performance on a professional level, placing them at high risk of developing eating disorders. Even after long-term therapy anorexic young women may still keep themselves thin and not resume menses. Relapse, crisis, hospitalization, and only partial recovery are common, and in spite of weight-for-height improvement in about 75% of the patients, menstrual cycles are often not maintained, ideas about food and weight remain disturbed, and psychosocial maladjustment is common.

If a pregnancy does occur, the clinical nutritionist on the special obstetrical care team works with the physicians and clinical psychologist in determining weight goals, assessing personal and pregnancy nutritional needs, calculating energy balances, and supporting the mother's efforts to eat. If sufficient oral feeding is not possible, the medical team may determine that parenteral nutrition is necessary. In this case the nutritionist monitors nutritional status and energy balances carefully to help the mother achieve sufficient weight gain to support a successful pregnancy course and outcome.

Bulimia nervosa. Bulimia nervosa is a more recently recognized psychophysiologic eating disorder that has similar roots to anorexia nervosa, but is characterized by uncontrolled intake of huge amounts of food (binges), followed by self-induced vomiting and laxative abuse. Usually the age at onset is older than that of anorexia nervosa, occurring in older adolescents and young women of college age, but bulimia also carries a deep weight phobia. Bulimics differ from anorexics in that they may not lose weight but do maintain their thin status, often making the eating problem more difficult to detect. Some estimate that as many as 20% of college women engage in at least mild bulimic habits.[69] In a sense, these persons with bulimia are "failed anorectics." Unable to go without eating, they secretly follow the characteristic binge-purge procedure.

Young women with bulimia report abnormal appetite and difficulty feeling a sense of satiety, which helps to account for the bingeing behavior with huge amounts of food. Thus recent research has centered on the search for an appropriate pharmacologic agent to aid in satiety. Prior work has indicated that persons with bulimia have a reduced meal-related secretion of cholecystokinin, the natural biologic agent shown to produce satiety in humans, so the use of such an agent to aid in overall long-term therapy is under further study.[23,29]

In general, compared with adolescents and young women with anorexia nervosa, older adolescents and young women with bulimia nervosa have less severe body image distortion and thus less restrictive weight goals. Because they do hold their weight at a more normal level, adolescents and young women with bulimia do not experience similar menstrual abnormalities and hence are more fertile. However, during pregnancy, bulimic behaviors may persist, causing an abnormal weight gain pattern, concern for both mother and fetus from the adverse biochemical environment resulting from the constant vomiting, and unrealistic ideas about nourishing herself and the fetus during the pregnancy and feeding the infant after birth.

Care of the bulimic mother during her pregnancy requires the same team of specialists described for the woman with anorexia nervosa. The clinical nutritionist again assesses nutritional status, determines nutrient needs according to recommended dietary allowance (RDA) standards and individual status, and calculates energy balances as the pregnancy progresses. However, continued individual counseling is needed. The team supports the mother's personal needs and her efforts to suppress bulimic behavior as much as possible to sustain a stable biochemical environment for maternal and fetal well-being. Then after the baby is born, the mother is helped to recognize natural hunger signals from the baby to guide her in developing sound infant feeding practices.

TOTAL PARENTERAL NUTRITION DURING PREGNANCY

Development

Pregnant women are not common candidates for total parenteral nutrition (TPN), but when it is indicated, this large central vein system of IV feeding may be life-saving for both mother and child. The feasibility of providing elemental nutrient substrates intravenously was first developed and demonstrated by Dudrick and his surgical colleagues, and their reports of its successful use in patients with chronic gastrointestinal disease soon followed in 1968.[14] The first report of TPN use during pregnancy appeared a few years later in 1972, when a malnourished young women with anorexia nervosa, in her 26th week of pregnancy, was successfully treated with a 3,000-kcalorie solution of protein, fat, carbohydrate, and electrolytes for 10 days.[45] In the intervening years since that first pregnancy use, products and procedures have advanced and TPN in obstetric practice has increased to meet critical nutritional needs. It has become an important mode of feeding for pregnant women when oral or enteral routes are not feasible and when restoring and maintaining an anabolic state is crucial for maternal health and fetal development.[34,78]

Indications for Use

TPN use in early gestation has been shown to supply adequate nutrition for women suffering from prolonged intractable hyperemesis gravidarum.[48] Long-term use has been associated with malabsorption problems resulting from

Crohn's disease, inflammatory bowel disease, or recurrent pancreatitis, and use during the second half of pregnancy for patients unable to tolerate oral or tube feeding.[78] Of the cases reported, term deliveries occurred in 38% and an appropriately sized rather than growth-retarded infant was delivered in 78%. Safe and effective TPN has been used throughout the pregnancy, or in the first, second, or third trimesters.

In general, TPN is recommended for pregnant adolescents or women who are unable to eat or tolerate enteral feeding to such an extent that malnutrition is a high risk, and maternal weight gain and fetal growth and development are impaired. Although each case must be carefully evaluated for TPN use, pregnancy itself presents no contraindications. Women identified at high risk for malnutrition during pregnancy include the following:[78]

- Underweight prepregnancy condition—10% or more below ideal BMI
- Adolescents—the younger the age, the greater the nutritional risk
- Obstetric history—high parity with short intervals between births, repeated delivery of low-birth-weight infants
- Low socioeconomic status
- Neuropsychiatric problems—depression, bizarre diet, eating disorders
- Prolonged gastrointestinal tract dysfunction—inflammatory bowel disease, infectious gastrointestinal disease, surgical short bowel syndrome, diabetic gastroenteropathy, intractable hyperemesis gravidarum

Nutrition Assessment

High risk patients should be identified immediately from initial assessment procedures so that if TPN is indicated it can be provided early in the pregnancy to minimize the effects of malnutrition on the maternal and fetal course and outcome. Of course, the basic indicator for use of TPN is an inaccessible or inadequate gastrointestinal route for any reason. Some additional assessment markers for maternal malnutrition include the following factors:[48,78]

- Total weight loss of 6 kg or more, or failure to gain weight
- Weight loss greater than 1 kg/wk for 4 consecutive weeks

- Underlying hypermetabolic chronic disease, prepregnancy malnutrition
- Biochemical flags: severe hypoalbuminemia less than 20 gm/100 ml, persistent ketosis, negative nitrogen balance
- Anthropometric indicators: low weight-for-height (BMI), poor growth rate shown by insufficient weight gain, delayed growth of adolescent
- Intrauterine growth retardation of fetus

Nutritional Therapy Goals

After the initial nutrition assessment is made and analyzed by the obstetrical care team, with referral to the nutrition support services and its team of therapists with special training in enteral and parenteral modes of feeding, a decision is made by the patient, family, and obstetrician in conjunction with the special support team as to the use of parenteral feedings. Once the decision has been made to start this course of therapy, basic nutritional goals guide the individual therapy:[59]

1. *Normal rate of weight gain.* Based on the mother's prepregnancy weight-for-height and calculated BMI, if she was underweight, about a 20% gain over prepregnancy BMI is established as an initial total goal, and adjustments made according to ongoing monitoring and pattern of gain.
2. *Positive nitrogen balance.* This goal is normally achieved if the recommended kcalorie and protein allowances are provided. Positive nitrogen accrual is essential to support fetal growth and development as well as the expanded blood volume of the mother.
3. *Safe and effective vitamin and mineral therapy.* RDA standards provide a baseline, with adaptations to meet individual needs reflected by regular monitoring.
4. *Avoidance of metabolic complications.* When blood levels are consistently monitored and concentrations of nutrients in the parenteral solutions are adjusted appropriately, metabolic complications are minimal. Since blood volume and plasma concentrations are altered by the pregnancy, the goal is to achieve levels appropriate for normal pregnancy, not laboratory values observed in nonpregnant women.
5. *Avoidance of sepsis.* Strict TPN protocols, followed carefully by all members of the hospital nutrition support services team, are designed to avoid complicating infection through meticulous catheter care and accurately calculated and formulated TPN solutions.

Nutritional Therapy to Meet Goals

The TPN team. The insertion of the central line catheter is a surgical procedure performed by the physician, usually at the bedside, following strict aseptic technique to avoid infection. Placement of the line in a larger central vein allows more concentrated nutrient solutions to be administered, usually via subclavian vein to superior vena cava. The nurse on the TPN team has special training in care of the patient on TPN and is responsible for administering the formula. Together with the team physicians, the clinical nutritionist on the team assesses initial and ongoing nutritional needs, determines individual TPN formulas, calculates responses in BMI and appropriate formula component adjustments, and provides nutrition counseling and education as needed for the mother and family. The team pharmacist serves as consultant to all team members and mixes the solutions indicated.

The TPN prescription: nutrition requirements. Requirements for kcalories and protein, as well as vitamins and trace elements, are increased in pregnancy as described in previous chapters. The RDAs for oral intake serve as baseline guides for determining TPN needs, but may not be adequate for pregnancy complicated by poor nutrition and underlying medical problems. Also, since micronutrients in TPN solutions are fed directly into the blood circulation, effectively bypassing the intestinal mucosal absorption barrier, some of them must be adjusted from their variable oral intake needs.

1. *Energy.* The kcalories required per day are based on: (1) basal energy expenditure (BEE), calculated by the Harris-Benedict equation for women (see p. 422), which accounts for both height and weight, (2) physical activity, (3) any underlying meta-

bolic stress factor associated with malnutrition, disease, or trauma, and (4) the pregnancy. The RDA estimate of an additional 300 kcal/day during the second and third trimesters of the pregnancy is based on the calculated average additional total caloric requirement of pregnancy (80,000 kcal), in a healthy, well-nourished woman. A malnourished pregnant woman requiring TPN would need additional kcalories in the first trimester also, whereas a woman with reduced activity as a result of underlying disease or injury may require less pregnancy allowance throughout. Typical case reports of TPN in pregnancy indicate a need for approximately 2,000 and 3,000 kcal/day, depending on the mother's BMI and medical condition, to supply sufficient energy intake for adequate maternal weight gain with needed fat storage, and for optimal fetal growth and development.[34,78]

2. *Carbohydrate.* The simple sugar dextrose (glucose) is the energy source commonly used in TPN formulations. It is well-tolerated by obstetric patients and with the larger central line route more hypertonic 50% solutions may be used in mixing formulas. However, strict glucose control is required to minimize concern for gestational diabetes in high-risk women.

3. *Fat.* Fat emulsions are usually prescribed to provide additional kcalories as well as the essential fatty acid, linoleic acid. Currently used products made from soybean oil (Intralipid) or a combination of 50% soy oil and 50% safflower oil (Liposyn II) are well-tolerated and have shown no maternal or fetal side effects.[2] Fat emulsions are used daily, or at least three times a week, in TPN therapy during pregnancy, restricted to no more than 40% of the total kcalories, usually starting with 10% and gradually increasing to 40%, according to continuing evaluation of need and toleration.[34,52]

Some interesting studies are investigating the use of alternative structured triglycerides as lipid sources for both enteral and parenteral nutrition that combine advantages of long-chain triglycerides (essential fatty acids) and medium-chain triglycerides (rapid oxidation and clearance).[4b] Such structured triglycerides may potentially provide enhanced metabolic and immune function for hospitalized maternal patients with more critical underlying hypermetabolic disease or trauma.

4. *Amino acids.* The increased protein required during pregnancy is supplied in TPN therapy by crystalline amino acids in 8.5% solution, using such commercial sources as Aminosyn, Freamine III, and Travenol products. The daily protein requirement during pregnancy is approximately 1.0-1.5 gm/kg, but patients in moderate to severe metabolic stress may need up to 2 gm/kg, with constant monitoring to evaluate responses. However, to minimize the potential for preterm labor, no more than 2 gm/kg should be used.[64a] Ongoing assessment should include total caloric intake and nitrogen balance to evaluate protein utilization in meeting maternal and fetal tissue growth needs.

5. *Vitamins, trace minerals, and electrolytes.* Standard electrolyte packages and vitamin and trace element packages meeting the guidelines of the American Medical Association (AMA) and the U.S. Food and Drug Administration (FDA) are commonly used.[78] For the most part, these guidelines meet RDA standards as well, with individual adjustments according to assessment needs.

TPN solution. Based on the nutritional requirements above, basic TPN solutions are formulated to meet these needs. For example, a typical daily TPN solution designed to meet these nutrition goals may be approximately two liters of hypertonic dextrose solution, prepared in the hospital pharmacy by combining a liter each of 50% dextrose solution and 8.5% amino acid solution with added vitamin, trace mineral, and electrolyte packages as indicated. In addition, a daily fat emulsion is given starting with 0.5 L of 10% emulsion. This daily feeding would provide approximately 2,585 kcalories and 85 gm protein.[52a]

Parenteral nutrition in pregnancy is not without risk and added cost. However, a careful

TPN program, provided by a hospital's Nutrition Support Services team of specialists, now has more complete products available, strict protocols for their use, and standardized solutions with which to work. Using appropriate nutritional, clinical, and laboratory assessment before and during TPN use, this team of skilled specialists has greatly reduced potential for metabolic or infectious complications. TPN use in pregnancy is now accepted as lifesaving when it is indicated, and prudent use minimizes both complications and cost.

Summary

Management of pregnancy complications and special disease conditions in the mother requires special nutritional care, usually provided by a clinical nutrition specialist serving on an interdisciplinary special care team. The most commonly encountered pregnancy-induced complication is potential anemia. Normal hemoglobin alterations in pregnancy, including increased circulating blood volume and total red blood cell mass, often lead to **iron-deficiency anemia,** which may be compounded by blood loss from hemorrhage. The "iron cost" of a pregnancy is high, and negative balances can easily occur. A less common megaloblastic anemia is caused by folate deficiency.

The cause of **pregnancy-induced hypertension,** a complication of late pregnancy, is not clearly understood but is clearly known to be associated with malnutrition and inadequate prenatal care. Nutrition factors involve insufficient protein, kcalories, minerals, and vitamins to support the increased nutritional demands of the pregnancy. Prevention through good prenatal care and sound nutrition is essential for all mothers.

Preexisting **diabetes mellitus** and **gestational diabetes,** pose added risks and require special care during pregnancy. Successful therapy is based on: (1) sound metabolic principles of both pregnancy and diabetes management; (2) close attention to the interacting components of diet, insulin, and exercise; (3) tight constant control of blood glucose levels, avoiding both hyperglycemia and hypoglycemia as well as ketonuria through a euglycemic diet and self-monitoring; (4) a close schedule of care to

❖ ❖ ❖

CASE STUDY

Carol is a 26-year-old woman with PKU, identified by newborn screening and started on treatment by 8 days of age, who has been followed by PKU Clinic since that time. She graduated from college, teaches at an elementary school, and married 2 years ago. She and her husband Bill had premarital counseling around the reproductive concerns of women with PKU. They came to PKU Clinic to meet with the team about pregnancy planning. Carol's blood phenylalanine levels have been consistently 360-480 μmol/L (6-8 mg/100 ml). She and Bill understand that these levels are reasonable for adult management of the disorder but pose a risk of maldevelopment for a fetus. They plan a period of pregnancy preparation before they make a final decision about conception. If Carol can reduce her plasma phenylalanine levels to 180 μmol/L (3 mg/100 ml) or less and maintain these levels while also maintaining her weight, positive at-

titude, and energy, they will attempt conception. If she is not able to achieve this, she and Bill, as a couple, will consider other options for building a family.

On her now more rigorous diet, Carol has found it somewhat difficult to increase her daily ingestion of phenylalanine-free formula enough to lower her blood phenylalanine levels. She also needs to emphasize planning family menus, and maintaining her employment, her social life, and her sports activities. Bill is very supportive.

After 5 months of faithful efforts, Carol's blood phenylalanine levels have been 180 μmol/L (3 mg/100 ml) or less for 6 continuous weeks. She feels very healthy and her iron status is normal. She has established a relationship with an obstetrician who specializes in high-risk pregnancy management. After significant discussion, Carol and Bill decide to attempt conceiving a child.

meet changes throughout gestation; and (5) adjustments for birth and postpartum needs. A team of expert specialists can best supply these needs for special care.

Similar approaches are required for other preexisting chronic diseases, such as maternal PKU, as well as complicating weight management conditions such as obesity and the psychophysiologic starvation of anorexia nervosa and bulimia nervosa. In critical situations of underlying maternal disease or trauma with malnutrition, special management with total parenteral nutrition (TPN) will need to be used. In each case, therapeutic principles of care include: (1) full knowledge of the respective physiologic adaptations to pregnancy and the underlying pathology and metabolism involved; (2) expert team care with frequent evaluation during the course of pregnancy; and (3) personalized individual care.

REVIEW QUESTIONS

1. Describe two ways U.S. health care is changing and relate these approaches to management of high-risk pregnancies. Give examples from the chapter discussions.
2. Describe three pregnancy-induced complications in terms of the nature of each condition, incidence, cause, symptoms, and nutritional management.
3. Identify the types of diabetes complicating pregnancies. Describe the changing metabolism through the course of gestation—first half, second half, and postpartum—and the alterations in diabetes management, especially the euglycemic diet, to meet these changes.
4. Select any one of the following conditions and describe its nature, relation to the course of pregnancy, and management during pregnancy, giving reasons for the special care: maternal PKU, obesity, anorexia nervosa or bulimia nervosa.
5. Explain the probable cause for mental retardation and congenital anomalies in infants whose mothers have PKU.
6. Describe the special mode of feeding providing total parenteral nutrition (TPN) in pregnancy. What are some indications for its use, its nutritional goals, products and solutions used to reach these goals, and the roles of each member of the special TPN team in the care process?

LEARNING ACTIVITIES

1. Speak with a pregnant woman with IDDM who is well along in her pregnancy to develop a feel for the course of a typical day.
2. Drink a glass of beverage used to screen for gestational diabetes. What do you think of it?
3. A 24-year-old woman with PKU is at 10 weeks gestation. Her phenylalanine concentration is 120 μmol/L (2 mg/100 ml) and her tyrosine level is normal. She has gained 2 kg in weight during gestation. Assess her weight gain using the tables in Chapter 8, and describe her need for energy and protein at this stage of pregnancy.
4. Plan an appropriate menu for a hospitalized woman coping with proteinuric preeclampsia.

REFERENCES

1. Abernathy RP: Body mass index, determination and use, *J Am Diet Assoc* 91:843, 1991.
2. Acosta PB: Nutritional support of maternal phenylketonuria, *Semin Perinatol* 19:182-190, 1995.
3. American Dietetic Association/American Diabetic Association: *Exchange lists for meal planning,* Chicago, 1995, ADA/ADA.
4. American Public Health Association: *Healthy communities 2000,* model standards, Washington, DC, 1991, APHA.
4a. Amato P, Quercia RA: A historical perspective and review of the safety of lipid emulsion in pregnancy, *Nutr Clin Pract* 6:189, 1991.
4b. Bell SJ et al: Alternative lipid sources for enteral and parenteral nutrition: long- and medium-chain triglycerides, structural triglycerides, and fish oils, *J Am Diet Assoc* 91:74, 1991.
5. Belizan JM et al: The relationship between calcium intake and pregnancy-induced hypertension, up-to-date evidence, *Am J Obstet Gynecol* 158:898, 1988.
6. Brech DM et al: Arkansas dietitians' practices in educating the patient with gestational diabetes, *J Am Diet Assoc* 94(5):551, 1994.
7. Brinch M et al: Anorexia nervosa and motherhood: reproductive pattern and mothering behavior of 50 women, *Acta Psychiatr Scand* 77:611, 1988.
8. Bruch H: *Eating disorders, obesity, anorexia nervosa, and the person within,* New York, 1973, Basic Books.

9. Bruch H: *The golden cage, the enigma of anorexia nervosa*, Cambridge, Mass, 1978, Harvard University Press.

10. Cartier L, Clow CL, Lippman-Hand A et al: Prevention of mental retardation in offspring of hyperphenylalaninemic mothers, *Am J Public Health* 72:1385, 1985.

11. Committee on Genetics, American Academy of Pediatrics: Maternal phenylketonuria, *Pediatrics* 88:1284, 1991.

12. Davidson DC, Isherwood DM, Ireland JT et al: Outcome of pregnancy in a phenylketonuric mother after low phenylalanine diet introduced from the ninth week of pregnancy, *Eur J Pediatr* 137:45, 1981.

13. Drogari E, Beasley M, Smith L, Lloyd JK: Timing of strict diet in relation to fetal damage in maternal phenylketonuria, *Lancet* 2:927, 1987.

14. Dudrick S et al: Long-term total parenteral nutrition with growth, development, and positive nitrogen balance, *Surgery* 64:134, 1968.

15. Erick M: Hyperolfaction as a factor in hyperemesis gravidarum: considerations for nutritional management, *Perspect Appl Nutr* 2(2):3, 1994.

16. Erick M: *No more morning sickness: a survival guide for pregnant women*, New York, 1993, Penguin/Plume Books.

17. Erick M, Hahn NI: Battling morning (noon and night) sickness: new approaches for treating an age-old problem, *J Am Diet Assoc* 94(2):147, 1994.

18. Fagen C et al: Nutrition management in women with gestational diabetes mellitus: a review by ADA's Diabetes Care and Education dietetic practice group, *J Am Diet Assoc* 95(4):460, 1995.

19. Ferris AM, Reece EA: Nutritional consequences of chronic maternal conditions during pregnancy and lactation: lupus and diabetes, *Am J Clin Nutr* 59(suppl, 2S):465S, 1994.

20. Fisch RO et al: Children of fathers with phenylketonuria and international survey, *J Pediatr* 118:739, 1991.

21. Fisch RO, Tagatz G, Stassart, JP: Gestational carrier—a reproductive haven for offspring of mothers with phenylketonuria (PKU): an alternative therapy for maternal PKU, *J Inher Metab Dis* 16:957-961, 1993.

22. Gardiner RM: Transport of amino acids across the blood brain barrier: implications for treatment of maternal phenylketonuria, *J Inherit Metab Dis* 13:627, 1990.

23. Geracioti TD, Liddle RA: Impaired cholecystokinin secretion in bulimia nervosa, *N Engl J Med* 319:683, 1988.

24. Gull WW: Anorexia nervosa, *Trans Clin Soc* (Lond) 7:22, 1874.

25. Guyton AC, Hall JE: *Textbook of medical physiology*, ed 9, Philadelphia, 1996, WB Saunders.

26. Hanley WB, Bell L: Maternal phenylketonuria: finding and treating women before conception, *Can Med Assoc J* 126:1289, 1982.

27. Harlan WR et al: Secular trends in body mass in the United States, *Am J Epidemiol* 128:1065, 1988.

28. Hazuda HP et al: Effects of acculturation and socioeconomic status on obesity and diabetes in Mexican Americans, *Am J Epidemiol* 128:1289, 1988.

29. Herzog DB, Copeland PH: Bulimia nervosa—psyche and satiety, *N Engl J Med* 319:716, 1988.

30. Jovanovic-Peterson L, Peterson CM: Diabetes and pregnancy, *Curr Ther Endocrinol Metab* 3:276, 1988.

31. Jovanovic-Peterson L, Peterson CM: Dietary manipulation as a primary treatment strategy for pregnancy complicated by diabetes, *J Am Coll Nutr* 9:320, 1990.

32. Jovanovic-Peterson L, Peterson CM: Is exercise safe or useful for gestational diabetic women? *Diabetes* 40(Suppl 2):150, 1991.

33. Kahn HS et al: Race and weight changes in U.S. women, the roles of socioeconomic and marital status, *Am J Public Health* 81:319, 1991.

34. Kirby DF et al: Intravenous nutritional support

35. Kirkman HN: Projections of a rebound frequency of mental retardation from phenylketonuria, *Appl Res Ment Retard* 3:319, 1982.

36. Kitzmiller JL et al: Preconception care of diabetes, glycemia control prevents congenital anomalies, *JAMA* 265:731, 1991.

37. Koch R, Friedman EG, Wenz E et al: Maternal phenylketonuria, *J Inherit Metab Dis* 9(Suppl 2):159, 1986.

38. Koch R, Hanley W et al: A preliminary report of the collaborative study of maternal phenylketonuria in the United States and Canada, *J Inherit Metab Dis* 13:641, 1990.

39. Koch R et al: The North American Collaborative Study of maternal phenylketonuria, Status report 1993, *Am J Dis Child* 147:1224-1230, 1993.

40. Koch R, Levy HL et al: The International Collaborative Study of Maternal Phenylketonuria: status report 1994, *Acta Paediatr* (suppl) 407: 111, 1994.

41. Kousen M: Treatment of nausea and vomiting in pregnancy, *Am Family Physician* 48:1279, 1994.

42. Krey SH et al: Eating disorders, the clinical dietitian's changing role, *J Am Diet Assoc* 89:41, 1989.

43. Krywawych S et al: Theoretical and practical aspects of preventing fetal damage in women with phenylketonuria. In Schaub J, Van hoof F, Vis HL, editors: *Inborn errors of metabolism,* Nestle' Nutrition Workshop Series #24, New York, 1991, Raven Press.

44. Kuczmarski RJ et al: Increasing prevalence of overweight among US adults: the National Health and Nutrition Examination Surveys, 1960 to 1991, *JAMA* 272(3):205, 1994.

45. Lakoff K, Felman J: Anorexia nervosa associated with pregnancy, *Obstet Gynecol* 39:699, 1972.

46. Larson BJ: Relationship of family communication patterns to Eating Disorder Inventory scores in adolescent girls, *J Am Diet Assoc* 91:1065, 1991.

47. Lenke RR, Levy HL: Maternal phenylketonuria and hyperphenylalaninemia: an international survey of the outcomes of untreated and treated pregnancies, *N Engl J Med* 303:1202, 1980.

48. Levine M, Esser D: Total parenteral nutrition for the treatment of severe hyperemesis gravidarum, maternal nutritional effects and fetal outcome, *Obstet Gynecol* 72:102, 1988.

49. Levy H et al: Paternal phenylketonuria, *J Pediatr* 118:741, 1991.

50. Levy HL, Waisbren SE, et al: Maternal mild hyperphenylalaninemia: an international survey of offspring outcome, *Lancet* 344:1589, Dec 10, 1994.

51. Lowitzer AC: Maternal phenylketonuria: cause for concern among women with PKU, *Res Dev Disabil* 8:1, 1987.

52. Luder AS, Greene CL: Maternal phenylketonuria and hyperphenylalaninemia: implications for medical practice in the United States, *Am J Obstet Gynecol* 161:1102, 1989.

52a. MacBurney M, Wilmore DW: Parenteral nutrition in pregnancy. In Rombeau JL and Caldwell MD, editors: *Parenteral nutrition,* Philadelphia, 1986, WB Saunders.

53. Manson J et al: Body weight and mortality among women, *N Engl J Med* 333(11):677, 1995.

54. Martin DW et al: *Harper's review of biochemistry,* ed 18, Los Altos, Calif, 1981, Lange.

55. Matalon R et al: Maternal PKU Collaborative Study: the effect of nutrient intake on pregnancy outcome, *J Inher Metab Dis* 14:371, 1991.

56. Matalon R et al: Maternal PKU Collaborative Study: pregnancy outcome and postnatal head growth, *J Inher Metab Dis* 17:353-355, 1994.

57. Maternal PKU Collaborative Study: *Maternal PKU Collaborative Study Protocol,* 1992.

58. National Academy of Sciences, Institute of Medicine: Nutrition during pregnancy, Washington, DC, 1990, National Academy Press.

59. Nelson MS, Jovanovic L: Pregnancy, diabetes, and Jewish dietary laws, *J Am Dietet Assoc* 87(8): 1054, 1987.

59a. Parenteral and Enteral Nutrition Team: *Parenteral and enteral nutrition manual,* Ann Arbor, Mich, 1988, University of Michigan Hospitals.

60. Preventing birth defects from phenylketonuria: the American Public Health Association Policy statement, *Am J Public Health* 80:228, 1990.

61. Rohr FJ et al: The New England Maternal PKU Project: prospective study of untreated and treated pregnancies and their outcomes, *J Pediatr* 110:391, 1986.

62. Rohr J: Maternal phenylketonuria: a new challenge in the dietary treatment of phenylketonuria, *Topics Clin Nutr* 2:44, 1987.

63. Rouse et al: Maternal phenylketonuria pregnancy outcome: a preliminary report of facial dysmorphology and major malformations, *J Inherit Metab Dis* 13:289, 1990.

64. Sanders SL, Greenspoon JS: New protocal to manage hyperemesis gravidarum (letter), *J Am Diet Assoc* 94(12):1367, 1994.

64a. Scott J et al: *Danforth's obstetrics and gynecology,* ed 6, Philadelphia, 1990, JB Lippincott.

65. Sharbaugh CO, ed: *Call to action: better nutrition for mothers, children, and families,* Washington, DC, 1991, National Center for Education in Maternal and Child Health.

66. Smith I, Erdohazi M, Macartney FJ et al: Fetal damage despite low phenylalanine diet introduced after conception in a phenylketonuric woman. *Lancet* 1:17, 1979.

67. Smith I, Glossop J et al: Fetal damage due to maternal phenylketonuria: effects of dietary treatment and maternal phenylalanine concentrations around the time of conception, *J Inherit Metab Dis* 13:651, 1990.

68. Steiger H et al: Relationship of body-image distortion to sex-role identification, irrational cognitions, and body weight in eating disordered families, *J Clin Psychol* 45:61, 1989.

69. Stein DM: The prevalence of bulimia: a review of the empirical research, *J Nutr Ed* 23;205, 1991.

70. Stevens-Simon C et al: Relationship of self-reported prepregnant weight and weight gain during pregnancy to maternal body habitus and age, *J Am Diet Assoc* 92:85, 1992.

71. Update: New exchange lists offer flexibility in meal-planning, *J Am Diet Assoc* 95(10):1088, 1995.

72. US Department of Health and Human Services, Public Health Service: *Healthy people 2000: National health promotion and disease prevention objectives*, PHS Pub. No. 79-55071, Washington, DC, 1990, Government Printing Office.

73. US Department of Health and Human Services, Public Health Service: *The surgeon general's report on nutrition and health*, PHS Pub No 88-50210, Washington, DC, 1988, Government Printing Office.

74. Waisbren SE et al: Psychological factors in maternal phenylketonuria: prevention of unplanned pregnancies, *Am J Public Health* 81:299, 1991.

75. Waisbren SE et al: Psychosocial factors in maternal phenylketonuria: women's adherence to medical recommendations. *Am J Pub Health* 85:1636-1641, 1995.

76. Williams SR: Nutrition and diet therapy, ed 8, St. Louis, 1997, Mosby.

77. Witte DJ et al: Relationship of self-concept to nutrient intake and eating patterns in young women, *J Am Diet Assoc* 91:1068, 1991.

78. Wolk RA, Rayburn WF: Parenteral nutrition in obstetric patients, *Nutr Clin Pract* 5:139, 1990.

79. Yankauer A: What infant mortality tells us, *Am J Pub Health* 80(6):653, 1990.

10

The Pregnant Adolescent: Special Concerns

Bonnie S. Worthington-Roberts
Jane Mitchell Rees

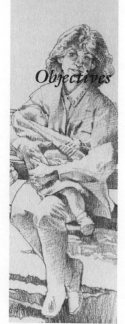

Objectives

+++

After completing this chapter, the student will be able to:

✓ *Describe recent trends in pregnancy rate and birth rate among adolescents in the United States.*

✓ *Define recent data on maternal mortality and morbidity among pregnant adolescents in the United States.*

✓ *Identify major concerns related to the offspring of adolescents.*

✓ *Outline major nutrition concerns related to pregnant adolescents.*

✓ *Suggest a method of predicting appropriate weight gain for pregnant adolescents.*

✓ *Describe appropriate characteristics of the nutrition component of comprehensive programs for pregnant adolescents.*

Introduction

Adolescent pregnancy is a topic of major concern to obstetricians, pediatricians, and other health care professionals. In 1990, there were an estimated 1 million pregnancies and 521,626 births to U.S. women ages 15 to 19 years (Fig. 10-1). During 1990, pregnancy rates ranged from 56 per 1,000 women ages 15 to 19 years (North Dakota) to 111 per 1,000 (Georgia). Birth rates ranged from 33 per 1,000 women (New Hampshire) to 81 per 1,000 (Mississippi).

In most states, birth rates increased from 1980 to 1990 because declines in abortion rates generally exceeded those of pregnancy rates. However, birth rates increased significantly in 29 states and Washington, D.C. Overall, despite national goals to reduce teenage pregnancy in the United States, pregnancy and birth rates exceeded those in most developed countries.[6,7]

The personal and societal impact of teen pregnancy in the United States is enormous; an estimated 86% of teenage pregnancies are unin-

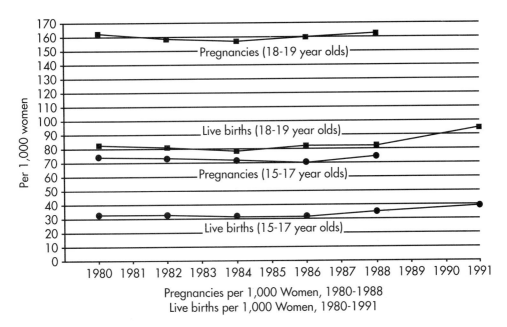

FIG. 10-1 Teen pregnancy.
From National Center for Health Statistics.

tended. From 1985 to 1990, the public costs related to teenage childbearing totaled $120.3 billion. Of this amount, an estimated $48.1 billion could have been saved if each birth had been postponed until the mother was at least 20 years old. Family planning services are essential for reducing teenage pregnancy.

Pregnancy in the teenage woman is especially distressing because she often demonstrates a variety of serious health and social problems. These basic problems may be further complicated by psychological, educational, nutritional and vocational difficulties, all of which need attention if the stress of pregnancy is to be minimized.

The pregnant adolescent is viewed as a high-risk patient, who is highly susceptible to suboptimal pregnancy outcome. Identification of needy pregnant adolescents and management of their problems and concerns should be a primary goal of community health organizations. Interdisciplinary programs designed to meet the adolescent's needs and those of her infant have operated with some success during the past two decades; such programs have served to improve prenatal conditions and prepare young mothers to cope with the problems of parenthood under adverse circumstances. Guidance in obtaining sufficient nourishment is an important component of successful programs for pregnant teenagers, and sincere efforts by skilled clinicians can help to improve the overall nutritional support available to both mother and child. Issues in adolescent pregnancy that influence nutritional well-being are shown on p. 303. These issues must be assessed and addressed in intervention strategies.

SCOPE OF THE PROBLEM
Demographic Considerations

A variety of factors are believed to be responsible for adolescent pregnancies. Significant among these factors are the following:

1. There was a sudden rise in the teenage population as an aftermath of the post-World War II "baby boom." From 1950 to 1969 the number of youths 15 to 19

years of age in the United States increased from 10.6 to 18.6 million. The percentage of the population who are teenagers has more recently begun to level off, and by the 1980s it had started to decrease.

2. Among females there was an apparent declining age of maturation. Tanner[97] observed that the age of maturation in the United States gradually dropped from about 14.25 years in 1900 to about 12.5 years in 1955. The average age of **menarche** is now 12.5 years of age and appears to have stabilized. Tanner et al. claim that the major factor responsible for the decline in age of menarche is an improvement in nutrition and health, which leads to an increase in rate of physical growth.

3. An increase in sexual freedom has occurred. By 1988 around 75% of young women had had sexual intercourse by the time they were 18 to 19, and 85% of young men were sexually active by age 19. It is generally believed that the changing attitudes of today's youth coupled with the so-called sexual revolution supported by the media have contributed in some degree to high numbers of adolescent pregnancies in all cultural, racial, and socioeconomic groups. These pregnancies occur in spite of the increasing availability of contraceptives, which are often ignored or are used ineffectually by teenagers.

Abortion is not considered an option by many teens. They often unrealistically feel the child will fill gaps in their lives, which otherwise lack long-term close relationships and future goals (Table 10-1).

Once they have been pregnant, adolescents often continue to reproduce. Continued efforts aimed both at delaying early sexual experience among adolescents and at encouraging the use of contraception among sexually active adolescents are necessary for further reduction in teenage pregnancy and birth rates in the United States.

Health professionals help to decrease the rates of unintended pregnancy and abortion as well as sexually transmitted diseases when they are able to contact adolescents. Counseling them about their sexuality, encouraging the use of effective contraceptive methods, and helping young people to develop positive self-images enables them to practice healthy sexual behaviors and make good decisions about reproduction.

Educational efforts to offset the human and economic costs that accompany adolescent pregnancies face formidable barriers. Marketing is one issue. Sexual attractiveness is coupled with everything from independence to worldly sophistication and pervades every aspect of commercial advertising. Sex gets the attention of adults and teenagers alike but adolescents are especially stimulated, since they are struggling with issues of identity and self-esteem. Another barrier to teenage pregnancy prevention is the concern that education outside the home addressing aspects of sexuality is inappropriate and serves to encourage early sexual activity.

Efforts to reduce teen pregnancy usually have taken one of two approaches: sex education programs aimed at knowledge, attitudes, and behavior (including abstinence); and contraceptive services. Recent studies show that a combination of both approaches is more successful at preventing pregnancy than either used alone.[35]

Most junior and senior high schools now offer sexuality education classes. Unfortunately, nearly half of teens initiate sexual intercourse before they ever attend the classes. Sexuality education programs generally are credited with increasing knowledge levels, and some have shown increased use of contraceptives when teenagers become sexually active. The impact of these programs on preventing pregnancy has been more difficult to measure.

Pregnancy prevention programs are becoming more targeted to respond to trends in reproductive behavior. The Federal Title X Family Planning Program's priorities include expanded clinic services and outreach to low-income women, adolescents, and persons at high risk of unintended pregnancy or infection with sexually transmitted diseases (STDs) who are not now receiving family planning services.

An emphasis on culturally relevant prevention strategies for black and Hispanic teens will be necessary to reduce the higher prevalence of pregnancies and births in these populations. Advocates are calling for comprehensive programs that include contraceptive education, risk reduction strategies for STDs and human immunode-

TABLE 10-1   Expectations vs. Reality

Expectation	Reality
Life with baby	
Life with baby will be wonderful.	Life with baby is not wonderful.
Baby will meet their emotional needs.	Baby doesn't meet their emotional needs. Baby may interfere with their own need-meeting.
They won't be lonely any more.	They may be even more lonely with the demands and limitations of baby.
Parenting	
Parenting is easy (based on their babysitting experiences). They will manage.	Parenting is not easy.
Others will help them: partner, family, etc.	Many are parenting alone. The 24-hour responsibility is overwhelming. There are few resources for teenage parents. They are not ready to accept help, education, role modeling, etc.
Self-esteem	
Self-esteem will increase with pregnancy and parenthood. They now have a role.	Self-conscious about body changes. Society disapproves. Self-esteem decreases. Baby takes attention away from them.
Relationships	
Her parents will be upset, then supportive. (They will care for the teen mom and her baby.)	Some have family support. Many parents reject them or do not support on their terms.
Relationship with partner will improve or he will come back.	Some live common-law or are married. Relationship with partner is often strained. He frequently leaves.
Friendships will continue as they are.	Life is different from peers. They become isolated from friends.
Finances	
Somebody will provide welfare.	Welfare, is not sufficient. They are unable to manage. Many are not interested in learning to budget.
Some plan to be self-sufficient (i.e., finish school, get a job).	Self-sufficiency takes a long time. Often they don't have energy and/or the organizational skills to continue or reenter school/work.
Housing	
Want to live on their own.	Vacancy rate is less than 1% in Toronto.
Want to find market housing at an affordable rent.	Much of what is available in housing market is inappropriate for young women and babies.
	Landlords are biased against single mothers, children, and tenants on welfare. Therefore housing is even less available.
	Market rent is impossible to manage.
Goals	
Motherhood will make life meaningful.	Life is no more meaningful.
Tend not to have long-term goals.	Difficult to follow through, even on short-term goals.

From Browne C, Urback M: Pregnant adolescents: expectations vs reality, *Canad J Pub Health* June 1989.

ficiency virus (HIV) infection, and access to health services, as well as encouragement for continuing postsecondary education and obtaining job training skills.

There also is growing attention to the role of males in preventing pregnancy. Pregnancy prevention has benefited from programs aimed at increasing condom use among males to prevent STDs and HIV. As males have increased use of condoms, risks for STDs and pregnancies have decreased.

Vincent, Clearie, and Schluchter[52] described a community-based program designed to prevent teen pregnancy. It involves the participation of multiple institutions and groups including schools, clergy, parents, and the media to create a supportive milieu for teens who must face decisions about their sexual activity. The school program provides education to ensure that adolescents have the knowledge and skills necessary to say "no" or, if deciding to say "yes," the knowledge and skills to protect themselves from becoming pregnant. The success of this program in reducing adolescent pregnancy is striking when compared with the control

counties, the nonintervention half of the county, and historical trends (Fig. 10-2). By themselves, the individual components of the program were not innovative. The innovation came from the sum of the parts: a well-coordinated and community-wide commitment to resolving a priority problem of common interest.

Healthy People 2000 calls for a 30% reduction in pregnancies among females ages 17 and younger, reducing to no more than 30% the proportion of all pregnancies that are unintended, and increasing to at least 90% the proportion of sexually active, unmarried persons ages 19 and younger who use contraception, especially combined method contraception that both effectively prevents pregnancy and provides protection against disease.

Based on current trends, meeting these objectives will be a challenge. The prospects for improvement are tied to society's ability to increase the life options available to youth. By having incentives to postponing pregnancy, teens will be able to choose alternatives to early parenthood that will allow them to be capable, responsible parents when adults.[35]

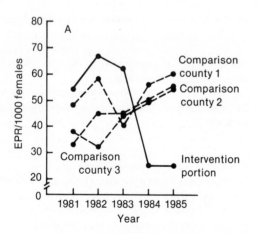 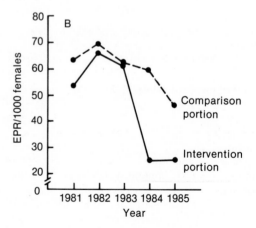

FIG. 10-2 **A,** Age-specific estimated pregnancy rates (EPRs) for the intervention portion of a South Carolina county and three other comparison South Carolina counties for females aged 14 to 17 years. **B,** Age-specific estimated pregnancy rates for intervention and comparison portions of a South Carolina county for females aged 14 to 17 years. EPR = live births plus fetal deaths plus induced abortions per 1000 female population.

From Vincent ML, Clearie AF, Schluchter MD: Reducing adolescent pregnancy through school and community-based education, *JAMA* 257:3382, 1987.

Adolescent Maternal Mortality

Maternal mortality rates for women under 20 years of age have declined more rapidly than for any other age group. In fact, current data indicate that women in this youngest category have the lowest maternal mortality rate of any age group in the United States (Table 10-2); this is true not only for whites but for blacks and other racial groups as well.

Reasons for the decline in adolescent maternal mortality in the United States are unclear. Improved access to prenatal care may be part of the explanation.[15] Among young women who did not survive the childbearing process, socioeconomic factors appear to have played a significant role. Most often the deaths were preventable. It is possible, however, that mortality among pregnant adolescents occurs largely in unsupervised settings; some of these deaths may go unreported. Although deaths from inappropriately performed abortions are less frequent than ever before, such phenomena still occur.

Maternal Morbidity

A number of problems have been described as common and significant for pregnant adolescents. Although psychosocial problems are of major significance, physical complications are also of concern. The most commonly mentioned complications include pregnancy-induced hypertension (PIH), **uterine dysfunction,** contracted pelvis, premature labor, prolonged labor, cephalopelvic disproportion, vagi-

nal infection, vaginal laceration, and heart disease. The most consistent high-risk characteristic, noted by virtually every observer of adolescent pregnancies, is PIH. Both preeclampsia and eclampsia occur with greater frequency in teenagers than in older women.

Although PIH may not seriously compromise the health of the infant, permanent damage may be done to the afflicted mother. The early (and often repeated) insult of PIH on the cardiovascular-renal system of a young woman may contribute substantially to the increased severity of PIH with subsequent pregnancies and the appearance of chronic disease later in life. Since pregnant teenagers are now known to be statistically destined to have more than the average number of pregnancies, the potential for repeated PIH is great, and the probability of development of long-term cardiovascular damage is sizable. It is obvious, therefore, that if the debilitating effects of frequent pregnancies are added to the nutritional burden already carried by the growing adolescent, the conditions are established for a rapid and irreversible slide from simple PIH to renal damage and hypertensive disease.

The Offspring

The outcome of a pregnancy cannot be measured in terms of maternal health alone. It is mandatory also to consider carefully the fate of the infant, and it is here that the greatest risks associated with adolescent pregnancy become glaringly apparent. Examination of the infant and perinatal mortality and morbidity in adolescent pregnancies strikingly points up the continuing excessive loss of human life in the form of pregnancy wastage. The majority of this wastage has preventable components, found mainly preconceptionally and/or prenatally.

In considering the offspring of adolescent mothers a major concern relates to the postnatal environment of the infant, especially if the infant was unplanned, unwanted, and is without the support of a parent who is knowledgeable in child care and home management. This set of adverse circumstances often prevails, and many times, a long list of related problems can also be developed. In dealing with the teenage mother, therefore, attention must be given not only to

TABLE 10-2 **Maternal Mortality Rates per 100,000 Births by Age: United States**

Age (yr)	Deaths
Under 20	6
20-24	7
25-29	7
30-34	9
35-39	18
40-44	42

From *The contraception report,* vol 3, no 2, 1992, p 5.

her medical, obstetrical, and nutritional problems but also to the wide range of social, financial, legal, educational, vocational, and other difficulties that exist. It is a well-known fact that success in management of the nutritional defects apparent in a pregnant adolescent *cannot* be achieved unless the health care professional or team is able to define and attend to the total needs of the patient through the establishment of priorities and definition of a systematic approach to optimizing the patient's circumstance.

Mercer[28] describes in *Nursing Care of Parents at Risk* the needs of parents who are "premature." She focuses on their strengths and weaknesses and points to these traits that seem to lead to successful management of an unplanned pregnancy during the already difficult period of adolescence. This is a useful resource for any clinician needing guidance in counseling pregnant teenagers and their partners. A brief summary of the characteristics of young mothers

---

❖

CHARACTERISTIC PROFILE OF THE ADOLESCENT GIRL WHOSE PREGNANCY OUTCOME IS BEST

1. Past experience in caring for, and positive feelings about, infants.
2. A supportive mate.
3. A mother who is able to acknowledge her capabilities and independence.
4. Level of hostility that is not excessive; for example, her verbal and nonverbal hostile expressions do not exceed expressed rewards and pleasures in mothers.
5. Family members available for support.
6. A cognitive level of functioning that permits recognition of and understanding of her infant's behavior.
7. An emotional level of maturity sufficient to delay her own gratification for the gratification of her infant and a willingness to do so.
8. Perception that her infant is above average in comparison to other infants.

Modified from Mercer RT: *Nursing care of patients at risk*, Thorofare, NJ, 1977, Charles B Slack.

---

who adapt best to pregnancy and whose infants do best in the early months of life is provided in box below.

IS BIOLOGICAL IMMATURITY OR "ENVIRONMENTAL" STRESS MORE CONTRIBUTORY TO PREGNANCY OUTCOME?

It has long been assumed that immature women probably have more low-birth-weight and preterm outcomes than older women because of their immature anatomy and physiology. However, a number of studies over the past 15 years have refuted this concept.[12,16,25,40] When researchers have controlled for sociodemographic factors, minimal differences in pregnancy outcomes have been reported between teens and women in their twenties. These observations have suggested that factors *associated with* young age, such as poverty, poor education, unmarried status and inadequate prenatal care, were more powerful influences on outcomes than maternal age. *There is no question about the relevance of these sociodemographic factors.*

A recent report, however, has reopened this controversy about biology vs. the environment. Fraser et al,[10] reporting in the New England Journal of Medicine, specifically addressed this question. Vital statistics from the state of Utah were used, providing data on 134,088 white mothers 13 to 24 years old. These mothers had delivered singleton, first-born children between 1970 and 1990. Age of mother and sociodemographic variables were examined. Among white married mothers who had educational levels appropriate for their ages and who received adequate prenatal care, teenage mothers (13 to 17 years of age) had a significantly higher risk than mothers age 20 to 24 years of delivering an infant who had low birth weight, or was premature or small-for-gestational age. Older teenage mothers (18 and 19 years of age) also had a significant increase in these risks. The researchers concluded that in white, middle-class women, a younger age conferred an increased risk of adverse pregnancy outcomes, which was independent of important sociodemographic factors.

They speculate that two features of biologic immaturity could play a role in this relationship: a young gynecologic age (defined as conception within 2 years after menarche) and the effect of an adolescent becoming pregnant before her own growth has ceased.

Growth of Young Mothers and the Competition for Nutrients

Growth patterns and the timing of menarche vary considerably from one young woman to another. The general sequence of events is similar but is not directly related to chronological age. Most young women begin their adolescent growth spurt between the ages of 10 and 14.[47] Peak height velocity is achieved within the following few years and menarche occurs after that time. Therefore by the time a young woman is capable of reproduction, her rate of growth has slowed considerably. It is to be emphasized, however, that the timing and levels of growth that occur in individual women vary significantly.[51]

Hence, do pregnant teens continue to grow? It has been tempting to conclude that if so, not much. Accurately assessing growth in stature during pregnancy is not an easy chore. Usual measures may underestimate it because of the tendency for compression of the spine and postural changes during pregnancy to cause apparent "shrinkage." A well-designed study by Scholl et al,[42] however, provided useful information. These researchers used a knee-height measuring device to track lower leg length during pregnancy in a group of teenagers in New Jersey. In this study, maternal growth during adolescent pregnancy was present in approximately 50% of the young women (both primiparas and multiparas). After controlling for a number of variables, like length of gestation, black ethnicity, smoking, prepregnant body mass index and weight gain, infants born to the young mothers who were growing weighed 156g less than infants of teens who were not growing; this was despite a significantly greater weight gain and less smoking.

Scholl et al. also examined the mothers themselves.[44] Body composition differences associated with maternal growth did not arise until after 28 weeks of gestation, when the growing teenagers continued to accrue fat, had larger gestational weight gains and retained more of this weight postpartum. Even so, these mothers had smaller babies. The researchers concluded that "despite an apparently sufficient weight gain and the accumulation of nutritional stores during pregnancy, young growing women appeared not to mobilize stores after 28 weeks' gestation reserving them instead for their own continued development."

This brings up the issue of competition for nutrients between mothers and fetuses. It has been proposed that fetal growth may be retarded in young mothers who are still growing since both are seeking a potentially limited source of nutrients; diminished placental transfer may account for this phenomenon.[46] Naeye[31] suggested this more than 15 years ago when he reported that fetuses grew more slowly in 10 to 16 year olds than in older women. Frisancho et al.[11] observed the same thing in a population of 400 Peruvian adolescents. Since a recent study in Black adolescents provided data to counter the notion of maternal/fetal competition for nutrients, this area remains controversial.[48] Biologically, however, it makes sense that available nutrients will only go so far. A fetus may reasonably suffer (in an immature mother) when the mother's needs are substantial.

In addition to considering growth in height and weight, maturational changes that continue after adult height has been achieved should be noted. A relevant example in the skeletal system are the bones of the pelvic girdle. Unlike growth in stature that decreases in rate following the menarche, the birth canal continues to grow slowly but continuously into late adolescence (Fig. 10-3). Those who mature earlier have smaller and less mature pelvises than do late maturers. The fact that women of low gynecologic ages have smaller pelvic basins may contribute to the higher incidence of physical complications during pregnancy in this group.[29] Whether a pregnancy at a young gynecologic age interferes with further development remains an interesting research question.

Weight Gain

As previously mentioned, low gestational weight gains have been associated with higher

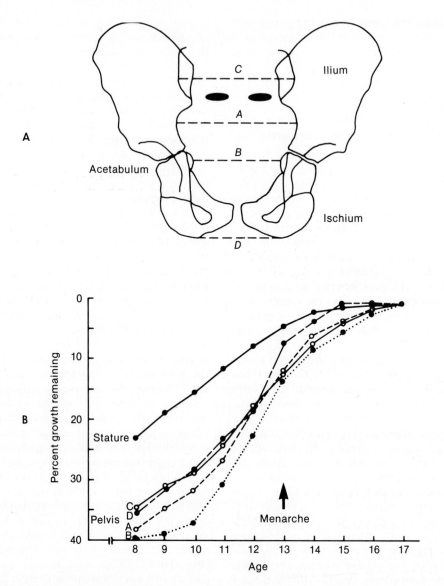

FIG. 10-3   **A,** Location of the four transverse measurements made of pelvic basin. All measurements were determined perpendicular to central axis of pelvis. **B,** Comparative slower growth of pelvic birth canal as compared with stature between ages 8 and 18. *Arrow,* Average menarcheal age of 12.7 years in this population sample of US adolescents.

From Moerman ML: Growth of the birth canal in adolescent girls, *Am J Obstet Gynecol* 143:528, 1982.

rates of low birth weight, small-for-gestational age infants, and prematurity, whereas higher gains reduce the risk of these adverse outcomes.[18]

In studies of weight gain in pregnant adolescents, continued gain in weight resulting from growth has been demonstrated by implication. That is, adolescents gain a mean of about 35 to 40 lbs, at the upper edge of the range of total weight gain provisionally recommended in the 1990 Institution of Medicine, National Academy of Sci-

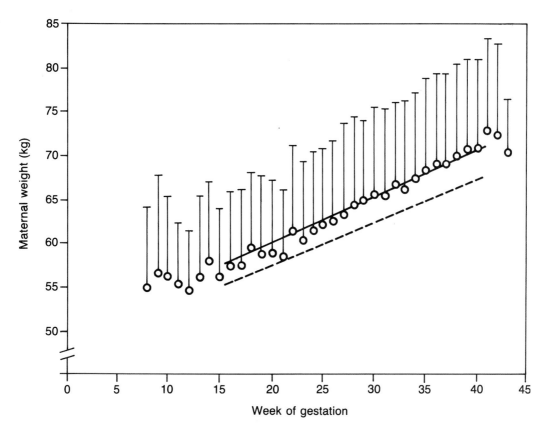

FIG. 10-4 Rate of weight gain of adolescent mothers of 3,000-4,000 gm (—) and <3,000 gm (--) infants described by regression statistics from 15 to 40 weeks' gestation (number of mothers in weeks 8 to 15 of pregnancy and after 40 too small to include in analysis). Means of weekly weight measures are shown for the total study population (○) and standard deviation (T). Symbols represent between 6 and 313 measures at a given week.

From Rees JM, Endres J, Worthington-Roberts BS: Position of the American Dietetic Association: teenage pregnancy and nutritional risks, *J Am Diet Assoc* 89:900, 1989.

ences report, *Nutrition during Pregnancy.*[18] A graph of a typical pattern of gain observed clinically is shown by the solid circles in Fig. 10-4.[37] Indeed it has been suggested that the amount usually gained at their stage of development be included in weight gain recommendations.[39] Data compiled from longitudinal studies define the amounts of expected weight gain in a particular postmenarcheal year (Table 10-3).

As discussed earlier, there is evidence that gestational weight gain in young, still-growing adolescents may have a greater impact on infant size than in older adolescents or mature women.

This makes sense from the standpoint that both mother and fetus are growing and if both are provided for, adequate growth of both can and may occur (see box p. 302). The pattern of gestational weight gain also appears to significantly affect fetal growth. In nearly 800 adolescents, early inadequate weight gain increased the risk of small-for-gestational age infants despite adequate total gains. Also, inadequate gains after 24 weeks of gestation increased the risk of preterm delivery in the same population.[44,43,15,14,49]

Until more formal guidelines are available on the amount and pattern of gestational weight

TABLE 10-3   *Approximate Increments in Weight of Postmenarcheal Women*

Postmenarcheal Year	lb	kg
1	10.12	4.6
2	6.16	2.8
3	2.42	1.1
4 and 5	1.76	0.8

✤

A SUGGESTED METHOD OF ESTIMATING APPROPRIATE WEIGHT GAIN FOR INDIVIDUAL PREGNANT TEENS

Add the following together:
1. The expected weight increase as a result of normal (nonpregnant) growth during the ninth month of pregnancy. (The weight increase will range from 7.7 lb during the first year after menarche to 1.3 lb 4 years after menarche.)   _____
2. A weight increase to support pregnancy (approximately 20% above standard weight for height using NCHS tables for normal weight adolescents).   _____
3. If underweight, a weight increase to achieve an average weight for height using NCHS tables.   _____

TOTAL ESTIMATED WEIGHT GAIN   _____

gain in young adolescents, use of the Institute of Medicine guidelines of 1990 seems appropriate.[18] It should be mentioned, however, that there are some who question the legitimacy of one of the recommendations, that is, young adolescents should strive for weight gains at the upper end of the newly recommended ranges during pregnancy.[18] The basis of this recommendation seems to be that there is a higher risk of young adolescents having smaller infants. The fact of the matter is that younger adolescents have smaller infants for a number of reasons; these include low income, lack of education, small prepregnancy size, cigarette smoking, cervical infections and psychosocial stress. Increased weight gain during pregnancy may compensate for their smaller prepregnancy size but may do little to ameliorate the adverse effects of cigarette smoking, cervical infections and psychosocial stress on their infants.[27]

In 1983, Garn and Petzold said, "Although it is true that larger weight gains during pregnancy do lead to increased birthweights and a lower incidence of prematurity, we do not urge a large weight gain for teenagers because this will lead to an elevated weight and an excess in body fat." Since the incidence of obesity has gradually increased in adolescents over time, this point may be well taken. This is especially true of high weight gains in young teens, which are associated with more macrosomic infants, more cesarean sections and more situations of birth asphyxia.[27]

Adolescent girls often question the need for a weight gain that exceeds the size of the baby. Their concern about body weight and body image is often substantial. Clear discussion of the components of weight gain is a desirable part of the health care process; visual materials are often helpful. Negative attitudes about weight gain were recently found to be most common among heavier adolescents and in those without family support.[50]

According to Story and Alton,[51] the promotion of appropriate weight gain patterns in pregnant adolescents may be facilitated by jointly setting weight gain goals with the adolescent, provision of a personal weight gain chart, involvement of family members and partner, and education regarding the importance of gestational weight gain to infant health. Monitoring of weight gain through pregnancy is appropriate and intervention with specific strategies when problems arise.

NUTRITIONAL CONCERNS

Adolescence is a time of great physical growth and development; to support its normal progress, substantial nutritional input is required (see box on p. 303). During adolescence,

ISSUES IN ADOLESCENT PREGNANCY THAT INFLUENCE NUTRITIONAL WELL-BEING

Acceptance of the pregnancy

Desire to carry out successful pregnancy

Acceptance of responsibility (even if child is to be relinquished)

Clarification of identity as mother separate from her own mother

Realistic acceptance versus fantasy and idealization

Food resources

Family meals (timing, quantity, quality, responsibility)

Self-reliance

School lunch

Fast-food outlets

Socially related eating

Food assistance (WIC programs and others)

Mobilization of all resources

Body image

Degree of acceptance of an adult body

Maturity in facing bodily changes throughout pregnancy

Living situation

Acceptance by living partners and extended family

Role expectations of living partners

Financial support

Facilities and resources

Ethnic group (religious, cultural, and social patterns)

Emancipation versus dependency

Support system vs. isolation

Relationship with the father of child

Presence or absence of father

Quality of relationship

Influence on decision making

Contribution to resources

Influence on mother's nutritional habits and general lifestyle

Understanding of physiologic processes

Tolerance of physical changes in pregnancy and physical needs of mother and child

Influence on child feeding

Peer relationships

Support from friends

Influence on nutritional knowledge and attitudes

Influence on general lifestyle

Nutritional state

Weight-for-height proportion

Maturational state

Tissue stores of nutrients

Reproductive and contraceptive history

Physical health

History of dietary patterns and nutritional status, including weight-losing schemes

Present eating habits

Complications of pregnancy (nausea and vomiting)

Substance use

Activity patterns

Need for intensive remediation

Prenatal care

Initiation of and compliance with prenatal care

Dependability of supporting resources

Identification of risk factors

Nutritional attitude and knowledge

Prior attitude toward nutrition

Understanding of role of nutrition in pregnancy

Knowledge of foods as sources of nutrients and of nutrients needed by the body

Desire to obtain adequate nutrition

Ability to obtain adequate nutrition and to control food supply

Preparation for child feeding

Knowledge of child-feeding practices

Attitude and decisions about child feeding

Responsibility for feeding

Understanding the importance of the bonding process

Support from family and friends

From Rees JM, Worthington-Roberts B: Adolescence, nutrition, and pregnancy: interrelationships. In Mahan LK, Rees JM: *Nutrition in adolescence,* St Louis, 1984, Mosby.

therefore, increased amounts of food are needed, and specific nutritional requirements relate directly to the time and degree of the pubertal growth spurt. As one would expect, nutritional demands are greatest when growth is most rapid; when growth rate slows down, nutritional needs gradually taper off. Because the pubertal acceleration in growth generally occurs in females (10½ to 13 years of age) before it occurs in males (12½ to 15 years of age), separate dietary recommendations are proposed for males and females after 9 years of age.

Character and timing of physical growth and sexual maturation differ greatly among individuals, but in general the adolescent female does not complete linear growth until 4 years postmenarche. Those who become pregnant at a low gynecologic age (2 years or less) are presently considered to be at high biologic risk because

they are anatomically and physiologically immature. In fact few will become pregnant at this stage because of the high incidence of anovulation in the first years following menarche. For these young women (who are the most likely to be still growing), nutritional requirements will exceed those of adults whose growth has stabilized.[25] Those who have achieved a gynecologic age of 4 years are considered physiologically mature and similar to other "adult" women in their nutritional demands for normal pregnancy.[11,37,38]

Since little information is available on nutritional needs of pregnant adolescents, *estimates* of needs are typically formulated by adding the difference between recommended dietary allowances (RDAs) for pregnant and nonpregnant adults to that for nonpregnant adolescents (Table 10-4). This method of approximation may overestimate total pregnancy requirements

TABLE 10-4 *Recommended Dietary Allowances for Pregnant Adolescents*

	Age (Reference Height)			
	11-14 yr (157 cm)		15-18 yr (163 cm)	
Nutrient	Total RDA	RDA/cm	Total RDA	RDA/cm
Energy (kcal)*	2,500	15.9	2500	15.3
Protein (gm)	60	0.38	58	0.36
Calcium (mg)	1,200	7.6	1,200	7.4
Phosphorus (mg)	1,200	7.6	1,200	7.4
Iron (mg)	30	0.19	30	0.18
Magnesium (mg)	320	2.0	340	2.1
Iodine (µg)	175	1.1	175	1.1
Zinc (mg)	15	0.09	15	0.09
Vitamin A (µg RE)	800	5.1	800	4.9
Vitamin D (µg)	10	0.06	10	0.06
Vitamin E (mg α-TE)	10	0.06	10	0.06
Ascorbic acid (mg)	60	0.38	70	0.43
Niacin (mg NE)	17	0.11	17	0.10
Riboflavin (mg)	1.6	0.01	1.6	0.01
Thiamin (mg)	1.5	0.01	1.5	0.01
Folate (µg)	370	2.3	400	2.5
Vitamin B_6 (mg)	2.0	0.01	2.1	0.01
Vitamin B_{12} (µg)	2.2	0.01	2.2	0.01

*Second and third trimester
Modified from Food and Nutrition Board, National Research Council: *Recommended dietary allowances,* ed 10, Washington, DC, 1989, National Academy of Sciences.

for some individuals. For example, the metabolic alterations promoted by pregnancy may increase the efficiency of nutrient absorption. Also, if reduction in the maternal physical activity level is substantial, energy needs may not differ greatly from those of nonpregnant adolescents. Recognizing all the potential variation that may exist in the aforementioned additive approximation of nutritional needs, the values in Table 10-4 are probably the best possible figures to use if the pregnant female is still growing. If, however, she is obviously mature, her nutritional requirements resemble more closely those of pregnant adults.

Energy

Since individual adolescents differ markedly in their growth patterns, body builds, and exercise routines, it is extremely difficult to predict energy requirements with great accuracy. The most sensible approach to the situation is to obtain information on body weight and height for each patient in question. Height data are helpful in predicting total energy needs, but weight information is also useful in reflecting both growth rate and body build. Prediction of energy requirements can be further improved by evaluating the changes in height and weight that the given adolescent has demonstrated over the entire childhood period. Such a practice allows the professional to *estimate* the present growth rate of the child and to plan for necessary energy needs with growth rate in mind. Since the growth spurt for females is relatively short, they typically demonstrate a rather rapid decrease in energy requirements *after* puberty.

The increased energy requirements during rapid growth are generally met without concentrated effort on the part of the adolescent. Appetite usually increases at this time, and increased food intake is a normal response to this circumstance. It is known, however, that young women proceeding through adolescence under today's pressures for maintenance of slim physique often limit their food consumption to levels significantly less than those required to meet demands for normal growth.[8]

The long-term effects of energy restriction by adolescent females in developed societies are still unknown, since strict control of weight gain in this population has existed for only several decades or thereabouts. The permanent effects on the individual will relate directly to the particular time during her growth period when serious restriction is imposed. Energy deprivation (below that required for basal metabolism and activity) during the period of rapid growth in height may compromise normal growth of the skeletal system. Under such circumstances long bones would be especially affected, and dimensions of the pelvic girdle may also be altered adversely. Energy restriction *after* the height spurt has been completed will not have such a devastating impact on normal growth processes in adolescent females. Under such conditions, however, nutritional status may deteriorate, and tolerance to stress, disease, and other insults may decline. Pregnancy under such adverse circumstances is accompanied by considerable risk to both mother and fetus.

In a study by Blackburn and Calloway[4] energy expenditure was assessed in pregnant adolescents. They found that during pregnancy, basal metabolic rate (BMR) was 1.11 kcal/min compared with 0.98 kcal/min at 6 to 10 weeks postpartum. Unexpectedly, however, when corrections were made for body weight, the differences in BMR between the two periods disappeared. These data suggest that the increase in body *mass* during pregnancy accounts for most of the increase in BMR. Blackburn and Calloway[4] confirmed this idea by measuring energy expenditure of pregnant adolescents during activities unrelated to body weight (quiet sitting, combing hair, cooking at stove, and so on) and compared these figures with energy expended in activities affected by body weight (treadmill running, sweeping, bedmaking, and so on). Results suggested that energy expenditure during the latter group of activities was significantly greater during pregnancy than in the nonpregnant state, whereas energy expenditure in the former activities varied little from one circumstance to the other. Energy needs during pregnancy therefore appear to relate directly to the cost of weight movement that accompanies increase in body mass. Since the typical woman increases body mass about 20% during pregnancy, activities that demand a lot of movement must require as much as 20% more energy to accomplish.

One further point of interest, however, is the modification in activity pattern typically demonstrated by pregnant adolescents. Blackburn and Calloway[4] recorded activity patterns of 12 pregnant teenagers and found that activity was distributed for most young women in the following categories:

Sleeping or lying in bed with magazine	40%
Quiet seated activities	40%
Eating	4%
Doing hair and other similar activities	5%
Light activities	9%
TOTAL	98%

It can be seen that most girls spent the vast majority of their time in sedentary activities. Although the most active girl in the group used 50 kcal/kg/day, 7 of the 12 girls observed expended approximately 38 kcal/kg/day. It is apparent, therefore, that energy expenditure may be highly variable from person to person, and assessment of this factor along with all others is necessary in approximating daily energy requirements for pregnant adolescents. The best assurance of adequate intake is a satisfactory weight gain over time.

Protein

Growth is accompanied by considerable nitrogen retention, and normal growth progress can be achieved only if adequate protein is provided in the diet. Protein deposition (and nitrogen retention) is greatest during the period of most active growth in the adolescent female; as growth slows down, protein deposition diminishes.

Protein intake by typical adolescent females has been studied by several researchers. It has been found that protein generally accounts for more than 10% of calories consumed, and often, the level of intake is even higher. Reports suggest that average protein intake of adolescent females exceeds recommended levels; daily protein intakes of 75 to 80 gm often are consumed by females in the 11- to 13-year-age group. Evaluation of dietary records clearly indicates that adolescent females prefer protein foods with a low energy value. In many circumstances representative diets are reasonably high in protein and low in energy such that some dietary protein is used for energy and less remains for building body tissues. Under conditions of rigorous energy restriction, the amount of protein available for production of lean body tissue may be inadequate, and retardation in physical growth may occur. For this reason adolescent females should be encouraged to ingest diets that contain enough energy to allow for use of an adequate amount of protein for tissue synthesis.

Clinical evaluations by King, Calloway, and Margen[21] involved estimation of protein requirements of pregnant adolescents. In this study nitrogen retention was measured in a group of pregnant females who resided in a metabolic research unit during the third trimester of their pregnancy. It was determined that when 15- to 19-year-olds were fed the 1968 National Research Council protein recommendation of 65 gm/day, they retained 1.4 gm/day of nitrogen (8.17 gm/day of protein). In addition, as nitrogen was increased from 9.3 to 20 gm/day (58 to 125 gm/day of protein) without variation of the energy input (43 kcal/kg), nitrogen retention increased linearly according to the following equation: nitrogen retention (gm/day) = 0.3 (nitrogen intake) − 1.73. King concluded from her findings that the 1968 National Research Council protein recommendation may not permit maximum protein storage during the third trimester in young primiparas. Taking those studies into consideration and using newer methods for calculating requirements led to the recommendation of a 66% reduction in protein allowance for the pregnant woman in the 1989 RDA. Studies reviewed by the Institute of Medicine indicated the mean protein intake of pregnant adolescents exceeds the recommendations, reaching levels suggested by the King studies, thereby reducing concern over the protein status of these young women.

Iron

Iron needs of the growing adolescent are sizable and relate to a requirement for iron by the enlarging muscle mass and blood volume. In addition, since the maintenance of adequate iron stores is considered desirable, extra iron is needed for this purpose. Because the adolescent female loses body iron each month during menstruation, this loss must also be made up for by provision of iron from exogenous sources. Early balance studies indicate that 11 to 13 mg/day of iron is needed to cover growth and menstrual losses. In 1989 the National Research Council recommended that adolescent and adult women consume 15 mg/day of iron[34]; it is generally believed that intake of iron at this level will allow for buildup of some iron stores, but low-level iron supplementation during pregnancy is considered desirable if the gastrointestinal side effects are not bothersome.

Many adolescents enter pregnancy with low iron stores. This may be a result of poor diet, recent rapid growth, heavy menstrual blood losses, or a combination of these factors. These young women are at high risk for development of iron deficiency anemia. Iron deficiency anemia in early gestation has been associated with a 200% to 300% increased risk for prematurity and low birth weight.[45] According to 1990 *Pregnancy Nutrition Surveillance* data, the prevalence of iron-deficiency anemia in pregnant adolescents was 11% during the first trimester, 16% during the second trimester, and 37% during the third trimester.[3]

Even though the efficiency of iron absorption is believed to increase progressively during pregnancy, an additional 15 mg of iron would likely be needed each day by the pregnant adolescent; thus the RDA is 30 mg per day during the second and third trimester, when the iron needs are highest. If anemia is present, it should be treated with a 60 to 120 mg/day supplement.[34]

Iron supplementation can be provided in several forms. Low-dose iron can be given alone or as part of a multivitamin-mineral supplement of appropriate composition for pregnancy. Liquid and chewable forms of iron are available if teenagers have trouble swallowing tablets or capsules. The most efficient absorption of iron occurs when the supplement is taken at bedtime or between meals with water or juice, not with milk, tea, or coffee. Diet should not be ignored; regular consumption of heme sources of iron are well-absorbed and ascorbic acid-containing foods or beverages should enhance the absorption of non-heme iron food sources.

Women of all ages, but especially adolescents, are notorious for their inconsistent attention to iron supplementation and dietary recommendations. It thus makes sense to monitor young women through pregnancy for the presence or absence of anemia. If anemia is found in the face of apparently faithful iron supplementation, other potential causes of the anemia should be sought; inflammation or excess hemodilution are possible explanations.[18,19]

Calcium

Balance studies with adolescents have shown that calcium absorption and retention increase before menarche and the growth spurt. According to a 1959 study by Ohlson and Stearns,[32] when calcium intakes range from 1 to 1.6 gm/day and vitamin D intakes are about 10 μg (400 IU)/day, retention of approximately 400 mg/day of calcium is allowed. Newer observations confirm that 50% of adult bone mass is accumulated in adolescence.[22-24] Studies among young women who restrict their food intake during this period show that they do so to the detriment of their skeletal system. Anorexic women have been shown to have 2 SD less lumbar vertebral and whole body bone density than age matched controls,[1] as well as reduced cortical bone density and a greater risk of fracture than normal women.[36] Reductions in cortical bone density were not rapidly reversed as subjects recovered. Thus dancers, gymnasts, and other athletes (along with young women who are influenced by fashion) who keep themselves in a state of semistarvation are at great risk for severe skeletal disorders later in life. Any of these adolescents who become pregnant face an even greater risk.

The need for extra calcium during pregnancy relates largely to the development of the fetal skeletal system. According to Hytten and Leitch,[17] approximately 28 gm of calcium are stored in the fetus at birth. In addition, variable quantities of calcium are deposited in the maternal skeleton and in supporting tissues and fluids. Overall, calcium deposition during pregnancy is about 30 gm. Since the healthy adolescent contains approximately 1,120 gm of calcium in her "body stores," the additional calcium required during pregnancy could likely be derived from this source if the dietary provisions were inadequate. Under such circumstances, however, demineralization of maternal bone is an inevitable consequence, and the possibility that this might prove detrimental to the young woman is worth recognizing.

In females whose calcium intakes have been low throughout childhood and adolescence, tissue stores of calcium may be insufficient to *optimally* meet the needs of both mother and fetus. If such a woman continues to consume a diet with inadequate calcium content, fetal skeletal development and/or maternal skeletal integrity may be compromised. Marginal calcium intake during pregnancy may also prevent adequate preparation of the maternal body for lactation.

The current RDA for calcium during pregnancy is 1,200 mg per day for women of all ages. The National Institutes of Health conference (1994) on Optimal Calcium Intakes recommended an increase in calcium intakes among adolescents to 1,200 to 1,500 mg/day.[33] However, low calcium intakes are well documented in adolescent females. It is recommended, therefore, that supplemental calcium be provided in such circumstances. A supplement providing 600 mg of elemental calcium is advised by the Institute of Medicine. Since regular prenatal vitamin/mineral supplements do not contain this much calcium, an additional supplement is needed. This supplement can be taken with meals since its absorption is enhanced under such circumstances.

Folate

Folate has been mentioned in previous discussions in this text and need not be addressed in detail again. It is important to recognize that the diets of adolescents are often marginal if not low in this vitamin. As with any woman of childbearing age, daily ingestion of 0.4 mg folic acid may be protective against fetal development of neural tube defects. Under the best of conditions, adolescents who are capable of pregnancy should be taking this level of folic acid daily before conception. Since conception in this population is often unplanned, unintended and undesired, this practice may seem unjustified, if the adolescent is aware of the recommendation at all. Following through with folic acid supplementation after pregnancy is diagnosed is desirable. However, this may be introduced at a time too late in pregnancy to affect embryonic development.

Other Nutrients

The restricted diets consumed by many adolescents contain inadequate amounts of vitamins and trace minerals. Attention to this problem during pregnancy is important if the maternal and fetal tissues are to receive sufficient amounts of each nutrient for maintenance of metabolic processes and support of normal growth. A low-dose vitamin-mineral supplement is recommended for adolescents who do not regularly consume a diet that meets the needs of pregnancy, are complete vegetarians, have a multiple gestation, or who smoke more than 20 cigarettes per day or abuse alcohol or drugs.[51]

ASSESSING NUTRITIONAL STATUS

Assessment of nutritional status of the pregnant adolescent is accomplished using methods applied to other populations. The more time available for the evaluation process, the more thorough the effort can be.[38] In reality, time may often be scarce and detailed dietary evaluation may be impossible. In such cases a screening process is helpful to provide a basis for counseling during present and future contacts. A clinical screen of nutritional status for the pregnant adolescent may be set up as follows:

Diet

Presence of protein source
  Animal
  Vegetable (product of protein complementation)
Presence of vitamin C source
Presence of some fresh fruits and/or vegetables
Presence of fiber source
Presence of calcium source in significant quantities
Presence of iron source(s)
Presence of inordinately large amounts of calorie-rich,
  nutrient-poor foods
Excessive use of dietary fats

Growth and physical condition

Gynecologic age
Prepregnancy height and weight progress
Weight gain during pregnancy
Physical signs of malnutrition
Hematologic indices

Activity patterns
Long-term medication
Presence of chronic disease or infection

Red flags suggesting nutritional problems

Disproportionate height/weight progress or sudden weight gain or loss before or during pregnancy
Abuse or avoidance of foods
Bizarre eating patterns
Psychological or economic problems interfering with nutrition
Unhealthful lifestyle, with or without substance abuse

In all situations, a skilled professional should be prepared to make appropriate recommendations for dietary improvement adapted to the lifestyle of the person without provoking undue stress on her or her family.

DIETARY PATTERNS IN THE ADOLESCENT

By the time a young girl has grown into adolescence, her dietary patterns are well-established. By and large, her general preferences and dislikes relate to family circumstances she has been exposed to throughout childhood. In addition, however, adolescent food patterns always are influenced by living habits, the preferences of peers, and exposure to the messages of the mass media.[30] Food is often purchased at "fast-food" outlets, where many selections have excess fat, sodium, and total energy value, coupled with inadequacies of folic acid and fiber. Because female adolescents often choose soft drinks in preference to milk when they eat convenience foods, they may also get less calcium, riboflavin, and vitamin A than they need.[13]

Attention to food may be excessive if the environment is food-oriented. Meals and eating, on the other hand, may be put off if the schedule or economic resources cannot accommodate them. Emotional problems commonly associated with adolescence may influence eating behavior in a variety of ways. Classic research has shown that young women who score best in emotional stability, conformity, adjustment to reality, and family relationships miss fewer meals, are familiar with a wider variety of foods, and have generally better diets than other young women. It was also found that females who mature late or early

often have emotional problems accompanying this developmental characteristic and many times, have poorer eating habits than those maturing at normal rates.

Irregular eating habits are now known to be characteristic of most adolescents. According to several surveys, as many as one fifth of all adolescent females skip breakfast, and another 50% have poor breakfasts. One report indicated that as students advanced from the seventh to the twelfth grade, the percentage who missed meals increased from 10% to 25%; in addition, twice as many missed breakfast in twelfth grade as in seventh grade. Many factors are involved in promoting alterations in meal patterns of the type described. For the adolescent girl, significant factors certainly include busy schedules and motivation for weight control.

It should be recognized that along with a pattern of skipping meals frequently comes the pattern of increased snacking. Snacking should be considered a normal practice among teenagers, and diet plans should be made with this in mind. As many as one fourth of the total daily energy consumption of adolescent females typically comes from snacks, and those who snack often (in moderation) are also likely to eat meals of good quality and to have overall good diets. In considering the diet for a pregnant adolescent, it should consequently be remembered that moderate snacking is not to be discouraged. On the contrary, a diet plan will be accepted by the young woman only if it fits her lifestyle closely; such a plan of necessity includes snacks, and the type of snack will be dictated by the environment in which it is obtained and/or consumed.

Most pregnant teens want to have healthy babies. The prenatal period is therefore a potential time to motivate young women toward dietary improvement. Some evidence does show that positive changes may occur. Schneck et al. reported that 60% of 99 low-income pregnant adolescents had made dietary changes, with 12% increasing consumption of fruits and vegetables, 8% increasing milk, and 16% decreasing non–nutrient-dense foods.[41]

Although nutritionists and other health professionals may place much time and effort in nutrition counseling of pregnant adolescents, changes in dietary patterns may not be observed in some young women. This is to be expected, and according to several researchers, food patterns of adolescent females are not related to their knowledge of nutrition or to the number of nutrition information resources to which they have access. Since adolescents ultimately determine their own behavioral patterns and since these behaviors develop from a number of motivational forces, one can only hope that the information they acquire is accurate and the adult examples to which they are exposed are sensible and of obvious merit. A competent clinician will intervene when possible to influence behavioral patterns and attitudes in a positive way. Development of intervention strategies is difficult but necessary in influencing the maturing child.

IMPROVING NUTRITION FOR PREGNANT TEENAGERS

Unfortunately, there is no secret formula for *motivating* adolescent females to adopt healthful dietary habits. First, however, it is essential to recognize the numerous factors that influence nutritional well-being in the adolescent (see p. 303). Then one must decide where attention should be focused in particular; how do the nutrition problems relate to the other difficulties with which the young woman must cope? Many approaches have proved successful in home and clinical circumstances, and every health professional and parent finds certain tactics superior to others. Of great importance in any consultation setting is the establishment of rapport with the teenager. Unless a relaxed and nonthreatening atmosphere is created for discussion, little successful interchange can take place.[36] It may develop that the concerns of the adolescent involve issues other than diet; the skilled health professional should stand prepared to provide guidance in important areas such as social skills, complexion management, hygiene, and figure control. Often, the pregnant adolescent is in great need of "an understanding friend to talk to." Health professionals who are not prepared to provide a listening ear may find that the specific "nutrition or diet goals" they are pushing are totally ignored by young women who see them as authoritarians rather than as understanding counselors.

Specific Counseling Issues[38]

The problems pregnant adolescents face will change from month to month as they react to the physical changes and psychological aspects of pregnancy. These changes can affect the dietary intake. Some prominent issues that generally are important throughout the prenatal counseling period can be delineated.

Basic nutrition guidelines. Pregnant adolescents are at high risk of being individuals who do not take care of themselves or attempt to control their physical environment. Imaginative individualized approaches are necessary in planning nutritional care and providing access to food to meet their needs.

Once it has been established that the adolescent has access to adequate food, the goal will be to ensure that it is as high in quality as possible. If the young woman is not obtaining sufficient food energy to maintain a satisfactory rate of weight gain or if nutrient-rich foods are missing, plans for obtaining those foods will be the focus of counseling sessions. Talking with her about foods she likes and is familiar with is the starting point. Efforts should be made to find some source of all important nutrients that she will eat regularly. When sources of certain nutrients are missing from the foods she normally eats, the attempt will be to find some source of those nutrients that she is willing to "add." When these goals are set realistically, there is a good probability of meeting them. Successfully adding a few new foods on a regular basis is much better than trying to urge the pregnant adolescent to "meet the RDA" in all nutrients or to eat a certain number of servings of each type of food daily. Failure usually results if the goal is not based on the reality of the young woman's actual food habits.

Because adolescent eating habits often do not follow a traditional meal pattern, the clinician should be ready to suggest valuable foods that pregnant adolescents can choose in many places and at any time. Although establishing a regular meal pattern may sound like a valuable goal, often it is not successful. As the counselor becomes more familiar with the patient's habits over time, suggestions can be more specific as to foods for particular times of day and for particular occasions.

A positive approach is more effective than a negative one that would put the clinician in the role of a disciplinarian and the adolescent in a position to rebel. This does not preclude labeling certain foods as ones that do not "give you what you need" or that "make you gain weight without giving you and your baby anything." For specialists in nutrition, counseling techniques can be quite detailed and related to specific nutrients. For clinicians whose time is limited to covering only the basics, primary points include the following:

- Dealing with issues that interfere with nourishment
- Providing support for obtaining resources
- Guidance for consuming the kind and amount of food energy to permit appropriate weight gain (including nutrient-rich foods)

Postpartum weight loss. Patterns of weight loss in teens are not well-documented. The suspicion is that they are highly variable and relate to the significant differentiation in growth status prepregnancy, gestational weight gain patterns, and a variety of cultural and lifestyle factors. No specific timeframe can be provided about the postpartum weight loss experience. However, since the young woman is still in the process of developing an adult body image, it will often be difficult for her to accept the changes in weight necessary to support pregnancy and perhaps lactation. Sensitive counseling by health care professionals will improve their acceptance and success in weight management.

Weight-related disorders. Some pregnant adolescents will suffer from eating disorders, including obesity and **bulimia.** Bulimia is becoming more common among teenagers across a relatively broad spectrum of socioeconomic levels. Bulimic females are often of near normal weight and are more likely to be fertile than are anorexic females.

Because bulimia is a relatively newly recognized phenomenon, research has not identified methods for clinically guiding pregnant bulimic females. It is therefore necessary to apply principles tested in related situations to identify the likely problems and design management strategies. The most outstanding problem theoretically is the possibility of a detrimental biochemical environment for the fetus, occurring as a result of an imbalanced state of nutriture following bingeing, and vomiting.

The bulimic female may be seriously threatened by the need to gain weight in support of her pregnancy while her instinct is to restrict gains. On the other hand, if she attempts to modify her bulimic behavior quickly, she may lose control over her weight so that she gains a great deal more than is recommended.

Management goals stemming from theoretical problems are to stabilize the biochemical environment as much as possible and to ensure at least adequate weight gain. Excessive gains, although not optimal, are less detrimental to the fetus than restriction or loss.

Of the methods for instilling in pregnant teenagers the motivation to consume adequate nourishment,[38] appealing to the desire of the bulimic young woman to produce a normal infant is probably the most effective. Education about the necessary foods will need to be provided, since most bulimic young women have a distorted view of physiologic needs. Appealing to her motivation to take care of herself is generally ineffective, since the young woman has overcome those instincts to carry out habits about which she feels guilt.

In practical terms, guidance will be directed toward helping her to delay vomiting until needed food has had the opportunity to be digested. If she is unable to avoid bingeing and vomiting totally, that activity should be held apart from the nourishing process that is in support of the fetus.

Cognitive restructuring, a psychotherapeutic technique whereby the person's basic cognitive concepts are examined and improved, has been used successfully in working with bulimic women. By this process a revised belief structure provides impetus for behavior change. For example, the bulimic woman may believe that her body can exist without taking in any food that she does not "burn off" with vigorous exercise. That is, she only eats because she is tempted, and eating is negative for her. As a result of cognitive restructuring, this belief will be replaced by the concept that her body and that of her unborn child is constantly undergoing change and needs ongoing nutritional support.

The manner in which consultation is given will depend on the openness of the young woman and her willingness or desire to make changes. If she is not ready to disclose her behavior, she will not take advantage of cognitive restructuring or other psychotherapeutic techniques. In that case, comments regarding the baby's growth as indicated by fundal height measurements will provide needed intervention. Messages such as "Your baby is growing—he is getting what he needs," or "Your baby is growing slowly—that shows she probably needs to be getting more nourishment," can motivate.

Undisclosed eating disorders can be confused with hyperemesis gravidarum. Distinction can usually be made on the basis of the person's response to hospital management of a crisis brought about by excessive vomiting. Management to control vomiting and correct fluid, electrolyte, and nutritional imbalances will generally suffice for the person who sincerely wants to eat and gain weight. Bulimic women either secretly or openly believe that they should not let themselves adopt the habit of gaining weight and will require additional psychological intervention to provide sufficient nourishment for their pregnancies.

Food resources. It is of primary importance to realize that pregnant adolescents will often lack a stable food supply. This is caused in part by their tenuous status in separating themselves from their families and establishing residences together with partners, friends, and relatives. In any of a variety of living situations, the amount of money they can spend on food may be small. For example, there may be a high degree of disorganization in the living group, or the pregnant adolescent may be in competition for food with other members of the household. This is the reality on which to base all messages about food intake.

The source, type, and amount of food available must be assessed, and suggestions made for mobilization of all possible resources. Helping adolescents to successfully stretch limited funds, obtain supplemental foods, find foods they can keep in a room without refrigeration, and choose wisely when buying prepared foods at a grocery or fast-food franchise become the standard focuses of the clinician serving this population. The total food knowledge and planning skill of the pregnant adolescent will generally need to be augmented.

Programs for pregnant adolescents that supply food along with nutritional counseling are especially effective resources for adolescents because they provide support in two most needed areas: (1) supplementation of resources and (2) guidance in the use of such resources. The design is appropriate to the most vulnerable of adolescents, with abstract nutritional principles being reinforced in a concrete sense with food.

Responsibility. Pregnant adolescents must take responsibility (often for the first time) for their own nourishment and for that of others. Helping patients to understand and carry out this responsibility will be one of the main objectives of nutritional counseling.

Social, emotional, and economic stress. Underlying all discussions with pregnant adolescents is the need to ascertain the degree of stress they are under as a result of their pregnancy. This stress must be taken into consideration in counseling them. Of prime importance is their decision to keep or relinquish their infant. Although the decision to give up a child is rare, the teenager may consider it when a supportive acquaintance or professional brings it up. The decision will determine whether messages about nutrition are directed toward a mother (or couple) bearing a child who will remain a part of her family or toward a woman who will only carry a child through its gestation. Because most adolescents are ambivalent about such a decision, it is important to phrase messages so they will not be judgmental of the apparent decision once it has been made. In some situations it will be important to leave the door open for her to change her mind. It is necessary to maintain communication with other members of the health-care team so as not to undermine their counseling efforts in this regard.

AN INTERNATIONAL PERSPECTIVE

The International Center for Research on Women has mounted a large campaign called *Investing in the Future: Six Principles for Promoting the Nutritional Status of Adolescent Girls in Developing Countries.*[20] A set of strategies is now in place, each of which relates to one of six principles. Although these strategies are program-oriented, they can provide policymakers a road map to the important issues in adolescent nutrition (see box below).

SPECIAL PROGRAMS FOR PREGNANT ADOLESCENTS

Since the pregnant teenager is considered "high risk" educationally, medically, socially, and nutritionally, a variety of comprehensive community programs have been developed with the intention of optimizing progress and well-being of mother and infant. A wide range of program models has been initiated, and each community has been responsible for defining its own pattern of operation and scope of services. Support for these programs has been handled in a variety of

ways, and the quality and scope of service and training provided in any setting are often determined by level of funding and requirements of funding agencies. Despite the variability in program design and individualized funding patterns, almost all programs have at least three common service components: (1) early and consistent prenatal care, (2) continuing education on a classroom basis, and (3) counseling on an individual or group basis. Sometimes all three services are provided by one community agency; more often, however, the services are offered through cooperative efforts of several organizations.

Most programs for pregnant adolescents have both long- and short-term goals and objectives. Long-range goals often aim at promoting competent motherhood, good health of the mother and infant, high school graduation, stable family life, maturity and independence, and avoidance

---

❖

SIX PRINCIPLES FOR PROMOTING THE NUTRITIONAL STATUS OF ADOLESCENT GIRLS IN DEVELOPING COUNTRIES[20]

Principle 1: improve adolescents' food intake
Strategies
- Increase household purchasing power
- Educate adolescents about nutrition
- Offer meals at schools or worksites
- Offer iron fortification or supplementation
- Discourage gender differences in food intake

Principle 2: keep girls in school
Strategies
- Ensure girls' safety and privacy at school
- Establish schools close to home
- Increase the proportion of female teachers
- Make school hours more flexible
- Offer an alternative to formal education
- Integrate food supplementation into school systems

Principle 3: postpone first births
Strategies
- Postpone age at marriage
- Offer appropriate family planning and reproductive health services for adolescents
- Provide family life education and life options
- Increase educational attainment for girls

Principle 4: reduce girls' workloads and improve work conditions
Strategies
- Introduce mechanisms to reduce girls' workloads
- Teach adolescents income-earning skills
- Build partnerships with employers

Principle 5: improve adolescents' health
Strategies
- Inform and educate adolescents about their health
- Design and provide health services for adolescents
- Develop effective communication strategies for adolescents

Principle 6: enhance girls' self-esteem
Strategies
- Increase knowledge and skills
- Provide opportunities for achievement
- Increase girls' awareness of opportunities for the future
- Establish means for communication

of further out-of-wedlock (or unwanted) pregnancies. While seeking to accomplish long-range goals, attention to immediate problems and needs may be necessary. Efforts are made to provide for continuation of regular education during pregnancy and reentry into regular school as soon as possible. Health care is provided during and after the pregnancy, and the expectant mother is taught how to care for the infant after birth. Counseling is offered as appropriate and necessary to help the young woman cope with the problems that led to or have been caused by her pregnancy.

Attention to the potential problem of recurring pregnancy should be of primary concern in programs for pregnant teenagers, since available data strongly suggest that the biologic and sociologic consequences of short interconception periods in the young woman are often highly unfavorable for both mother and offspring. The plan in programs for pregnant adolescents is to deal with pressing problems first and then move to more general goals. General goals relate basically to management of medical, social, and educational circumstances that will determine the long-range health and welfare of mother and child. Among the many issues requiring attention is the role of diet (or nutrition) in promoting growth and health in mother and baby. The pregnant adolescent should leave the program with an appreciation for the important part she plays in providing satisfactory nutritional support to the young family for which she is responsible.

In most situations where good programs have been established, efforts are ongoing to upgrade and improve program design and to campaign vigorously for continued financial support from private and public sources. The number of young women and men served annually by such programs has risen gradually over the past 20 years. It is still apparent, however, that considerable variability exists from one community to another, and in many areas the establishment of minimal services has not yet been accomplished. Available data strongly suggest that improvement of discrepant conditions around the United States is needed. The challenge of the future for most communities is to describe community strengths and deficits and to establish interdisciplinary services in accordance with needs of the population served.

Specific effects of established programs are being studied. Conclusions will lead to new designs and techniques to improve clinical services. In some cases clinics will be reorganized to be more attractive and approachable to adolescents or to use new resources such as volunteer workers. New services may be directed to specific problems such as preterm births or pregnancy preventing preconceptional care or to groups at high risk, including the homeless and prostituting teenager and teenage fathers. The primary goals of contacts with young males are to improve their ability to support themselves and their pregnant partners (and children), as well as their ability to make decisions about future reproduction.

Unfortunately, adolescent health in general has received low priority in the traditional health care system of the United States. The particular problem of adolescent pregnancy must not be limited to any one health agency or social sector; it is the responsibility of many different health professionals, educators, the community, and the teenager's family and peer groups. All must work together and devise programs to reduce physical, mental, and socioeconomic threats that teenage pregnancy poses to the health of young people and to the health of society itself.

The adolescent population provides a unique challenge to the health care providers, teachers and family members who work with them. Faught has pointed out the qualities of individuals who seem unusually effective in working with this population.[9] These observations have been identified in *Working with Pregnant and Parenting Teens/Resource Guide/Teacher's Edition: Teenage Pregnancy: A New Beginning*[2]: Qualities included are as follows:

1. *Understanding, compassion, empathy*
   A warm approach that says, "I care about you."
2. *Good self-image*
   A good self-image radiates confidence. Confidence is catching! And it allows you to be natural.
3. *Enthusiasm and friendliness*
   Both create an excitement for learning and growing.

4. *Nonjudgmental approach*
   Acceptance is critical to a strong, open relationship.
5. *Sense of humor*
   Humor is a valuable stress reducer. Help them to see the beauty in their situations.
6. *Patience*
   Patience is a virtue to be demonstrated and modeled.
7. *Ability to refrain from giving advice*
   Our role is to empower them to accept and respond to the challenges they face. Our responsibility is to provide accurate, objective information to assist them in their decision making.
8. *Recognition of your own values*
   Identifying your beliefs assures that your values will stay your values and will not unduly influence the teens or negatively affect your relationship.
9. *Be concerned, not emotionally involved*
   Being concerned without becoming emotionally involved preserves your own emotional health and creates a supportive relationship that allows the young people you teach to become competent and self-reliant.

The importance of nurturing the "mother-infant dyad" has been emphasized by McAnarney and Lawrence.[26] They point out that young adolescent mothers may successfully finish school, obtain jobs, and achieve financial independence during their children's formative years. At the same time, these children have more cognitive and behavioral problems, both short-term and long-term, than do children of adult mothers. They go on to stress that if, for some young mothers to succeed, their children receive inadequate nurturing, minimal care, and little-to-no supervision, resulting in adverse developmental outcome, then the price of these mothers' success is unacceptably high for their children, for them, and for society. It obviously makes sense to provide these mother-child pairs with an environment in which both can flourish.

Day-care programs for young mothers and their children provide an appropriate setting, if they are located close to mothers' high schools and jobs. Young, inexperienced mothers need to learn about the development of children at different ages. They also need to be taught how to communicate both verbally and nonverbally with their children in mutually satisfying ways.

There are now sufficient data to provide targeted interventions for teenagers and their children and to build on adolescents' assets. First, adolescent mothers often lack knowledge of child development even though they may have previous experience babysitting other people's children. Young mothers should be given basic information about child development, focused on the specific age and stage of their children. Second, young mothers must learn to delay their own needs and place their children's needs above their own. Third, young mothers need to accept without frustration that their children may not respond immediately to their well-meaning overtures. Fourth, skilled older women might teach young mothers how to verbalize with their infants and children. Fifth, young people should be taught about nonverbal communication. They need to learn how to read their children's nonverbal signals and how to respond to them. Children's response to their mothers' nonverbal communication can be positively reinforcing if the mothers learn to read their infants' signals and response accordingly.

The best time to intervene with young mothers and their children is early in the children's lives. Thus ideally, young mothers and their infants should start a day-care program together. Every effort should be made to keep young mothers and their children together in supervised settings. *We have the opportunity to mold the young mother's behavior while she is still young and flexible by involving both her and her child in the program.*[26]

Summary

Although pregnant adolescents vary considerably in their biological maturity and psychosocial circumstances, each presents some degree of challenge to the health care provider. The nutritional needs of this diverse population are poorly understood, but it is generally believed that the simultaneous demands for both adolescent growth and pregnancy produce an increment in nutrient requirements that markedly exceeds that of the mature pregnant woman. Just how

❖ ❖ ❖

CASE STUDY

Adolescent Chapter

Margo is a 16-year-old who has come for prenatal care during her fourth month of pregnancy. Her main concern is weight gain—she
is afraid she will "get fat" and wants to know
how she can control her weight gain. She
seems to want the baby but is much more concerned about her weight and relationship with
the baby's father than the health of the "soon-
to-come" infant. She is considering the option
of adoption but is still undecided. She asks the
clinic staff to help her resolve these difficult
decisions she has to make.
1. Where do you begin with this challenge?
2. Nutritionally, what advice should be given?
3. Where are you "out of your element" when
   it comes to counseling?
4. What are your strengths and limitations in
   this situation?

true this concept is for the typical pregnant
teenager is the subject of debate; in reality most
young women who conceive during adolescence
have completed almost all of their physical
growth. It is therefore necessary to develop
counseling strategies that allow for attention to
individual needs. It is also essential that focus be
given to the development of satisfactory parenting skills in young parents. Special clinical programs for pregnant adolescents can serve as a
base for management of this high-risk situation.
Ultimately, however, connections need to be established with educational and health care agencies who can provide for ongoing support of the
young family.

REVIEW QUESTIONS

1. Compared with a decade ago, what changes have
   occurred in adolescent pregnancy rates, adolescent
   maternal morbidity and mortality, low-birth-
   weight rate among pregnant adolescents, and
   neonatal and postneonatal mortality rates in offspring of adolescents?
2. Describe a suitable method for estimating weight
   gain for an individual pregnant adolescent.

3. Define "red flags" suggesting nutritional problems
   in an adolescent population.
4. Describe desirable elements of the nutrition component of an interdisciplinary program for pregnant adolescents.

LEARNING ACTIVITIES

1. Sit in on a nutrition counseling session involving a
   pregnant adolescent.
2. Evaluate the dietary characteristics of several pregnant teens.
3. Review a series of charts related to weight gain of
   pregnant adolescents and summarize the usual
   pattern seen.
4. Visit a school-based program for pregnant teens
   and observe the activities (especially related to nutrition) that occur.

REFERENCES

1. Bachrach LK et al: Decreased bone density in
   adolescent girls with anorexia nervosa, *Pediatrics*
   86:440, 1990.
2. Barr L, Monserrat C: Working with pregnant and
   parenting teens: resource edition: teenage pregnancy: a new beginning. Albequerque, NM, New
   Futures.
3. Beard JL: Iron deficiency: assessment during
   pregnancy and its importance in pregnant adolescents, *Am J Clin Nutr* 59(suppl):502S, 1994.
4. Blackburn ML, Calloway OH: Energy expenditure and pregnant adolescents. In *Protein
   requirements of pregnant teenagers, final report
   to National Institutes of Health, Division of
   Research Grants,* Grant No HD 05246,
   Bethesda, Md, 1973, National Institutes of
   Health.
5. Browne C, Urback M: Pregnant adolescents: expectations vs reality, *Can J Public Health,* June
   1989.
6. Centers for Disease Control and Prevention:
   Morbidity and Mortality World Report. State-
   specific pregnancy and birth rates among
   teenagers—United States, 1991-1992, *JAMA*
   274:1501, 1995.
7. Centers for Disease Control. *MMWR.* (October
   1, 1993). *Teenage pregnancy and birth rates—
   United States, 1990,* US Department of Health
   and Human Services, PHS.

8. Endres J et al: Older pregnant women and adolescents: nutrition data after enrollment in WIC, *J Am Diet Assoc* 87:1011, 1987.

9. Faught P: Special people, special needs: the adolescent challenge. *Intern J Childbirth Educ* 10:15, 1994.

10. Fraser AM, Brockert JE, Ward RH: Associa-tion of young maternal age with adverse reproductive outcomes, *N Engl J Med* 332:1113, 1995.

11. Frisancho AR, Matos J, Flegel P: Maternal nutritional status and adolescent pregnancy outcome, *Am J Clin Nutr* 38:739, 1983.

12. Geronimus AT, Korenman S: Maternal youth or family background. On the health disadvantages of infants with teenage mothers, *Am J Epidemiol* 137:213, 1993.

13. Guenther PM: Beverages in the diets of American teenagers, *J Am Diet Assoc* 86:493, 1986.

14. Hediger ML et al: Patterns of weight gain in adolescent pregnancy: effects of birth weight and preterm deliver, *Obstet Gynecol* 74:6, 1989.

15. Hediger ML et al: Rate and amount of weight gain during adolescent pregnancy: associations with maternal weight-for-height and birth weight, *Am J Clin Nutr* 52:793, 1990.

16. Horon IL, Strobina DM, MacDonald HM: Birthweight among infants born to adolescent and young adult women, *Am J Obstet Gynec* 146:444, 1983.

17. Hytten FE, Leitch I: *The physiology of human pregnancy,* ed 2, Oxford, 1971, Blackwell Scientific Publications.

18. Institute of Medicine, National Academy of Sciences: *Nutrition during pregnancy,* Washington, DC, 1990, National Academy Press.

19. Institute of Medicine, National Academy of Sciences, Food and Nutrition Board: *Nutrition during pregnancy and lactation. An implementation guide,* Washington DC, 1992, National Academy Press.

20. International Center for Research on Women: *Investing in the future: six principles for promoting the nutritional status of adolescent girls in developing countries,* 1994.

21. King JC, Calloway DH, Margen S: Nitrogen retention, total body ^{40}K and weight gain in teenage pregnant girls, *J Nutr* 103:772, 1973.

22. Kreipe RE, Forbes GB: Osteoporosis: a "new morbidity" for dieting female adolescents? *Pediatrics* 86:478, 1990.

23. Matkovic V et al: Factors that influence peak bone mass formation: a study of calcium balance and the inheritance of bone mass in adolescent females, *Am J Clin Nutr* 52:878, 1990.

24. Matkovic V et al: Influence of calcium on peak bone mass: a pilot study, *J Bone Miner Res* 1:168 (Supp), 1986.

25. McAnarney ER: Young maternal age and adverse neonatal outcome, *Am J Dis Child* 141:1053, 1987.

26. McAnarney ER, Lawrence RA: Day care and teenage mothers: nurturing the mother-child dyad, *Pediatrics* 91:202, 1993.

27. McAnarney ER, Stevens-Simon C: First, do no harm, *Am J Dis Child* 147:983, 1993.

28. Mercer RT: *Nursing care of parents at risk,* Thorofare NJ, 1977, Charles B Slack.

29. Moerman ML: Growth of the birth canal in adolescent girls, *Am J Obstet Gynecol* 143:528, 1982.

30. Morton HN: A survey of the television viewing habits, food behaviors and perception of food advertisements among South Australian year 8 high school students, *J Home Econ Assoc Aust* 22:34, 1990.

31. Naeye RL: Teenaged and pre-teenaged pregnancies: consequences of the fetal-maternal competition for nutrients, *Pediatrics* 67:146, 1981.

32. Ohlson MA, Stearns G: Calcium intake of children and adults, *Fed Proc* 18:1076, 1959.

33. Porter D. Washington Update. Optimal calcium intake. NIH consensus development consensus. *Nutr Today* 29:39, 1994.

34. *Recommended dietary allowances,* ed 10, Washington, DC, 1989, National Academy of Sciences, National Research Council.

35. Reducing teenage pregnancy increases life options for youth, *Prevent Rep,* US Public Health Service, April/May, 1994, pp. 1-3.

36. Rees JM: Nutritional counseling in adolescence. In Mahan LK, Rees JM: *Nutrition in adolescence,* St Louis, 1984, Mosby.

37. Rees JM et al: Weight gain in adolescents during pregnancy: rate related to birthweight outcome, *Am J Clin Nutr,* 56: 868, 1992.

38. Rees JM, Worthington-Roberts B: Adolescence, nutrition, and pregnancy: interrelationships. In Mahan LK, Rees JM: *Nutrition in adolescence,* St Louis, 1984, Mosby.

39. Rosso P, Lederman SA: Nutrition in the pregnant adolescent. In Winick M, editor: *Adolescent nutrition,* New York, 1982, John Wiley & Sons.

40. Satin AJ et al: Maternal youth and pregnancy outcomes: middle school vs high school age groups compared with women beyond the teenage years, *Am J Obstet Gynecol* 171:184, 1994.

41. Schneck ME, Sideras KS, Fox RA: Low income pregnant adolescents: dietary findings and their health outcomes, *J Am Diet Assoc* 90:555, 1990.

42. Scholl TO, Hediger ML, Ances IG et al: Growth during early teenage pregnancies, *Lancet* 1:701, 1988.

43. Scholl TO et al: Weight gain during pregnancy in adolescence: predictive ability of early weight gain, *Obstet Gynecol* 75:948, 1990.

44. Scholl TO, Hediger ML: A review of the epidemiology of nutrition and adolescent pregnancy and its effect on the fetus, *J Am Coll Nutr* 12:101, 1993.

45. Scholl TO et al: Anemia vs iron deficiency: increased risk of preterm delivery in a prospective study, *Am J Clin Nutr* 55:985, 1992.

46. Scholl TO et al: Maternal growth during pregnancy and lactation, *Horm Res* 39S:59, 1993.

47. Scholl TO et al: Maternal growth during pregnancy and the competition for nutrients, *Am J Clin Nutr* 60:183, 1994.

48. Stevens-Simon C, McAnarney ER, Roghmann KI: Adolescent gestational weight gain and birth weight, *Pediatrics* 92:805, 1993.

49. Stevens-Simon C, McAnarney ER: Adolescent maternal weight gain and low birth weight: a multifactorial model, *Am J Clin Nutr* 47:948, 1988.

50. Stevens-Simon C, Nakashima II, Andrews D: Weight gain attitudes among pregnant adolescents, *J Adolesc Health Care* 14:369, 1993.

51. Story M, Alton I: Nutrition issues and adolescent pregnancy, *Nutr Today* 30:142, 1995.

52. Vincent ML, Clearie AF, Schluchter MD: Reducing adolescent pregnancy through school and community-based education, *JAMA* 257:3382, 1987.

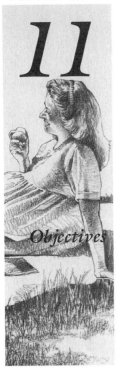

11

Lactation: Basic Considerations

Bonnie S. Worthington-Roberts

Objectives

✦✦✦

After completing this chapter, the student will be able to:

✓ *Describe the anatomy of the mammary glands.*

✓ *Discuss the development of the mammary glands from immature structures to mature, functional organs.*

✓ *Describe the process of milk production and secretion.*

Introduction

Lactation is an ancient physiologic process accomplished by females since the origin of mammals. Today, as in times past, the process of breastfeeding is successfully initiated by at least 99% of women who try. All that is required of the lactating mother is an intact mammary gland (or preferably two) and the presence and operation of appropriate physiologic mechanisms that allow for adequate milk production and release. The establishment and maintenance of lactation in the human are determined by at least three factors:

1. The anatomical structure of the mammary tissue and the adequate development of alveoli, ducts, and nipples
2. The initiation and maintenance of milk secretion
3. The ejection or propulsion of milk from the alveoli to the nipple

A thorough understanding of each of these factors is essential for proper and effective lactation management and for prevention of lactation failure of today's inexperienced mother.

ANATOMY OF THE MAMMARY GLAND

The mammary gland of the human female consists of milk-producing cells (glandular epithelium) and a duct system embedded in connective tissue and fat (Fig. 11-1). The size of the breast is variable, but in most instances it extends from the second through the sixth rib and from the sternum to the **anterior axillary line.** The mammary tissue lies directly over the pectoralis major muscle and is separated from this muscle by a layer of fat, which is continuous with the fatty tissue of the gland itself.

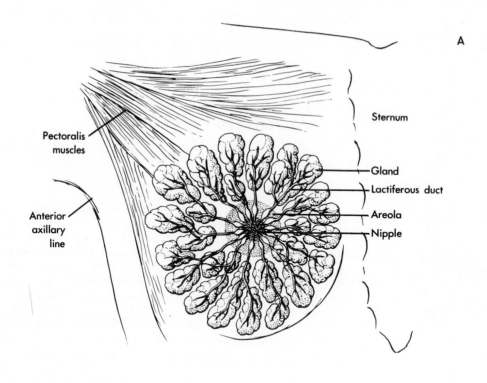

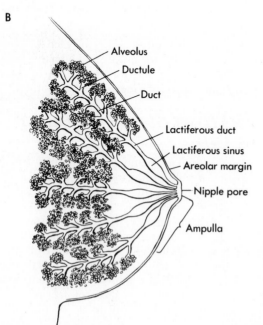

FIG. 11-1   **A,** General anatomical features of the human breast showing its location on anterior region of thorax between sternum and anterior axillary line. **B,** Detailed structural features of human mammary gland showing terminal glandular (alveolar) tissue of each lobule leading into duct system, which eventually enlarges into lactiferous duct and lactiferous sinus. Lactiferous sinuses rest beneath areola and converge at nipple pore.

The center of the fully developed breast in the adult woman is marked by the **areola,** a circular pigmented skin area from 1.5 to 2.5 cm in diameter. The surface of the areola appears rough because of the presence of large, somewhat modified sebaceous (fluid-producing) glands, which are located directly beneath the skin in the thin subcutaneous tissue layer. The fatty secretion of these glands is believed to lubricate the nipple. Bundles of smooth muscle fibers in the areolar tissue serve to stiffen the nipple for a better grasp by the suckling infant.

The nipple is elevated above the breast and contains 15 to 20 **lactiferous ducts** surrounded by modified muscle cells and covered by wrinkled skin. Partly within this compartment of the nipple and partly below its base, these ducts expand to form the short **lactiferous sinuses** in which milk may be stored. The sinuses are the continuations of the mammary ducts, which extend outward from the nipple toward the chest wall with numerous secondary branches. The ducts end in epithelial masses, which form subsections, or lobules, of the breast (Fig. 11-1). The number of tubules and size of the acinar structures vary greatly in different women and at different ages. In general, the terminal tubules and glandular structures are most numerous during the childbearing period and reach their full physiologic development only during pregnancy and lactation.

During adolescence the breasts of the female enlarge to their adult size; one is often slightly larger than the other, but this difference is usually unnoticeable. In a nonpregnant woman the average mature breast weighs approximately 200 gm. During pregnancy there is some increase in size and weight such that by term, the breast may weigh between 400 and 600 gm. During lactation this weight increases to between 600 and 800 gm.

Wide variation in the structural composition of the human breasts has been observed in women after childbirth. Some breasts contain little secretory tissue; some large breasts contain less glandular tissue than much smaller organs. One researcher reported that in a series of 26 lactating breasts, only 16 showed what appeared to be adequate amounts of alveolar tissue. It is well known, however, that neither size nor structural composition of the breast significantly influences lactation success in the average woman. Almost all women who want to breastfeed find that they can.

BREAST DEVELOPMENT

Mammogenesis begins in early fetal life and is not complete in the woman until after **parturition.** The precise hormonal contributions to this process are not well-understood, although estrogens, progesterone, and lactogenic hormones appear to be involved.

In the human newborn the mammary glands are developed sufficiently to appear as distinct, round elevations, that feel like movable soft masses. Under the microscope, the future milk ducts and glandular lobules can be easily recognized. These early glandular structures can produce a milklike secretion ("witch's milk"), starting 2 or 3 days after birth. All of these neonatal phenomena related to the mammary glands probably result from the intensive developmental processes that occur in the last stages of intrauterine life; usually they subside in the first few weeks after birth. Some shrinkage, or **involution,** in the breast then takes place, and this is followed by the "quiescent" period of mammary growth and activity during infancy and childhood.

With the onset of puberty and during adolescence, ovarian maturation and follicular stimulation are accomplished by an increased output of estrogenic hormone (Fig. 11-2, *A*). As a result of the response, the mammary ducts elongate, and their lining epithelium reduplicates and proliferates at the ends of the mammary tubules. The growth of the ductal epithelium is accompanied by growth of periductal fibrous and fatty tissue, which is largely responsible for the increasing size and firmness of the adolescent female gland. During this period the areola and nipple also grow and become pigmented.

BREAST MATURATION

As the developing woman matures and ovulation patterns become established, the regular development of progesterone-producing corpora lutea in the ovaries promotes the second

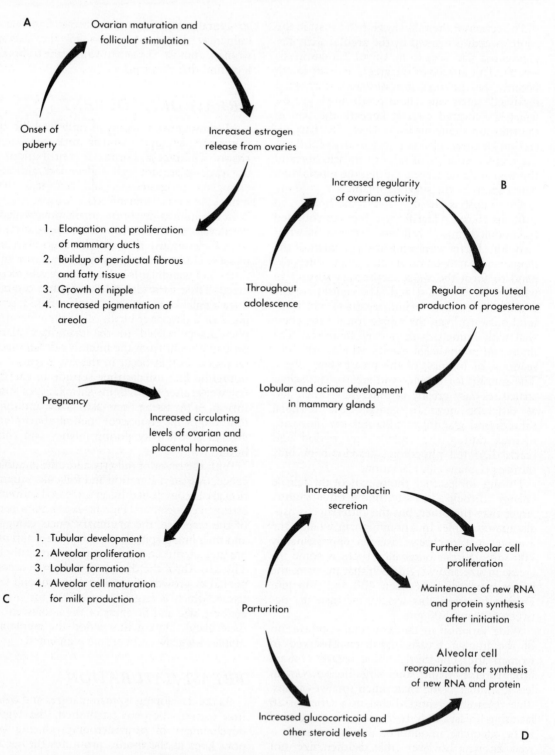

A

Ovarian maturation and
follicular stimulation

Onset of
puberty

Increased estrogen
release from ovaries

Increased regularity
of ovarian activity

B

1. Elongation and proliferation
   of mammary ducts
2. Buildup of periductal fibrous
   and fatty tissue
3. Growth of nipple
4. Increased pigmentation of
   areola

Throughout
adolescence

Regular corpus luteal
production of progesterone

Pregnancy

Increased circulating
levels of ovarian and
placental hormones

Lobular and acinar development
in mammary glands

Increased prolactin
secretion

1. Tubular development
2. Alveolar proliferation
3. Lobular formation
4. Alveolar cell maturation
   for milk production

C

Further alveolar cell
proliferation

Maintenance of new RNA
and protein synthesis
after initiation

Parturition

Alveolar cell
reorganization for synthesis
of new RNA and protein

Increased glucocorticoid and
other steroid levels

D

FIG. 11-2 Events in breast development.

stage of mammary development (Fig. 11-2, *B*). Lobules and acinar structures gradually appear, giving the mammary gland the characteristic lobular structure found during the childbearing period. This differentiation into a lobular gland is finished approximately 12 to 18 months after the first menstruation, but further acinar development continues in proportion to the intensity of the hormonal stimuli during each menstrual cycle and especially during pregnancies. Fat deposition and formation of fibrous connective tissue contribute to the increasing size of the gland in the adolescent period.

Cyclical changes in the adult mammary gland are associated with the hormonal changes that occur during the menstrual cycle. The ovary releases estrogen during the early part of the cycle, and this compound stimulates proliferation of the glandular tissue with formation of epithelial sprouts. This hyperplastic activity continues into the latter part or secretory phase of the menstrual cycle when the corpus luteum provides increased amounts of estrogen and progesterone. Lobular edema may occur at this time, along with thickening of the epithelial basement membrane and deposition of secretory material in the alveolar lumen. Lymphoid and plasma cells infiltrate the stroma, and mammary blood flow also increases. This set of events is experienced by women as fullness, heaviness, and turgescence; the breast may appear somewhat "nodular" at times, but this should not be cause for alarm.

After the onset of menstrual flow the reduced circulating sex hormone levels rapidly promote changes in the breasts. Degeneration of the glandular cells is seen along with loss of proliferation tissue and edema fluid. The size of the breast is noticeably reduced, although complete regression of the glandular-alveolar growth is not complete after each cycle until about 30 years of age.

Some young women may enter reproductive life with insufficient functional mammary tissue to produce enough milk for their baby's total nourishment. In some cases this relates to underdevelopment of the mammary ductwork associated with periodic amenorrhea or very late menarche. In addition, there are women who have surgery to remove cysts, tumors, or other growths; others have undergone surgery for breast reduction or reconstruction. For whatever reason, circumstances exist in which functional mammary tissue is insufficient to support a nursing infant fully; fortunately these circumstances are rare.

The mammary gland of a nonpregnant woman is inadequately prepared for secretory activity. Only during pregnancy do the changes occur that make satisfactory milk production possible (Fig. 11-2, *C*). In the first trimester of pregnancy the terminal tubules sprouting from the mammary ducts proliferate to create a maximum number of epithelial elements for future acinar formation. In the midtrimester the reduplicated terminal tubules group together to form large lobules. Their lumina begin to dilate, and the acinar structures thus formed are lined by cuboidal epithelium. In the last trimester the existent clumps of milk-producing cells progressively dilate in final preparation for the lactation process.

As the glandular and duct tissue proliferates during pregnancy, the adipose tissue appears to diminish. During this time there is increased infiltration of the interstitial tissue with lymphocytes, plasma cells, and eosinophils. In the last trimester any enlargement of the breast is the result of enlargement of the milk-producing cells and distention of the alveoli with early colostrum. The microscopic appearance of the gland is variable, ranging from dilated ducts with thin-walled alveolar cells to narrow-lumened, thick-walled glandular tissue. The lumen of each alveolus is crowded with fine granular material and lipid droplets, the latter of which are similar to the droplets or blebs protruding from the surface of adjacent alveolar cells. In the pregnant woman, the breasts are capable of milk secretion beginning sometime in the second trimester.[24]

The placenta has been found to play an important role in mammary growth in pregnancy. It is known that in some animals **hypophysectomy, ovariectomy,** or both can be performed after a certain stage of gestation without interrupting pregnancy and mammary development. The placenta has been found to secrete ovarian-like hormones in large quantities. Placental lactogen, prolactin, and chorionic gonadotropin have been identified as contributors to mam-

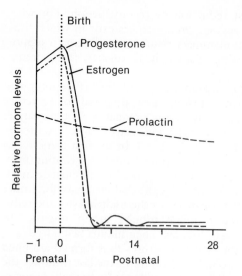

FIG. 11-3   Relative hormone production before and after delivery of human baby.

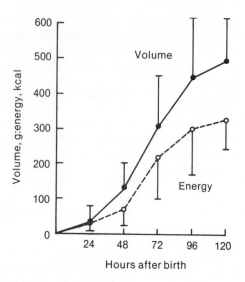

FIG. 11-4   Daily intakes of milk and energy by breast-fed infants in first 5 days after birth. Each point is total (mean ±SD) for preceeding 24-hour period.

From Casey CE et al: Nutrient intake by breast-fed infants during the first five days after birth, *Am J Dis Child* 140:933, 1986.

mary gland growth. Human chorionic so-matomammotropin has been found to promote mammary growth and lactation in experimental animals and presumably is secreted in sufficient amounts to act with placental progesterone and estradiol to stimulate breast development in pregnancy.

Although mammary growth and development occur rapidly throughout pregnancy, additional proliferation of parenchymal cells takes place shortly after parturition (Fig. 11-2, *D*). The proliferation of epithelial cells that begins just before parturition results in daughter cells with a new complement of enzymes. The expression of new enzyme activities is the result of production of a new species of messenger RNA. A glucocorticoid is required for the synthesis of several enzymes involved in carbohydrate metabolism. An adrenocortical steroid is necessary also for redistribution of free ribosomes into the rough endoplasmic reticulum (RER). Once the RER is formed, prolactin is required for sustained RNA synthesis and subsequent casein synthesis.

Lactogenesis generally refers to the onset of copious milk secretion around parturition. The hormonal mechanisms that bring about lactogenesis have long been the subject of controversy.

It now seems clear that this process is triggered by a fall in plasma progesterone levels under conditions in which mammary development and plasma prolactin levels are sufficient to promote milk secretion (Fig. 11-3).

THE PHYSIOLOGY OF LACTATION

Full lactation does not begin as soon as the baby is born (Fig. 11-4). During the first 2 or 3 days after birth, a small amount of colostrum is secreted. In subsequent days a rapid increase in milk secretion occurs, and in usual cases lactation has become reasonably well-established by the end of the first week. In first-time mothers (primiparas), however, the establishment of lactation may be delayed until the third week or even later. Generally, therefore, the first 2 or 3 days is a period of rapid lactation initiation, and this is followed by the longer period of maintenance of lactation. These two phases are not caused by precisely the same stimuli, but the basic physiologic mechanisms that are operative are similar in both cases.[8]

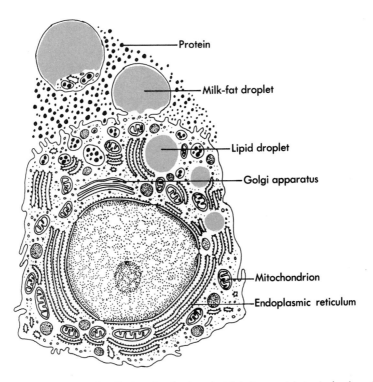

Protein

Milk-fat droplet

Lipid droplet

Golgi apparatus

Mitochondrion

Endoplasmic reticulum

FIG. 11-5 Mammary gland cell, showing basic cuboidal shape with typical microvillus border and basal nucleus. Cytoplasmic organization is characteristic of cells undergoing active protein synthesis and secretion. Synthetic apparatus consists of many free ribosomes and extensive system of rough endoplasmic reticulum. Large Golgi body is located above nucleus, and associated with it are some vacuoles containing fibrillar or particulate material that condenses into central core or granule. Toward apex granules become progressively larger and contain more-dense protein granules. Vacuoles fuse with surface membrane and liberate their contents intact into lumen. Fat droplets are found throughout cell but are largest near apex. They protrude into lumen and appear to pinch off from cell proper along with small bit of cytoplasm. Other cytoplasmic structures include large mitochondria with closely packed cristae, lysosomes, and small number of smooth membranous tubules and vesicles.

Modified from Lentz TL: *Cell fine structure: an atlas of drawings of whole cell-structure,* Philadelphia, 1971, WB Saunders.

Initiation and maintenance of lactation comprise a complex neuroendocrine process. It involves the sensory nerves in the nipples and adjacent skin of the breast and chest wall, the spinal cord, the hypothalamus, and the pituitary gland with its various hormones, particularly prolactin, adrenocorticotropic hormone (ACTH), glucocorticoids, growth hormone, and oxytocin. The process of milk production occurs in two distinct stages, including the stage of secretion of milk into the alveolar lumen and the stage of propulsion, or ejection, whereby the milk passes along the duct system. Although the two events are closely related and often occur simultaneously in the nursing mother, they are best discussed separately for greatest clarity.

The secretion of milk involves both the synthesis of the milk components and the passage of the formed product into the alveolar lumen (Fig. 11-5). These events may be under independent control, since the accumulation of both lipid and protein, as observed by electron microscopy, reaches a high level during the latter part of pregnancy. Shortly before parturition the accumulated secretory products begin to be passed into the lumen, leaving the epithelial cells essentially devoid of biosynthetic products. The secretory process is activated again by the sucking stimulus of the infant.

In general, each milk-producing alveolar cell proceeds through a secretory process that is preceded and followed by a resting stage (Fig. 11-6). The cytoplasm is finely granular during the resting phase but striated (microscopically) as milk secretion begins. Milk synthesis is most active during the suckling period but occurs at lower levels at other times. The secretory cells are cuboidal but change to a cylindrical shape just before milk secretion, whereas cellular water uptake is increased. As secretion commences, the enlarged cell with its thickened apical membrane becomes clublike in shape. The tip pinches off leaving the cell intact; the milk constituents are then free in the secreted solution, and the cell retains a cap of membrane. Between periods of active milk secretion, alveolar cells return to their characteristic resting state.

During the process of weaning, lactating women gradually decrease their milk volume, deliberately replacing breastfeedings with supplemental foods. Women who have not yet be-gun to wean their infants may add some solids to the babies diet but maintain the usual number of breastfeedings. The difference between these two groups in the volume of milk production is substantial (Fig. 11-7).[34]

Mechanisms for Milk Synthesis and Secretion[35]

Four secretory processes are synchronized in the alveolar cell to produce milk: **exocytosis,** fat synthesis and secretion, secretion of ions and water, and immunoglobulin transfer from the **extracellular** space (Fig. 11-8). A fifth process, the **paracellular** pathway, is a transit route for plasma components and leukocytes. Briefly, the following points are relevant:

1. *Exocytosis*—Proteins, lactose, calcium, phosphate, and citrate are packaged into secretory vesicles and secreted by exocytosis. Proteins deriving from the endoplasmic reticulum are transferred to the Golgi system for further processing and sorting. Calcium, phosphate, and citrate are transported into the Golgi vesicles from the cytoplasm. Large aggregates called *micelles* are formed. Lactose is synthesized and, because it cannot escape from the Golgi apparatus, water is drawn into the Golgi vesicles. Secretory vesicles bud off from the Golgi complex and move toward the apical portion of the cell, where they fuse with

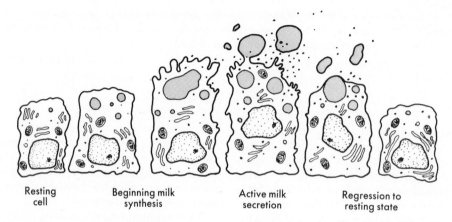

Resting   Beginning milk   Active milk   Regression to
cell   synthesis   secretion   resting state

FIG. 11-6   Cycle of changes that occur in secretory cells of alveoli from resting stage through milk production and secretion, with eventual return to resting stage.

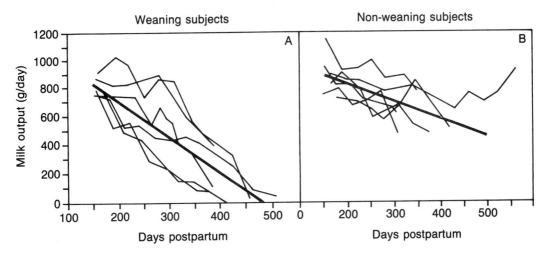

FIG. 11-7 Changes in milk production during weaning as compared with nonweaning.

From Neville MC, Allen JC, Archer PC et al: Studies in human lactation: milk volume and nutrient composition during weaning and lactogenesis, *Am J Clin Nutr* 54:81, 1991.

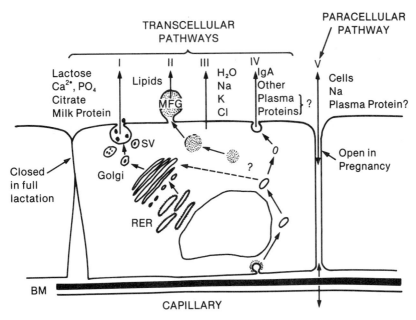

FIG. 11-8 Pathways for milk synthesis and secretion in mammary alveolus. **I,** Exocytosis of milk protein and lactose in Golgi-derived secretory vesicles. **II,** Milk fat secretion via milk-fat globule. **III,** Secretion of ions and water across apical membrane. **IV,** Pinocytosis-exocytosis of immunoglobulins. **V,** Paracellular pathway for plasma components and leukocytes. SV = secretory vesicle; RER = rough endoplasmic reticulum; BM = basement membrane; MFG = milk-fat globule.

Redrawn from Neville MC, Allen JC, Watters C: The mechanisms of milk secretion. In Neville MC, Neifert MR, ed: *Lactation: physiology, nutrition and breast-feeding,* New York, 1983, Plenum Press.

the apical membrane and release their contents into the alveolar lumina.

2. *Lipid synthesis and secretion*—Triglycerides, synthesized in the cytoplasm and smooth endoplasmic reticulum, coalesce into large droplets that gradually make their way to the top of the alveolar cell, where they are enveloped in apical plasma membrane. The milk fat globule finally separates from the cell, occasionally taking with it a segment of cytoplasm.

3. *Secretion of **monovalent** ions and water*—Sodium, potassium, and water appear to permeate the Golgi, secretory vesicles, and apical membrane freely. Water moves across these membranes in response to the osmotic gradient set up by lactose; electrolytes follow water.

4. *Immunoglobulin secretion*—Immunoglobulin A (and maybe other plasma proteins) attaches to receptors on the **basolateral membrane** of the alveolar cell, where it is internalized through endocytosis and then transported either to the apical membrane or to the Golgi apparatus for subsequent release into milk.

5. *The paracellular pathway*—The passage of substances through the spaces between the alveolar cells is normally prevented by the tight junctions between the adjacent cells. Sometimes these junctions become leaky (during pregnancy and when breasts are **mastitic** or involuting), allowing plasma constituents to pass directly into milk. Milk produced under these circumstances tends to be high in sodium and chloride and lower in concentrations of lactose and potassium. Leukocytes may also pass through these "gaps" in the mucosal lining.

Fat synthesis. Fat synthesis takes place from precursor compounds synthesized intracellularly or imported from the maternal circulation. Alveolar cells are able to synthesize short-chain fatty acids, which are derived predominantly from available acetate. Long-chain fatty acids and triglycerides are derived from maternal plasma, but the fatty acids are predominantly used for the synthesis of milk fat. Synthesis of triglyceride from intracellular carbohydrate also plays a predominant role in fat production for human milk.

Two enzymes responsible for synthesis of fat (lipoprotein lipase and palmitoyl-coenzyme A L-glycerol-3-phosphate palmitoyl transferase) are known to increase markedly in alveolar cells after delivery. Lipoprotein lipase acts in the walls of the capillaries to catalyze the hydrolysis of triglycerides in circulating lipoproteins such that fatty acids and glycerol are available for uptake into epithelial cells; the transferase enzyme catalyzes triglyceride synthesis within alveolar tissue. It is believed that the significant increase in lipase and transferase during lactation is stimulated by prolactin. Hormonal control of the glycerol precursors and the enzymatic release of fatty acids (leading to the formation of triglycerides) has been associated not only with prolactin but also with insulin, which stimulates the uptake of glucose into the mammary cells.

Protein synthesis. The vast majority of proteins present in normal milk are specific to mammary secretions and are not identified in any quantity elsewhere in nature. The formation of milk protein and mammary enzymes is induced by prolactin and further stimulated by insulin and cortisol.

The proteins in milk are derived from two sources: some are synthesized de novo in the mammary gland, and others are derived as such from plasma. Inclusion of plasma-derived proteins in the milk secretion occurs primarily in the early secretory product colostrum. Thereafter the three main proteins in milk (casein, α-lactalbumin, and β-lactalbumin) are synthesized within the gland from amino acid precursors. All the essential and some of the nonessential amino acids are taken up directly from plasma, but some of the nonessential amino acids are synthesized by the alveolar cells of the gland.

Carbohydrate synthesis and release. The predominant carbohydrate in milk is lactose, and its synthesis occurs in association with the Golgi apparatus of the alveolar cell. The synthesis of lactose combines glucose and galactose, the latter originating from glucose-6-phosphate (Fig. 11-9). Most of the intracellular glucose is derived continually from circulating blood glucose. A specific whey protein, α-lactalbumin, is a major component of the lactose-synthesizing

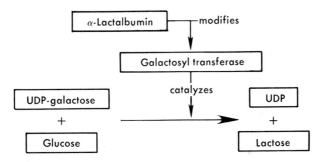

FIG. 11-9 Synthesis of lactose in human mammary glands.

enzyme galactosyl transferase. The availability of this protein serves as a rate-limiting step in the overall process of lactose synthesis. Synthesis of α-lactalbumin is inhibited by progesterone during pregnancy, but with a drop in estrogen and progesterone levels after the removal of the placenta at delivery (Fig. 11-4), the relatively high levels of prolactin become very significant. The synthesis of α-lactalbumin then becomes greater, and large amounts of lactose are produced from glucose.

Because of the constancy of concentration of lactose in milk, it has been suggested that the lactose concentration cannot vary under physiologic conditions and therefore must play a decisive role in the control of the volume of milk secretion. Progesterone apparently inhibits milk secretion by inhibiting one component of lactose synthetase.

The role of hormones. The stimulus for active milk secretion derives largely from the hormone prolactin (Fig. 11-10),[23] which acts on mammary alveolar cells and promotes continual milk production and release. The effect of suckling on serum prolactin levels is quite dramatic (Fig. 11-11) and apparently related to the intensity of nipple stimulation; this was demonstrated when the prolactin rise doubled after two infants were put to the breast simultaneously.[47] Maintenance of milk secretion, however, requires other **galactopoietic factors** from the anterior pituitary. If sucking is discontinued during the lactation period, pituitary release of the necessary hormones falls and milk secretion usually stops in the following few days, with accompanying atrophy and sloughing of alveolar cells.

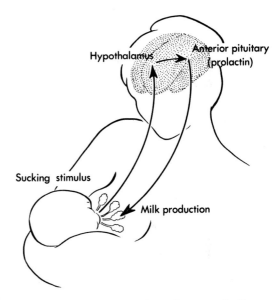

FIG. 11-10 Basic physiologic features of milk production. Sucking stimulus provided by baby sends message to hypothalamus. Hypothalamus stimulates anterior pituitary to release prolactin, the hormone that promotes milk production by alveolar cells of mammary glands.

Efforts have been made to compare the hormonal patterns of women with adequate and inadequate lactation. Geissler, Margen, and Calloway[19] studied urban Iranian women from low and middle socioeconomic groups. Growth hormone level was significantly lower in subjects with adequate lactation than in those with inadequate or ceased lactation; cortisol values

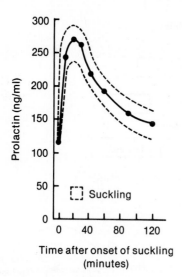

FIG. 11-11 Effect of suckling on serum prolactin levels; average values for 20 breast-feeding women suckling 10 minutes on days 5 and 6 of puerperium. Dashed lines represent standard error of the mean.

From Howie PW et al: The relationship between suckling-induced prolactin response and lactogenesis, *J Clin Endocrinol Metab* 50:670, 1980.

showed the same trend. In view of the role of growth hormone and cortisol in stress and malnutrition and some evidence of a reciprocal relationship between growth hormone and prolactin, these hormones may be a link in the chain between the urban environment, malnutrition, and lactation failure.

A variety of other hormones and exogenous stimuli are known to affect the process of milk secretion in humans (Table 11-1). Estrogens, for example, affect milk secretion, probably by acting through the pituitary. The type of effect promoted by estrogens, however, has been shown to relate to the level of estrogens in the blood. When the blood estrogen level is low, as in the virgin, there is no prolactin secretion. If the blood level is suitable, as occurs in parturition, the pituitary gland can discharge prolactin. When the estrogen level is raised beyond the point of adequacy, as occurs in pregnancy, the output of prolactin is inhibited. For this reason estrogens were once used to arrest lactation when it is undesirable, as in the case of severe engorgement of the breast. The inhibitory effects of estrogens on milk production are less in the period of established lactation than in the early weeks of the initiation period.

Studies of the use of combined estrogen-progestin contraceptive pills (usually containing 30 to 50 μg of ethinyl estradiol or 50 to 100 μg of mestranol) indicate that lactation is not inhibited in women who wish to nurse their infants as long as the pill is not used in the immediate postpartum period.[1] However, some dose-related suppression of the quantity of milk produced and the duration of lactation is found with extended use. Even though several reports suggest that measurable compositional changes occur in the milk produced by women taking combined oral contraceptive agents, results are inconsistent and largely viewed as insignificant. One well-designed study of the effects of two combination pills and one progestin-only pill emphasizes that the composition and volume of breast milk vary considerably in the absence of steroidal contraception and that whereas changes in these values occur in association with contraceptive use, they tend to remain within normal ranges.[31] *No unique effect of steroidal contraceptives on nursing mothers has been confirmed.*

During lactation there is a profound suppression of the production of luteinizing hormone. This appears to be related to inhibition of the release of gonadotropin-releasing hormone. With complete weaning, the follicular phase of ovulation is established. Before this time, however, there is a gradual return of luteinizing hormone secretion, obviously increasing the risk of pregnancy occurring.[21,27,39]

The "let-down" reflex. Once milk production and secretion have been accomplished, the baby may then obtain this milk by promoting its "ejection" from the alveoli and ducts. The "milk ejection," or "let-down," reflex is a mechanism involving both nerves and hormones, regulated in part by central nervous system factors (Fig. 11-12). The primary stimulus is sucking on the nipple, which triggers the discharge of oxytocin from the posterior pituitary. Oxytocin is carried in the bloodstream to the myoepithelial cells around the alveoli, causing them to contract; contraction of these small musclelike cells pushes the milk out of the alveoli and along the

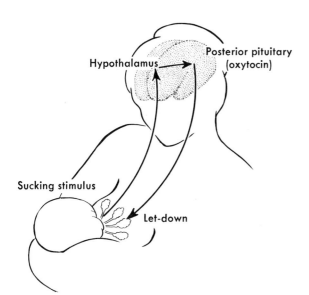

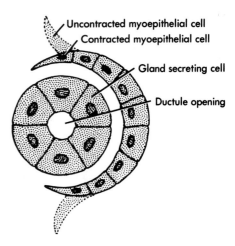

FIG. 11-12 Basic features of "let-down reflex." The sucking stimulus arrives at hypothalamus, which promotes release of oxytocin from posterior pituitary. Oxytocin stimulates contraction of myoepithelial cells around alveoli in mammary glands. Contraction of these musclelike cells causes milk to be propelled through duct system and into lactiferous sinuses, where it becomes available to nursing infant.

FIG. 11-13 Mammary alveolus surrounded by long, thin myoepithelial cell. Contraction of myoepithelial cell promotes "squeezing" pressure on gland cells so milk is forced to move along attached duct system.

duct system, where it is easily available to the nursing baby (Fig. 11-13).

The milk ejection reflex appears to be sensitive to a variety of environmental and emotional factors, although the mechanisms involved are poorly understood; unfortunately, these phenomena may influence the degree to which breast milk is "released" to the baby. The psychological importance of the milk ejection reflex in humans has been demonstrated by numerous case histories, which illustrate the fact that milk ejection can be inhibited by embarrassment or stress and can be "set off" by the mere thought of the baby or the sound of his or her cry. This observation has been confirmed by experimental stimulation (or inhibition) of the milk ejection reflex so that it is now known to be easily accomplished. Signs of successful let-down are easily recognized by the nursing mother. Common and significant occurrences include (1)

milk dripping from the breasts before the baby starts nursing, (2) milk dripping from the breast opposite to the one being nursed, (3) contraction of the uterus during breastfeeding, often causing slight pain or discomfort, and (4) a tingling sensation in the breast.

Occasionally a woman will experience an overactive let-down. Although not of concern to the health of the mother, it may be bothersome. Andrusiak and Larose-Kuzenko[4] have provided some management suggestions for an overactive let-down.

Maintenance of Lactation

Sucking stimulation is widely accepted as the most effective means of maintaining adequate lactation. It is believed to be of even greater significance than the milk ejection reflex itself. There is considerable evidence in human subjects that the restriction of sucking significantly inhibits lactation. Artificial sucking stimulation in the form of manual expression or a breast pump has repeatedly been recommended as a means of increasing milk yield or maintaining yield in the absence of the baby. Evidence suggests that feeding on demand optimally stimulates the lactation process.

TABLE 11-1   Hormonal Contributions to Breast Development and Lactation

Hormone	Origin	Function	
		Before and During Pregnancy	After Delivery
Prolactin	Anterior pituitary	Serum level rises, but estrogen suppresses its effect during pregnancy	Stimulates alveolar cells to produce milk; is probably of primary importance in initiating lactation but of secondary importance in maintaining lactation; may also cause lactation infertility by suppressing release of follicle-stimulating hormone and luteinizing hormone from pituitary or by causing ovaries to be unresponsive to gonadotropins; levels rise in response to various psychogenic factors, stress, anesthesia, surgery, high serum osmolality, exercise, nipple stimulation, and sexual intercourse
Prolactin-inhibiting factor (PIF)	Hypothalamus	Suppresses release of prolactin into blood; release stimulated by dopaminergic impulses (i.e., catecholamines)	Suppresses release of prolactin from anterior pituitary; agents that increase prolactin by decreasing catecholamines and thus PIF include phenothiazides and reserpine
Oxytocin	Posterior pituitary	Generally no effect on mammary function; sensitivity of myoepithelial cells to oxytocin increases during pregnancy	Causes myoepithelial cells to contract, leading to "milk ejection"; release is inhibited by stresses such as fear, anxiety, embarrassment, and distraction; also causes uterine contraction and postpartum involution of the uterus
Estrogen	Ovary and placenta	Stimulates proliferation of glandular tissue and ducts in breast; probably stimulates pituitary to secrete prolactin but inhibits its prolactin effects at the mammary cell level	Blood level drops at parturition, which aids in initiating lactation; not important to lactation thereafter

Hormone	Source	Effect on mammary growth / pregnancy	Effect on lactation
Progesterone	Ovary and placenta	With estrogen, stimulates proliferation of glandular tissue and ducts in breast; inhibits milk secretion	Blood level drops at parturition, which aids in initiating lactation; probably unimportant to lactation thereafter
Growth hormone	Anterior pituitary		May act with prolactin in initiating lactation but appears to be most important in maintaining established lactation
ACTH	Anterior pituitary	Gradually increases in blood during pregnancy; stimulates adrenals to release corticosteroids	High level is believed necessary for maintenance of lactation
Placental lactogen	Placenta	Like growth hormone in structure; stimulates mammary growth; associated with mobilization of free fatty acids and inhibition of peripheral glucose utilization and lactogenic action	
Human chorionic gonadotropin	Placenta	Contributes to mammary gland growth during pregnancy	
Placental lactogen	Placenta	Contributes to mammary gland growth during pregnancy	
Human chorionic somatomammotropin	Placenta	Contributes to mammary gland growth during pregnancy	
Thyroxine	Thyroid	Normally no direct effect on lactation	Appears to be important in maintaining lactation either through some direct effect on the mammary glands or by control of metabolism
Thyrotropin-releasing hormone	Hypothalamus	Normally no effect on lactation	Stimulates release of prolactin; can be used to maintain established lactation

Local and cultural patterns of infant feeding are of great significance in determining the duration of breastfeeding for a given mother. Although successful lactation can continue as long as adequate sucking stimulation is maintained (see box below), a gradual fall in the amount of milk produced generally develops after 12 months. This drop in milk output largely relates to reduction of demand and cessation of recurrent stimulation of the nipple by the infant. In a survey of 46 preliterate cultures Ford[17] found that in none of them did weaning occur before 6 months of age. In 31 of the cultures the earliest recorded age of weaning any infant from the breast was 2 or 3 years. It is clear from these and many other observations that the potential duration of lactation in most women is significantly greater than the actual period.

Induced Lactation

The phenomenon of lactation without pregnancy has been recognized as possible for many centuries. The Talmud describes a poor man whose wife died in childbirth leaving him without a means of feeding the infant. Miraculously he grew breasts and nursed the child through infancy. Other case studies have periodically appeared in the literature involving lactation by virgin girls and nonpuerperal women who have responded to vigorous suckling by infants with the resulting mammary growth and lactation. In these interesting cases it is likely that the ovarian or testicular hormones were present in sufficient amounts to prepare the mammary glands for lactation.

Induced lactation in nonpuerperal women is still, in some areas, a well-recognized and accepted method of feeding infants whose moth-

---

SUGGESTIONS FOR SUCCESSFUL BREASTFEEDING

Newborn to three months old

1. Encourage frequent nursing.
2. Suggest that the mother nurse on only one breast at a feeding.
3. Encourage the mother to nurse the baby before he or she is fully awake.
4. If the baby wants to nurse shortly after a feeding, encourage the mother to offer the least-full breast.
5. Suggest that the mother nurse during the fussy period with a minimum of breast switching.
6. Encourage the mother to use various nursing positions, especially those that allow the baby to lie on his side.
7. Encourage the mother to burp the baby often, and show her how to do it effectively.
8. Suggest that the mother avoid giving the baby a pacifier.
9. Suggest that the mother avoid supplementing her milk with other fluids or solid food.

10. Encourage the mother by telling her that she can continue to nurse and comfort the baby.

Three to six months old

1. Encourage the mother to offer the breast before the baby is fully awake.
2. Have the mother determine where, when, and what positions the baby favors for nursing.
3. Suggest that the mother take advantage of the times when the baby nurses well, without forcing the issue.
4. Suggest that the mother nurse on only one breast at each feeding.
5. Help the mother and baby to experience skin-to-skin touching and comfort at the breast without asking the baby to suckle.
6. Encourage the mother to obtain regular evaluations of the baby's weight gain.
7. Advise the mother that supplementation may be necessary if the baby is not nursing often.

ers could not breastfeed or who died in childbirth. Breastfeeding of adopted children has been successfully carried out by mothers in the United States, Australia, and other parts of the world. Many cases of lactation persisting for long periods after pregnancy result from continued stimulation of the breasts. This phenomenon has been recognized since the Middle Ages, when grandmothers often maintained employment as wet nurses by putting suckling puppies to their breasts between jobs.

DIET FOR THE NURSING MOTHER

The Committee on Recommended Dietary Allowances of the Food and Nutrition Board considers the optimal diet for the lactating woman to be one that supplies somewhat more of each nutrient than that recommended for the nonpregnant female (Table 11-2).[16] Obviously, the needs of specific women relate directly to the volume of milk produced daily. Observations of completely breastfed babies who appear to be thriving suggest that daily volume of breast milk consumption ranges from 340 to over 1,000 ml per day (Fig. 11-14); the mean falls between 600 and 900 ml daily at least for representative North American women.[1] Mothers of twins or triplets may show an enhanced capacity for milk production (Fig. 11-15). Australian researchers have reported the milk yield for three mothers of twins who were fully breastfeeding and four mothers who were partially breastfeeding at 6 months postpartum.[40] Full breastfeeding was associated with production of 0.84 to 2.16 kg of milk per 24 hours; partial breastfeeding allowed for the release of 0.42 to 1.39 kg of milk per 24 hours. The milk yield of one mother fully breastfeeding two 5-month-old triplets was 3.08 kg per 24 hours. One might conclude that the maximum potential milk yield for women may be higher than normally assumed.

During pregnancy, most women store approximately 2 to 4 kg of body fat, which can be mobilized to supply a portion of the additional energy for lactation. It is estimated that storage fat will provide 100-200 kcal per day during a lactation period of 3 months; this amount of energy represents only part of the energy cost to produce milk. The remainder of the energy needs should derive from the daily diet during the first 3 months of lactation. During this time lactation can be successfully supported, and readjustment of maternal fat stores can take place. If lactation continues beyond the initial 3 months or if maternal weight falls below the ideal weight for height, the daily extra energy allowance may need to be increased accordingly. If more than one infant is nursed during the first few months of life, maternal calorie stores will be more quickly used, and daily supplemental energy needs may double when maternal stores are depleted.[2]

TABLE 11-2 *Recommended Daily Dietary Allowances for Lactation*

	First 6 Months	Second 6 Months
Energy (kcal)	+500	+500
Protein (gm)	65	62
Vitamin A (RE*)	1,300	1,200
Vitamin D (μg)	10	10
Vitamin E activity (mg αTE)†	12	11
Ascorbic acid (mg)	95	90
Folacin (μg)	280	260
Niacin (mg‡)	20	20
Riboflavin (mg)	1.8	1.7
Thiamin (mg)	1.6	1.6
Vitamin B_6 (mg)	2.1	2.1
Vitamin B_{12} (μg)	2.6	2.6
Calcium (mg)	1,200	1,200
Phosphorus (mg)	1,200	1,200
Iodine (μg)	200	200
Iron (mg)	15	15
Magnesium (mg)	355	340
Zinc (mg)	19	16

*RE = retinol equivalent.
†α-Tocopherol equivalents: 1 mg d-α-tocopherol = 1 αTE.
‡Although allowances are expressed as niacin, it is recognized that on the average, 1 mg of niacin is derived from 60 mg of dietary tryptophan.
Modified from Food and Nutrition Board, National Research Council: *Recommended dietary allowances,* ed 10, Washington, DC, 1989, Government Printing Office.

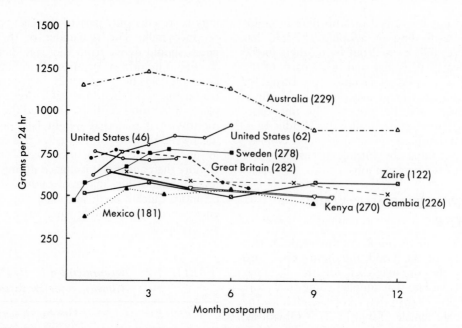

FIG. 11-14 Daily breast milk outputs of lactating women in various parts of the world. Methods used to determine milk yield were variable and therefore cannot be easily compared but should be considered as estimates.

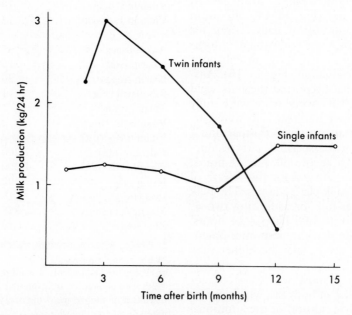

FIG. 11-15 Milk outputs of western Australian women breastfeeding twins and exclusively breastfeeding single babies.

From Hartmann PE et al: Breastfeeding and reproduction in women in Western Australia—a review, *Birth Family J* 8:215, 1981.

Some controversy remains about the energy cost of lactation. English and Hitchcock[14] compared the energy intake of 16 nursing mothers to 10 nonnursing mothers and found that the energy intake of breastfeeders in the sixth and eighth postpartum week was 2,460 kcal. The energy intake of nonnursing mothers during the same postpartum period was 1880 calories—a difference of 580 calories. In a later study by Thomson, Hytten, and Billewicz,[45] lactating women were found to ingest 2,716 kcal per day and nonnursing mothers 2125 kcal per day—a difference resulting from nursing of 590 kcal. By adding the assumed energy equivalents of body weight being lost, total energy available to the two groups was about 2,977 and 2,364 kcal per day, respectively. If one assumes that the energy requirements for basal metabolism and activity are equivalent for the two groups, the energy needed for daily milk production is close to 560 kcal; the production efficiency of human milk is therefore about 90%.

Other observations of lactating women, however, have led some researchers to propose that energy needs have been overestimated. Butte et al.[7,18] found that typical lactating women who were producing about 750 ml of milk per day had a mean daily energy consumption of 2,171 ± 545 kcal per day. Observations of postpartum weight-loss patterns and subsequent calculations of energy balance led to an estimation of 80% efficiency in energy utilization for milk production. When energy available from the diet (2,171 kcal per day) was added to the energy derived from tissue mobilization (315 kcal per day) and the caloric equivalent of the milk was subtracted (597 kcal per day), a net balance of 1889 kcal per day was left for maintenance and activity. These findings suggest that successful lactation is compatible with gradual weight reduction and attainable with energy intakes less than current recommendations.

Similarly, Manning-Dalton and Allen[33] evaluated postpartum weight-loss patterns, breastfeeding completeness, and daily kcalorie intakes of well-nourished North American women. In spite of low mean kcalorie intakes (2,178 kcal per day), breastfeeding was successful, and weight loss during the 12 to 90 days postpartum averaged only 2.0 kg for the entire sample and 1.6 kg for the solely breastfeeding women.

To discover how much daily caloric restriction it takes before milk production is impaired, researchers studied lactating baboons.[38] Three different diets were fed, and milk production was measured after each. The first diet was completely unrestricted; the second diet was 80% of the caloric level of the first diet; and the third diet was 60% of the caloric level of the first diet. As seen in Fig. 11-16, milk volume was not adversely affected until caloric provisions were dropped to 60% of the desired level.

More recent efforts to evaluate the energy cost of lactation provide additional information. Dutch investigators examined a group of healthy lactating women and reported the following[48]

Estimated cost of lactation	630 kcal per day
Energy cost was met by:	
Eating more food	415 kcal per day
Tissue mobilization	35 kcal per day
Reducing energy expenditure	180 kcal per day

Researchers in the United Kingdom measured energy intake, basal metabolic rate (BMR), total energy expenditure (TEE), physical activity plus thermogenesis (TEE-BMR), changes in body fat stores, and milk energy transfer. The energy-balancing strategies adopted by different women varied markedly. Overall, energy costs and expenditures were the following[20]:

Energy content of milk	534 kcal per day
Estimated cost of milk synthesis	106
Energy costs met by:	
Eating more food	306 to 418 kcal per day
Reduction in basal metabolic rate	minimal
Reduction in physical activity	165 to 227 kcal per day
Use of stored fat	minimal

Piers et al. observed in well-nourished Indian women that the energy costs of lactation were largely met by increases in energy intake rather than in any metabolic economy or fat mobilization.[36]

It is apparent that there is more than one way to satisfy the energy costs of lactation. The flexibility in this regard likely explains the ability of almost all women to maintain satisfactory milk production under a variety of dietary and lifestyle circumstances.

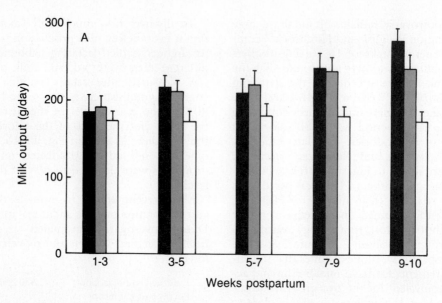

FIG. 11-16 Milk output of lactating baboons fed ad libitum (■), or ad libitum until 2 weeks postpartum and thereafter with 80% (■) or 60% (□) of their own voluntary intake. Values are means ± SEM.

From Roberts SB, Coward WA: Lactational performance in relation to energy intake in the baboon, *Am J Clin Nutr* 41:1270, 1985.

Dieting

For many women the usual slow rate of weight loss after childbirth may not satisfy their desires for immediate return to prepregnancy body weight. It is therefore likely that dietary restriction may be instituted, even though it is discouraged by health care professionals. It is important to recognize, however, that moderate to severe restriction of calorie intake during lactation will compromise the woman's ability to synthesize milk. This is especially significant in the early weeks of lactation initiation before the process is firmly established. As a result of this effect of calorie restriction on milk production, lactating women should be advised to accept a gradual rate of weight loss in the first 6 months after

More modest weight reduction efforts after lactation is well-established may not hamper milk output, at least if the caloric restriction is short term. This was demonstrated by Strode, Dewey, and Lonnerdal[44] using 22 well-nourished lactating women. Nutrient intake and milk

volume and composition were evaluated over a 3-week period. Mean maternal energy intakes were 2,316 (week 1), 1,591 (week 2) and about 2,100 (thereafter). Milk intake was not reduced by those infants nursing during the "short-term diet."

Recently, other researchers addressed the question of dieting by following 22 healthy, well-nourished lactating women.[13] These women with established lactation reduced their daily calorie intake by more than 500 calories. Mean daily milk production was assessed before the "dieting" period and after 10 weeks, mean daily milk production was 759 ml/day at baseline and 802 ml/day at week 10. Percent milk fat and protein were unchanged. These findings suggest that modest weight loss by healthy breastfeeding women does not adversely affect either quantity or quality of milk consumed by their infants.

With regard to postpartum weight loss, the notion has been proposed that breastfeeding speeds the rate of weight loss, compared with the rate of loss experienced by women choosing formula feeding. In general, this is not the case.[6,12,37] Examination of the rate of weight loss in both groups suggests that there is very little difference. Lactating women, however, are able to consume more calories each day while demonstrating a gradual decline in stored fat.

Exercise

Observations in lactating animals provide mixed data on the impact of exercise on the process of lactation. Cows exposed to treadmill walking at different levels of intensity and duration showed some depression in milk output.[29,30] Mice with access to running wheels were not significantly different from sedentary controls in milk yield, mammary gland weight, or offspring body weight.[26] Rats trained to swim 2 hours per day, 5 days a week with a 3% tail weight showed no significant reduction in milk yield or offspring weight to day 15.[46]

Recent observations in lactating women suggest that vigorous exercise does not interfere with the process of lactation. In one study, eight exercising women were compared with eight sedentary controls.[32] Measures of fitness, diet, energy expenditure and milk production were made. The exercising women demonstrated a higher level of fitness, a lower level of percent body fat (21.7% vs. 27.9%), a higher level of energy expenditure (3,169 kcal per day vs. 2,398 kcal per day), and a higher level of energy intake (2,739 kcal per day vs. 2,051 kcal per day). There was no difference between the groups in plasma hormones or milk energy, lipid, protein, or lactose content. Exercising women tended to have higher milk volume (839 gm per day vs. 776 gm per day). These findings show that there is no apparent adverse effect of vigorous exercise on lactation performance in humans.

The same conclusion was drawn in a follow-up study in which 33 sedentary women whose infants were being exclusively breastfed were randomly assigned to an exercise group or a control group.[11] The exercise program consisted of supervised aerobic exercise (at a level of 60 to 70% of the heart rate reserve) for 45 minutes per day, 5 days per week, for 12 weeks. Energy expenditure, dietary intake, body composition and the volume and composition of breast milk were assessed at 6, 8, 12-14, and 18-20

weeks postpartum. The women in the exercise group expended about 400 calories per day in the exercise sessions but compensated for this energy expenditure with a higher energy intake than that recorded for the control women (2,497 kcal/day vs. 2,168 kcal/day). There were no significant differences between the two groups in maternal body weight or fat loss, the volume or composition of the breast milk, or the infant's weight gain during the 12-week study. Hence there was no adverse effect on the process of lactation and the cardiovascular fitness of the exercising mothers improved.

Protein

Along with the recommended energy increment, a 12- to 15-gm increase in daily protein intake is advised for lactating women. The extra protein is believed to be necessary to cover the requirement for milk production with an allowance of 70% efficiency in protein utilization. The increased needs for energy and protein can be easily met by consumption of about 3 to 3½ extra cups of milk per day. This will provide the needed protein and energy but will not cover the increased recommendations for ascorbic acid, vitamin E, and folic acid. It is therefore recommended that other foods such as citrus fruits, vegetable oils, and leafy green vegetables be increased slightly in the daily diet.

Maintenance of lactation while consuming a vegetarian diet can be managed nicely, providing all the basic principles of sensible vegetarian eating are followed carefully.[15] The nutritional needs of the lactating vegetarian woman are the same as those of the lactating woman with a more traditional diet. Appropriate extra sources of calories and protein must be clearly defined; if dairy products are acceptable in the chosen dietary regimen, extra milk consumption is applicable here, as previously mentioned. If dairy products are not included in the accepted list of foods, extra energy and high-quality protein and calcium must be obtained from appropriately combined vegetables, grains, nuts, and other such sources. Dietary supplements may be unacceptable, and thus intelligent diet planning on a daily basis is of utmost importance for maintenance of successful lactation and health of the vegetarian mother.

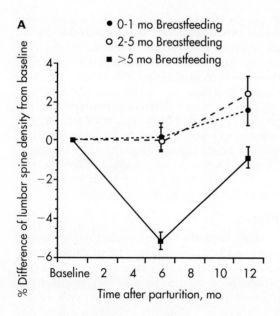

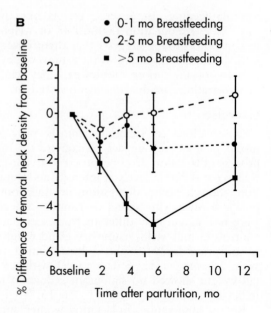

FIG. 11-17   Changes in lumbar spine. **A,** and femoral neck, **B,** bone mineral density observed across 12 months.

From Sowers M et al. Changes in bone density with lactation, *JAMA* 269:3130, 1993.

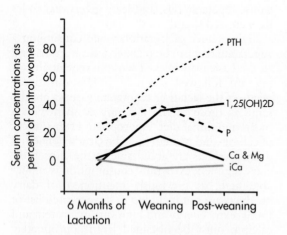

FIG. 11-18   Changes in calcium homeostasis as a function of lactation and weaning. PTH = parathyroid hormone, P = phosphorus, iCa = ionized calcium.

From Specker BL, Tsang RC, Ho ML: Changes in calcium homeostasis over the first year postpartum: effect of lactation and weaning, *Obstet Gynecol* 78:56, 1991.

Supplementation

Although lactation increases a woman's requirement for nearly all nutrients, these increased needs can be provided by a well-balanced diet. For this reason, nutritional supplements are generally unnecessary except when there is a deficient intake of one or more nutrients. It is true, for example, if the lactating woman is intolerant of milk, that calcium supplementation (as well as alternative calorie and protein sources) would help to prevent unnecessary calcium loss from bones.

Calcium: A Special Concern

Whereas there is no evidence that calcium composition of human milk can be influenced by dietary intake of calcium, it is believed that dietary calcium deficiency promotes mobilization of calcium from bones to maintain milk calcium levels.[49] Other clinical literature documents cases of osteomalacia and tetany in mothers who nursed for long periods while on inadequate diets.[3,5]

❖ ❖ ❖

Questions About Breastfeeding

Georgeanne P. Syler, PhD, Southeast Missouri State University

Community Hospital provides an 8-week pre-natal education class for all expectant mothers and fathers who plan to deliver at this hospital. Jan S., a dietitian employed at the hospital, has just completed a presentation to the class about breastfeeding: basic considerations, advantages, and benefits to the infant and mother. When the class dismisses for the evening, two women stay behind to talk with Jan.

The first woman, Vanessa, who is 3 months pregnant, asks Jan several questions. Vanessa describes herself as having had anorexia ner-vosa during her adolescence. She experienced amenorrhea from age 15 through 21 because of low body fat, low weight, and extensive ex-ercise. She is still very thin, with small breasts, and continues to be very conscious of her body image. Exercise is still an important part of her life; she has been a jogger for years and has continued to jog thus far during her preg-nancy. How should Jan answer the following questions for Vanessa?

1. Will the fact that I had anorexia, or my small breast size, mean that I won't be able to breastfeed?

2. I'm happy to be pregnant, and I want to do what is best for the baby, but will breast-feeding make me gain additional weight after the baby comes or keep me from losing the weight I gained while I was pregnant? I'm okay with eating what I should eat while I'm pregnant, but I don't know about eating extra to breastfeed.

3. What about dieting while breastfeeding? Would that affect my breast milk or affect my baby?

The second woman appears to be very close to her due date. She introduces herself as Sarah, and tells Jan she is carrying twins. Sarah would like to breastfeed, but she also has ques-tions. How should Jan answer the following questions for Sarah?

1. Will I have enough milk for two babies? Will breastfeeding twins be to much trouble?

2. Wouldn't it be better to bottle-feed, so my husband could help with the feeding?

3. Can I use oral contraceptives while I breastfeed? I understand that breastfeeding is not a foolproof method of contraception, and I sure don't want another pregnancy any time soon after having twins!

Recent research has focused on the changes that occur in bone during and after the process of lactation. Sowers et al.[41] measured bone den-sity in the femur and lumbar spine in nursing mothers at 2 weeks, 6 months and 12 months after birth in a longitudinal study. Bone density was not compromised in nonnursing mothers or a group of mothers who breastfed for up to 5 months. Bone density was significantly reduced in the extended lactation group (>6 months). However, evidence supported the concept that recovery of bone density occurs after the wean-ing process (Fig. 11-17).

This phenomenon of bone loss during lacta-tion and recovery after weaning has since been documented by other researchers.[9,10,25,43] In the face of adequate calcium nutrition, bone re-modeling during lactation and postweaning ap-pears to be a normal biological phenomenon and does not appear to adversely affect bone health. The physiological explanation for this process has been examined. Observed increases during weaning of parathyroid hormone and 1, 25 dihydroxy vitamin D may be responsible for bone recovery (Fig. 11-18).[9] Should pregnancy occur again before the recovery process is com-plete, one wonders whether the lactation bone loss is permanent.

Assuming that bone mineral density recovers during the weaning process, the health of mater-nal bone should not differ from that of women who never lactated. Support for this concept has been provided in a study of postmenopausal women whose reproductive history was evaluated.[28] Bone mineral density among 741 white postmenopausal women age 60 to 89 years indicated that the bone mineral density of the wrist, radius, and hip was not related to the number of pregnancies or lactation experiences.

It has been proposed that the relatively high incidence of osteomalacia and osteoporosis in the United States is partially related to the waning intake of milk and dietary calcium by adult women. Whether this is the case is still unknown. It stands to reason, however, that prolonged lactation accompanied by poor calcium intake may significantly compromise the calcium status of the skeletal system and increase its susceptibility to fractures and other forms of trauma.

Cost Considerations

The cost of providing adequate nutritional support to the lactating mother depends heavily on what foods she selects to meet her nutritional needs. Some older studies suggest that human milk costs more than bottle-feeding because of the extra nutrients the mother must consume. It is clear, however, in examining the costs of appropriate extra foods for the lactating mother that human milk is cheaper than proprietary cow's milk formulas if economical food choices are made. The present difference between the cost of commercially prepared cow's milk formulas and human milk undoubtedly will continue to increase in coming years, since the price of "double-cycle" animal products (including cow's milk) continues to escalate. Beyond the price consideration, however, it is hard to justify "wastage" of human milk and the resultant unnecessary draw on the precious supply of other animal protein available to the world's population. Human milk represents a vital national resource, which if used to its fullest extent, could markedly improve not only the health and nutritional status of today's children but also the "natural resource base" of many underdeveloped countries.

Summary

Human milk is designed for human infants, and the process of lactation has maintained the human race since its origin. The mammary glands develop during the embryonic period but most of the growth and differentiation takes place during the postmenarcheal years, with the final events occurring during pregnancy. Lactation occurs through a sequence of neuroendocrine phenomena; interference with any of the steps in the pathway may compromise milk delivery to the infant. The major impact of maternal malnutrition on lactation is reduction in the total volume of milk produced. Almost all women can breastfeed if they choose to do so; good maternal nutrition optimizes the quality and quantity of milk production while maintaining health of the mother.

REVIEW QUESTIONS

1. Diagram the anatomy of a mammary gland.
2. Discuss the development of the mammary glands.
3. Outline the basic steps in the physiology of lactation.
4. Summarize basic nutritional requirements for the healthy lactating woman.
5. Compare the cost of lactating with the cost of purchasing commercial infant formula.

LEARNING ACTIVITIES

1. Diagram the process of milk production and let-down.
2. Design a dietary pattern appropriate for a typical lactating woman.
3. Ask a local pharmacist about current recommendations for drug use or nonuse during lactation.
4. Evaluate locally available teaching materials that have to do with the physiology of lactation.

REFERENCES

1. American Academy of Pediatrics, Committee on Drugs: Breast-feeding and contraception, *Pediatrics* 68:138, 1981.
2. American Academy of Pediatrics, Committee on Nutrition: Nutrition and lactation, *Pediatrics* 68:435, 1981.
3. Anderson AB, Brown A: Tetany following prolonged lactation on a deficient diet, *Lancet* 2: 482, 1941.
4. Andrusiak F, Larose-Kuzenko: *Lactation consultant series,* 1987.
5. Atkinson PJ, West RR: Loss of skeletal calcium in lactating women, *J Obstet Gynaecol Br Commonw* 77:555, 1970.

6. Brewer MM et al: Postpartum changes in maternal weight and body fat in lactating and nonlactating women, *Am J Clin Nutr* 49:259, 1989.

7. Butte NF et al: Maternal energy balance during lactation, *Fed Proc* 42:922, 1983.

8. Casey CE: Nutrient intake by breastfed infants during the first five days after birth, *Am J Dis Child* 140:933, 1986.

9. Cross NA et al: Calcium homeostasis and bone metabolism during pregnancy, lactation, and postweaning: a longitudinal study, *Am J Clin Nutr* 61:514, 1995.

10. Cross NA et al: Changes in bone mineral density and markers of bone remodeling during lactation and postweaning in women consuming high amounts of calcium, *J Bone Mineral Res* 10:1312, 1995.

11. Dewey KG et al: A randomized study of the effects of aerobic exercise by lactating women on breast milk volume, *N Engl J Med* 330:449, 1994.

12. Dugdale AE, Evans JE: The effect of lactation and other factors on postpartum changes in body weight and triceps skinfold thickness, *Br J Nutr* 61:149, 1989.

13. Dusdieker LB, Hemingway DL, Stumbo PJ: Is milk production impaired by dieting during lactation? *Am J Clin Nutr* 59:833, 1994.

14. English RM, Hitchcock NE: Nutrient intakes during pregnancy, lactation, and after the cessation of lactation in a group of Australian women, *Br J Nutr* 22:615, 1968.

15. Finley DA et al: Food choices of vegetarians and nonvegetarians during pregnancy and lactation, *J Am Diet Assoc* 85:678, 1985.

16. Food and Nutrition Board, National Research Council: *Recommended dietary allowances,* ed 10, Washington, DC, 1989, Government Printing Office.

17. Ford CSA: *Comparative study of human reproduction,* New Haven, 1945, Yale University Press.

18. Garza C, Butte N: The effect of maternal nutrition on lactational performance. In Kretchmer N, ed: *Frontiers in clinical nutrition.* Rockville, Md, 1986, Aspen Systems.

19. Geissler C, Margen S, Calloway DH: Lactation and pregnancy in Iran: III. Hormonal factors, *Am J Clin Nutr* 32:1097, 1979.

20. Goldberg GR et al: Longitudinal assessment of the components of energy balance in well-nourished lactating women, *Am J Clin Nutr* 54:788, 1991.

21. Gray RH et al: Risk of ovulation during lactation, *Lancet* 335:25, 1990.

22. Hartmann PE: Breastfeeding and reproduction in women in Western Australia—a review, *Birth Family J* 8:215, 1981.

23. Howie PW: The relationship between suckling-induced prolactin response and lactogenesis, *J Clin Endocrinol Metab* 50:670, 1980.

24. Institute of Medicine: *Nutrition during lactation,* Washington, DC, 1991, National Academy of Sciences.

25. Kalkwarf HJ, Specker BL: Bone mineral loss during lactation and recovery after weaning, *Obstet Gynecol* 86:26, 1995.

26. Karasawa K, Suwa J, Kimura S: Voluntary exercise during pregnancy and lactation and its effects on lactational performance in mice, *J Nutr Sci Vitam* 27:333, 1981.

27. Kennedy KI, Visness CM: Contraception efficacy of lactational amenorrhea, *Lancet* 339:227, 1992.

28. Kritz-Silverstein D, Barrett-Connor E, Hollenbach KA: Pregnancy and lactation as determinants of bone mineral density in postmenopausal women, *Am J Epid* 136:1052, 1992.

29. Lamb R, Anderson M, Walters J: Effects of forced exercise on two-year-old Holstein heifers, *J Dairy Sci* 62:1791, 1979.

30. Lamb R, Anderson M, Walters J: Forced walking prepartum for dairy cows of different ages, *J Dairy Sci* 64:2017, 1981.

31. Lonnerdal B, Forsum E, Hambraeus L: Effect of oral contraceptives on composition and volume of breast milk, *Am J Clin Nutr* 33:816, 1980.

32. Lovelady CA, Lonnerdal B, Dewey KG: Lactation performance of exercising women, *Am J Clin Nutr* 52:103, 1990.

33. Manning-Dalton C, Allen LH: The effects of lactation on energy and protein consumption, postpartum weight change and body composition of well nourished North American women, *Nutr Res* 3:293, 1983.

34. Neville MC, Allen JC, Archer PC et al: Studies in human lactation: milk volume and nutrient consumption during weaning and lactogenesis, *Am J Clin Nutr* 54:81, 1991.

35. Neville MC, Allen JC, Watters C: The mechanisms of milk secretion. In Neville MC, Neifert MR, editors: *Lactation: physiology, nutrition and breast-feeding*, New York, 1983, Plenum Press.

36. Piers LS et al: Changes in energy expenditure, anthropometry and energy intake during the course of pregnancy and lactation in well-nourished Indian women, *Am J Clin Nutr* 61:501, 1995.

37. Potter S et al: Does infant feeding method influence maternal postpartum weight loss? *J Am Diet Assoc* 91:441, 1991.

38. Roberts SB, Coward WA: Lactational performance in relation to energy intake in the baboon, *Am J Clin Nutr* 41:1270, 1985.

39. Rosner AE, Schulman SK: Birth interval among breast-feeding women not using contraceptives, *Pediatrics* 86:747, 1990.

40. Saint L, Maggiore P, Hartmann PE: Yield and nutrient content of milk in eight women breast-feeding twins and one woman breast-feeding triplets, *Br J Nutr* 56:49, 1986.

41. Sowers M et al: Changes in bone density with lactation, *JAMA* 269:3130, 1993.

42. Specker B et al: Changes in calcium homeostasis over the first year postpartum: effect of lactation and weaning, *Obstet Gynecol* 78:56, 1991.

43. Specker BL et al: Calcium kinetics in lactating women with low and high calcium intakes, *Am J Clin Nutr* 59:593, 1994.

44. Strode MA, Dewey KG, Lonnerdal B: Effects of short-term caloric restriction on lactational performance of well-nourished women, *Acta Paediatr Scand* 75:222, 1986.

45. Thomson AM, Hytten FE, Billewicz WZ: The energy cost of human lactation, *Br J Nutr* 24:565, 1970.

46. Treadway JL, Lederman SA: The effects of exercise on milk yield, milk composition and offspring growth in rats, *Am J Clin Nutr* 44:481, 1986.

47. Tyson JE: Nursing and prolactin secretion: principal determinants in the mediation of puerperal infertility. In Crosignani PG, Robyn C, eds: *Prolactin and human reproduction*, New York, 1977, Academic Press.

48. van Raaij JMA et al: Energy cost of lactation and energy balances of well nourished Dutch lactating women, reapproval of the extra energy of lactation, *Am J Clin Nutr* 53: 612, 1991

49. Wong KN et al: Effect of lactation and calcium deficiency and of fluoride intake of bone turnover in rats: isotopic measurements on bone reabsorption and formation, *J Nutr* 111:1848, 1981.

CHAPTER

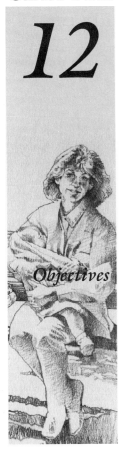

12

Human Milk Composition and Infant Growth and Development

Bonnie S. Worthington-Roberts

Objectives

✦✦✦

After completing this chapter, the student will be able to:

✓ *Compare the composition of human milk with that of cow's milk.*

✓ *Discuss the impact of maternal diet upon the quality and quantity of milk production.*

✓ *Compare the composition of term milk with that of preterm milk.*

✓ *Define what is meant by fortified human milk and discuss its impact on growth of preterm infants.*

Introduction

Human milk was designed for human infants, and its composition is unique to the needs of our species. In addition to containing the necessary macronutrients, it also is endowed with the full spectrum of vitamins and minerals. Attention has been given to the array of nonnutrient growth factors, hormones, and protective factors such as immunoglobulins; there may be other important substances in human milk that have yet to be identified. Unfortunately, compounds enter human milk that may adversely affect the nursing infant; however, their numbers are few and their concentrations generally low. The value of human milk for the health and

growth of the baby is undisputed; rarely does breastfeeding need to be discouraged.

COMPOSITION OF HUMAN MILK

Large numbers of investigations over more than 25 years have been aimed at defining the biochemical and nutritional properties of different types of mammalian milk (Table 12-1). It is clear from these efforts that each type of milk is unique and consists of a highly complex mixture of organic and inorganic compounds. It is likely that the characteristics of mammalian milks relate directly to variable mother-child relationships that take place in infancy. Shaul[171] found

TABLE 12-1 **Composition of Milk from Representative Mammals**

Mammalian Species	Total Protein (gm/100 gm)	Casein (gm/100 gm)	Total Fat (gm/100 gm)	Lactose (gm/100 ml)	Ash (gm/100 gm)
Man	1.2-1.5*	0.4	3.8	7.0	0.2
Baboon	1.6	—	5.0	7.3	0.3
Black bear	—	8.8	24.5	0.4	1.8
California sea lion	13.8	—	36.5	0.0	0.6
Black rhinoceros	—	1.1	0.0	6.1	0.3
Domestic dog	—	5.8	12.9	3.1	1.2
Norway rat	—	6.4	10.3	2.6	1.3
Whitetail jackrabbit	—	19.7	13.9	1.7	1.5

*Recent Swedish studies have shown the "true protein content" of human milk to be only 0.8 to 0.9 mg/100 ml in apparently well-nourished women when determined by amino acid analysis; the above figures were derived by calculation from assayed nitrogen content, which overestimates the protein content because about 25% of the nitrogen in human milk is nonprotein nitrogen. From Hambraeus L: Proprietary milk versus human breast milk in infant feeding: a critical appraisal from the nutritional point of view, *Pediatr Clin North Am* 24:17, 1977.
Modified from Jenness R and Sloan RE: Composition of milk. In Larson BL and Smith VR, editors: *Lactation. III. Nutrition and biochemistry of milk/maintenance,* New York, 1974, Academic Press.

support for this idea while examining five groups of wild animals. Group 1 consists of marsupials and animals that bear their young while in hibernation; in these animals the mother is available at all times, and the milk produced is dilute and low in fat. Group 2 consists of animals born in a relatively mature state that follow or are carried by their mothers at all times. Here the maternal attentiveness is high, and the milk produced is dilute and rather low in fat. (The low fat content is often seen in animals that nurse frequently.) Group 3 consists of animals that leave their young in a secluded place and return to nurse them at widely spaced intervals; the lioness is a good example, but in all cases this group of animals has very concentrated milk that is high in fat. Group 4 consists of animals born in a relatively immature state and that remain for a considerable time in nests or burrows. The mother must leave for several hours at a time, and nursing is inclined to be "on schedule" rather than "on demand." Group 5 consists of animals that spend much time in cold water or, when on land, are often made wet by the mother returning from the water. In all cases the fat content of milk is extremely high and the milk very concentrated.

Human milk is dilute and thus resembles the milk of the marsupials and hibernating bears whose offspring feed constantly.[93] It is therefore not surprising, as mentioned by Gerrard,[63] that the human baby demands to be fed often, and for this reason, in many parts of the world, the mother carries the baby where she goes at all times.

Reports during the past 25 years on the biochemical composition of human milk have included hundreds of publications; new components continue to be characterized such that more than a hundred constituents are now recognized.[25] Basically, human milk consists of a solution of protein, sugar, and salts in which a variety of fatty compounds are suspended (Table 12-2). The composition varies from one human to another, from one period of lactation to the next, and even hourly during the day. The composition of a given milk sample is related not only to the amount secreted and the stage of lactation but also to the timing of its withdrawal and to individual variations among lactating mothers. These latter variations may be affected by such variables as maternal age, parity, health, and social class. Gestational age of the infant may also make a difference in that analyses of milk from mothers of premature infants indicate

TABLE 12-2   *Composition of Human Colostrum and Mature Breast Milk*

Constituent (per 100 ml)	Colostrum, 1-5 Days	Mature Milk, >30 Days
Energy (kcal)	58	70
Total solids (gm)	12.8	12.0
Lactose (gm)	5.3	7.3
Total nitrogen (mg)	360	171.
Protein nitrogen (mg)	313	129
Nonprotein nitrogen (mg)	47	42
Total protein (gm)	2.3	0.9
Casein (mg)	140	187
α-Lactalbumin (mg)	218	161
Lactoferrin (mg)	330	167
IgA (mg)	364	142
Amino acids (total)		
Alanine (mg)	—	52
Arginine (mg)	126	49
Aspartate (mg)	—	110
Cystine (mg)	—	25
Glutamate (mg)	—	196
Glycine (mg)	—	27
Histidine (mg)	57	31
Isoleucine (mg)	121	67
Leucine (mg)	221	110
Lysine (mg)	163	79
Methionine (mg)	33	19
Phenylalanine (mg)	105	44
Proline (mg)	—	89
Serine (mg)	—	54
Threonine (mg)	148	58
Tryptophan (mg)	52	25
Tyrosine (mg)	—	38
Valine (mg)	169	90
Taurine (free) (mg)	—	8
Urea (mg)	10	30
Creatine (mg)	—	3.3
Total fat (gm)	2.9	4.2
Fatty acids (% total fat)		
12:0 lauric	1.8	5.8
14:0 myristic	3.8	8.6
16:0 palmitic	26.2	21.0
18:0 stearic	8.8	8.0
18:1 oleic	36.6	35.5
18:2, n-6 linoleic	6.8	7.2
18:3, n-3 linolenic	—	1.0
C_{20} and C_{22} polyunsaturated	10.2	2.9

From Casey CE, Hambidge KM: Nutritional aspects of human lactation. In Neville MC, Neifert MR, editors: *Lactation: physiology, nutrition and breast-feeding,* New York, 1983, Plenum Press. (A very detailed summary of the numerous studies focused on human milk composition is found in the appendix of the report from the Institute of Medicine: *Nutrition during lactation,* Washington DC, 1991, National Academy of Sciences.)

TABLE 12-2 *Composition of Human Colostrum and Mature Breast Milk—cont'd*

Constituent (per 100 ml)	Colostrum, 1-5 Days	Mature Milk, >30 Days
Cholesterol (mg)	27	16
Vitamins		
Fat soluble		
Vitamin A (retinol equivalents) (μg)	89	47
β-Carotene (μg)	112	23
Vitamin D (μg)	—	0.04
Vitamin E (total tocopherols) (μg)	1,280	315
Vitamin K_1 (μg)	0.23	0.21
Water soluble		
Thiamin (μg)	15	16
Riboflavin (μg)	25	35
Niacin (μg)	75	200
Folic acid (μg)	—	5.2
Vitamin B_6 (μg)	12	28
Biotin (μg)	0.1	0.6
Pantothenic acid (μg)	183	225
Vitamin B_{12} (ng)	200	26
Ascorbic acid (mg)	4.4	4.0
Minerals		
Calcium (mg)	23	28
Magnesium (mg)	3.4	3.0
Sodium (mg)	48	15
Potassium (mg)	74	58
Chlorine (mg)	91	40
Phosphorus (mg)	14	15
Sulphur (mg)	22	14
Trace elements		
Chromium (ng)	—	39
Cobalt (μg)	—	1
Copper (μg)	46	35
Fluorine (μg)	—	7
Iodine (μg)	12	7
Iron (μg)	45	40
Manganese (μg)	—	0.4,1.5
Nickel (μg)	—	2
Selenium (μg)	—	2.0
Zinc (μg)	540	166

higher concentrations of some nutrients than in similar samples from mothers of term infants.

Although much data have been recorded on the differences in samples of human milk, the general picture is the same throughout the world. Except for vitamin and fat content, the composition of human milk appears to be largely independent of the state of nutrition of the mother, at least until malnutrition becomes severe. Even after prolonged lactation for 2 years or more, the quality of milk produced by Indian and African women appears to be rela-

TABLE 12-3   *Content of Selected Nutrients in Mature Human Milk from Well-Nourished and Poorly Nourished Communities*[97]

Country	Fat (gm/100 ml)	Lactose (gm/100 ml)	Protein (gm/100 ml)	Calcium (gm/100 ml)
Well-nourished				
American	4.5	6.8	1.1	34.0
American (middle/upper class)	3.8	—	1.1	—
British	4.78	6.95	1.16	29.9
Australian	—	—	—	28.6-30.7
Poorly nourished				
India	3.42	7.51	1.06	34.2
Bantu, South Africa	3.9	7.10	1.35	28.7
New Guinea Highlands	2.36	7.34	1.01	—
Alexandria, Egypt				
Healthy	4.43	6.65	1.09	—
Malnourished	4.01	6.48	0.93	—
Brazil				
High income	3.9	6.8	1.3	20.8
Low income	4.2	6.5	1.3	25.7
Ibadan, Nigeria	4.05	7.67	1.22	—
Wuppertal, Germany (post–World War II)	3.59	—	1.2	—
Guatemala	3.2	—	1.1	—
Pakistan	2.7	—	1.2	—
Burma	3.6	—	1.1	—
Ivory Coast	3.1	—	1.0	—
American (Navajo)	—	—	1.4	—

From Jelliffe DB, Jelliffe EFP: The uniqueness of human milk, *Am J Clin Nutr* 31:492, 1978; and Garza C, Butte N: The effect of maternal nutrition on lactational performance. In Kretchmer N, ed: *Frontiers in clinical nutrition*, Rockville, Md, 1986, Aspen.

tively well-maintained, although the quantity may be small (Table 12-3). It is also well-known that severely undernourished women during time of famine often manage to feed their babies reasonably well.

Colostrum

In the first few days after birth of the baby the mammary glands secrete a small amount of thick fluid called *colostrum*. The volume varies between 2 and 10 ml per feeding per day in the first 3 days, related in part to the parity of the mother. Women who have had other pregnancies, particularly those who have nursed babies previously, usually demonstrate colostrum output sooner and in greater volume than other women. Colostrum is typically yellow, a feature associated with its relatively high carotene content. It is also transparent and contains more protein, less sugar, and much less fat than milk produced thereafter. As might be expected from these compositional differences, it is lower in calories than mature milk (58 vs. 70 kcal/100 ml). The ash content of colostrum is high, and concentrations of sodium, potassium, and chloride are greater than in mature milk. The few compositional analyses of human colostrum that have been reported show striking variability during any one day and from day to day; it is likely that this circumstance partially reflects the unstable secretory patterns that exist in the mammary apparatus as it begins active production, secretion, and ejection of milk.

A benefit believed to be associated with colostrum is its reported ability to facilitate the establishment of "bifidus flora" in the digestive tract. Colostrum also may facilitate the passage of meconium, the dark-green, mucilaginous material in the intestine of the newborn. **Meconium** contains an essential growth factor for *Lactobacillus bifidus* and is the first culture medium in the sterile intestinal lumen of the infant. The abundance of antibodies found in colostrum may also assist in providing protection against various gastrointestinal-tract infections.[150]

Colostrum changes to transitional milk between the third and sixth day, at which time the protein content is still rather high. By the tenth day the major changes have been completed, and by the end of the first month the protein content reaches a consistent level, which does not fall significantly thereafter. As the content of protein falls, the content of lactose progressively rises. This is also the case for fat, which increases to typical levels as lactation becomes more firmly established.

Mature Milk

Protein. It is well-known that different animals show different rates of growth, and this appears to be related to the composition of their milk. The slowest rate of growth is found in humans, and human milk contains the least protein. The major proteins found in breast milk are casein (curd protein) and α-lactalbumin, lactoferrin, and secretory IgA (whey proteins). It also contains a number of other proteins, such as serum albumin, β-lactoglobulins, other immunoglobulins, and various glycoproteins.[123] A listing of individual human milk proteins is provided in Table 12-4. Overall, mature milk contains about 0.7 to 0.9 gm of protein per 100 ml of whole milk as compared with 3.5 gm in cow's milk. This level of protein found in human milk is lower than the previously accepted value of 1.5 gm/100 ml that was determined by calculation from analyzed nitrogen content. Since human milk has been found to contain more than 25% of its nitrogen in nonprotein compounds,

TABLE 12-4 *Concentration of Individual Proteins in Human Milk*

Protein	Molecular Weight	Concentration (mg/ml)
Casein		2-3
β-Casein	24,000	—
κ-Casein	38,000	—
Lactoferrin	77,000	1-3
α-Lactalbumin	14,100	2-3
Secretory IgA	420,000	0.5-1.0
Secretory component	86,000	0.2-0.3
IgA	160,000	0.1
IgM	900,000	0.02
IgG	150,000	0.01
Serum albumin	68,000	0.3
Lysozyme	15,000	0.05-0.25
Bile-salt stimulated lipase	90,000	0.1
Lipoprotein lipase	72,600	—
α-Amylase	60,000	—
Galactosyltransferase	55,000	—
Sulfhydryl oxidase	89,000	—
Lactoperoxidase	85,000	<0.0001
α_1-Antitrypsin	50,000	0.01
α_1-Antichymotrypsin	70,000	0.01
Folate-binding protein	26,000	0.007
Vitamin B_{12}-binding protein	102,000	—
Thyroxine-binding protein	36,500	—
Corticosteroid-binding protein	93,000	0.1

From Lonnerdal B: Biochemistry and physiological function of human milk proteins, *Am J Clin Nutr* 42:1299, 1985.

the lower protein concentration is now accepted as the "true" amount.[24]

A major difference between human milk and cow's milk is the concentration of casein and **whey** proteins (lactalbumins). The ratio of whey proteins to casein is 1.5 for breast milk and 0.2 for cow's milk; this means that 40% of human milk protein is casein and 60% whey proteins, whereas cow's milk contains 80% casein and 20% whey proteins. Casein is the group of milk-specific proteins that form sizable curds when exposed to heat, pH changes, or enzymes; under these circumstances the casein is transformed into an insoluble calcium caseinate-calcium phosphate complex. Human milk with its low casein content forms a flocculent suspension with a curd tension of 0. These small curds are easily digested and consequently better tolerated by the neonate.

The major whey protein is α-lactalbumin, a specific protein component of the enzyme lactose synthetase. Lactoferrin is an iron-binding protein that has been observed to inhibit the growth of certain iron-dependent bacteria in the gastrointestinal tract. It has been suggested that lactoferrin helps protect against certain gastrointestinal-tract infections in breastfed infants. Investigations by Lonnerdal, Forsum, and Hambraeus[124] have shown many unexplained variations in healthy, well-fed women in milk concentration of specific proteins such as α-lactalbumin and lactoferrin.

Immunoglobulins are found in breast milk, and these are distinct from those found in serum. By far the major component in this class of proteins is secretory IgA (sIgA), with monomeric IgA, IgG, and IgM being minor components. Major research efforts have concentrated on sIgA. It is synthesized by the mammary gland from two IgA units and two other proteins. The concentration of sIgA is very high in colostrum but declines to low levels by the fourteenth day. Since sIgA is very stable at low pH and resistant to **proteolytic enzymes,** it survives in the intestine of the breastfed infant and provides a protective defense against infection by retarding viral and bacterial invasion of the mucosa.

Milk from women who have not been pregnant or who have initiated lactation long after a pregnancy has been completed is somewhat different in its protein content from milk of typical lactating women. Researchers evaluated milk samples from five women who had adopted their infants and who had induced lactation by having their infants suckle; two of the five had delivered normal infants in the past. For all donors, lactation was achieved within 11 days of first putting the infant to the breast, and the first secretions expressed were sent for analysis. Control milk samples were collected from five normal women who had uncomplicated pregnancies. Comparison of the biologic mother's milk with the nonbiologic mother's milk showed that concentrations of certain whey proteins and total protein were similar in amount to values obtained from transitional milk and mature milk collected after the fifth day postpartum from biologic mothers; the milk was also lower in IgA and higher in α-lactalbumin than in colostrum (Fig. 12-1). These differences should probably be taken into account when discussing the nutritional and protective values of human milk for different groups of infants with widely different requirements, such as premature infants, and those beyond the neonatal period.[106]

Amino acids. The amino acid content of human milk is recognized as ideal for the human infant (Table 12-5). It is relatively low in several amino acids that are known to be detrimental if found in the bloodstream at high levels (e.g., phenylalanine); it is also high in other amino acids that the infant cannot synthesize well, such as cystine and taurine. Some of the positive features about amino acid composition of human milk are summarized in Table 12-6. These characteristics are especially useful to infants whose biochemical capabilities are underdeveloped at birth.

One study was undertaken to determine changes in amino acid composition of human milk over time as well as daily amino acid intakes of breastfed babies.[36] Both total amino acid and nitrogen intakes declined by approximately 34% during the first 8 weeks postpartum, primarily because of a 20% decline in concentration of individual amino acids (Fig. 12-2). Intakes of seven of nine essential amino acids studied were less than requirements specified by the Food and Agricultural Association (FAO) and World Health Organization (WHO) at both 4 and 8 weeks of age. These data suggest that FAO/WHO estimates of amino acid requirements may be inflated, at least for some of the essential amino acids.

Of interest with regard to amino acid composition is a study by Stegnick, Filer, and Baker,[180] who administered significant amounts of aspartame* to lactating women. Serum, red-cell, and milk phenylalanine levels were assessed to determine the potential spillage of phenylalanine

---

*Aspartame is a dipeptide sweetener that contains aspartic acid and phenylalanine.

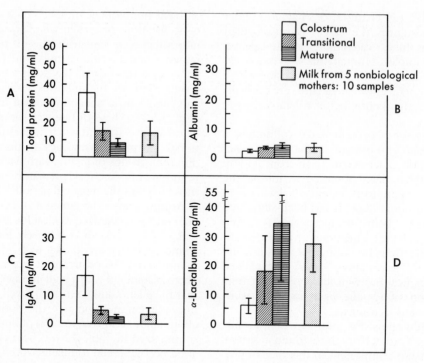

FIG. 12-1 Protein changes in human milk with time (±SD) in bioligic mothers as compared with protein concentrations in nonbiologic mothers during the first 5 days of lactation.

From Kleinman R et al: Protein values of milk samples from mothers without biologic pregnancies, *J Pediatr* 97:612, 1980.

FIG. 12-2 Decline in human milk total nitrogen and total amino acid concentrations from 2 to 8 weeks of lactation. Total amino acids include phenylalanine, tyrosine, methionine, threonine, valine, leucine, lysine, histidine, isoleucine, arginine, glutamate, proline, aspartate, serine, alanine, and glycine.

From Janas LM, Picciano MF: Quantities of amino acids ingested by human milk-fed infants, *J Pediatr* 109:802, 1986.

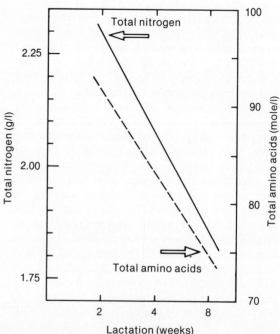

TABLE 12-5 *Amino Acid Content of Human and Cow's Milk*

Amino Acid	Human Milk*		Cow's Milk†	
	% of Protein	mg/100 gm Fluid Milk	% of Protein	mg/100 gm Fluid Milk
Tryptophan	1.7	17	1.4	46
Threonine	4.5	46	4.5	148
Isoleucine	5.4	56	6.0	198
Leucine	9.2	95	9.7	321
Lysine	6.6	68	7.9	260
Phenylalanine	4.5	46	4.8	158
Tyrosine	5.1	53	4.8	158
Valine	6.1	63	6.7	220
Methionine	2.0	21	2.5	82
Cystine	1.8	19	0.9	30
Histidine	2.2	23	2.7	89
Arginine	4.2	43	3.6	119
Alanine	3.5	36	3.4	113
Aspartic acid	8.0	82	7.5	249
Glutamic acid	16.3	168	20.8	687
Glycine	2.5	26	2.1	69
Proline	8.0	82	9.7	318
Serine	4.2	43	5.4	178

*Based on 1.03% protein.
†Based on 3.3% protein.
From U.S. Department of Agriculture, Agricultural Research Center: *Agricultural handbook no 8-1 (revised)*, Washington, DC, 1976, U.S. Department of Agriculture.

TABLE 12-6 *Significant Characteristics of the Amino Acid Composition of Human Milk*

Characteristic	Explanation
Lower in methionine and rich in cystine	An enzyme, cystathionase, is late to develop in the fetus; this impairs optimal conversion of methionine to cystine, which is needed for growth and development; methionine may increase in the bloodstream of an infant fed cow's milk but not one fed human milk; hypermethioninemia may damage the central nervous system
Lower in phenylalanine and tyrosine	The enzymes tyrosine aminotransferase and parahydroxyphenyl pyruvate oxidase are late in developing: cow's milk-fed babies may develop hyperphenylalaninemia and hypertyrosinemia, which may adversely affect development of the central nervous system, especially in the premature infant; breast milk offers much less problem
Rich in taurine	Breast milk provides taurine for bile acid conjugation, and it may also be a neurotransmitter or neuromodulator in the brain and retina; humans cannot synthesize taurine well; cow's milk contains little taurine; the requirement for taurine in the developing neonate is uncertain

from aspartame into human milk. Whereas maternal plasma phenylalanine levels increased approximately fourfold after aspartame ingestion, milk levels of phenylalanine, aspartate, and tyrosine were elevated only slightly. The mammary gland appears to regulate the migration of some amino acids from the mother's circulation to her milk. Given these observations, it seems unreasonable to worry about aspartame consumption by lactating women.[62]

For many years it was generally assumed that the protein found in human milk was nutritionally superior to that of cow's milk. Lactalbumin (in whey) was thought to have a higher biologic value than casein (in curd), largely because it contained more methionine and cystine. Amino acid analyses of the two milks, however, have revealed that they are similar, and both adults and babies have been kept in nitrogen balance when fed equivalent amounts of both casein and lactalbumin. However, 1-day-old breast-fed infants demonstrate a mean serum albumin concentration that is higher than that of evaporated milk-fed babies. Some researchers maintain that human milk protein may indeed be superior and that serum albumin concentration may be a more sensitive index of protein quality than nitrogen balance studies or standard growth-rate parameters.

With chronic protein undernutrition, breast milk composition may change. The effects of prolonged lactation on the quantity of protein and patterns of amino acids in breast milk were evaluated in Thai women at various times during lactation. Protein levels decreased from 1.56% during the first week to a low of about 0.6% from 180 to 270 days and then rose to about 0.7%. Using these data, one can calculate that a 3-month-old infant in the fiftieth percentile for weight would require about 1,250 ml of milk per day to meet protein needs. Since few infants in developing countries would receive this volume of milk daily and since supplemental sources of protein are scarce, the protein status of such infants could be significantly compromised.

The effect of maternal protein supplementation has not been examined to an adequate degree. One protein supplementation study indicated increased milk production with a corresponding fall in protein concentration; overall protein output in 24 hours was not significantly altered. One must remember, however, in evaluations of this type that only milk volume and composition are considered. The condition of the mother should also be assessed, and deterioration in nutritional status should be anticipated when maintenance of "quality" milk production is a physiologic priority. A nutritional supplement may not alter the milk, but it may support retention of maternal health and well-being.[39,68,69]

Nonprotein nitrogen[40]. The total amount of nonprotein nitrogen (NPN) in human milk is at least 25% of all nitrogen and is significantly higher than that found in cow's milk (about 5%). NPN consists of a variety of organic and trace amounts of inorganic compounds shed into the milk supply. Among these compounds are **peptides** and free amino acids, the latter of which may provide a nutritional advantage to the infant. NPN also includes urea, creatinine, and sugar amines. Since each species of mammal seems to carry a characteristic pattern of free amino acids in NPN, scientists have speculated that this is of nutritional significance.

Much discussion has centered on taurine. Since taurine is found in particularly high levels in fetal brain tissue, it has been proposed that it may play a role in the development of the brain. In addition, taurine is associated with bile acid and thus plays an important role in digestion and may function in the management of cholesterol in the body. Since human milk contains much more taurine than does cow's milk, it has been speculated that the breastfed infant might profit significantly from the higher taurine intake. Interestingly, however, observations show that breastfed babies maintain plasma taurine levels that are similar to those of formula-fed infants. It would appear that taurine is not an essential amino acid for term infants.[187]

Lipids. The total lipid content of milk varies considerably from one woman to another and is even affected by parity and season of the year (Fig. 12-3). Separate observations by different investigators around the world give the following average levels of fat in human milk: 2.02%, 3.1%, 3.2%, 3.27%, 3.95%, 4.5%, and 5.3%. Data from the U.S. Department of Agriculture survey of 1976 place the average at 4.4%. Sampling methods may affect fat content, since the first milk (fore-milk) is low in fat and the last milk

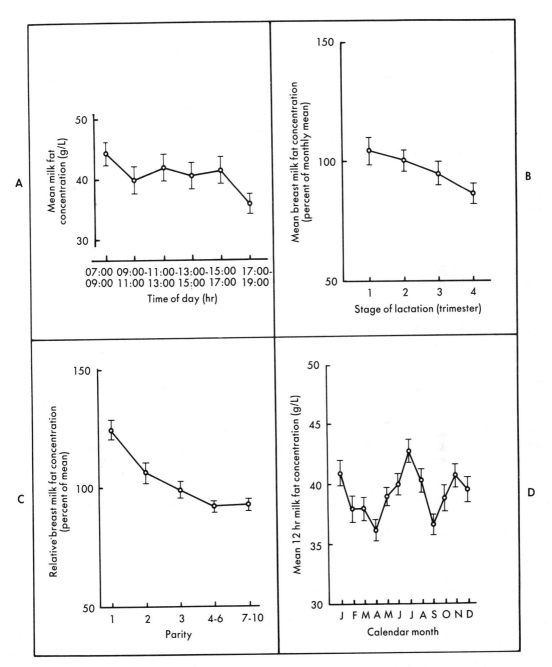

FIG. 12-3   Variations in breast milk fat concentrations in rural African women **A,** during a 12-hour period, **B,** during stages of lactation in first year postpartum (seasonally corrected), **C,** in women with different parity, and **D,** during different seasons of the year.

(hind-milk) shows about three times an increase in fat content (Fig. 12-4).

Nearly 90% of the lipid in human milk is present in the form of triglycerides, but small amounts of phospholipids, cholesterol, diglycerides, monoglycerides, **glycolipids,** sterol esters, and free fatty acids are also found. The fatty acid composition of human milk differs greatly from that of cow's milk. The content of the essential fatty acid linoleic acid is considerably greater in human milk than in cow's milk; the content of oleic acid is also greater in human milk, whereas the content of shorter-chain saturated fatty acids (C_4 to C_8) is greater in cow's milk. Of equal interest is the observation that human milk contains more cholesterol than cow's milk and much more cholesterol than commercial infant formulas. A beneficial effect of this higher cholesterol level has been suggested on grounds that (1) it is needed by the rapidly growing central nervous system for **myelin** synthesis, and (2) it stimulates in early life the development of enzymes necessary later for cholesterol degradation. Whether this dietary constituent should be considered essential remains to be determined; in any case its presence in breast milk is significant.

Data reported by Harzer et al.[80] showed changing patterns of human milk lipids during the course of lactation. Triglyceride content was found to increase (mainly during the first postpartum week), cholesterol concentration declined, and phospholipid content remained the same (Fig. 12-5). After an ordinary period of milk release about 20% of the milk remains in the gland, and this milk contains 50% of the fat. This phenomenon may result from the adsorption of the fat globules to the surface of the alveolar cells. It has been suggested that this changing fat composition of human milk during a feed may be one of the mechanisms of aiding appetite control of infants. The higher fat composition of the hind-milk in comparison with the fore-milk may serve to signal satiety in infants and gradually motivate them to withdraw from the breast and cease feeding. This intriguing idea has not been supported, however, by several researchers. In one study assessing milk intake and six parameters of sucking, there was no indication that high-fat milk acted as a cue to babies to slow or stop feeding.[42,148] On the contrary, babies appeared to feed more actively on the high-fat milk in that they sucked in longer bursts for it and spent a smaller proportion of the test period resting. Similar observations were made by several other groups of researchers.[41,192]

Evidence suggests that the fat content of breast milk may be reduced to as low as 1 gm/100 ml. Under these circumstances the kcalorie content of the milk may be much decreased with significant lessening of available energy for the infant. The basis for low-fat milk composition is believed to be related not only to diet during lactation but also to inadequate energy intake in pregnancy with an inadequate subcutaneous "fat bank."[18,162]

Just because a mother's milk is low in fat does not mean that the infant will necessarily suffer. Tyson et al.[182] studied two groups of mother-infant pairs. One group of mothers produced high-fat milk and the other produced low-fat milk. Growth of the infants, mother-infant interaction and maternal satisfaction were assessed. Babies receiving the low-fat milk seemed to adapt to their situation; they spent more time

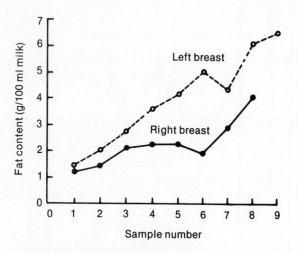

FIG. 12-4   Variation in fat content of human milk during a single feeding. Data are from successive samples from one woman obtained by breast pump.

From Neville MC, Allen JC, Watters C: The mechanisms of milk secretion. In Neville MC, Neifert MR, editors: *Lactation: physiology, nutrition, and breast-feeding,* New York, 1983, Plenum Press.

per feeding and had more complete emptying of the breast. Growth was comparable to that of the infants receiving high-fat milk. Mothers producing the low-fat milk had no adverse maternal satisfaction or maternal-infant interaction during feeding. The researchers point out, however, that in the case of low-fat milk production,

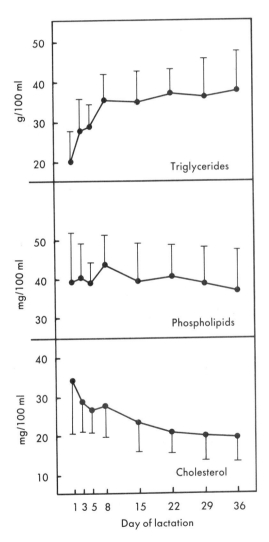

FIG. 12-5 Changing patterns of human milk lipids as lactation progresses (means ±SD).

From Harzer G et al: Changing patters of human milk lipids in the course of the lactation and during the day, *Am J Clin Nutr* 37:612, 1983.

there is little reserve if milk production diminishes.

Women accustomed to low fat intake tend to adapt to such diets and produce milk that is lower in fat than that of women following high-fat regimens. It has been proposed that in the presence of a habitually low fat intake, prolonged lactation might have a hypolipidemic effect. One study of African women did not support this idea[188]; serum lipid levels did not differ significantly among long-lactating mothers, nonlactating mothers, and nulliparous women. The investigators suggest that this lack of hypolipidemic effect reflects the adaptability and the homeostatic capacity of the lactating women who were examined.

Fatty acids[43]. The composition of the fat in human milk varies significantly with the diet of the mother. The fatty acid pattern of human milk can be changed significantly by modifying energy intake and fatty acid composition of dietary fat. Lactating women fed a diet rich in polyunsaturated fats, such as corn and cottonseed oil, produce milk with an increased content of polyunsaturated fats. This is best seen by comparing total vegetarians with nonvegetarians,[58,168] as is seen in Table 12-7. It is also illustrated by providing lactating women with fish oil supplements and evaluating changes in ω-3 fatty acid concentration in their milk (Fig. 12-6).[79] Over the years, as dietary unsaturated fat intake has increased in the United States, the fatty acid composition of breast milk samples has reflected this change.

When calorie intake is severely restricted, fatty acid composition of human milk resembles that of depot fat. This circumstance is to be expected and represents fat mobilization in response to the reduction in energy intake. A substantial increase in the proportion of dietary kcalories from carbohydrate will result in an increase in milk content of lauric and myristic acids. The significance of this latter observation is unknown, but Sinclair and Crawford[174] reported increased mortality and reduced body size and brain cell number among rats nourished by dams whose milk contained a high content of short- and medium-chain fatty acids.

At present, there is much interest in the importance of long-chain polyunsaturated fatty acids in human milk.[37,115,127-130] Data from

TABLE 12-7 *Mean Breast Milk Fatty Acid Concentration in Vegetarians (Vegans) and Nonvegetarians (Controls)*

Methyl Esters	Vegans*	Controls*
Lauric ($C_{12:0}$)	39	33
Myristic ($C_{14:0}$)	68	80
Palmitic ($C_{16:0}$)	166	276
Stearic ($C_{18:0}$)	52	108
Palmitoleic ($C_{16:1}$)	12	36
Oleic ($C_{18:1}$)	313	353
Linoleic ($C_{18:2}$)	317	69
Linolenic ($C_{18:3}$)	15	8

*Mean values expressed as milligrams per gram total methyl esters detected for four vegans and four controls (nonvegetarians).

Modified from Sanders TAB et al: Studies of vegans: the fatty acid composition of plasma cholinephosphoglycerides, erythrocytes, adipose tissue and breast milk and some indicators of susceptibility to ischemic heart disease in vegans and omnivore controls, *Am J Clin Nutr* 31:805, 1978.

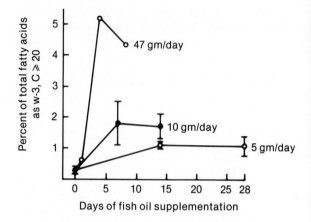

FIG. 12-6 Effects of various levels of fish oil on levels of ω-3 fatty acids of chain length C_{20} and above in human milk. Respective intake levels are indicated adjacent to the curves.

Modified from Harris WS, Connor WE, Lindsey S: Will dietary ω-3 fatty acid change the composition of human milk? *Am J Clin Nutr* 40:780, 1984.

many sources indicate an essential role of docosahexaenoic (DHA) for early human development. In utero, the placenta appears to supply DHA and other long-chain polyunsaturated fatty acids to the fetus. After birth, breast milk does so, providing an especially rich source of DHA and arachidonic acid (AA). Structural lipids in brain and nervous tissue contain large amounts of these fatty acids. Currently available infant formulas do not provide these important compounds.

Lucas et al. have provided impressive data that supports the value of human milk in neurological development.[127] These researchers followed 926 premature infants from birth to 7½ to 8 years of age. Some of them were provided human milk in the neonatal period and some were provided formula. Assessment of IQ at 7½ to 8 years of age indicated that human milk-fed babies had significantly higher IQs (8.3 points); this was true after controlling for social class, mother's education, and maternal-infant contact. The authors theorize that the DHA in human milk may explain the difference.

Similar results were reported by Lanting et al.[115] who assessed neurological status of about 500 9 year olds. Some of them had been breastfed and others had been provided formula. An advantageous effect of breastfeeding was observed and the DHA and AA contributions from human milk were suggested to explain the outcome. Additionally, there is evidence that supplementation of preterm babies with DHA improves visual function.[14] Differences in visual performance between breastfed and formula-fed term infants have also been reported.[15,129] Finally, breastfed infants demonstrate a higher concentration of DHA in both erythrocytes and brain.[128] Animal models support these clinical observations and suggest that dietary deficiency of ω-3 fatty acids results in altered brain composition and function.

Cholesterol. The cholesterol content of human milk ranges from about 10 to 20 mg/100 ml with an approximately daily consumption by the infant of 100 mg. The amount of cholesterol drops as lactation progresses, even though the fat content may rise. The cholesterol content of milk is not altered by diet; however, a fall in plasma cholesterol level of the infant is associated with an increase in linoleic acid concentration of the milk. There is no evidence that consumption of breast milk as an infant provides for more efficient metabolism of cholesterol as an adult or that endogenous synthesis is inadequate for the infant's requirements.

Lipases. Of interest is the finding that human milk contains several fat-digesting enzymes or lipases. One is a serum-stimulated lipase (lipoprotein lipase) that may appear in the milk as a result of leakage from the mammary tissue. Another lipolytic milk enzyme is similar to the activity of pancreatic lipase, breaking down triglycerides to free fatty acids and glycerol. This enzyme is present in the fat fraction and appears to be inhibited by bile salts. It probably is responsible for lipolysis of milk refrigerated or frozen for later use. Additional lipases in the skim milk fraction are inactive until they encounter bile. These lipases, the bile-salt-stimulated lipases, are believed to be present only in the milk of primates and are thought to complement the digestive activity of pancreatic lipase.

Since the bile-salt–stimulated lipases have been clearly shown to be stable and active in the intestines of infants, they can contribute significantly to the hydrolysis of milk triglycerides and partly account for the greater ease in fat digestion that is commonly demonstrated by breast-fed babies.

Carnitine. Carnitine plays an important role in the oxidation of long-chain fatty acids by facilitating their transport across the mitochondrial membrane. It also helps regulate **thermogenesis** in brown adipose tissue and functions together with malonyl-coenzyme A in the initiation of **ketogenesis**. The body's supply of carnitine is derived in part by ingestion of dietary carnitine and in part by endogenous synthesis from the essential amino acids lysine and methionine.

Newborns are especially in need of carnitine since fat provides a major source of energy. It has been suggested that carnitine may be an essential nutrient for the newborn since infants may have a limited carnitine synthetic capacity, especially those born prematurely. Human milk contains about 50 to 100 nmol/ml. Formula products based on milk or beef contain 50 to 656 nmol/ml. Those prepared from soy isolate

(and specialized formulations from egg white and casein) carry an amount equal to or less than 4 nmol/ml. Whether infants using any of these formulas or provided human milk require additional carnitine has been the subject of some debate. However, data from both term and preterm infants indicate that serum carnitine concentrations do not correlate with carnitine intake. Supplemental carnitine appears unnecessary for the vast majority of neonates.[166]

Carbohydrate. Lactose is the main carbohydrate in human milk, and for a long time it was considered to be the only one present. **Chromatographic** processing of human milk samples, however, has revealed trace amounts of glucose, galactose, glucosamines, and other nitrogen-containing oligosaccharides. The role or significance of these minor carbohydrates has not been defined, but it is possible that one or more of them could contribute to the gut colonization by specific microorganisms with potentially beneficial effects to the infant.[35] The nitrogen-containing oligosaccharides, for example, have a *L. bifidus*-promoting activity. This organism has the property of breaking down lactose into lactic acid and acetic acid, and thus it is responsible for the acid reaction of the intestinal contents of breastfed infants that may interfere with the growth of many **enteropathogenic organisms.**

The lactose found in human milk occurs in two forms, α-lactose and β-lactose. It is relatively insoluble and is slowly digested and absorbed in the small intestine. The presence of lactose in the gut of the infant stimulates the growth of microorganisms, which produce organic acids and synthesize many of the B vitamins. It is believed that the acid milieu that is created helps to check the growth of undesirable bacteria in the infant's gut and to improve the absorption of calcium, phosphorus, magnesium, and other metals. Since human milk contains much more lactose than cow's milk (7% and 4.8%, respectively), these gut-associated benefits of lactose are more significant in the breastfed than in the bottle-fed infant.

Lactose levels are quite constant throughout the day in a given mother's milk. Even in poorly nourished mothers the levels of lactose do not vary. Since lactose is influential in controlling volume, the total output for the day may be diminished, but the concentration of lactose in human milk will be 6.2 to 7.2 gm/100 ml.

Normal term infants are able to digest lactose, but observations by Lifschitz et al.[119,120] suggest that lactase sufficiency develops more slowly in some infants than previously suspected. Undigested lactose moves into the lower bowel, where bacterial fermentation of the available sugars takes place with liberation of measurable hydrogen gas.* This phenomenon is not associated with either fermentative diarrhea or impaired growth. Gradually lactase levels in the small bowel increase, and hydrogen production in the lower bowel is markedly reduced.

The rare infant with **congenital lactase deficiency** may actually be able to profit from the use of human milk. Although such infants require a lactose-free diet, human milk can be used for these infants, providing the lactose is first broken down. This can be achieved by adding three drops of lactase to each 200-ml bottle of human milk; removal of lactose by fermentation with *Saccharomyces fragilis* has also been reported.[46] After the milk is stored at 4° C for 24 hours, the percentage of lactose decreases from 6.9 gm/100 ml to 1.1 gm/100 ml. Similä et al.[173a] found that lactase-deficient infants provided with hydrolyzed human milk showed good growth and development with only a small increase in looseness of stools.

Although human milk does not contain much complex carbohydrate, it does contain a starch-digesting enzyme, amylase, which is quite stable at pH levels found in the stomach and small bowel.[85] This enzyme may provide an alternative pathway for digestion of glucose polymers and starches in early infancy when pancreatic amylase is low or absent in duodenal fluid. The physiologic importance of mammary amylase may be analogous to that of the bile salt-stimulated lipase found in human milk.

Minerals. One of the most striking differences between human and cow's milk lies in the mineral composition. As with protein, it is believed that this difference may be related to the rate of growth of the species for which the milk

---

*Degree of bacterial liberation of hydrogen in the lower bowel can be estimated by the **hydrogen breath test**.

TABLE 12-8   *Renal Solute Load Provided by Various Milks*

Feed	Approximate Renal Solute Load (mOsml/100 kcal)
Human milk	10
Commercial formula	20
Cow's milk	40
Skim milk	70
Mixed diet	60

was intended. According to typical estimations, there is six times more phosphorus, four times more calcium, three times more total ash, and three times more protein in cow's milk than in human milk. The high mineral and protein composition of cow's milk distinctly affects the solute or osmolar load provided to the kidney (Table 12-8). One might speculate that the kidney of the newborn infant is prepared to handle the solute load derived from breast milk but is "stressed" unduly by the requirements placed on it when cow's milk (especially nonfat milk) is selected as an alternative.

The major minerals found in mature human milk are potassium, calcium, phosphorus, chlorine, and sodium. Iron, copper, and manganese are found in only trace amounts, and since these elements are required for normal red-cell synthesis, infants fed too long on milk alone may become anemic. Minute amounts of zinc, magnesium, aluminum, iodine, chromium, selenium, and fluorine are also found in breast milk. Infants who are not provided with fluoridated water in addition to breast milk may benefit from a daily oral fluoride supplement of regulated dosage predetermined by the physician and pharmacist. Providing the lactating woman with a fluoride supplement does not significantly alter her milk output of fluoride (Fig. 12-7).[48,49]

The total mineral content of human milk is fairly constant, but the specific amounts of individual minerals may vary with the status of the mother and the stage of lactation. Observations from several laboratories have shown declining concentrations of several minerals over the weeks and months following the onset of lactation (Fig.

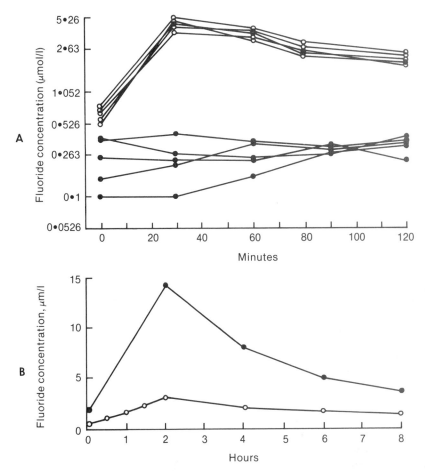

FIG. 12-7   Plasma (open symbols) and breast milk (closed symbols) fluoride concentrations after oral dose of fluoride. **A,** Dose of 1.5 mg of fluoride as sodium fluoride solution. **B,** Dose of 11.25 mg of fluoride as sodium fluoride tablets.

From Ekstrand J: No evidence of transfer of fluoride from plasma to breast milk, *BMJ* 283:761, 1981; and Ekstrand J et al: Distribution of fluoride to human breast milk, *Caries Res* 18:93, 1984.

12-8). It has also been shown that during a single nursing,[155] mineral concentration may change significantly. Of substantial interest are other reports in which dietary intake and supplementation habits of mothers were compared with mineral composition of milk; in most situations no relationship was found between maternal mineral intake and milk mineral content.*

Some minerals are more easily absorbed from breast milk than from cow's milk or commercial formulas. It has been reported that nearly 50% of the iron in human milk is absorbed, whereas availability of iron from cow's milk and iron-fortified formulas is only 10% and 4%, respectively. More recently, it was found that iron absorption from human milk may be much higher than 50% during the first 3 months of life. An explanation for this improved absorption has not been found, but the presence of considerable

*References 21, 38, 53, 54, 74, 104, 155, 156, and 163.

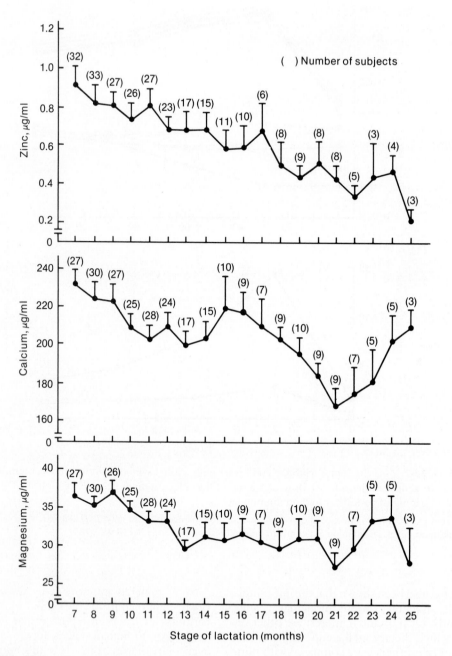

FIG. 12-8 Concentrations of zinc, calcium, and magnesium in milk samples collected at morning feeding from 7 to 25 months of lactation. Vertical bars represent SEM.

From Karra MV et al: Changes in specific nutrients in breast milk during extended lactation, *Am J Clin Nutr* 43:495, 1986.

amounts of inosine 5'-monophosphate in milk has led several investigators[52] to speculate that this factor is responsible, since inosine and its metabolite have been shown to enhance iron absorption in the rat.

Whether breastfed infants should receive iron supplements is still the subject of much debate.[23,157] Several studies suggest that infants who are breast-fed during the first 6 months of life and receive little or no dietary iron other than that in human milk appear to be iron sufficient at age 6 months.[152] However, based on changes in total body iron determined by body weights and hemoglobin and ferritin concentrations, it has been concluded that some nonsupplemented breastfed infants are in negative iron balance between age 3 and 6 months.

So when, if ever, should an exclusively breastfed infant be given an iron supplement? In the study by Siimes, Salmenpera, and Perheentopa,[173] infants were observed for a period of 9 months. At 6 months of age, one of the infants met laboratory criteria for iron deficiency but was not anemic. By age 7½ months, an additional five infants met the criteria for iron deficiency. The authors concluded that the majority of exclusively breastfed infants remain iron sufficient for the first 9 months of life. In contrast to the previous recommendation,[60] these authors feel that it is safe to defer any iron supplements in the exclusively breastfed infants until at least 6 months. The data from one researcher support this recommendation but reinforce the point that iron stores are significantly reduced in breastfed infants by the middle of the first year of life (Fig. 12-9). Oski[151] suggests, however, that if solid foods are introduced before 6 months of age, it may be necessary to provide an iron supplement unless the foods introduced are good sources of iron, such as iron-fortified cereals.

Like iron, the bioavailability of zinc from human milk is substantially better than from alternative preparations.[26,102] In one study the bioavailability of zinc fed to rats in various milk solutions was 59.2% for human milk, 42% for cow's milk, and 26.8% to 39% for commercial formulas.[98] In other work, human subjects demonstrated better absorption of zinc from human milk than from cow's milk or selected in-

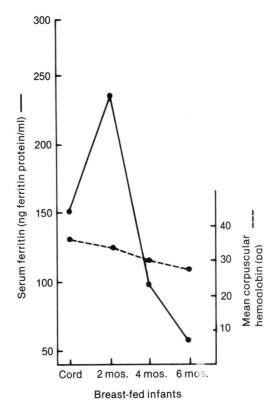

FIG. 12-9   Changes in mean values of serum ferritin and mean corpuscular hemoglobin in breastfed infants from birth to 6 months.

From Duncan B et al: *J Pediatr Gastroenterol Nutr* 4:421, 1985.

fant formulas (Fig. 12-10).[26] An explanation for the better absorbability of zinc from human milk is still being sought; it has been suggested, however, that the unique distribution and binding of zinc (and some other elements) to high- and low-molecular-weight fractions of milk very likely are related to the differences in bioavailability that have now been demonstrated by a number of investigators.[45,148] At least three different absorption facilitators have been proposed, including citrate, picolinic acid, and a biologically active 12,500 molecular weight human milk protein.[44]

The impact of maternal zinc supplementation on the zinc content of human milk has recently

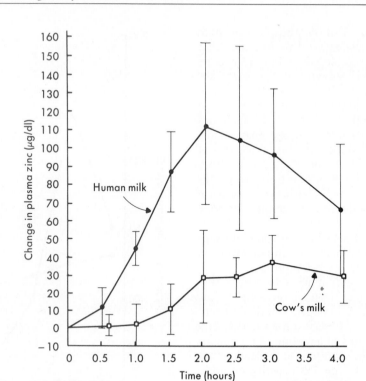

FIG. 12-10   Changes in plasma zinc concentration after ingestion of 25 mg of zinc with human milk (5 subjects) and cow's milk (7 subjects). Points represent means ±SD from baseline value.

From Case CE, Walravens PA, Hambidge KM: Availability of zinc: loading tests with human milk, cow's milk and infant formulas, *Pediatrics* 68:394, 1981. © American Academy of Pediatrics, 1981.

been reevaluated[141,189] through more than 7 months of lactation in 71 women. Dietary intake of zinc in the nonsupplemented group was 13.0 mg/day; diet plus supplemental zinc intake of the supplement group was 25.7 mg/day. Although the supplemented group demonstrated a higher mean serum zinc concentration throughout the study, milk zinc concentrations did not differ between the groups. In both groups, a gradual decline in milk zinc concentration occurred. At least in the case of this relatively healthy population, zinc supplementation did not affect milk zinc level.

Of interest, however, is the observation that in a low-income population in Paris,[111,189] zinc supplementation of breastfed babies improved their growth. Supplemented and nonsupplemented babies were monitored for a 3-month period. The superior growth in the supple-

mented group was due mainly to greater linear growth of boys. The authors conclude that among infants breastfed for longer than 4 months, decreases in growth velocity result partly from inadequate zinc intake.

In rare situations lactating women have been found to produce milk that is potentially harmful to their infants because of a high or low concentration of specific nutrients.[10,88,105,144] For example, several babies have reportedly developed hypernatremia caused by ingestion of breast milk that is abnormally high in sodium. The etiologic factors of increased breast milk sodium concentration is unclear in some cases, since maternal dietary sodium level is unrelated to milk sodium concentration. However, mastitis and lesions of the nipple may cause elevation of sodium concentration of milk. Other possible explanations include a delay in maturation of milk, an effect of the mother's "dieting program," or some unrecognized defects in milk secretion. Whatever the case, increased breast milk sodium concentrations should be considered among the causes of neonatal hypernatremia.

With regard to sodium concentration in human milk, a recent study suggests that a normal drop in sodium concentration is highly predictive of successful lactation but a prolonged elevation in breast milk sodium level signifies impaired lactation with a high rate of failure.[140] This observation was made in 130 nursing mothers who were monitored between the third and eighth months of lactation. In general, those who failed in lactation tended to have higher initial sodium levels. The longer the sodium remained elevated, the lower the success rate. The mechanism behind this phenomenon is unknown.

As far as other minerals are concerned, little work has been done on human milk.[61] Fluorine, iodine,[161] and selenium show a geographic variation in cow's milk and there is reason to believe that the same occurs in human milk. Work on the selenium content of human milk strongly indicates its relationship to maternal selenium status.[1] Data from both Finnish and American women suggest that typical milk concentration of chromium in human milk is 30 to 40 ng/100 ml.[5] Variable levels of manganese have been observed in samples of human milk from different laboratories; some data suggest a mean concentration of 3.5 to 3.7 µg/L. Finally, molybdenum and nickel levels in humans have now been assessed; results indicate that mature human milk contains about 1 to 2 ng/ml of molybdenum and 1.2 ng/ml of nickel.

Vitamins. All the vitamins required for good nutrition and health are supplied in breast milk, but the amounts vary markedly from one person to another. Several reasons may account for this observation; genetic differences likely are important, but diet and drug use by individual women also influences vitamin composition of milk.

The vitamin content of human milk may be seen to change dramatically in some instances over the first few days of lactation. Generally, the level of water-soluble vitamins goes up and the level of fat-soluble vitamins declines. However, exceptions exist. None of the normal variations poses any risk to the infant.

❖

CASES OF RICKETS IN BREASTFED BABIES NOT RECEIVING VITAMIN D SUPPLEMENTS

1. Four cases of rickets caused by vitamin D deficiency in breast-fed babies were reported in 1991; all four babies were black. These babies were all from the southern part of the United States. (Browmick SK, Rettig KR: Rickets caused by vitamin D deficiency in breast-fed infants in Southern United States, *Am J Dis Child* 145:127, 1991.)[19]

2. Nutritional rickets was diagnosed in 18 infants aged 8 to 24 months; all cases were diagnosed in an urban clinic in Seattle. All of the mothers breast-fed their infants, and none provided their infants vitamin D supplements. (Feldman KW et al: Nutritional rickets, *J Am Acad Fam Pract* 42-1311, 1990.)[55]

3. Vitamin D metabolism in breast-fed infants and their mothers was assessed. Judged by the plasma 25-OHD levels, the vitamin D stores of most children born to mothers with normal vitamin D status are depleted approximately 8 weeks after delivery. This suggests that an appropriate dose of vitamin D should be provided shortly after birth, especially in the winter. (Hoogendaezem T et al: Vitamin D metabolism in breast-fed infants and their mothers, *Pediatr Res* 25:623, 1989.)[90]

The amount of biologically active *vitamin D* in human milk has been found to be low (40 to 50 IU/L).[87] 25-Hydroxyvitamin D_3 accounts for about 75% of the biologic activity, with vitamin D_2 and vitamin D_3 accounting for the majority of the remainder.[89] The fact that the majority of the activity in human milk is in the form of 25-hydroxyvitamin D (25-OHD) may be an advantage for the breastfed neonate because hepatic hydroxylase for the conversion of vitamin D to 25-OHD may be underdeveloped.[90] In addition, 25-OHD in milk may provide the infant with a form of vitamin D that is most readily used (see box above).

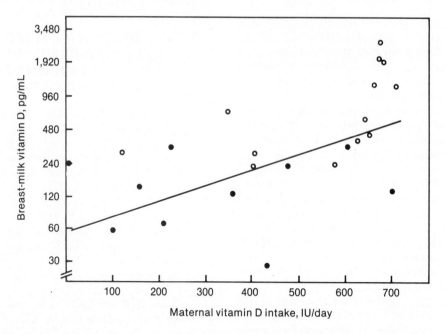

FIG. 12-11   Relationship between breast milk vitamin D and vitamin D intake (IU/day). Open and closed circles indicate white and black patients, respectively. Breast milk vitamin D was significantly correlated with vitamin D intake (r = 0.57; *p* = 0.005).

From Specker BL, Tsang RC, Hollis BW: Effects of race and diet on human-milk vitamin D and 25-hydroxyvitamin D, *Am J Dis Child* 139:1134, 1985.

There is evidence that vitamin D activity in human milk is influenced by maternal vitamin D intake (Fig. 12-11). Polskin, Kramer, and Sobel[159] demonstrated that when mothers were given large doses of fish liver oil, the vitamin D content of milk increased. Others[179] also found that increased vitamin D intake resulted in large increases of vitamin D in breast milk. Similar results were found with ingestion of things such as garlic (see box on p. 367). A shorter regimen of oral vitamin D supplementation (60 µg of vitamin D_2 per day for 2 weeks) raised the level of vitamin D_2 in the milk of a lactating woman 40 times.[113]

Maternal exposure to ultraviolet light also affects breast milk vitamin D content. This has been demonstrated on a number of occasions in which breast milk vitamin D levels have been measured during winter and summer months; routinely, breast milk vitamin D is higher during the summer.[108,131,133,177,178] In addition, expo-

sure to ultraviolet phototherapy quickly raises the levels of the vitamin D sterols in both plasma and milk.[72]

A question remains regarding the need for vitamin D supplementation in the term, exclusively breastfed infant. Although some clinicians do not believe it is necessary, the bulk of data support the practice. Greer et al.[70,71] found low serum 25-OHD concentrations and early decreases in bone mineral content in breastfed infants not receiving supplemental vitamin D. Several groups reported low serum 25-OHD levels at 1 month of age in breastfed infants not supplemented with vitamin D. Markestad[132] demonstrated a significant drop in vitamin D sterols between 4 days and 6 weeks of age in exclusively breastfed infants. In some of the sunniest parts of the world, such as the Middle East, rickets is common in certain breastfed infants because cultural practices keep the babies well clothed and indoors for the first year. Even in

❖

HOW DOES GARLIC IN THE MOTHER'S DIET AFFECT THE NURSING INFANT?

One recent study investigated the effects of garlic ingestion by the mother on the odor of her breast milk and the suckling behavior of her infant. Evaluation of the milk samples by a sensory panel revealed garlic ingestion significantly and consistently increased the perceived intensity of the milk odor; this increase in odor intensity peaked in strength 2 hours after ingestion. That the nursing infant detected these changes in mother's milk is suggested by the finding that infants were attached to the breast for longer periods of time and sucked more when the milk smelled like garlic. There was a tendency for infants to ingest more milk as well. Does this mean that babies love garlic?

From Mennella JA, Beauchamp GK: Maternal diet alters the sensory qualities of human milk and the nursing behavior, *Pediatrics* 88:737, 1991.

the United States, reports of resurgence in rickets among breastfed infants provoke considerable concern.[11,47] Since no harm is associated with vitamin D supplementation at 400 IU/day and since expense and inconvenience are trivial, support of this practice seems justifiable. For light-skinned suburban populations in sunny regions and seasons, one may worry less about compliance with this recommendation. Estimates of the amount of sunlight exposure necessary to maintain serum 25-OHD above the lower limits of the normal range (11 ng/ml) have been determined.[177] Conservatively, these estimates are 30 minutes per week wearing only a diaper or 2 hours a week fully clothed without a hat.

Milk is a good source of *vitamin A* and its precursors.[184] Its concentration in human milk is strongly influenced by the quality and quantity of the dietary elements consumed by the mother. The vitamin A content of breast milk is reportedly much lower in some developing countries than in the West; maternal serum vitamin A levels in these same regions are also typi-

cally low. Vitamin A (or carotene) intake of some Western mothers is higher in the spring and summer months because of greater supplies of green leafy and yellow vegetables; modern methods of preservation, however, have extended the length of seasons for many vegetables and fruits so that dietary differences from season to season may be minimal for many women with access to supermarkets, home freezers, and other such luxuries of modern society.

Vitamin A is present in human milk as retinol, retinyl esters, and beta carotene. The retinyl esters of human milk are a significant source of retinol for the infant. There is efficient hydrolysis of retinyl esters by bile-salt–stimulated lipase in breast milk and subsequent absorption of the retinol. More than 85% of the vitamin A in human milk may be in the form of esters. Thus both the adequacy of vitamin A supplied by human milk and the hydrolysis of retinyl esters by bile-salt–stimulated lipase may explain the lack of vitamin A deficiency in breastfed infants in affluent societies.

Vitamin E levels in human milk are substantially greater than those in cow's milk.[96]

Colostrum	1.00 mg/100 ml
Transitional human milk	0.48 mg/100 ml
Mature human milk	0.32 mg/100 ml
Cow's milk	0.07 mg/100 ml

As might be expected, serum levels of vitamin E rise quickly in breastfed infants and are maintained at normal levels without much fluctuation. Cow's milk-fed babies demonstrate, instead, depressed circulating levels of vitamin E unless supplemented. Fortunately, manufacturers of infant formulas have increased their levels of vitamin E fortification to avoid potential deficiency.

There is a large variation in the data on the vitamin E content of human milk. Factors contributing to the variation include differences in stage of lactation, maternal dietary habits, and biochemical methodology used for assessment. It has been shown, however, that milk contains tocopherol isomers other than α-tocopherol. In fact, β- and γ-tocopherol levels are highest in mature milk.[96] Dietary γ-tocopherol is likely an important contributor to the content of this isomer in human milk since its presence in the American food supply has increased greatly over the past several decades.[184]

Vitamin K is present in human milk at a level of 0.21 μg/100 ml[81]; cow's milk contains much more than this, with a typical reported value of 1.0 to 2.0 μg/100 ml. Based on this reported value, the suggested intake of 12 μg/day would not be supplied by mature breast milk.[24] Vitamin K is produced by the intestinal flora, but it takes several days for the sterile infant gut to establish an effective microbe population. Even then, onset of hemorrhagic disease, with bleeding as late as 4 to 8 weeks after delivery, has been associated with breastfeeding with no vitamin K given at birth.[149,171] It is recommended, therefore, that all newborn infants receive vitamin K, ideally at birth and later in the first month of life.[142] Both oral and intramuscular administration are acceptable.[143] Administration beyond the neonatal period is not necessary.[73]

The levels of *water-soluble vitamins* in human milk are more likely to reflect maternal dietary or supplement intake than most other ingested compounds. Maternal dietary supplementation with most of these vitamins has been shown to increase their content in breast milk (Fig. 12-12). This is especially true in women whose dietary patterns or nutritional status is suboptimal.

Sneed, Zane, and Thomas[175] demonstrated in lactating women of low socioeconomic status that supplementation with ascorbic acid, folate, vitamin B_{12}, and vitamin B_6 significantly increased milk levels of each vitamin, except ascorbic acid. A similar study involving well-nourished women showed that vitamin supplementation did not affect the breast milk concentration or the nutritional status of the subjects.[181] It appears that with some vitamins a plateau may be reached where increased intake has no further impact on milk composition. This idea was nicely demonstrated when varying levels of supplemental ascorbic acid were provided to lactating women.[22] With comparable diets, women consuming either 90 or 250 mg/day of ascorbic acid produced milk with similar concentration of this vitamin; women taking 1,000 mg of ascorbic acid per day produced milk that was only slightly higher in its ascorbic acid content (Fig. 12-13).

Felice and Kirksey have provided evidence that milk concentration of vitamin B_6 may be a sensitive indicator of vitamin B_6 status of the mother.[56] They further suggest that the majority of lactating women produce milk with a vitamin B_6 content that is substantially less than that recommended for good health and growth of infants.[100,101] In one report, mothers receiving

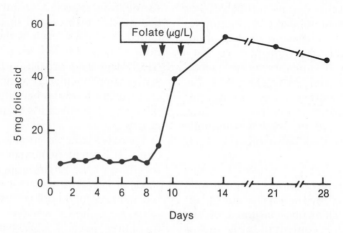

FIG. 12-12   Effect of folic acid supplementation on the milk folate level of a folic-acid–deficient nursing mother.

Modified from Cooperman JM et al: The folate in human milk, *Am J Clin Nutr* 36:576, 1982.

2.5 mg per day of supplemental vitamin B_6 failed to supply their breastfeeding infants with 0.3 mg of vitamin B_6 per day, which is the recommended dietary allowance (RDA) for young infants.[17]

The vitamin B_{12} content of human milk has been reevaluated. The content of 19 samples of milk ranged from 0.33 to 3.2 ng/ml (mean 0.97 ng/ml), and ingestion of supplemental cyanocobalamin did not significantly affect milk content. Human milk from well-fed mothers was found to contain adequate amounts of cobalamin; its availability, however, depends on the sufficiency of proteolytic enzymes to release it from its bound form.

There are a number of reports concerning vitamin B_{12} deficiency in breastfed infants of vegan and malnourished mothers.[86,112,135,176] Higginbottom et al.[86] described a severely affected infant with progressive multisystem disease secondary to vitamin B_{12} deficiency; in this case the mother was a strict vegetarian with low serum and milk vitamin B_{12} concentrations. Another infant examined by Johnson and Roloff[99] was breastfed by a mother having neither dietary idiosyncracy nor hematologic abnormality. Significant hematologic and neurologic abnormalities were recorded, and evidence of serious vitamin B_{12} deficiency was obtained. In this situation it was ultimately found that the mother had

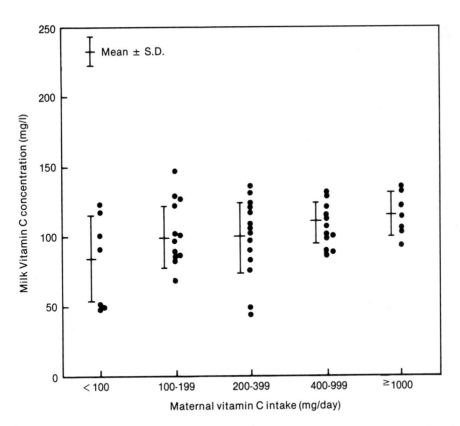

FIG. 12-13 Vitamn C concentration of milk in relation to different levels of maternal intake of vitamin C.

From Byerly LO, Kirksey A: Effects of different levels of vitamin C intake on the vitamin C concentration in human milk and the vitamin C intakes of breast-fed infants, *Am J Clin Nutr* 41:665, 1985.

latent pernicious anemia; review of the literature provides other examples of megaloblastic anemia in breastfeeding infants of mothers with this disease.[84,114,193]

As with most other micronutrients, the levels of water-soluble vitamins in breast milk decline as lactation progresses (Fig. 12-14).[103] The exception is folacin, which remains unaltered throughout all stages of lactation. It has been proposed that folacin in milk is bound to a folate-binding protein that enhances its absorption. Support for this concept has been provided by Colman, Hettiarchchy, and Herbert,[32] who found that the uptake of bound folate by isolated mucosal cells from the rat small intestine was twice that of free folate. These researchers suggest that this milk factor is of substantial clinical importance in reducing the risk of folate deficiency and megaloblastic anemia in young infants. Support for this concept has been provided by a number of investigators.

Resistance factors.[67] A thorough discussion of the composition of breast milk must include mention of the beneficial components of human milk that are not classified as nutrients (Table 12-9).* One of the earliest resistance factors to be described in human milk was the bifidus factor, which may be a nitrogen-containing polysaccharide that favors the growth of *L. bifidus*. Its uniqueness to human milk has been confirmed.[12] *L. bifidus* confers a protective effect against invasive enteropathogenic organisms. This results from the accumulation of bacterial metabolites, among them, short-chain fatty acids, which create an intestinal milieu antagonistic to invasive enteric bacteria and protozoa. The striking resistance of breastfed infants to colonization by coliforms, enteropathogenic *Escherichia coli*, *Shigella* species, and protozoa, even in environments in which the risk of infec-

*References 16, 20, 26, 73, 83, 146, 158, 174.

TABLE 12-9 **Antiinfectious Factors in Human Milk**

Factor	Function
Bifidus factor	Stimulates growth of bifidobacteria, which antagonizes the survival of enterobacteria
Secretory IgA (sIgA), IgM, IgE, IgD, and IgG	Act against bacterial invasion of the mucosa and/or colonization of the gut (show bacterial and viral neutralizing capacity; activate alternative complement pathway)
Antistaphylococcus factor	Inhibits systemic staphylococcal infection
Lactoferrin	Binds iron and inhibits bacterial multiplication
Lactoperoxidase	Kills streptococci and enteric bacteria
Complement (C3, C4)	Promotes opsonization (the rendering of bacteria and other cells susceptible to phagocytosis)
Interferon	Inhibits intracellular viral replication
Lysozyme	Lyses bacteria through destruction of the cell wall
B_{12}-binding protein	Renders vitamin B_{12} unavailable for bacterial growth
Bile-salt-stimulated lipase	Aids in the production of antiparasitic lipids
Low-molecular-weight glycosides and oligosaccharides	Inhibit heat-stable and heat-labile toxins from *Escherichia coli*; prevent bacterial adhesion to epithelial cells by acting as receptor analogs
Low-molecular-weight peptides	Display antiviral activity by interfering with virus attachment onto target cells
Lymphocytes	Synthesize secretory IgA; may have other roles
Macrophages	Synthesize complement, lactoferrin, lysozyme, and other factors; carry out phagocytosis and probably other functions

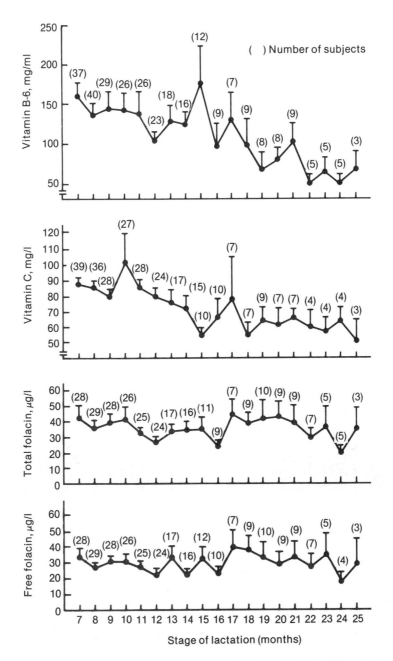

FIG. 12-14 Concentrations of vitamins B$_6$, vitamin C, and free and total folacin in milk samples collected at a morning feeding from 7 to 25 months of lactation. Vertical bars represent SEM.

From Karra MV et al: Changes in specific nutrients in breast milk during extended lactation, *Am J Clin Nutr* 43:495, 1986.

tion is high has been conclusively demonstrated in a rural setting.

Various immunoglobulins are present in human milk, including IgM, IgA, IgG, IgD, and IgE. Although IgG appears to migrate from maternal serum into milk, evidence suggests that IgA, IgD, and IgE are produced locally in mammary tissue. A variety of studies support the idea of migration of lymphoblasts from maternal gut-associated lymphoid tissue to the mammary glands followed by local production of immunoglobulins at this site and secretion of them into the milk.[66,76,83] This mechanism allows for maternal lymphoblasts to obtain antigenic exposure from distant sites and carry this experience to the mammary tissue, where synthesis of appropriate antibodies can occur for protection of the suckling infant (Fig. 12-15).

Secretory IgA (sIgA) is the predominant immunoglobulin in human milk; it is found in large amounts in colostrum and in smaller, but still significant, levels in mature breast milk (Fig. 12-16, *A*). Secretory immunoglobulins have been shown to be a major host resistance factor against organisms that infect the gastrointestinal tract, in particular *E. coli* and the enteroviruses. In addition, a protective effect against other organisms has been demonstrated, and human milk clearly can be said to exhibit a prophylactic effect against septicemia of the newborn.

The precise mechanisms by which sIgA protect the neonatal gastrointestinal tract from infectious organisms are unresolved at present. The antibody may bind to the mucosal surface and serve as a proteolytically resistant "antiseptic paint," preventing pathogenic invasion of the gut epithelium. The virus-neutralizing capability of sIgA, its capacity to agglutinate bacteria, and its ability to activate the alternative pathway of complement fixation are all undoubtedly prominent facets of the role of sIgA in the protective process.

It has been proposed that the human neonate may absorb IgA into the circulation, where it might act as humoral antibody. Reports concerning permeability of the neonatal intestine to human milk immunoglobulins are contradictory. In several studies, gut permeability for colostrum, milk, and serum immunoglobulins was demonstrated, whereas in others it was not.

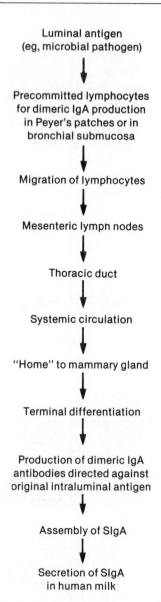

FIG. 12-15   Enteromammary and bronchomammary pathways.

Some of the other host resistance factors in breast milk are also worthy of mention. Lysozyme (Fig. 12-16, *B*), an antimicrobial enzyme, occurs at 300 times the concentration found in cow's milk. Lactoferrin (Fig. 12-16, *C*) has been described as a compound with a

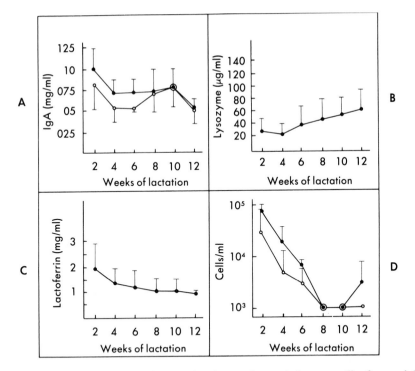

FIG. 12-16 Longitudinal study of selected resistance factors in human milk of normal American women. **A,** Total (•) and secretory (○) IgA. **B,** Lysozyme. **C,** Lactoferrin. **D,** Macrophages-neutrophils (•——•) and lymphocytes (○——○).

Modified from Goldman AS et al: Immunologic factors in human milk during the first year of lactation, *J Pediatr* 100:563, 1982.

"monilia-static" effect against *Candida albicans;* it inhibits the growth of staphylococci and *E. coli* by binding iron, which the bacteria require to proliferate.[59] Lactoperoxidase, which has been shown in vitro to act with other substances in combatting streptococci, is also found in human milk. Specific **prostaglandins** have also been defined, and these may protect the integrity of the gastrointestinal-tract epithelium against noxious substances.

Of additional interest is the discovery that the lymphocytes in human milk produce the antiviral substance interferon. Macrophages are also found in colostrum and mature milk; 21,000/mm reportedly are present in a typical colostrum specimen. Macrophages are motile and phagocytic and have been shown to produce complement, lactoferrin, lysozyme, and other factors. The full role of the macrophages is still under investigation, but they undoubtedly have a protective function, both within the mammary lacteals and subsequently within the baby.

Studies of the activities of lymphocytes in milk have been carried out by a number of investigators. Milk samples from lactating mothers have been collected at various times postpartum and examined for cell types present and in vitro activities of the various identified cells. The greatest number of cells appear in colostrum with numbers dropping significantly during the following 8 weeks (Fig. 12-16, *D*). Analysis of cell-mediated immunity to microbial antigens shows milk lymphocytes are limited in their ability to recognize and respond to certain infectious agents (as compared with lymphocytes from the peripheral circulation). This is believed to be an intracellular action and not caused by lack of external factors.

Lymphocytes collected from human milk appear to have unique reactivities not seen by comparable cells in peripheral blood. Goldblum et al.[64] showed a response in human colostrum to *E. coli* given orally that was not accompanied by a systemic response in the mother. This suggests that milk provides a site for local humoral or cell-mediated immunity induced at a distant site such as the gut with the reactive lymphoid cells migrating to the breast. This proposal has been further refined to suggest that IgA and IgM in colostrum may represent products of specific antibody-producing cells that migrate from the gut lymphoid tissue (specifically, **Peyer's patches**) to the mammary glands; here they infiltrate the glands and their secretions and serve as immune cells capable of selected immune responses.

Such host resistance factors as those described clearly have greatest significance in countries where infections are common and hygienic background is poor. Nevertheless, benefits have been observed in breastfed infants in the so-called developed countries. In these areas the protective effects of human milk seem substantiated for **necrotizing enterocolitis, acrodermatitis enteropathica,** intractable diarrhea, and pathogenic *E. coli* infection. The incidence of these problems reportedly is greater in babies who are not breastfed.[6,7,92,125,160,167]

As one might expect, maternal malnutrition adversely affects not only the nutritional composition of human milk but also its content of immunologic substances. Observations of malnourished Colombian women have shown that colostrum contained only one-third the normal concentration of IgG and less than half the normal level of albumin; significant reductions in colostrum levels of IgA and the fourth component of complement (C4) were also observed. The differences noted tended to disappear in mature milk, concomitant with improvement in the nutritional status of the malnourished mothers during the first several weeks postpartum. The authors concluded that the protective qualities of colostrum and milk may be significantly influenced by maternal nutritional status.

One final word about protective factors relates to their integrity when milk is stored. Although little change occurs with short-term refrigeration, storage and processing of human milk adversely affect its content of cells and proteinaceous compounds. Freezing of milk is the best method of preservation, since only the immune cells are destroyed as a result of membrane breakdown. Other treatments, such as **pasteurization** and **lyophilization,** destroy most protective factors in addition to cells.[121]

Hormones.[50] The presence of hormones in human milk was described many years ago but only lately have methodologic advances allowed for thorough research in this area. Table 12-10 lists the hormones that have been identified in

TABLE 12-10 *Hormones and Hormone-Like Substances in Human Milk*

Pituitary Hormones	Steroids
Prolactin	Estradiol
Growth hormone	Estriol
Thyroid-stimulating hormone	Progesterone
Follicle-stimulating hormone	Testosterone
Luteinizing hormone	17-ketosteroids
Adrenocorticotropin	Corticosterone
Oxytocin	Vitamin D
Neurotensin	

Brain-Gut Peptides	Nonsteroids
Thyrotropin-releasing hormone	Thyroxin
Growth hormone-releasing hormone	Triiodothyroxin
	Prostaglandins
Vasoactive intestinal peptide	(E2 and F2α)
Bombesin	cAMP
Luteinizing hormone-releasing hormone	cGMP
	Melatonin
Cholecystokinin	
Gastrin	
Gastric inhibitory peptide	

Growth Factors
Epidermal growth factor
Insulin-like growth factors (I and II)
Neural growth factor

human milk thus far. Some have been found to be absorbed from the gastrointestinal tract, but their true physiologic significance for the infant is largely unknown.[110] However, a variety of growth factors have been identified in human milk; they are believed to be of significance in, among other things, inducing maturation of the gut. Much more remains to be learned about these nonnutritional components of human milk and their impact on health and development of the infant.[109,134,208]

Contaminants. The lactating woman is often exposed to a variety of nonnutritional substances that may be transferred to her milk.[147] Such substances include drugs, environmental pollutants, caffeine, alcohol, and food allergens. Although moderate amounts of many of these agents are believed to pose no risk to nursing infants, some substances provoke concern because of known or suspected adverse reactions.[116]

Drugs. Much research has focused on the release of drugs into the milk of lactating women.[2] Whether the mother drinks it, eats it, sniffs it, inserts it as an anal or vaginal suppository, or injects it, some level of the active agents in the drug enters the maternal tissues and blood and finally migrates to the breast milk. The difference in method of administration determines the amount of drug that finally enters the blood and the speed with which it reaches the capillaries of the breast. In general the amount of a drug excreted in milk is not more than 1% to 2% of the maternal dose.

Although concern exists about the amount of a given drug in the breast milk, of greater concern is the amount that actually reaches the infant's bloodstream. Unfortunately, there is no accurate way to measure this because other factors also affect the level in the infant's bloodstream. The tolerance of the chemical to the pH of the stomach and the enzymatic activity of the intestinal tract is significant. The volume of milk consumed by the infant is a factor as well.

In 1989 the American Academy of Pediatrics issued a statement about transfer of drugs into breast milk.[2] In this study, lists of the pharmacologic agents transferred into human breast milk and their possible effects on the infant or on lactation are provided. These tables are meant to assist the clinician in counseling a patient regarding breastfeeding when the patient has a condition for which a drug is medically indicated. The impact of a number of drugs on infant well-being is unknown; physicians who encounter adverse effects in breastfed infants as a result of exposure to drugs are urged to document the effects in a communication to the Committee on Drugs of the American Academy of Pediatrics. Drugs that are contraindicated during breastfeeding or that warrant temporary cessation of breastfeeding are listed in Table 12-11.

Some drugs appear in human milk in sufficient quantities to be harmful to the infant.[2] Sedatives used to relieve tension may produce drowsiness in the baby as well as in the mother. Several anticoagulants may cause bleeding problems in nursing infants. **Valium** residuals in mother's milk induce lethargy in breastfed babies. Lithium carbonate, a drug prescribed for relief of manic depression, may induce lowered body temperature, loss of muscle tone, and bluish skin in the nursing infant. Both **cyclophosphamide** and **methotrexate** cause bone marrow depression when ingested by infants. A variety of disorders follow intake by infants of breast milk contaminated with antimicrobial agents of one kind or another. Penicillin in breast milk may produce an allergic reaction in a sensitive infant; other antibiotics may produce similar reactions, as well as sleepiness, vomiting, and refusal to eat. Radioactive thyroid medications may damage the thyroid gland. Bowel problems in infants may result from maternal consumption of some laxatives (e.g., anthraquinone, aloes, cascara, emodin, and rheum [rhubarb]); safe laxatives include magnesia, castor oil, mineral oil, bisacodyl (Dulcolax), senna phenolphthalein or nonprescription Ex-Lax, and fecal softeners. Heroin or the painkiller dextropropoxyphene (Darvon) can lead to infant addiction.

If a mother needs a specific medication and the hazards to the infant are believed to be small, the following important adjustments can be made to minimize the effects:

1. Do not use the long-acting form of the drug because the infant has even more difficulty than the mother does in excreting these agents, which usually require detoxi-

TABLE 12-11   Drugs that Are Contraindicated during Breastfeeding

Drug	Reported Sign or Symptom in Infant or Effect on Lactation
Amphetamine	Irritability, poor sleep pattern
Bromocriptine	Suppresses lactation
Cocaine	Cocaine intoxication
Cyclophosphamide	Possible immunosuppression; unknown effect on growth or association with carcinogenesis; neutropenia
Cyclosporine	Possible immunosuppression; unknown effect on growth or association with carcinogenesis
Doxorubicin*	Possible immunosuppression; unknown effect on growth or association with carcinogenesis
Ergotamine	Vomiting, diarrhea, convulsions (doses used in migraine medications)
Heroin	Tremors, restlessness, vomiting, poor feeding
Lithium	1/3 to 1/2 therapeutic blood concentration in infants
Marijuana	Only one report in literature; no effect mentioned
Methotrexate	Possible immunosuppression; unknown effect on growth or association with carcinogenesis, neutropenia
Nicotine (smoking)	Shock, vomiting, diarrhea, rapid heart rate, restlessness; decreased milk production
Phencyclidine (PCP)	Potent hallucinogen
Phenindione	Anticoagulant; increased prothrombin and partial thromboplastin time in 1 infant (not used in United States)

*Drug is concentrated in human milk.
From American Academy of Pediatrics, Committee on Drugs: The transfer of drugs and other chemicals into human breast milk, *Pediatrics* 93:137, 1994.

fication in the liver. Accumulation in the infant is then a genuine concern.

2. Schedule the doses so the least amount gets into the milk. Given the usual absorption rates and peak blood levels of most drugs, having the mother take the medication immediately after breastfeeding is the safest time for the infant.
3. Watch the infant for any unusual signs or symptoms such as change in feeding pattern or sleeping habits, fussiness, or rash.
4. When possible, choose the drug that produces the lowest level of the drug in the milk.

The increasing use of cocaine in the United States and elsewhere has provoked considerable concern about the potential consequences of this practice both for the developing fetus and the breastfeeding infant. Pregnancies of cocaine-using women are subject to multiple complications, including an increased rate of abruptio placentae and premature delivery.[29,30] Neonates exposed in utero to cocaine are often of low birth weight and demonstrate neurobehavioral abnormalities with marked tremulousness and irritability and deficiencies in mood control and interactive behavior.[30] Two cases of breastfeeding infants affected by cocaine have been described. The infant in the first case was 2 weeks old and demonstrated clinical manifestations of cocaine intoxication (tachycardia, tachypnea, hypertension, irritability, and tremulousness) following ingestion of her mother's milk.[28] From the information given by the mother, the infant showed symptoms of cocaine intoxication within 3 hours after her mother began intranasal use. In the second case, an infant developed apnea and seizures from direct ingestion of cocaine used as a topical anesthetic for nipple soreness.[27]

Environmental pollutants. The current concern over pesticide residues, industrial wastes, and other environmental contaminants is not without cause. Many of these compounds have accidentally contaminated food and water supplies around the world. In general the chemical contaminants that appear in breast milk have high lipid solubility, resistance to physical degradation or biologic metabolism, wide distribution in the environment, and slow or absent excretion rates. Of greatest concern among such chemicals are the **organohalides** such as PCBs and dichlordiphenyltrichloroethane (DDT). Long-term low-level exposure to the organohalides results in a gradual accumulation of residues in fat, including the fat of breast milk. Lactation is the only way in which large amounts of such residues can be excreted.

As pointed out by Rogan, Bagniewska, and Damstra,[165] reports of organohalide concentrations in breast milk must be interpreted with caution. Breast milk varies widely in its fat content, so levels of chemical may not be comparable from study to study unless the concentration is given on a fat basis or adjusted for fat content. Concentrations in fat will usually be about 30 times higher than concentrations in whole milk.

An example of the kinds of studies reported is by Savage et al.,[169] which focused on levels of chlorinated hydrocarbon insecticide residues in nearly 1,500 human milk samples around the United States. The majority of samples showed low but detectable levels of most of these insecticides or their metabolites, but significant differences were found among the five geographical regions. The southeastern United States had the highest mean residue levels, whereas the Northwest had the lowest. The factor deemed the most significant in raising residue levels in the Southeast was chemical treatment of homes for protection against termites. The same situation has been found in western Australia.

Table 12-12 summarizes available information about major pollutants in human milk and their probable significance. It is clear that human milk is a variable source of these agents, but it is difficult to define a "safe" level of exposure to these compounds. However, both the WHO and the Food and Drug Administration (FDA) have set "regulatory" or "allowable" levels for daily intake of several organohalides. These standards provide a large margin of safety, so the fact that a given infant exceeds the level does not

mean that such exposure is toxic. Much remains to be learned about the significance of chemical contamination of human milk. Meanwhile, it is heartening to know that very few case reports of illnesses caused by transmission of environmental chemicals through breast milk have appeared.

Alcohol. Ethanol has been shown to reach human milk in a similar concentration to that in maternal blood. Interestingly, however, the major breakdown product of ethanol, acetaldehyde, does not appear in human milk even though considerable amounts may be measured in maternal blood. The role of the mammary gland in eliminating acetaldehyde may be similar to that of the placenta; in the pregnant rat acetaldehyde may be observed in the blood although none is apparent in the rat fetus. Since acetaldehyde is a highly toxic substance, producing sympathomimetic changes in blood pressure and heart, it is crucial that maternal metabolism be able to protect the fetus and suckling infant.

If human milk contains large amounts of ethanol, the nursing infant may develop a pseudo-Cushing syndrome as described by Binkiewicz, Robinson, and Senior.[13] The 4-month-old infant they describe (Fig. 12-17) was breastfed by a mother who consumed at least 50 12-oz cans of beer weekly, plus generous amounts of other more-concentrated alcoholic drinks. When the mother stopped drinking but continued to nurse, the infant's growth rate promptly increased and her appearance gradually returned to normal. (The mother also noted that the baby did not sleep as well as she used to.)

Of interest is a report on the development of babies whose mothers consumed the equivalent of about two standard drinks or more daily during lactation.[122] The progress of these babies was compared with that of breastfed babies whose mothers consumed no or little alcohol and babies who were fed commercial infant formula. When evaluated at 1 year of age, the babies whose mothers were lactating and consuming the higher levels of alcohol daily had significantly poorer scores on measures of psychomotor development. Whether this finding is indicative of any long-term effects could not be determined. It suggests, however, that moderation in use of alcohol during lactation is in order.

TABLE 12-12   *Representative Data on Human Milk Contamination by Environmental Pollutants and Its Proposed Significance*

Contaminant	Population Studied	Years	Comments
DDT (and its major metabolite DDE)	Diverse groups in the United States	1950-1975	Contamination results from ambient rather than specific occupational exposure; adverse effects in infants have not been reported
PCBs (polychlorinated biphenyls)	Women in Japan	1968-1970	Pregnant and lactating women consumed contaminated rice oil; 13 children were born to exposed women: 1 was stillborn, 4 were small for gestational age, 10 had dark skin pigmentation, 4 had pigmented gums, 9 had conjunctivitis, and 8 had neonatal jaundice; PCBs were found in breast milk, and breastfed infants had higher serum levels than controls; 9-year follow-up of some of these children showed slight but clinically important neurologic and developmental impairment
	U.S. residents (by the Environmental Protection Agency)	1975	Of 1038 samples, 1% had no contamination, 69% had low but detectable levels, and 30% had higher levels; of the latter group, 20% had levels above 0.1 ppm
	Nursing mothers in Michigan	1977-1978	All 1057 samples contained PCB residues ranging from trace amounts to 5.1 ppm; half the total study population had PCB levels nearly equal to or greater than the present FDA tolerance limit for cow's milk; effects on breastfed infants were not assessed; so far, there have been no case reports of illnesses caused by contamination of PCBs through breast milk
	Female rhesus monkeys, perinatal exposure to PCBs (2.5 ppm)	1976-1993	Offspring demonstrated low birth weight; breastfeeding led to skin changes; developmental testing yielded abnormal results; early mortality was increased; infants demonstrated hyperactivity, but as adolescents they became hypoactive; relevance of these data to human circumstances is unknown
PCBs (polychlorinated biphenyls)	Residents of Franklin, Idaho	1983	In 1979 accidental leakage of PCBs from a transformer occurred in a hog-slaughtering plant in Montana; chicken and egg food products were contaminated; breast milk PCB levels were directly correlated with amount of egg consumption; effects on breastfed infants were not evaluated

TABLE 12-12   *Representative Data on Human Milk Contamination by Environmental Pollutants and Its Proposed Significance—cont'd*

Contaminant	Population Studied	Years	Comments
PBBs (polybrominated biphenyls)	Residents of Michigan	1978-1994	About 50% of the samples contained PBBs; 19 exposed children were studied between ages 2½ and 4 years; children with higher body burdens of PBB scored significantly lower than exposed children with lower body burdens; later observations between 4 and 6 years of age showed no significant differences in performance on an array of examinations
Other chlorinated pesticides (dieldrin, heptachlor epoxide, PCBs)	Diverse groups in the United States	1974-1977	Widespread presence in human milk samples; effects on nursing infants unknown

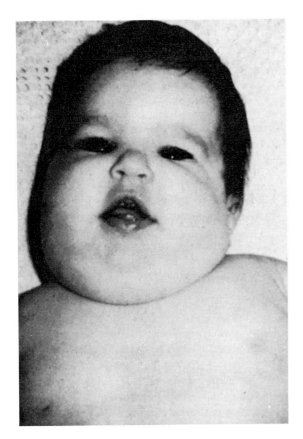

FIG. 12-17   Cushingoid appearance in a 4-month-old infant whose mother consumed at least 50 cans of beer weekly in addition to significant portions of other more-concentrated alcoholic beverages.

From Binkiewicz A, Robinson MJ, Senior B: Pseudo-Cushing syndrome caused by alcohol in breast milk, *J Pediatr* 93:965, 1978.

Several additional reports related to maternal drinking and lactation involved an attempt to determine (1) if milk produced after alcohol consumption had a significantly different odor as assessed by trained adults and (2) if sucking behavior was any different when nursing babies were exposed to alcohol-containing milk.[137,138] Results indicated that the odor of the milk was perceived to be more alcohol-intense when collected within 30 minutes to 1 hour after alcohol consumption. Also, infants' feeding behavior changed. Within the first minute after exposure to alcohol-containing milk, infants sucked more often. Thereafter, however they slowed down and the total volume of milk consumed by the end of the feed was significantly less than that of a feed with unexposed milk. Long-term effects of these observations remain to be determined.

Lead and mercury, both heavy metals, are transferred placentally to the fetus and also to the infant through the maternal milk. Studies in rats[205] have shown that lactation increases lead absorption from the gut, which leads ultimately to an increased level of lead excretion through the milk. The exact mechanism for this phenomenon is not known; however, lactose may play a dominant role, since it is known to facilitate the absorption of calcium, other trace elements, and lead. There is also evidence that bone-deposition lead in the mouse is mobilized during lactation along with calcium. If the mother is exposed to lead while nursing, the amount of lead transferred to the infant is further increased.

Nicotine enters the milk of humans and can cause nicotine poisoning of the breastfed infant. Infants 3 to 4 days of age whose mothers smoked 6 to 16 cigarettes were reported to refuse to suckle, become apathetic, vomit, and retain urine and feces. In a chain-smoking mother the nicotine content of milk reached 75 µg/L. In the case of mothers who smoke very little it is likely that the amount of nicotine the infant would get from breathing cigarette smoke in the immediate environment would be more significant than that obtained from milk.[51,57,107,126,153,191]

Cigarette smoke also contains cancer-causing compounds, and one of these, benzopyrene, has been found to enter the milk supply of lactating mice when introduced to the animals through the trachea.[154] Marijuana is even worse, with 50%

more carcinogens than tobacco smoke. To date, however, no work has been done to determine the amount of carcinogens that reach the milk supply of a nursing mother who smokes marijuana. Some evidence suggests, nevertheless, that tetrahydrocannabinols are present in the breast milk of women who smoke marijuana, and these compounds can be absorbed by nursing infants. The effect of these compounds on the growth and development of the neonate is unknown.

Caffeine. Caffeine is excreted into breast milk, and milk:plasma ratios of 0.5 and 0.76 have been reported. Following ingestion of coffee or tea containing known amounts of caffeine, peak milk caffeine levels occur at 1 hour. Estimates suggest that a nursing infant would receive 1.5 to 3.1 mg of caffeine after the mother drinks a single cup of coffee. This amount is probably too low to be clinically significant. However, accumulation may occur in infants whose mothers use moderate to heavy amounts of caffeinated beverages.[118] The elimination half-life of caffeine is approximately 80 hours in term newborns and 97.5 hours in premature babies. Irritability and poor sleeping patterns have been observed in nursing infants during periods of heavy maternal use of caffeine.

Viruses. In 1986 it was reported that a newborn infant apparently contracted the acquired immunodeficiency syndrome (AIDS) virus through breast milk from his mother.[190] The child was delivered by cesarean section and the mother contracted the AIDS virus after blood transfusion given in conjunction with her cesarean section. In this case, the blood transfusion was given after delivery, and the baby was breastfed for 6 weeks. Thirteen months later, AIDS developed in the donor of one of the units of blood used for transfusion, resulting in testing of the mother and the child. Both the mother and the child were found to be positive for the virus. The mother had AIDS-related complex. The baby had a transient episode of failure to thrive and then developed lymphadenopathy and eczema but was otherwise well. The spouse and siblings were seronegative.

A subsequent study involved observation of 212 mother-infant pairs who were negative for human immunodeficiency virus Type I (HIV-1) at delivery. All of the infants were breastfed.

Mothers were followed for 3 months; those who became positive for HIV-1 were compared with those who did not; comparisons were completed after 16.6 months of further evaluation. Results indicated that HIV-1 infection can be transmitted from mother to infants during the postnatal period. Colostrum and breast milk were considered to be efficient routes for the transmission of HIV-1 from recently infected mothers to their infants.[117,185,186]

The Centers for Disease Control and Prevention (CDC) in the United States has issued the statement that "infected women should be advised against breastfeeding to avoid postnatal transmission to a child who may not be infected." However, WHO has taken a different stand; the following statement was issued in 1992[33]:

In view of the importance of breast milk and breast-feeding for the health of infants and young children, the increasing prevalence of human immunodeficiency virus (HIV) infection around the world, and recent data concerning HIV transmission through breast-milk, a Consultation on HIV Transmission and Breast-feeding was held by WHO and UNICEF from 30 April to 1 May 1992. Its purpose was to review currently available information on the risk of HIV transmission through breast milk and to make recommendations on breastfeeding.

Based on the various studies conducted to date, roughly one-third of the babies born worldwide to HIV-infected women become infected themselves, with the rates varying widely in different populations. Much of this mother-to-infant transmission occurs during pregnancy and delivery, and recent data confirm that some occurs through breast-feeding. However, the large majority of babies breast-fed by HIV-infected mothers do not become infected through breast milk. Recent evidence suggests that the risk of HIV transmission through breast-feeding (a) is substantial among women who become infected during the breast-feeding period, and (b) is lower among women already infected at the time of delivery. However, further research is needed to quantify the risk of HIV transmission through breast-feeding and determine the associated risk factors in both of these circumstances.

Studies continue to show that breast-feeding saves lives. It provides impressive nutritional, immunological, psychosocial and child-spacing benefits. Breast-feeding helps protect children from dying of diarrhoeal diseases, pneumonia and other infections. For example, artificial or inappropriate feeding is a major

contributing factor in the 1.5 million annual infant deaths from diarrhoeal diseases. Moreover, breast-feeding can prolong the interval between births and thus make a further contribution to child survival, as well as enhancing maternal health.

It is therefore important that the baby's risk of HIV infection through breast-feeding be weighed realistically against its risk of dying of other causes if it is denied breast-feeding. In each country, specific guidelines should be developed to facilitate the assessment of the circumstances of the individual woman.

Recommendations

1. In all populations, irrespective of HIV infection rates, breast-feeding should continue to be protected, promoted and supported.

2. Where the primary causes of infant deaths are infectious diseases and malnutrition, infants who are not breast-fed run a particularly high risk of dying from these conditions. In these settings, breast-feeding should remain the standard advice to pregnant women, including those who are known to be HIV-infected, because their baby's risk of becoming infected through breast-milk is likely to be lower than its risk of dying from other causes if deprived of breast-feeding. The higher a baby's risk of dying during infancy, the more protective breast-feeding is and the more important it is that the mother be advised to breast-feed. Women living in these settings whose particular circumstances would make alternative feeding an appropriate option might wish to know their HIV status to help guide their decision about breast-feeding. In such cases, voluntary and confidential HIV testing accompanied in all cases by pre- and post-test counselling could be made available where feasible and affordable.

3. In settings where infectious diseases are not the primary causes of death during infancy, pregnant women known to be infected with HIV should be advised not to breast-feed but to use a safe feeding alternative for their babies. Women whose infection status is unknown should be advised to breast-feed. In these settings, where feasible and affordable, voluntary and confidential HIV testing should be made available to women along with pre- and post-test counselling, and they should be advised to seek such testing before delivery.

4. When a baby is artificially fed, the choice of substitute feeding method and product should not be influenced by commercial pressures. Companies are called on to respect this principle in

keeping with the International Code of Marketing of Breast-milk Substitutes and all relevant World Health Assembly resolutions. It is essential that all countries give effect to the principles and aim of the International Code. If donor milk is to be used, it must first be pasteurized and, where possible, donors should be tested for HIV. When wet-nursing is the chosen alternative, care should be taken to select a wet-nurse who is at low risk for HIV infection and, where possible, known to be HIV-negative.

5. HIV-infected women and men have broad concerns, including maintaining their own health and well-being, managing their economic affairs, and making future provision for their children, and therefore require counselling and guidance on a number of important issues. Specific issues to be covered by counselling include infant feeding practices, the risk of HIV transmission to the offspring if the woman becomes pregnant, and the transmission risk from or to others through sexual intercourse or blood. All HIV-infected adults who wish to avoid childbearing should have ready access to family planning information and services.

6. In all countries, the first and overriding priority in preventing HIV transmission from mother to infant is to prevent women of childbearing age from becoming infected with HIV in the first place. Priority activities are (a) educating both women and men about how to avoid HIV infection for their own sake and that of their future children; (b) ensuring their ready access to condoms; (c) providing prevention and appropriate care for sexually transmitted diseases, which increase the risk of HIV transmission; and (d) otherwise supporting women in their efforts to remain uninfected."

Concern about the AIDS virus in human milk has led to considerable stress in the milk-banking arena. Existent milk banks take great care to appropriately pasteurize their samples; this process destroys the virus. However, since the awareness of the virus intensified in the late 1980s, the volume of breast milk submitted to milk banks around the United States has dropped markedly (Fig. 12-18).[136]

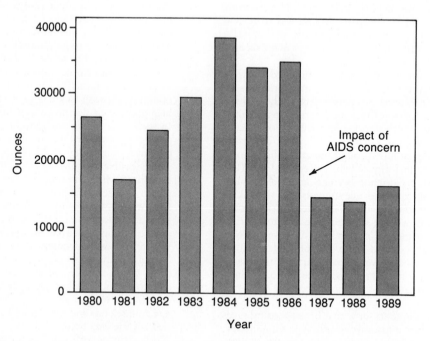

FIG. 12-18 Human milk banking and the AIDS virus: Georgetown University Hospital.

From Mehta NR, Subramanian KNS: Human milk banking: current concepts, *Indian J Pediatr* 57:361, 1990.

Preterm Milk

With the renewed interest in the feeding of human milk to preterm infants, substantial attention has been focused on the composition of milk produced by mothers who deliver prematurely.* Early reports suggested that the protein and nonprotein nitrogen content of preterm milk was higher than that of term milk; additional observations revealed that preterm milk might also be higher in its concentration of calcium, IgA, immune cells,[94] sodium, potassium, chloride, phosphorus, magnesium, medium-chain and polyunsaturated long-chain fatty acids, and total lipid but lower in its lactose level than term milk. The opinion thus developed that premature infants who are fed their own mothers' milk might demonstrate superior growth and development to that observed in premature infants fed banked human milk.[3,4,75,76] In general this suspicion has proven to be true for very-low-birth-weight infants as reported by researchers who have completed appropriate comparisons.[31] It appears, however, that commercial infant formulas designed for low-birth-weight infants may also be superior to banked human milk in supporting growth of these babies.[75]

Although discussion about the superiority of preterm milk has mounted among researchers and clinicians, the question has remained whether an infant receiving preterm milk would actually acquire more nutrition during the first 2 weeks postpartum if provided 24-hour milk collections from mothers delivering prematurely as opposed to 24-hour milk collections of mothers delivering at term. Anderson et al.[3] focused on this question and measured the nutrient composition of 24-hour milk collections obtained over the first 14 days postpartum from mothers who delivered either at-term or prematurely. Term milk volume was greater than preterm volume; volume was therefore controlled for in comparing composition of the milks. Nutrient values of term and preterm milk were compared with each other and to nutrient values measured in donor milk collected after 6 or more months of lactation. No specific differences in specific nutrient or energy content were demonstrated between term and preterm milk. The nutrient and energy content of spot donor milk was highly variable and often different from term and preterm milk. These data indicate that milk from mothers who deliver prematurely does not contain significantly different concentrations of nutrients or energy than milk from mothers delivered at term. The differences previously noted between the two groups may have related to differences in 24-hour milk volume.

With regard to the nutritional adequacy of human milk for the very-low-birth-weight infant, controversy still exists. Although observations have suggested that premature infants can thrive on milk from their own mothers,[31,75] it is known that protein and sodium concentrations are marginal and calcium and phosphate levels are too low to support optimal development of the skeleton.[9] Vitamin content is variable but in general suboptimal for maintenance of growth and health in the very-low-birth-weight infant.[82,183,184] In the face of immature gastrointestinal-tract and renal function and poor nutrient stores, the very-low-birth-weight infant who is provided human milk will often profit from an organized supplementation program.[78,138,194]

It is even possible to supplement human milk with a powdered* or liquid† product designed to improve nutritional adequacy for very-low-birth-weight infants. The powdered fortifier contains protein and carbohydrate and increases the caloric density of breast milk to about 24 kcal/oz. The product is sold in premeasured packets; one packet is designed for addition to 25 ml of human milk. The liquid fortifier is designed to be mixed with human milk or fed alternately with human milk. It is relatively similar to the powdered product in the nutritional additions; it has the same composition as Similac Special Care 24 (a formula designed for low-birth-weight infants) except that the liquid contains additional calcium and phosphorus. Several groups of researchers have demonstrated the effectiveness of fortified human milk for promotion of good growth and development in low-birth-weight infants.

---

*Enfamil Human Milk Fortifier, Mead Johnson.
†Similac Natural Care, Ross Laboratories

CASE STUDY

More Questions About Breastfeeding

Georgeanne Syler, PhD, Southeast Missouri State University

You are a WIC nutritionist. Betsy S., a pregnant college student majoring in nursing, has come in for counseling. She is intelligent, understands basic physiology and nutrition, and wants to provide "the best" for her baby. Your job is to convince Betsy that she should choose to breastfeed. In addition to providing the optimum nutritional care for her infant, you know that Betsy's successful breastfeeding experience will make her a breastfeeding proponent for many of the women with whom she will be working as a registered nurse.

You begin by explaining how breast milk differs from formula. Even though formula is designed to duplicate breast milk, it does not provide colostrum, immunoglobulins, bifidus factor, or lactoferrin. What would you tell Betsy about each of these substances?

You also explain that the macronutrient composition of breast milk differs from formula made either from the milk of another animal species or from soy. You specifically explain the variations in types of proteins, how fatty acid composition differs (including higher cholesterol and long-chain fatty acid

and DHA content) and the effect on enteropathogens of the different types of lactose present. How would you explain the differences in each of these macronutrients to Betsy?

You also want Betsy to understand that breastmilk is unique to the specific mother/infant dyad. If her child is of low birth weight or premature, her breast milk will be specific for her infant's needs, because the composition of breast milk changes as the infant grows and develops; it even changes during a single breastfeeding. What would you tell Betsy about each of these topics? How *specifically* does the milk change as the infant's needs change?

Betsy also has some questions. If she breastfeeds, will she have to continue the lifestyle changes she has made? These include: taking a prenatal vitamin-mineral supplement, avoiding alcohol, not smoking (although she formerly smoked two packs per week), and cutting her caffeine intake severely from the 4 to 5 cups of coffee sweetened with aspartame (Equal or NutraSweet). How would you answer Betsy's questions concerning her personal habits and their effect on breastmilk composition?

Summary

The composition of human milk has been examined thoroughly during the past 50 years with major attention given to this effort since about 1970. The nutrient composition is well-understood, although it is possible that there are additional components to identify. The array of protective factors has been defined but true action of each of them is less well-understood. Hormones, growth factors, and other nonnutrients are now the focus of much attention; functions of these substances are even less clear but it is presumed that they function for the good of the infant. Unfortunately, human milk is "contaminated" with undesirable compounds to which the mother is exposed; rarely, however, is it necessary to discourage breastfeeding. For the majority of lactating mothers and their infants, the benefits of breastfeeding outweigh the possible disadvantages.

REVIEW QUESTIONS

1. Summarize important features about the composition of human milk.
2. Define the role that maternal diet plays in influencing the quantity and composition of human milk.
3. Discuss the pros and cons of providing preterm infants with human milk.

LEARNING ACTIVITIES

1. Examine a variety of samples of human milk to see the differences (particularly in color) that are common.

2. Visit a unit that stores and processes human milk and ask about the precautions that are taken to ensure safety.

3. Interview a mature lactating woman and a lactating adolescent to determine what they know about the composition of human milk.

REFERENCES

1. Alaejos M, Romero C: Selenium in human lactation, *Nutr Rev* 53:159, 1995.

2. American Academy of Pediatrics, Committee on Drugs: The transfer of drugs and other chemicals into human breast milk, *Pediatrics* 93:137, 1994.

3. Anderson DM et al: Length of gestation and nutritional composition of human milk, *Am J Clin Nutr* 37:810, 1983.

4. Anderson GH, Atkinson SA, Bryan MH: Energy and macronutrient content of human milk during early lactation from mothers giving birth prematurely and at term, *Am J Clin Nutr* 34:258, 1981.

5. Anderson RA et al: Breast milk chromium and its association with chromium intake, chromium excretion and serum chromium, *Am J Clin Nutr* 57:519, 1993.

6. Argeanas S, Harrill I: Nutrient intake of lactating women participating in the Colorado WIC program, *Nutr Rep Int* 20:805, 1979.

7. Ashraf RN, Jalil F, Zaman S et al: Breastfeeding and protection against neonatal sepsis in a high risk population, *Arch Dis Child* 66:488, 1991.

8. Atkinson SA, Bryan MH, Anderson GH: Human milk: differences in nitrogen concentration in milk from mothers of term and premature infants, *J Pediatr* 93:67, 1978.

9. Atkinson SA, Radde IC, Anderson GH: Macromineral balances in premature infants fed their own mothers' milk or formula, *J Pediatr* 102:99, 1983.

10. Atkinson SA, Whelan D, Whyte RK et al: Abnormal zinc content in human milk, *Am J Dis Child* 143:608, 1989.

11. Bachrach S, Fisher J, Parks JS: An outbreak of vitamin D deficiency rickets in a susceptible population, *Pediatrics* 64:871, 1979.

12. Beerens H, Romond C, Neut C: Influence of breast-feeding on the bifid flora of the newborn intestine, *Am J Clin Nutr* 33:2434, 1980.

13. Binkiewicy A, Robinson MJ, Senior B: Pseudo-Cushing syndrome caused by alcohol in breast milk, *J Pediatr* 93:965, 1978.

14. Birch DG et al: Dietary essential fatty acid supply and visual acuity development, *Invest Opthamol Vis Sci* 33:3242, 1992.

15. Birch E et al: Breast feeding and optimal visual development, *J Pediatr Opthamol Strabis* 30:33, 1993.

16. Boorman KE, Dodd BE, Gunther M: A consideration of colostrum and milk as sources of antibodies which may be transferred to the newborn baby, *Arch Dis Child* 33:24, 1958.

17. Borschel MW, Kirksey A: Relationship of plasma pyridoxal phosphate levels to vitamin B_6 intakes during the first six months, *Fed Proc* 42:1331, 1983.

18. Brown KH, Akhtar NA, Robertson AD et al: Lactational capacity of marginally nourished poshers: relationships between maternal nutritional status and quantity and proximate composition of milk, *Pediatrics* 78:909, 1986.

19. Brownick SK, Rettig KR: Rickets caused by vitamin D deficiency in breastfed infants in Southern United States, *Am J Dis Child* 145:127, 1991.

20. Buts J et al: Polyamine profiles in human milk, infant artificial formulas and semi-elemental diets, *J Pediatr Gastroent Nutr* 21:44, 1995.

21. Butte NF et al: Macro- and trace-mineral intakes of exclusively breast-fed infants, *Am J Clin Nutr* 45:42, 1987.

22. Byerly LO, Kirksey A: Effects of different levels of vitamin C intake on the vitamin C concentration in human milk and the vitamin C intakes of breast-fed infants, *Am J Clin Nutr* 41:665, 1985.

23. Calvo EB, Galindo A, Aspres NB: Iron status in exclusively breast-fed infants, *Pediatrics* 90:375, 1992.

24. Canfield LM et al: Vitamin K in colostrum and mature human milk over the lactation period—a cross-sectional study, *Am J Clin Nutr* 53:730, 1991.

25. Casey CE, Hambidge KM: The nutritional and immunological significance of mammary secretions. In Neville MC, Neifert MR, eds: *Lactation: physiology, nutrition and breast-feeding,* New York, 1983, Plenum Press.

26. Casey CE, Walravens PA, Hambidge KM: Availability of zinc: loading tests with human milk, cow's milk and infant formulas, *Pediatrics* 68:394, 1981.

27. Chaney NE, Franke J, Wadlington WB: Cocaine convulsions in a breast-feeding baby, *J Pediatr* 112:134, 1988.

28. Chasnoff IJ, Lewis DE, Squires L: Cocaine intoxication in a breast-fed infant, *Pediatrics* 80:836, 1987.

29. Chasnoff IJ: Cocaine use in pregnancy: perinatal morbidity and mortality, *Neurotoxicol Teratol* 9:291, 1987.

30. Chasnoff IJ et al: Cocaine use in pregnancy, *N Engl J Med* 313:666, 1985.

31. Chessex P et al: Quality of growth in premature infants fed their own mothers' milk, *J Pediatr* 102:107, 1983.

32. Colman N, Hettiarchchy N, Herbert V: Detection of a milk factor that facilitates folate uptake by intestinal cells, *Science* 211:1427, 1981.

33. Consensus statement from the consultation in HIV transmission and breastfeeding, *J Hum Lac* 8:173, 1992.

34. Cooperman JM et al: The folate in human milk, *Am J Clin Nutr* 36:576, 1982.

35. Coppa G et al: Change sin carbohydrate composition in human milk over 4 months of lactation, *Pediatrics* 91:637, 1993.

36. Davis TA et al: Amino acid composition of human and other milks, *J Nutr* 95:1126, 1994.

37. Decsi T, Thiel I, Koletzko B: Essential fatty acids in full term infants feed breast milk or formula. *Arch Dis Child* 72:F23, 1995.

38. De Filippi JP, Kaanders H, Hofman A: Sodium in diet and milk of breast-feeding women, *Acta Paediatr Scand* 70:417, 1981.

39. DeSantiago S et al: Protein requirements of marginally nourished lactating women, *Am J Clin Nutr* 62:364, 1995.

40. Donovan SM et al: Postprandial changes in the content and composition of nonprotein nitrogen in human milk, *Am J Clin Nutr* 54:1017, 1991.

41. Dorea JG et al: Correlation between changeable human milk constituents and milk intake in breast-fed babies, *J Pediatr* 101:80, 1982.

42. Drewett RF: Returning to the suckled breast: a further test of Hall's hypothesis, *Early Hum Dev* 6:161, 1982.

43. Drury PJ, Crawford MA: Essential fatty acids in human milk. In *Clinical nutrition of the young child*, New York, 1990, Raven Press.

44. Eckhert CD: Isolation of a protein from human milk that enhances zinc absorption in humans, *Biochem Biophys Res Commun* 130:264, 1985.

45. Eckhert CD: Zinc binding: a difference between human and bovine milk, *Science* 195:789, 1977.

46. Edelstein D, Ebbesen F, Hertel J: The removal of lactose from human milk by fermentation with *Saccharomyces fragilis, Milchwissenschaft* 34:733, 1979.

47. Edidin DV et al: Resurgence of nutritional rickets associated with breastfeeding and special dietary practices, *Pediatrics* 65:232, 1980.

48. Ekstrand J: No evidence of transfer of fluoride from plasma to breast milk, *BMJ* 283:761, 1981.

49. Ekstrand J et al: Distribution of fluoride to human breast milk, *Caries Res* 18:93, 1984.

50. Ellis LA, Picciano MF: Milk-borne hormones: regulators of development in neonates, *Nutr Today* Sept/Oct,:6, 1992.

51. Ey JL et al: Passive smoke exposure and otitis media in the first year of life, *Pediatrics* 95:670, 1995.

52. Faelli A, Esposito G: Effect of inosine and its metabolites on intestinal iron absorption in the rat, *Biochem Pharmacol* 19:2551, 1970.

53. Feeley RM et al: Calcium, phosphorus and magnesium contents of human milk during early lactation, *J Pediatr Gastroenterol Nutr* 2:262, 1983.

54. Feeley RM et al: Copper, iron and zinc contents of human milk at early stages of lactation, *Am J Clin Nutr* 37:443, 1983.

55. Feldman KW: Nutritional rickets, *J Am Fam Pract* 42:1311, 1990.

56. Felice JH, Kirksey A: Effects of vitamin B_6 deficiency during lactation on the vitamin B_6 content of milk, liver, and muscle of rats, *J Nutr* 111:610, 1981.

57. Ferguson BB, Wilson DS, Schaffner W: Determination of nicotine concentrations in human milk, *Am J Dis Child* 130:837, 1976.

58. Finley DA et al: Breast milk composition: fat content and fatty acid composition in vegetarians and nonvegetarians, *Am J Clin Nutr* 41:787, 1985.

59. Fleet JC: The new role of lactoferrin: DNA binding and transcription activation, *Nutr Rev* 53:226, 1995.

60. Fomon SJ, Strauss RG: Nutrient deficiencies in breast-fed infants, *N Engl J Med* 299:355, 1978.

61. Fransson G, Lonnerdal B: Zinc, copper, calcium and magnesium in human milk, *J Pediatr* 101:504, 1982.

62. Franz M: Is it safe to consume aspartame during pregnancy? A review, *Diabetes Educ* 12:145, 1986.

63. Gerrard JW: Wild animal milks, *Pediatrics* 66:819, 1980.

64. Goldblum RM et al: Antibody-forming cells in human colostrum after oral immunization, *Nature* 257:797, 1975.

65. Goldman RM et al: Effects of prematurity on the immunological system in human milk, *J Pediatr* 101:901, 1982.

66. Goldman AS et al: Immunologic factors in human milk during the first year of lactation, *J Pediatr* 100:563, 1982.

67. Goldman AS: The immune system of human milk: antimicrobial, anti-inflammatory and immunomodulating properties, *Breastfeeding Rev* 2:422, 1994.

68. Gopalan C: Studies on lactation in poor Indian communities, *J Trop Pediatr* 4:87, 1958.

69. Gopalan C, Belavady B: Nutrition and lactation, *Fed Proc* 20:177, 1961.

70. Greer FR et al: Bone mineral content and serum 25-hydroxyvitamin D concentration in breast-fed infants with and without supplemental vitamin D, *J Pediatr* 98:696, 1981.

71. Greer FR et al: Bone mineral content and serum 25-hydroxyvitamin D concentrations in breast-fed infants with and without supplemental vitamin D: one year follow-up, *J Pediatr* 100:919, 1982.

72. Greer FR et al: Effects of maternal ultraviolet B irradiation on vitamin D content of human milk, *J Pediatr* 105:431, 1984.

73. Greer FR et al: Vitamin K status of lactating mothers, human milk, and breastfeeding infants, *Pediatrics* 88:751, 1991.

74. Greer FR, Steichen JJ, Tsang RC: Calcium and phosphate supplements in breast milk—related rickets, *Am J Dis Child* 136:581, 1982.

75. Gross SJ: Growth and biochemical response of preterm infants fed human milk or modified infant formula, *N Engl J Med* 308:237, 1983.

76. Gross SJ, Geller J, Tomarelli RM: Composition of breast milk from mothers of preterm infants, *Pediatrics* 68:490, 1981.

77. Guerrini P et al: Human milk: relationship of fat content with gestational age, *Early Hum Dev* 5:187, 1981.

78. Hagelberg S et al: The protein tolerance of very low-birth-weight infants fed human milk protein enriched mother's milk, *Acta Paediatr Scand* 71:597, 1982.

79. Harris WS, Connor WE, Lindsey S: Will dietary ω-3 fatty acid change the composition of human milk? *Am J Clin Nutr* 40:780, 1984.

80. Harzer G et al: Changing patterns of human milk lipids in the course of the lactation and during the day, *Am J Clin Nutr* 37:612, 1983.

81. Haroon Y et al: The content of phylloquinone (vitamin K_1) in human milk, cow's milk and infant formula foods determined by high performance liquid chromatography, *J Nutr* 112:1105, 1982.

82. Haug M et al: Vitamin E in human milk from mothers of preterm and term infants, *J Pediatr Gastroenterol Nutr* 6:605, 1987.

83. Head JR: Immunobiology of lactation, *Semin Perinatol* 1:195, 1987.

84. Heaton D: Another case of megaloblastic anemia of infancy due to maternal pernicious anemia, *N Engl J Med* 300:202, 1979.

85. Heitlinger LA et al: Mammary amylase: a possible alternate pathway of carbohydrate digestion in infancy, *Pediatr Res* 17:15, 1983.

86. Higginbottom MC, Sweetman L, Nyhan WL: A syndrome of methylmalonic aciduria homocystinuria, megaloblastic anemia and neurologic abnormalities in a vitamin B_{12}-deficient breast-fed infant of a strict vegetarian, *N Engl J Med* 299:317, 1978.

87. Hoff N et al: Serum concentrations of 25-hydroxyvitamin D in rickets of extremely premature infants, *J Pediatr* 94:460, 1979.

88. Hoffman B, Lonnerdal B: Distribution of trace elements and minerals in infant formulas, *Fed Proc* 42:1329, 1983.

89. Hollis BW: Individual quantitation of vitamin D_2, vitamin D_3, 25-hydroxyvitamin D_2, and 25-hydroxyvitamin D_3 in human milk, *Ann Biochem* 131:211, 1983.

90. Hoogendauzem T: Vitamin D metabolism in breast-fed infants and their mothers, *Pediatr Res* 25:623, 1989.

91. Hopkinson JM et al: Milk production by mothers of premature infants: influence of cigarette smoking, *Pediatrics* 90:934, 1992.

92. Howie PW, Forsyth JS, Ogston SA et al: Protective effect of breastfeeding against infection, *BMJ* 300:11, 1990.

93. Hytten FE, Thomson AM: Nutrition of the lactating woman. In Kon SK, Cowie AT, eds: *Milk: the mammary gland and its secretions,* vol 2, New York, 1961, Academic Press.

94. Jain N, Mathur NB, Sharma VK et al: Cellular composition including lymphocyte subsets in preterm and full term human colostrum and milk, *Acta Pediatr Scand* 80:395, 1991.

95. Janas LM, Picciano MF: Quantities of amino acids ingested by human milk-fed infants, *J Pediatr* 109:802, 1986.

96. Jansson L, Akesson B, Holmberg L: Vitamin E and fatty acid composition of human milk, *Am J Clin Nutr* 334:8, 1981.

97. Jelliffe DB, Jelliffe EFP: The uniqueness of human milk, *Am J Clin Nutr* 24:968, 1971.

98. Johnson PE, Evans GW: Relative zinc availability in human breast milk, infant formulas and cow's milk, *Am J Clin Nutr* 31:416, 1978.

99. Johnson PR, Roloff JS: Vitamin B_{12} deficiency in an infant strictly breast-fed by a mother with latent pernicious anemia, *J Pediatr* 100:917, 1982.

100. Kang-Yoon S et al: Vitamin B-6 adequacy in neonatal nutrition associations with preterm delivery, type of feeding and vitamin B-6 supplementation, *Am J Clin Nutr* 62:932, 1995.

101. Kang-Yoon S et al: Vitamin B-6 status of breast-fed neonates: influence of pyridoxine supplementation on mothers and neonates, *Am J Clin Nutr* 56:548, 1992.

102. Karra M, Kirksey A, Galal O: Effect of oral zinc supplementation on the concentration of zinc in milk from American and Egyptian women, *Nutr Res* 9:471, 1989.

103. Karra MV et al: Changes in specific nutrients in breast milk during extended lactation, *Am J Clin Nutr* 43:495, 1986.

104. Kenan BS et al: Diurnal and longitudinal variations in human milk sodium and potassium: implication for nutrition and physiology, *Am J Clin Nutr* 35:527, 1982.

105. Khoshoo V: Zinc deficiency in a full term breast fed infant: unusual presentation, *Pediatr* 89:1094, 1992.

106. Kleinman R et al: Protein values of milk samples from mothers without biologic pregnancies, *J Pediatr* 97:612, 1980.

107. Klonoff-Cohen H, Edelstein S, Lefkowitz E: The effect of passive smoking and tobacco exposure through breast milk on sudden infant death syndrome, *JAMA* 273:795, 1995.

108. Kokkonen J, Koivisto M, Kirkinen P: Seasonal variation in serum-25-OH-D in mothers and newborn infants in northern Finland, *Acta Paediatr Scand* 72:93, 1983.

109. Koldovsky O, Bedrick A, Rao R: Role of milk-borne prostaglandins and epidermal growth factor for the suckling mammal, *J Am Coll Nutr* 10:17, 1991.

110. Koldovsky O, Thornburg W: Hormones in milk, *J Pediatr Gastroenterol Nutr* 6:172, 1987.

111. Krebs NF et al: Zinc supplementation during lactation: effects on maternal status and milk zinc concentrations, *Am J Clin Nutr* 61:1030, 1995.

112. Kuhne T, Bubl R, Baumgartner R: Maternal vegan diet causing a serious infantile neurological disorder due to vitamin B_{12} deficiency, *Eur J Pediatr* 150:205, 1991.

113. Lammi-Keefe CJ, Jensen RG: Fat-soluble vitamins in human milk, *Nutr Rev* 42:365, 1984.

114. Lampkin BC, Shore NA, Chadwick D: Megaloblastic anemia of infancy secondary to maternal pernicious anemia, *N Engl J Med* 274:1168, 1966.

115. Lanting CI et al: Neurological differences between 9-year-old children fed breast milk or formula milk as babies, *Lancet* 344:1319, 1994.

116. Lederman SA: Breast milk contaminants: substance abuse, infection and the environment, *Clin Nutr* 8:120, 1989.

117. Lederman SA: Estimating infant mortality from human immunodeficiency virus and other causes in breastfeeding and bottle-feeding populations, *Pediatr* 89:290, 1992.

118. Le Guennec JC, Billon B: Delay in caffeine elimination in breast-fed infants, *Pediatrics* 79:264, 1987.

119. Lifschitz CH, Smith EO, Garza C: Delayed complete functional lactase sufficiency in breast-fed infants, *J Pediatr Gastroenterol Nutr* 2:478, 1983.

120. Lifschitz CH et al: Colonic metabolism of malabsorbed lactose in breast-fed infants, *Am J Clin Nutr* 35:849, 1982.

121. Liebhaber M et al: Alterations of lymphocytes and of antibody content of human milk after processing, *J Pediatr* 91:897, 1977.

122. Little RE, Anderson K, Ervin CH et al: Maternal alcohol use during breastfeeding and infant mental and motor development at one year, *N Engl J Med* 321:425, 1989.

123. Lonnerdal B: Biochemistry and physiological function of human milk proteins, *Am J Clin Nutr* 42:1299, 1985.

124. Lonnerdal B, Forsum E, Hambreaus L: The protein content of human milk. In *Proceedings of the 10th International Congress on Nutrition*, Kyoto, Japan, 1976, Victory-sha Press.

125. Lucas A, Cole TJ: Breast milk and neonatal necrotising enterocolitis, *Lancet* 336:1519, 1990.

126. Luck W, Nau H: Nicotine and cotinine concentrations in serum and urine of infants exposed via passive smoking or milk from smoking mothers, *J Pediatr* 107:816, 1985.

127. Lucas A et al: Breast milk and subsequent intelligence quotient in children born preterm, *Lancet* 39:261, 1992.

128. Makrides M et al: Fatty acid composition of brain, retina and erythrocytes in breast- and formula-fed infants, *Am J Clin Nutr* 60:189, 1994.

129. Makrides M et al: Erythrocyte docosahexaenoic acid correlates with visual response of healthy term infants, *Pediatr Res* 33:425, 1993.

130. Makrides M et al: Changes in the polyunsaturated fatty acids of breast milk from mothers of full term infants over 30 week of lactation, *Am J Clin Nutr* 61:1231, 1995.

131. Markestad T: Effect of season and vitamin D supplementation on plasma concentrations of 25-hydroxyvitamin D in Norwegian infants, *Acta Paediatr Scand* 72:817, 1983.

132. Markestad T: Plasma concentrations of vitamin D metabolites in unsupplemented breast-fed infants, *Eur J Pediatr* 141:77, 1983.

133. Markestad T et al: Serum concentrations of vitamin D metabolites in exclusively breast-fed infants at 70° north, *Acta Paediatr Scand* 73:29, 1984.

134. McCleary MJ: Epidermal growth factor: an important constituent in human milk, *J Hum Lact* 7:123, 1991.

135. McPhee AJ, Davidson GP, Leahy M et al: Vitamin B_{12} deficiency in a breastfed infant, *Arch Dis Child* 63:921, 1988.

136. Mehta NR, Subramanian KNS: Human milk banking: current concepts, *Indian J Pediatr* 57:361, 1990.

137. Mennela JA, Beauchamp GK: Effects of beer on breast-fed infants, *JAMA* 269:1637, 1993.

138. Mennella JA, Beauchamp GK: The transfer of alcohol to human milk: effects on flavor and infant's behavior, *N Engl J Med* 325:981, 1991.

139. Mendelson RA, Bryan MH, Anderson GH: Trace mineral balances in preterm infants fed their own mother's milk, *J Pediatr Gastroenterol Nutr* 2:256, 1983.

140. Morton JA: The clinical usefulness of breast milk sodium in the assessment of lactogenesis, *Pediatrics* 93:802, 1994.

141. Moser-Veillon P and Reynolds RD: A longitudinal study of pyridoxine and zinc supplementation of lactating women, *Am J Clin Nutr* 52:135, 1990.

142. Motohara K et al: Relationship of milk intake and vitamin K supplementation to vitamin status in newborns, *Pediatrics* 84:90, 1989.

143. Motohara K, Endo F, Matsuda I: Vitamin K deficiency in breast-fed infants at one month of age, *J Pediatr Gastroenterol Nutr* 5:931, 1986.

144. Munro CS, Lazaro C, Lawrence CM: Symptomatic zinc deficiency in breast-fed premature infants, *Br J Dermatol* 121:773, 1989.

145. Murphy JF, Neale ML, Matthews N: Antimicrobial properties of preterm breast milk cells, *Arch Dis Child* 58:198, 1983.

146. Nail PA, Thomas MR, Eakin R: The effect of thiamin and riboflavin supplementation on the level of those vitamins in human breast milk and urine, *Am J Clin Nutr* 33:198, 1980.

147. Neville MC, Walsh CI: Effects of xenobiotics on milk secretion and composition, *Am J Clin Nutr* 61(suppl):687S, 1995.

148. Nysenbaum AN, Smart JL: Sucking behavior and milk intake of neonates in relation to milk fat content, *Early Hum Dev* 6:205, 1982.

149. O'Connor ME et al: Vitamin K deficiency and breast-feeding, *Am J Dis Child* 137:601, 1983.

150. Ogra SS, Ogra PL: Immunological aspects of human colostrum and milk. I: Distribution characteristics and concentrations of immunoglobulins at different times after the onset of lactation, *J Pediatr* 92:550, 1978.

151. Oski FA, Landaw SA: Inhibition of iron absorption human milk by baby food, *Am J Dis Child* 134:459, 1980.

152. Owen GM et al: Iron nutriture of infants exclusively breast-fed the first five months, *J Pediatr* 99:237, 1981.

153. Packard VS: *Human milk and infant formula,* New York, 1982, Academic Press.

154. Parmelay MJ, Beer AE: Colostral cell-mediated immunity and the concept of a common secretory immune system, *J Dairy Sci* 60:655, 1977.

155. Picciano MF: Mineral content of human milk during a single nursing, *Nutr Rep Int* 18:5, 1978.

156. Picciano MF, Guthrie HA: Copper, iron and zinc contents of mature human milk, *Am J Clin Nutr* 29:242, 1976.

157. Pisacane A et al: Iron status of breast-fed infants. *J Pediatr* 127:429, 1995.

158. Pollack PF, Koldovsky O, Nishioka K: Polyamines in human and rat milk and in infant formulas, *Am J Clin Nutr* 56:371, 1992.

159. Polskin LJ, Kramer B, Sobel AE: Secretion of vitamin D in milks of women fed fish liver oil, *J Nutr* 30:452, 1947.

160. Popkin BM, Adair L, Akin JS, et al: Breastfeeding and diarrheal morbidity, *Pediatrics* 86:874, 1990.

161. Postellon D, Aronow R: Iodine in mother's milk, *JAMA* 247:463, 1982.

162. Prentice AM et al: Long-term energy balance in child-bearing Gambian women, *Am J Clin Nutr* 34:2790, 1981.

163. Prentice A et al: Calcium requirements of lactating mothers, *Am J Clin Nutr* 62:58, 1995.

164. Rivera-Calimbim L: Drugs to influence lactation, *Drug Ther,* December:20, 1977.

165. Rogan WG, Bagniewska A, Damstra T: Pollutants in breast milk, *N Engl J Med* 302:1450, 1980.

166. Rovamo LM et al: Carnitine during prolonged breast feeding, *Pediatr Res* 20:806, 1986.

167. Ruiz-Palacios GM, Calva JJ, Pickering LK et al: Protection of breastfed infants against campylobacter diarrhea by antibodies in human milk, *J Pediatr* 116:707, 1990.

168. Sanders TAB et al: Studies of vegans: the fatty acid composition of plasma cholinephosphoglycerides, erythrocytes, adipose tissue and breast milk and some indicators of susceptibility to ischemic heart disease in vegans and omnivore controls, *Am J Clin Nutr* 31:895, 1978.

169. Savage EP et al: National study of chlorinated hydrocarbon insecticide residues in human milk, USA, *Am J Epidemiol* 113:413, 1981.

170. Schanler RJ, Oh W: Composition of breast milk obtained from mothers of premature infants as compared to breast milk obtained from donors, *J Pediatr* 96:679, 1980.

171. Shaul DMB: The composition of milk from wild animals, *Int Year Zoo Book* 4:333, 1962.

172. Sheard NF, Walker WA: The role of breast milk in the development of the gastrointestinal tract, *Nutr Rev* 46:1, 1988.

173. Siimes MA, Salmenpera L, Perheentopa J: Exclusive breast-feeding for 9 months: risk of iron deficiency, *J Pediatr* 104:196, 1984.

173a. Similä S, Kokkonen J, Kouvalainen K: Use of lactose-hydrolyzed human milk in congenital lactose deficiency, *J Pediatr* 101:584, 1982.

174. Sinclair AJ, Crawford MA: The effect of low fat maternal diet on neonatal rats, *Br J Nutr* 29:127, 1973.

175. Sneed SM, Zane C, Thomas MR: The effects of ascorbic acid, vitamin B_6, vitamin B_{12} and folic acid supplementation on the breast milk and maternal nutritional status of low socioeconomic lactating women, *Am J Clin Nutr* 34:1338, 1981.

176. Specker BL, Black A, Allen L et al: Vitamin B_{12}: low milk concentrations are related to low serum concentrations in vegetarian women and to methylmalonic aciduria in their infants, *Am J Clin Nutr* 52:1073, 1990.

177. Specker BL et al: Sunshine exposure and serum 25-hydroxyvitamin D concentrations in exclusively breast-fed infants, *J Pediatr* 107:372, 1985.

178. Specker BL, Tsang RC: Cyclical serum 25-hydroxyvitamin D concentrations paralleling sunshine exposure in exclusively breast-fed infants, *J Pediatr* 110:744, 1987.

179. Specker BL, Tsang RC, Hollis BW: Effect of race and diet on human-milk vitamin D and 25-hydroxyvitamin D, *Am J Dis Child* 139:1134, 1985.

180. Stegnink LD, Filer LJ, Baker GL: Plasma erythrocyte and human milk levels of free amino acids in lactating women administered aspartame or lactose, *J Nutr* 109:2173, 1979.

181. Thomas MR et al: The effects of vitamin C, vitamin B$_6$, vitamin B$_{12}$, folic acid, riboflavin and thiamin on the breast milk and maternal status of well-nourished women at 6 months postpartum, *Am J Clin Nutr* 33:2151, 1980.

182. Tyson J et al: Adaptation of feeding to a low fat yield in breast milk, *Pediatrics* 89:215, 1992.

183. Udipi SA et al: Vitamin B$_6$, vitamin C and folacin levels in milk from mothers of term and preterm infants during the neonatal period, *Am J Clin Nutr* 42:522, 1985.

184. Vaisman N, Mogilner BM, Sklan D: Vitamin A and E content of preterm and term milk, *Nutr Res* 5:931, 1985.

185. Van de Perre P: Postnatal transmission of human immunodeficiency virus type 1. The breastfeeding dilemma, *Am J Obstet Gynecol* 173:483, 1995.

186. Van de Perre P et al: Postnatal transmission of human immunodeficiency virus Type I from mother to infant, *N Engl J Med* 325:593, 1991.

187. Volz VR, Book LS, Churella HR: Growth and plasma amino acid concentrations in term infants fed either whey predominant formula or human milk, *J Pediatr* 102:27, 1983.

188. Walker ARP et al: Serum lipids in long-lactating African mothers habituated to a low-fat intake, *Atherosclerosis* 44:175, 1986.

189. Walravens PA et al: Zinc supplements in breast-fed infants, *Lancet* 340:683, 1992.

190. Wasserberger J, Ordog GJ, Stroh JJ: AIDS in breast milk, *JAMA* 255:464, 1986.

191. Woodward A, Grgurinovich N, Philiprgan A: Breast-feeding and smoking hygiene, *J Epidemiol Community Health* 40:309, 1986.

192. Woolridge MW, Baum JD, Drewett RF: Does a change in the composition of human milk affect sucking patterns and milk intake? *Lancet* 2:1292, 1980.

193. Zetterstrom R, Franyen S: Megaloblastic anemia in infancy, *Acta Paediatr* 43:379, 1954.

194. Ziegler EE, Biga RL, Fomon SJ: Nutritional requirements of the premature infant. In Suskind RM, editor: *Textbook of pediatric nutrition*, New York, 1981, Raven Press.

Promotion and Support of Breastfeeding

Angela M. Jacobi
Meta L . Levin

Affordable health care begins with breastfeeding.
A. Jacobi, *Journal of Human Lactation,* December 1992

Objectives

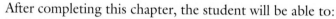

After completing this chapter, the student will be able to:

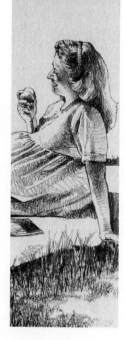

- ✓ *Discuss the rise of artificial infant feeding in the industrialized world and developing countries.*
- ✓ *List the advantages of breastfeeding for the mother and for the baby.*
- ✓ *Describe low-cost strategies for breastfeeding promotion.*
- ✓ *List the breastfeeding concepts that should be shared in the prenatal and postpartal periods.*
- ✓ *List the most commonly cited breastfeeding concerns.*
- ✓ *Describe methods of prevention, management, and evaluation for the most commonly cited breastfeeding concerns.*
- ✓ *Identify the essential strategies for maintaining lactation during short-term separation from the infant.*
- ✓ *Identify the essential strategies for maintaining lactation during prolonged separation.*
- ✓ *List the most important concepts in maintaining lactation when returning to work or school.*
- ✓ *Identify sources of support for breastfeeding and promotion on the local, national, and international levels.*

Introduction

Eve breastfed Cain and Abel. She had no support other than Adam and only the animals as role models. Successive generations of women were better off. They had mothers, sisters, and other women to help and guide them. Then artificial feeding became popular in the developed world, and more and more women began using it. Within a generation or two there were no more grandmothers who had breastfed to help their daughters nurse their grandchildren.[7] And mothers need support to breastfeed a baby successfully.

Before artificial feeding became the norm, those who did not breastfeed usually hired **wet nurses,** who breastfed the infants. At first this practice was limited to noblewomen,[45] but by the early eighteenth century, it spread to the middle classes.[83] Two things happened in the early part of this century to change the custom of giving human infants primarily human milk: (1) a high infant mortality rate (especially in the cities) was thought to be caused primarily by poor diet, and (2) pediatrics was gaining popularity as a medical specialty. Pediatricians followed the accepted belief that poor diet was the cause of most infant morbidity and mortality, and made infant feeding an important part of their practices.[147]

This meant controlling diet. In the early part of this century breastfeeding was still recommended, but when mother's milk was not available, women had trouble finding suitable wet nurses. In these cases, doctors recommended artificial infant foods; they found success with these formulas in their own practices, whether or not the results were backed up by raw data.[7]

By the 1950s, artificial infant feeding was the norm in the United States (Fig. 13-1). It was then that five mothers who needed support and information sat together at a church picnic nursing their babies. La Leche League, which grew out of that picnic, and similar support groups were primarily responsible for the start of the rise in breastfeeding in this country,[7] which started in the 1970s, peaked in the mid-1980s,[46] and seems to be in decline again.[143]

The role of teaching breastfeeding now falls primarily to health professionals: **lactation consultants,** nurses, dietitians, physicians, peer counselors, physical and occupational therapists, and pharmacists. These individuals must all work together to supply the information and support these women need.

Most women begin breastfeeding for all the right reasons: the health and welfare of the baby.

❖

BENEFITS OF BREASTFEEDING

Best for baby
Designed exclusively for human infants
Nutritionally superior to any alternative
Bacteriologically safe and always fresh
Provides immunity to viral and bacterial diseases
Stimulates the infants own immunologic defenses
Decreases risk of respiratory and diarrheal diseases
Prevents or reduces the risk of allergy
Promotes correct development of jaws, teeth, and speech patterns
Decreases tendency toward childhood obesity
Promotes frequent tender physical contact with mother

Best for mother
Promotes physiologic recovery from pregnancy:
•Promotes **uterine involution**
•Decreases risk of **postpartum** hemorrhage
•Increases period of postpartum **anovulation**
Promotes psychological attachment
Facilitates positive self-esteem in maternal role
Allows for daily rest periods
Eliminates need to mix, prepare, use, and wash feeding equipment
Saves money not spent on formula and equipment
Decreases risk of breast cancer and ovarian cancer

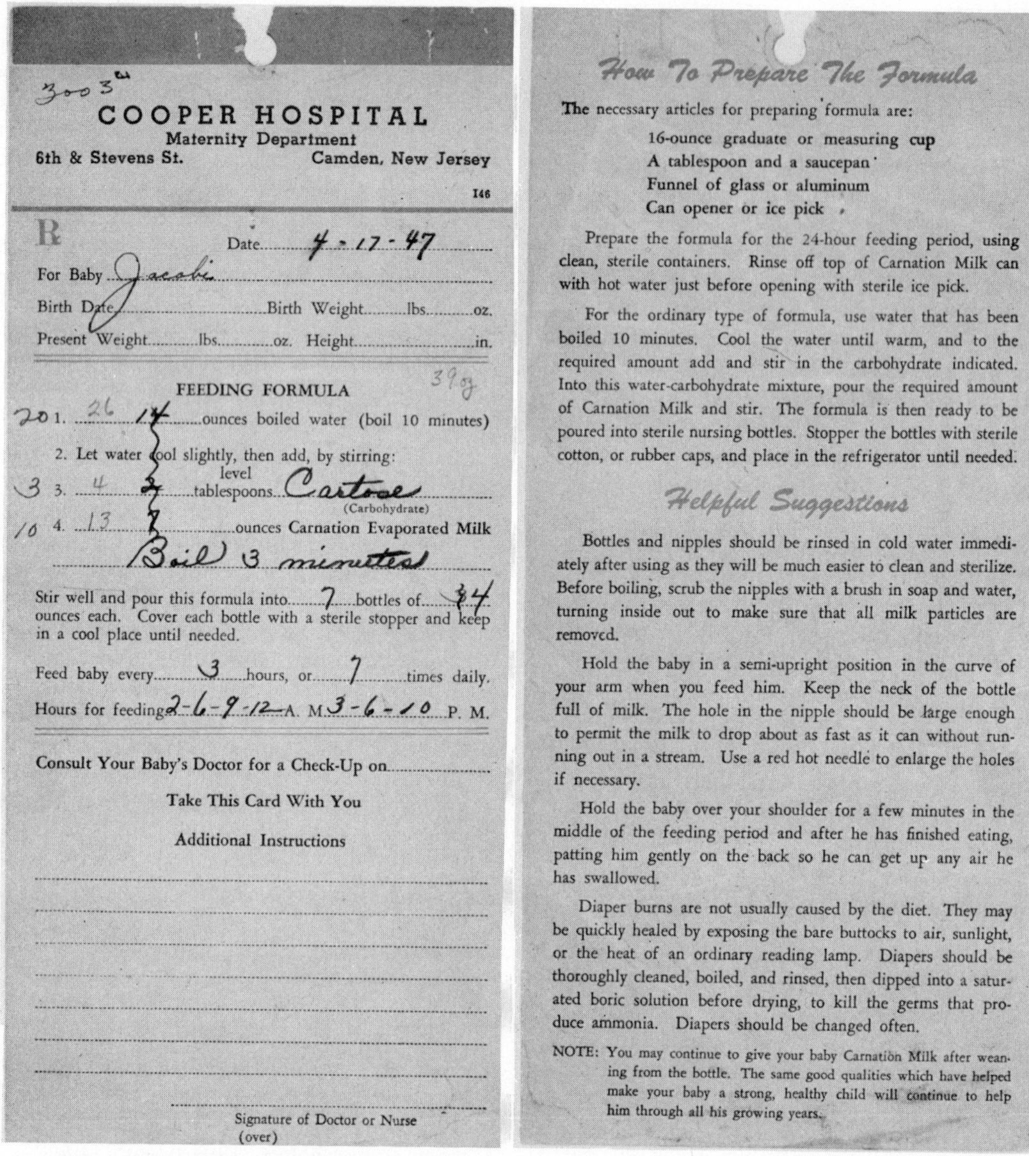

3003

COOPER HOSPITAL
Maternity Department
6th & Stevens St. Camden, New Jersey
146

R Date 4-17-47
For Baby Jacobi
Birth Date .... Birth Weight .... lbs .... oz.
Present Weight .... lbs .... oz. Height .... in.

FEEDING FORMULA 39 oz

1. 26 14 ounces boiled water (boil 10 minutes)
2. Let water cool slightly, then add, by stirring:
3. 4 2 level tablespoons Cartose (Carbohydrate)
4. 13 ounces Carnation Evaporated Milk

Boil 3 minutes

Stir well and pour this formula into 7 bottles of 34 ounces each. Cover each bottle with a sterile stopper and keep in a cool place until needed.

Feed baby every 3 hours, or 7 times daily.
Hours for feeding 2-6-9-12 A. M. 3-6-10 P. M.

Consult Your Baby's Doctor for a Check-Up on ....

Take This Card With You

Additional Instructions

Signature of Doctor or Nurse
(over)

How To Prepare The Formula

The necessary articles for preparing formula are:

16-ounce graduate or measuring cup
A tablespoon and a saucepan
Funnel of glass or aluminum
Can opener or ice pick

Prepare the formula for the 24-hour feeding period, using clean, sterile containers. Rinse off top of Carnation Milk can with hot water just before opening with sterile ice pick.

For the ordinary type of formula, use water that has been boiled 10 minutes. Cool the water until warm, and to the required amount add and stir in the carbohydrate indicated. Into this water-carbohydrate mixture, pour the required amount of Carnation Milk and stir. The formula is then ready to be poured into sterile nursing bottles. Stopper the bottles with sterile cotton, or rubber caps, and place in the refrigerator until needed.

Helpful Suggestions

Bottles and nipples should be rinsed in cold water immediately after using as they will be much easier to clean and sterilize. Before boiling, scrub the nipples with a brush in soap and water, turning inside out to make sure that all milk particles are removed.

Hold the baby in a semi-upright position in the curve of your arm when you feed him. Keep the neck of the bottle full of milk. The hole in the nipple should be large enough to permit the milk to drop about as fast as it can without running out in a stream. Use a red hot needle to enlarge the holes if necessary.

Hold the baby over your shoulder for a few minutes in the middle of the feeding period and after he has finished eating, patting him gently on the back so he can get up any air he has swallowed.

Diaper burns are not usually caused by the diet. They may be quickly healed by exposing the bare buttocks to air, sunlight, or the heat of an ordinary reading lamp. Diapers should be thoroughly cleaned, boiled, and rinsed, then dipped into a saturated boric solution before drying, to kill the germs that produce ammonia. Diapers should be changed often.

NOTE: You may continue to give your baby Carnation Milk after weaning from the bottle. The same good qualities which have helped make your baby a strong, healthy child will continue to help him through all his growing years.

FIG. 13-1 Instructions given to new mothers in post-World War II United States assumed that the baby would be bottle-fed.

From *1947 feeding instructions,* Cooper Hospital, Camden, NJ.

Those who continue, do so because they like it. The box above summarizes benefits of breastfeeding for both baby and mother. Breastfed babies look different, feel different, and are different from their bottle-fed counterparts. This should be an indication that there is a difference, despite artificial baby milk or formula manufacturers's claim that their products are equal or similar to breast milk.[59]

Human milk is designed for human infants. Research has shown human milk to be a living tissue, with almost the same number of live cells as blood.[113] It has been linked with decreases in diarrhea and acute gastrointestinal-tract infections, as well as the number and severity of other illnesses in infants. Nutrients in breast milk are more easily used by the infant. For instance, in the case of iron, breast milk is known to have smaller quantities than artificial baby milk. However, human milk contains a transfer factor for iron. This allows the baby to absorb and use the iron more efficiently.[108] Artificial baby milk, on the other hand, must be fortified with excessive amounts of iron, which causes constipation in many babies. The artificial milk needs to be overfortified with the iron because so little can be absorbed by the baby.

The ready availability of formula in western countries, and methods used to advertise it to consumers and the medical profession all over the world, have caused some women to doubt their ability to nourish their babies adequately. Helsing and King[59] state:

Women fear that their milk is of poor quality, because their diet is simple, so they think it is inadequate for "good" milk production. Some women learn this from well-meaning but misinformed health workers, and some from the baby-food advertisements. . . . It is important to convince women on simple diets that their bodies are quite capable of making high quality milk out of the cereals . . . which they eat. It is not necessary to eat eggs, meat, or even drink milk in order to produce good milk themselves.

GASTROINTESTINAL BENEFITS

One of the biggest problems worldwide, especially in developing countries, is severe diarrhea in infants. Rotaviruses are now recognized as the most common cause of gastroenteritis in young children, evidenced by the detection of rotavirus in nearly 50% of cases of diarrhea in hospitals in developed and developing countries.[60]

In 1990 in the United States alone, at least 500 babies under 1 year old died as a result of diarrhea from rotavirus.[53] Another 200,000 were treated in hospitals at a cost of more than $500 million. An estimated 1.4 million were treated at home for the same condition.

Popkin et al. suggest that "global promotion of breastfeeding could reduce diarrheal morbidity rates 8% to 20% for infants up to the age of 6 months."[133] The study focused on infants from the Cebu region of the Philippines and was controlled for other environmental causes of diarrhea. It showed that benefits of exclusive breastfeeding were greatest during the first 6 months, and lessened during the next 6 months. Interestingly, the study also showed that combining breast milk with either nonnutritive liquids or nutritive foods increased the likelihood of diarrhea in infants up to age 6 months. For nonnutritive liquids, the risk tripled, and for nutritive foods it was 6 to 20 times as great in an urban sample. The effect was smaller, but still significant in a rural sample.[133]

In Henry and Bartholomew's study in St. Lucia, West Indies, breastfed children had lower rates of rotavirus infections than those using bottles or combined breast milk and other fluids or foods. This was true in the 0-to-5-month age group, as well as in the 6-to-11-month population.[60]

The reason for less diarrhea in exclusively breastfed babies remains unclear. Studies have suggested that the protection may not have anything to do with antibodies. One pointed at a **bile-salt-stimulated lipase (BSSL),** which destroyed *Giardia lamblia,* a protozoan parasite, which induces giardiasis, a common cause of diarrhea in children.[125] BSSL is not found in cow's milk, the basis for many infant formulas. Finally, breastfeeding seems to be most protective against the most life-threatening persistent or severe diarrheas.[42]

ANTIINFECTIVE PROPERTIES

Immunologists and cell biologists have found an increasing number of protective factors in human milk.[36] Cunningham et al. noted that breastfeeding is "associated with significant reductions in nongastrointestinal infections, including pneumonia, bacteremia, and meningitis, and with a reduced frequency of chronic diseases later in life."[36]

Hospitalization for respiratory infections is more common in bottle-fed infants,[36] as is the incidence of respiratory illnesses in the same group. Cunningham et al. estimate that as many as 7% of all infants are hospitalized for respiratory infections, primarily because of the added risk of bottlefeeding. When breast-fed infants do develop respiratory illnesses, they are much less severe. Cunningham estimates that the risk of bacterial infections in breastfed infants was 10 times less than in their bottle-fed counterparts.[35] These outcomes are not limited to developing countries. A study done in the Netherlands found an inverse relationship between breastfeeding and morbidity in the first 3 years of life. This was strongest during the first year, but also was present during the second and third years.[157] For records of early childhood feeding, this study relied on questionnaires sent home to the mother. When compared with accounts from one well-baby clinic that kept such records, all but one of the questionnaires matched exactly.[157] Instances of morbidity were collected from the Continuous Morbidity Registration in Nijmegen, the Netherlands. Most of the children were from the middle and lower social classes. About two thirds of the 1,347 children in this study were breastfed. The results showed:

> When the duration of breastfeeding was considered, generally morbidity was lower with increasing length of breastfeeding, especially when it was continued for longer than 90 days. These trends were found for both the first year and the first three years of life.[157]

When factors such as birth year, gender, number of siblings, birth weight, social class, allergic history in family, parental smoking habits, and illness behavior of the mother were taken into account, breastfed infants were more likely to have episodes of throat and/or nose diseases and less likely to have gastroenteritis than nonbreastfed infants. However, during the first 3 years of life, breastfed children had lower rates of serious disease, laryngitis, and acute bronchitis than did nonbreastfed children. Those breastfed for longer than 90 days had fewer incidences of morbidity, lower rates of gastroenteritis, skin disorders, and skin infections during the first year, and lower rates of moderately serious illness, respiratory-tract illness, acute bronchitis, and gastroenteritis during the first 3 years of life. The authors also note that breastfeeding may be associated with other behaviors that affect

health.[157] Leventhal et al., studying infants in the Yale-New Haven area, found that while breastfeeding had some protective effect for infectious illness, its advantage may be more in reducing the severity of the illness and preventing hospitalization.[90] However, studies from developing countries do show that breastfeeding decreases rates of respiratory-tract infections, diarrhea, and infant death.

REDUCED RISK OF ATOPIC DISEASES

There is some controversy about how breastfeeding is protective against allergies. What seems to be certain is that breastfeeding at least delays the onset, and reduces the severity in children for whom there is a family history of allergies.

Strimas and Chi found that allergy symptoms occurred more often in formula-fed infants between 0 and 6 months of age than in their breastfed counterparts.[154] Of the 83 infants, 33 in this study were initially breastfed. The researchers found that infants who were breastfed for 6 months or more had significantly fewer allergies than those on formula or who were nursed for less than 6 months.

In a literature review, Broadbent and Sampson found evidence that breastfeeding exclusively for at least 4 months reduces the incidence of **atopic dermatitis** in the infants of parents with this problem.[24] These infants are considered most at risk. They cited a study done by Fergusson et al. that showed that the condition developed in 23% of infants from parents with atopic dermatitis. However, of those exclusively breastfed for at least 4 months, atopic dermatitis developed in only 12%. Atopic dermatitis developed in 24% of the formula-fed infants in the group. If solids had been introduced to the breastfed infants in the first 4 months, the rate of atopic dermatitis jumped to 28%.[44]

Many breastfeeding mothers can confirm the results of another study cited by Broadbent and Sampson, showing that infants can react to food antigens transmitted in their mother's breast milk.[71]

In their own study, Broadbent and Sampson noted that six exclusively breastfed infants, in whom atopic dermatitis developed, had positive skin-prick tests for egg. These babies' skin cleared completely when their mothers stayed on an egg-free diet. Four underwent an in-hospital challenge, and symptoms developed within 4 to 36 hours after their mothers ate eggs.[24] Cow's milk is another common allergen. A study by Machtinger and Moss suggests that secretory immunoglobulin A (sIgA) may protect against the development of atopic disease from cow's milk.[99] In this study, Machtinger and Moss had presumed that sIgA in breast milk decreases antigen entry across the gastrointestinal mucosa while the newborn's mucosal defense mechanisms are maturing. They studied 57 exclusively breastfeeding mother-infant pairs in the first 6 months of life. The 11 infants who scored high on an allergy symptom scale, received breast milk with total and cow's–milk-specific sIgA antibody concentrations below the median value.[99] These authors believe that inadequate quantities of maternal IgA antibodies to food allergens may play more of a role in the development of allergy symptoms in breastfed babies than does the parents' having allergic disease.[99]

Broadbent and Sampson note that "the institution of prophylactic measures, such as exclusive breastfeeding, has been shown to be effective in preventing atopic symptoms in young infants."[24] A study by Miskelly et al. showed that breast-feeding was associated with cutting the incidence of wheezing by half and with a "significant" reduction in diarrhea in allergy-prone children. [115]

NUTRITIONAL PROPERTIES

Breast milk provides everything a baby needs nutritionally, as well as the proper amount of liquid, at least for the first 4 to 6 months.[144] Saini et al. believe that "variability of breast milk composition is responsible for wide variations in growth rate of breastfed infants."[144] However, others believe that this is caused more by family growth patterns.

Infant demand regulates milk production[121]; therefore an otherwise healthy, normal infant allowed to nurse on demand will take, and stimulate his mother to produce, the amount of milk

necessary to meet his needs and growth pattern. Growth rates of breast- vs. bottle-fed infants appear to be different. Neville found that the mean growth rate of exclusively breastfed infants was higher than their bottle-fed counterparts for the first 4 weeks, was similar in the second month, then fell gradually so that by 6 months it was 70% of the artificially fed infants.[122] There are still unanswered questions as to why there is this difference. Some pediatric specialists feel that the slower rate of growth among older breastfed infants represents the pattern for optimal health. It has even been suggested that the National Center of Health Statistics standards are not appropriate for evaluating the growth performance of breastfed infants and that growth curves based exclusively on breastfed infants should be used for that purpose.

Milk secreted in early lactation has higher concentrations of protein, calcium, zinc, and other nutrients. It has been suggested that this is better able to support rapid infant growth and development than milk from later lactation. In later months, exclusively breastfed infants get less protein than artificially fed babies.[122]

Researchers also are intrigued by the levels of cholesterol in human milk. Average breast milk contains 40% to 50% of its kcalories as fat, and about 150 mg per deciliter of cholesterol.[12] Many infant formulas contain lower cholesterol but similar fat levels. Formation of membranes particularly nerve lipids, requires cholesterol. Therefore it may be risky to feed an infant artificial milk with lower levels. This is an area deserving of further research in light of the risk of cardiovascular disease in the United States.

COGNITIVE DEVELOPMENT

To say that breastfeeding will make a child more intelligent is bound to be controversial. However, there have been a few studies attempting to compare the IQ of artificially fed children vs. breastfed children.

Data by Lucas seemed to show that a cohort of breastfed children had higher developmental scores at 18 months.[96] This study attempted to measure neurodevelopment. The authors followed the same children and reported similar results for children ages 7½ to 8 years old.[96] In this study 300 children were tested with an abbreviated version of the Weschler Intelligence Scale for Children (revised Anglicized).

Those who had been given breast milk in the early weeks of life had a significantly higher IQ at this age than those who received no breast milk.[96] The babies in this study had been born preterm. The author acknowledges that social class and the mother's education may have been a factor in the decision to provide breast milk and might also have contributed to the difference in the IQ scores. However, he also found that children of mothers who planned to provide breast milk, but then failed to do so, had scores nearly the same as those from mothers who never intended to provide breast milk. The IQ advantage also was seen in babies who received breast milk only through a nasogastric tube while hospitalized, but not later, so mother-child interaction while nursing was ruled out as a factor. Lucas[96] notes that the benefit found is larger than in similar studies done with infants born at full term. This finding has important implications for promoting breast milk for preterm infants who are less likely to be breastfed because of the extended separation from their mothers resulting from their long hospitalization.

OTHER PROTECTIVE BENEFITS

An array of other advantages for babies have been proposed to be associated with breastfeeding. Two studies, one done in Finland and one in Galway County, Ireland, seem to show that breastfeeding at least delays the onset of symptoms of coeliac disease.[102] Studies of the effect of breast milk on preterm infants are beginning to show some evidence that it may protect against necrotizing enterocolitis, which causes a significant amount of morbidity in this group of babies.[20]

There is some evidence that exclusive breastfeeding for at least 6 months confers protection from certain types of childhood cancer.[37] In a case-control study to assess whether inadequate exposure to immunologic benefits of human milk may affect infants' response to infection and make them more susceptible to childhood malignancies, a group from the National Institutes of Health (NIH) found higher risk for childhood cancers in children who were breastfed less than 6 months or who were artificially fed. Some studies have related artificial feeding and early introduction of solid foods with obesity in later life. One study showed that exclusive breastfeeding did seem to keep infants in a normal weight range through the first 6 months of life.[1] However, results were inconclusive for older infants and children.

Research is beginning to indicate a protective effect against Crohn's disease and insulin-dependent diabetes mellitus. Support for these and other hypotheses is limited, but future observations may confirm their validity.

Mothers start breastfeeding because they believe it is good for the baby, but they continue because they like it. Nature fixed it that way to ensure the continuation of the species. She also tucked in some benefits for the mother. The most obvious one is the tender physical contact, which helps form a special attachment between mother and child.

This attachment also is the basis for a long and important relationship, allowing the mother to recognize and respond to subtle behavior cues quickly.[93] In addition, the closeness allows the newborn to feel secure in the warm, loving arms of its mother.[86]

Breastfeeding may also contribute to maternal security. Virden studied 60 first-time mothers from a large urban area in California.[158] She found that at 1-month postpartum, breastfeeding mothers had less anxiety and more mother-infant harmony than women who were bottle-feeding their infants. Further analysis shows that mothers who breastfed patterned their touch and talking to the infant's activity more than did the bottle-feeding mothers. Virden found that "during feeding, the breastfeeding mother was more engrossed in the interaction than the bottle-feeding mother."[158] Dr. Ashley Montague emphasized the importance of this in his book *Touching*:

What is established in the breast-feeding relationship constitutes the foundation for the development of all human social relationships, and the communications the infant receives through the warmth of the mother's skin constitute the first of the socializing experiences of life.[116]

The onset of lactation is a spontaneous part of the "fourth **trimester** of pregnancy." There is a sense of harmony to the idea that the gradual rise of the hormones of pregnancy should, as a corollary, gradually reduce over the period of lactation. To prevent a newly delivered woman from lactating is like trying to hold back a sneeze. Each is a normal physiologic process that serves a useful purpose to the body and that must be forcibly repressed or it will proceed spontaneously. The urge to lactate is strong, just as is the urge to sneeze.

Breastfeeding immediately after birth has more immediate physical advantages for the mother than for the infant. The infant's suckling stimulates the release of **oxytocin,** which, in turn, stimulates uterine contractions, helping both to expel the placenta and reduce maternal blood loss.[93] Continued breastfeeding also helps the uterus return to its nonpregnant state.

There is some evidence that breastfeeding reduces the risk of later breast cancer in the mother. One study found lower levels of estrogens in breast fluids of women who had nursed at least one child, which the researchers theorized may provide some protection.[130] A study of Chinese women in Shanghai, who normally nurse for prolonged periods, showed a clear beneficial effect on breast cancer risk.[173] The study showed a lower incidence of breast cancer in the women who had breastfed, independent of age or menopausal status.

In addition, research on ovarian cancer showed a lower risk for women who had breastfed than for those who had not.[150] Human lactation has long been cited as a way of inducing prolonged **anovulation,** and thus as an important way to space pregnancies. In other words, breastfeeding can be used for a form of birth control—and is in many countries.[56] However, the duration of anovulation varies with the mother and with other factors, and can range from 3 months to 20 to 24 months.[53] Prolonged cessation of ovulation occurred most often when the infants suckled frequently, and small amounts of solid foods were not introduced until the babies were at least 6 months old.[69] Although breastfeeding should not be relied on as the sole source of contraception, there is evidence that if the baby is breastfed on de-

mand day and night for the first 6 months without the use of pacifiers or supplemental feedings, if solid or other foods are gradually introduced in small amounts beginning at 6 months, and if nursing continues as the primary food source for the first year, there will be a longer instance of **amenorrhea** and possibly anovulation in the mother.

Many women are worried about the weight they gain during pregnancy. Breastfeeding may play an integral part here, too. A few small studies seem to indicate that breastfeeding a baby for 6 to 12 months can help a mother reduce fat stores, including those on her thighs, better than if she chooses to bottle-feed.

Breast milk itself may have some curative powers. There is anecdotal evidence that mothers in some countries routinely apply breast milk to minor eye infections in their children. A study in Great Britain showed that when nursing mothers applied breast milk to their cracked nipples, it promoted healing.[138] The women were on a postpartum ward and were instructed to apply expressed breast milk to their nipples and let it air dry following each feeding. They were paired with a ward in which the mothers used other methods.

However, little is ever said about the hazards of suppressing lactation. There is evidence that the drug used to inhibit lactation (**bromocriptine**) can actually induce postpartum depression in some women.[27] Canterbury et al. followed two women who were given bromocriptine in low doses to inhibit lactation. Both exhibited psychosis severe enough for hospitalization, which subsided after the drug was discontinued. In a second study, the bromocriptine was thought to exacerbate an already existing condition, which again improved after the drug was discontinued.[87]

Parents also have found that formula-feeding is expensive. La Leche League often cites an estimate by one father that the money saved by breastfeeding one year can equal the cost of a major appliance.[86] A 1987 U.S. Department of Agriculture report estimated that $30 million in formula costs could be saved each year if half the mothers in the Women Infants and Children (WIC) program would breastfeed for just 1 month (Lazaroff M: personal communication).

Most women who choose to breastfeed do not consider the benefits to themselves. They think of their children, but nature clearly had the mothers in mind when she provided this source of ready nourishment.

Formula companies spend millions on promoting and advertising their product. Advertisements and news stories inform the public about major artificial baby milk companies to the extent that one of the most easily recognized symbols for a baby is a bottle.

The clinician will find plenty of free literature, samples, and incentives, such as toys or infant care and parenting videos, available from the formula companies. As a nutrition and health educator, information about artificial baby milk as an option is readily available.

However, most groups promoting breastfeeding do not have the resources to do the same. A growing body of information is available to promote breastfeeding among a varied population of women. With little of it available for free, this poses a problem for programs operating on a limited budget. Formula companies do publish breastfeeding information brochures and booklets, and offer them free of charge. However, many of these contain either inaccurate information or imply that breastfeeding is

---

❖

BREASTFEEDING PROMOTION

When promoting breastfeeding, remember this:

- Most American women have never seen a mother breastfeeding a baby.
- Pregnant women are adult learners.
- Formula companies have vast resources to promote their product, but breastfeeding advocates do not.
- Breastfeeding promotion must be across the board and consistent throughout your agency/facility.
- Promotion must be based on knowledge and current research.
- Cultural and ethnic variances must be respected.
- Breastfeeding is a family affair.

---

difficult or often unsuccessful. The difference between information and promotion often is subtle, and it is easy for formula companies to imply that their product is best. Written information, posters, and booklets are not enough to promote breastfeeding successfully. Breastfeeding promotion and support must be facility-wide, and women must feel that they will be supported constantly, consistently, and comprehensively. (See the box below for tips to remember when promoting breastfeeding.)

Methods for promoting breastfeeding must account for dealing with an adult population. Even teenagers who become mothers see themselves as adults and want to be treated that way. Few, if any, of these women have seen a baby breastfeed. Even the most enthusiastic probably do not know how to breastfeed.[28] In an earlier era, they would have looked to mothers, sisters, grandmothers, and other women in their family and community as role models, but the role models are gone; they have been sacrificed to a combination of noble and not so noble causes. Nearly all American and Canadian mothers breastfed their babies as recently as the turn of the century.[51] However, those who did not breastfeed employed wet nurses, so the babies were indeed breastfed.

As early as the late 1860s, Baron von Liebig was promoting his "soluble food" as the "most perfect substitute for mother's milk," under the banner headline, "No More Wet Nurses!"[7] In the early 1870s, Henri Nestlé, a Swiss chemist, began to distribute his Milk Food in Europe, Australia, and the Americas. Others saw a market and joined, including Mellin, Hawley, Borden and Horlick. Most of the advertising was aimed at mothers, although Nestlé attempted to aim some of his at physicians.[7] This did not create a revolution; what happened came slowly.

There was a high infant mortality rate in cities around the turn of the century.[7] Many physicians argued that poor diet was the most common cause of those deaths. Although most still recommended breastfeeding, they often had trouble finding suitable wet nurses for women who could or would not nurse their own infants. Others found reasons that a mother's milk was not suitable—often because of the woman's lifestyle. The door was open for artificial infant milk. At the same time a new medical specialty was gaining popularity—pediatrics. Infant feeding was made the foundation of this new medical practice.[7] Most of the popular artificial baby milk relied on complex formulas, supposedly determined individually for each infant by the doctor. Baby milk laboratories began to advertise their products directly to the physician, and they, in turn, found it advantageous to have mothers and babies tied so closely to their practice.

In the early 1930s, 88% of mothers began breastfeeding their babies, but by 1965 that number had dropped to only 31%.[74] Not long after that, breastfeeding rates began to improve.

Breastfeeding began to rise again in the 1970s and peaked in the mid-1980s. Ironically, now that such groups as the American Academy of Pediatrics, the Surgeon General of the United States, the United Nations World Health Organization (WHO), and the American Dietetic Association all endorse and promote breastfeeding, its use in the western hemisphere is on the decline again (Fig. 13-2). This is especially true in low-income groups. Faced with the current decline, health care professionals are more important than ever in the fight to encourage women to breastfeed their babies. Most studies of women enrolled in the WIC program show they are influenced to breast- or bottle-feed by the baby's maternal grandmother, father, and other female relatives. If the mother's own mother breastfed and actively supports her daughter doing so, then she is less vulnerable to pressure from bottle-feeding peers.[25]

However, results of focus group interviews by Bryant et al. with African- and Anglo-American teens and women enrolled in the WIC and Maternal and Child Health (Title V) clinics, showed that these mothers and mothers-to-be placed a high value on health care professionals' advice.[25] Nurses and nutritionists had provided them with most of the information they had received on breastfeeding. A sample of this type of information is shown in Fig. 13-3.

Bryant et al. further found that much of the information had reinforced fears and lack of confidence about breastfeeding. Materials typi-

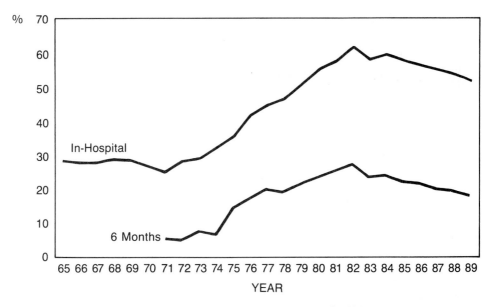

FIG. 13-2 Trends in breast feeding in the United States, 1965-1989.

From Lawrence R et al: Recent declines in breastfeeding in the United States, 1984 through 1989, *Pediatrics* 88:719, 1991.

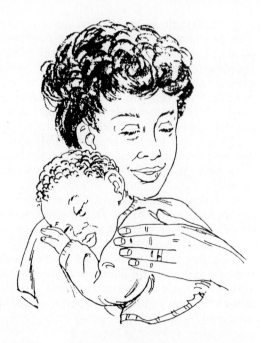

Question: **What if I get upset or nervous?**
Answer: Some women have been told that their milk will spoil if they get upset or nervous. This isn't true. In fact, nursing will help you feel more relaxed and in control. Even if you do get worried, sad or angry, these feelings will not change your breast milk.

One last thing to remember is that most women with health problems can still breastfeed their babies successfully.

FIG. 13-3 Simple information is the most helpful. From Best Start, developed with funds from the Kentucky WIC Program.

cally depicted attractive, well-dressed women, who the respondents believed to have the emotional, social, and financial resources to succeed at breastfeeding. In addition, many cited information from health professionals and educational materials perceived as cautioning that nursing a baby requires sacrifice and a stringent lifestyle. This included the necessity to eat a complicated diet of the right foods. Hence, what can a dietitian, childbirth instructor, or other health care professional do to promote breastfeeding? Walker's strategies for improving classes are as follows[160]:

1. Provide written materials without formula advertising.
2. Provide a list of resources in the community for finding help.
3. Use slides, charts, and cloth models for visual reinforcement and clarity.
4. Avoid making breastfeeding seem difficult.
5. Correct misinformation and myths.
6. Refer parents to breastfeeding classes.
7. Have a breastfeeding couple visit the class.
8. Describe and show breastfeeding devices that may be helpful.
9. Discourage separation immediately after birth.
10. Encourage the father's involvement.

The most important part is first to listen to your client. Understand the mother's fears, concerns, and cultural biases, then try to meet these on a positive level. One successful program to do this has been using peer counselors.[81] **Peer counselors** are mothers from the same ethnic and socioeconomic group who have breastfed a baby and have been trained to help other women.

In the lower socioeconomic communities, cultural differences between clients and health care providers are great. It is in these areas that peer counselors seem to offer the most advantages.[81] Peer support, such as that traditionally offered by La Leche League International, has proved to be effective in helping middle-income women initiate and continue to breastfeed their babies.

The peer counselors in the study by Kistin et al. were trained in breastfeeding promotion and management, nutrition, basic infant growth and development, common infant illnesses with emphasis on when medical intervention may be needed, counseling techniques, procedures for making referrals to community resources, and how to identify problems beyond their scope and refer to professionals.[81] Counselor self-esteem and empowerment also were reinforced.

The study compared two groups of breastfeeding women: those who wanted counselors and for whom they were available and those for whom there was no peer counselor available. Of the first group, 93% breastfed, but in the second, only 70% did. Of those who had counselors, 77% exclusively breastfed for some length of time, but in the no-counselor group, only 40% did so. In the category with counselors, the mean number of weeks of exclusive breastfeeding was 8, but of those without, the mean was 4. The mean number of weeks of any breastfeeding (exclusive or not) of those with counselors was 15, whereas those without was 8.

The study was conducted at Cook County Hospital, a large public hospital in Chicago, which serves an uninsured, multicultural population of Cook County, Illinois. Previous intervention by health care professionals in this hospital had resulted in little exclusive breastfeeding and rapid declines in the rates within a few weeks postpartum. Clearly, continued support by peers has now been demonstrated as being important in promoting breastfeeding, and should be a part of any breastfeeding program.

Choosing educational and promotional materials must be done with a careful eye toward communicating with a particular client population. Samples of various types of promotional material currently in use are pictured throughout this chapter. They range from pamphlets available through programs aimed at low-income and low-education-level women, to materials targeting specific ethnic groups.

As an example: the La Crosse, Wis., Health Department proudly displays posters of Hmong women receiving prenatal care and breastfeeding. These women are Southeast Asians who settled in La Crosse and elsewhere. A peer counselor at La Crosse saw that none of the promotional materials at the office depicted the Hmong lifestyle, so she wrote to relatives in Hmong refugee camps in Thailand who sent handstitched banners (Fig. 13-4) depicting breastfeeding practices at home. The result has been an increase in breastfeeding by the Hmong women who now see that their ways are honored and respected by the La Crosse Department of Health workers (Lee L: personal communication).

It is important to avoid printed and visual materials that send a double message. For in-

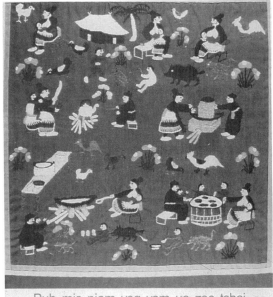

Pub mis niam yog yam ua zoo tshaj rau koj thiab koj tus menyuam
Breastfeeding is best for you and your baby

Produced by La Crosse County WIC Program and the Wisconsin WIC Program 1990

FIG. 13-4 Culturally sensitive promotional poster representing traditions of Southeast Asian women.
From LaCrosse County, WI WIC Program.

stance, many formula companies offer posters, pamphlets, notepads and other items supposedly promoting breastfeeding, but including large amounts of artificial baby milk advertising or company logos. In addition, the breastfeeding pictures on these materials are sometimes—intentionally or not—offensive to certain groups of people. A good example of this is a mother nursing a baby with her nursing bra exposed. Parents from cultures where modesty in dress is important, or shy people, might conclude that breastfeeding is not right for them if they have to expose themselves in public.

In one study of primarily Mexican-American migrant farm workers, one of the most common reasons given for not breastfeeding was embarrassment.[172] These women would be discouraged by a poster showing a woman exposing herself while nursing a baby. A culturally sensitive alternative is shown in Fig. 13-5. Big busi-

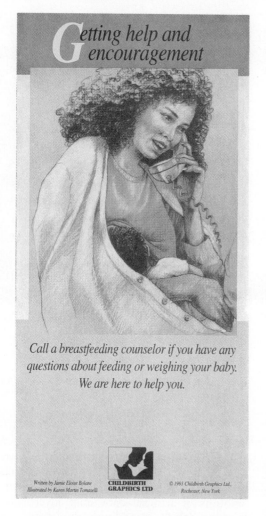

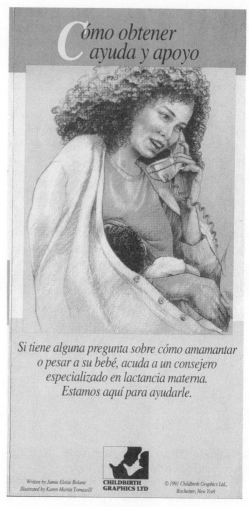

FIG. 13-5 Both verbal and nonverbal messages are sent by this pamphlet directed to Spanish-speaking women. The nonverbal messages include that breastfeeding can be done modestly and that you can do other things at the same time.

Copyright 1991 Childbirth Graphics Ltd., Rochester, NY.

ness has long known that offers of incentives often help promote a product. Sometimes this can work to induce women to at least attend a breastfeeding class. In one study of migrant women, researchers found that many did not have adequate clothing, diapers, or other items for their babies.[172] WIC workers made lists of basic layette items and distributed them to church groups involved in migrant ministries in the area. These groups supplied the items,

which then were used as incentives for women to attend a breastfeeding class.

Involving other family members often is a good promotional tool. A study of 1,525 women showed that, if the woman is married, her husband's opinion is a strong influence on her decision to breastfeed. There also was a strong association between the child's grandmothers' method of feeding and her own. Outside influence can also be subtle. Encouraging

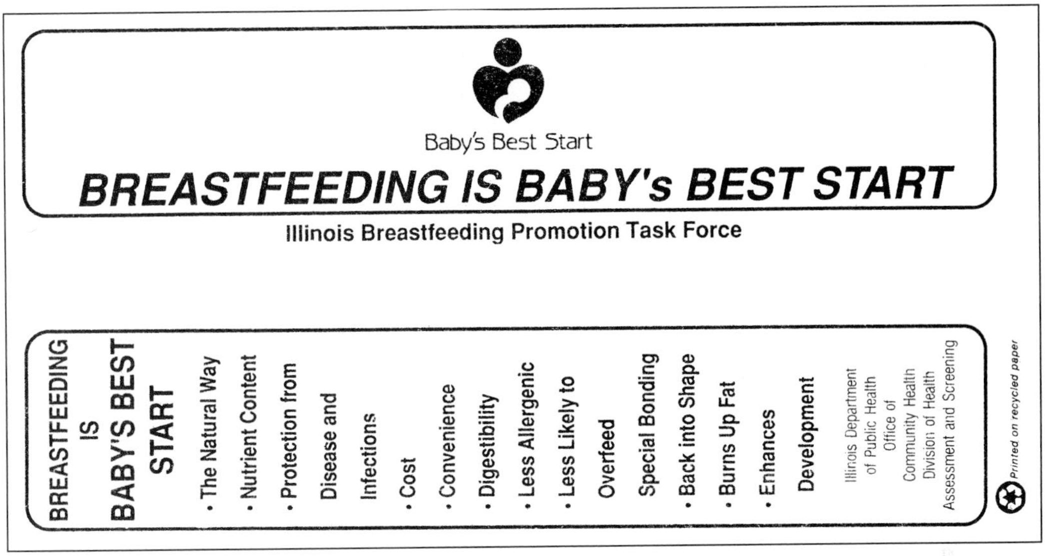

Baby's Best Start

BREASTFEEDING IS BABY's BEST START

Illinois Breastfeeding Promotion Task Force

BREASTFEEDING IS BABY'S BEST START

- The Natural Way
- Nutrient Content
- Protection from Disease and Infections
- Cost
- Convenience
- Digestibility
- Less Allergenic
- Less Likely to Overfeed
- Special Bonding
- Back into Shape
- Burns Up Fat
- Enhances Development

Illinois Department of Public Health
Office of Community Health
Division of Health Assessment and Screening

Printed on recycled paper

FIG. 13-6 An example of breastfeeding promotion, this bookmark can be used by health care personnel or distributed with breastfeeding literature.

Reprinted with permission from the Illinois Department of Public Health.

staff to wear pro-breastfeeding buttons and to use bookmarks (Fig. 13-6) and notepads with breastfeeding slogans (and without formula advertising), and integrating conveniences such as a private breastfeeding or pumping room into the regular scheme of things sends a powerful message: *We support the breastfeeding family.*

Historically, health care workers were encouraged to be neutral in discussions of infant feeding. The idea was that if a health care worker supported breastfeeding, it might make a bottle-feeding mother feel guilty. However, Maureen Minchin feels that bottle-feeding mothers aren't feeling guilty, but rather very angry with health professionals for not having disclosed the facts that would have given them a stronger motivation to begin or to continue breastfeeding. Women fail to breastfeed because professional persons have failed to take this major physiologic process seriously, and so often provide inaccurate diagnoses and inappropriate advice.[112]

However, health care workers might ask what has been done to breastfeeding mothers because of the profession's neutrality. Mothers have gotten the message that the health care profession does not support breastfeeding, denying them the opportunity to breastfeed and denying their babies breast milk. Humans are the only mammalian species to do that voluntarily. What has been gained?

PRECONCEPTION AND PRENATAL PERIOD

In another time, breastfeeding was a part of life. Women learned about it as girls and knew long before contemplating pregnancy that their babies would be nourished this way. Declines in breastfeeding rates suggest that the advantages and techniques of nursing a baby at the breast should be taught early.

Some studies indicate that the infant-feeding decision is made early in pregnancy,[15,146] whereas other research shows that it is actually influenced by what was seen and heard in the family as an individual grew up.[78] If health care professionals are to encourage clients to breastfeed, these health care professionals must understand it themselves. However, many of today's medical, nursing, and dietetic students who were raised in the United States, never saw an infant breastfed at home or at family gatherings. As children of the 1960s and early 1970s, when breastfeeding was at its lowest rate in America, they and their siblings were bottle-fed. Nonverbal reinforcement of bottle-feeding was seen in dolls packaged with baby bottles rubber-banded to their wrists. Breastfeeding was not discussed, or when it was, it was done in a negative way. Many of these same students actually admit to having no idea at all as to how they or their siblings were fed.

Conversely, international students, even male Muslims, speak of having been breastfed and of witnessing siblings breastfeeding within the privacy of the home. African and Asian students, male and female alike, tell of seeing women breastfeeding comfortably, both at home and in public, in their countries of origin. They often are mystified by the dichotomy between the proliferation of breasts in American advertising, and the American discomfort with the idea of breastfeeding.

Although people in the United States may be uncomfortable talking about breastfeeding, teenagers, young adults, and prospective parents are curious about childbirth and parenting. This is a perfect opening to introduce human lactation and breastfeeding. Women and their partners perceive themselves as adult learners when it comes to childbirth education, regardless of their age or educational level.[34,66] They need to be treated this way when teaching about lactation and breastfeeding. If not, the message will be lost. Table 13-1 offers information on teaching adult learners.

Pregnant women are beginning to mentally explore the role of mother and consider which behaviors fit with their perceptions of themselves.[142] For this reason, the instructor must be up-to-date and present accurate information on breastfeeding to the client.

There are a few common breastfeeding concerns that most prospective mothers have (see box above). By treating them seriously, honestly, and respectfully, breastfeeding will be effectively promoted.

QUESTIONS WOMEN TYPICALLY ASK ABOUT BREASTFEEDING

- How does it feel?
- Does it hurt?
- How long should I breastfeed?
- What if the baby gets hungry in public?
- What happens when I return to work?
- What about sex?

New parents are frustrated by the disagreement between professionals on how to breastfeed. Part of the conflict over breastfeeding instruction comes from the profession's own lack of accurate education on the principles of breastfeeding. Lactation and breastfeeding is not afforded much, if any, time in most health care curricula. It cannot be taught as a procedure, like giving an injection, or preparing a recipe, because a procedure or recipe has a straightforward set of steps and is an easily mastered technical skill. Breastfeeding is an interactive process that occurs between a mother and an infant, and each mother-baby couple provides a different set of variables.

Fortunately, there are some concepts that apply to all mother-baby couples, and these can be shared with prospective parents so that they are prepared to breastfeed. These concepts lay the foundation on which the individual differences between mother-baby couples can be built. Techniques that work for one mother may not for another, and there can be considerable variation between the two. The same can be said for differences between siblings who were breastfed. What worked with the first or second baby may not work with the third. Therefore it is important to stick to the basics when presenting material on breastfeeding in the prenatal period, as follows:

1. Benefits of breastfeeding to mother and baby
2. Prenatal assessment and preparation of nipples
3. How breastfeeding works
4. Assessing a "baby-friendly" hospital

Experience in breastfeeding education shows that 99% of prenatal preparation for breastfeed-

TABLE 13-1 Teaching Adult Learners

Characteristics of Adult Learners	Application to Breastfeeding Mothers	
	Do	**Don't**
Like to be actively involved in learning	Use samples (i.e., breast pumps), allow her to handle, manipulate, take apart; structure teaching around an actual feeding episode to allow more infant-mother interaction.	Lecture at/to mother Leave printed materials at bedside without interaction
Life-tasks and challenges produce a desire to learn	Determine who made decision to breast-feed (new mom, husband, mother, mother-in-law.) If her decision, use as an example of life-task to be accomplished, encourage, support, reaffirm. If someone else's decision, acknowledge challenge, affirm her capabilities.	Overlook an opportunity to acknowledge her desire to learn new information or techniques
Learn best in environment that is less formal, more relaxed	Establish a relationship before beginning to teach, she must be ready to learn or the effort is wasted; call her by her first name every time you see her, not just when teaching; use interactive learning exchanges. If in group, rather than one on one, place chairs so you can see all faces during class—makes mother realize you care.	Place clients in straight row of chairs, in small/crowded room Talk down to clients as if you are the expert with all the answers
Prefer to "reason through" a problem rather than be told an answer; generally rational thinkers	Ask questions—lead her to a decision	Provide all the information for them
Would rather identify need themselves than be told they have a problem	Ask what they are interested in learning/knowing about breastfeeding—it may not be what you feel is their real need, but use their input to lead to points you wish to discuss	Appear to know it all and have the answers to all problems
Prefer to focus on principles/concepts rather than learn/memorize minutiae	Talk about the normal relationship of food/fluid intake on quality/quantity of milk	Give printed materials that you expect to be memorized (i.e., physiology of "let-down" or constituents of breast vs. cows' milk)
Have many responsibilities, resent someone wasting their time	Come to teaching episode well prepared; know about client's previous breastfeeding history; have a pre-planned objective in mind—accomplish it or revise expectation; plan to teach in small, manageable segments (10-15 min) rather than in hours	Expect everything to be learned at one time (especially when tired following labor and delivery)

Continued.

TABLE 13-1 Teaching Adult Learners—cont'd

Characteristics of Adult Learners	Application to Breastfeeding Mothers	
	Do	**Don't**
Internally motivated to learn but like to have accomplishments acknowledged	Provide constant praise, even for small improvements; provide inexpensive certificate of accomplishment for successful breastfeeding. Compliment small quantity of pumped milk for preemies	Provide reinforcement for negative responses at initial breastfeeding attempts

Developed by Barbara C. Woodring, RN, EdD.

ing takes place in the head and only 1% in the nipples. Breastfeeding information is only part of the overall preparation for the baby's arrival. As such, it should be integrated into all prenatal care and education. Every prenatal contact is an opportunity to reinforce the choice to breast-feed.

The first contact with a pregnant woman is the appropriate time to ask about her plans for breastfeeding. Open-ended questions such as, "How are you planning to feed your baby?" provide an opportunity for the client to express herself. If she plans to bottle-feed, she should be asked how she came to that decision. She should be encouraged to reconsider her decision in light of your information about the benefits of breastfeeding and how the clinical staff will support her while she breastfeeds.

If she is adamant about bottle-feeding, then it is important to close the discussion on a positive note and move on to other business. However, if she expresses interest in learning more about breastfeeding, a clinician should find out what her immediate concerns are, respond to them, and refer her to sources for further information.

Health care providers should assess the breasts and nipples at the first prenatal visit. This is another opportune moment to ask how the client plans to feed her baby. It also is a good time to encourage breastfeeding. Breast assessment should begin with a visual inspection. Assure the client that any minor size differences are normal. Anyone with palpable lumps or cysts should be referred for evaluation. Anyone with a history of breast augmentation or reduction

surgery should also be referred to a lactation specialist for follow-up after delivery, since the extent of lactation function can only be evaluated after the baby is nursing. Significant breast size discrepancies may also indicate the need for **postpartum** follow-up for lactation adequacy.[41,88,89]

Next, the nipples should be inspected. Overtly **everted** nipples are ready for breastfeeding. Less than fully everted nipples should be monitored for spontaneous eversion, which usually occurs during pregnancy (Fig. 13-7).

Moderate manipulation of the breasts and nipples as a natural part of lovemaking can assist in everting the nipples.[86] In addition, the mother can use gentle outward manipulation of the nipples or the Hoffman technique to help nipples turn outward.[9] Nipples that remain inverted into the third trimester can be helped by wearing breast cups during the day (Fig. 13-8). There is one contraindication to nipple stimulation during pregnancy: women who are at risk for preterm labor are advised to refrain from any form of nipple stimulation, as this could cause the onset of contractions leading to preterm labor and preterm birth.[126]

Prenatal breast care has become simplified as more is learned about successful lactation. The old techniques designed to "toughen" the nipples were not only unnecessary, but counterproductive, and have given way to a more gentle approach. The Montgomery glands of the areola secrete lanolin, which lubricates the nipple and areola, to keep them soft and pliable. Therefore soap should be avoided, since it will remove the lanolin.

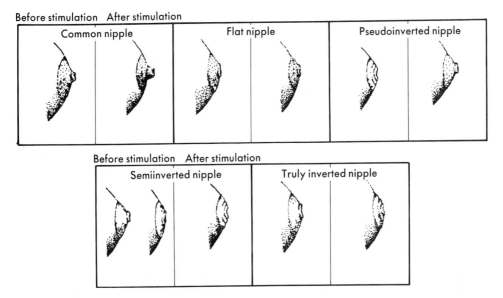

FIG. 13-7 Five types of nipples and their responses to stimulation.

From Lauwers J, Woessner C: *Counseling the nursing mother: a reference handbook for health care providers and lay counselors,* Garden City Park, NY, 1989, Avery. Reprinted with permission.

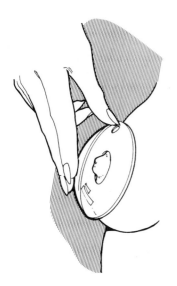

FIG. 13-8 Breast cup in place.

Tangible ongoing support in the form of accessible prenatal classes on breastfeeding, as well as referrals to dietitians and lactation consultants, are an important part of prenatal breastfeeding promotion efforts. Appropriate pamphlets, posters, and videos posted at the office will give clients a clear message that you support breastfeeding.

However, the strongest message that can be given in support of breastfeeding is to provide a clean, quiet, comfortable place for mothers to nurse and pump while at the health care facility. To the mother, this not only shows support for breastfeeding during pregnancy, but also proves the facility and staff will assist them in it after the baby arrives.

BREASTFEEDING IN THE POSTPARTUM PERIOD

In an ideal world, putting the baby to breast immediately would be part of the birthing process. It is truly beautiful to watch a newborn infant, who has been placed cheek to breast im-

---

IS YOUR HOSPITAL "BABY-FRIENDLY?"

WHO/UNICEF has jointly launched a new initiative aimed at promoting breastfeeding through the creation of "baby-friendly" hospitals. Institutions that adopt and apply the "10 steps to successful breast-feeding" will be designated as "Baby-Friendly" and will receive a plaque or other award of public recognition.

Every health facility providing maternity services and care for newborn infants should

1. Have a written breast-feeding policy that is routinely communicated to all health care staff.
2. Train all health care staff in skills necessary to implement this policy.
3. Inform all pregnant women about the benefits and management of breastfeeding.
4. Help mothers initiate breastfeeding within half an hour of birth.
5. Show mothers how to breastfeed and how to maintain lactation even if they are separated from their infants.
6. Give newborn infants no food or drink other than breast milk, unless medically indicated.
7. Practice rooming-in—allow mothers and infants to remain together—24 hours a day.
8. Encourage breastfeeding on demand.
9. Give no artificial teats or pacifiers (also called dummies or soothers) to breastfeeding infants.
10. Foster the establishment of breastfeeding support groups and refer mothers to them on discharge from the hospital or clinic.

Representatives of the International Paediatric Association, at whose meeting the "Baby Friendly" campaign was introduced, ask for the assistance of all health professionals as partners in this initiative. The UNICEF resolution also calls on "manufacturers and distributors of breast-milk substitutes to end free and low-cost supplies of infant formula to maternity wards and hospitals by December 1992," to reduce their detrimental effect on breastfeeding.

From WHO Unicef, *J Hum Lact 7*:196, 1991.

---

mediately after birth, try to rouse itself as if from sleep. Given time, and proximity of lips to nipple, the infant will begin to make mouthing and licking motions. Some will actually search for the breast and latch on to it. It is a special time for the baby and its family.

Current American hospital policies vary widely regarding the way a woman and her infant are treated during the days and hours surrounding birth. Some hospitals still have policies that make breastfeeding initiation very difficult, and some have just started to make changes to support breastfeeding. Still others have reached the point at which personnel and policies are truly supportive (see box above).

It is important that the client understand the concepts involved in initiating breastfeeding so that she can be better prepared to handle the va-

riety of experiences she may encounter during her hospitalization. A clinician should become familiar with the hospitals most often used by clients, so that instruction and support can be tailored appropriately. No matter how supportive the hospital personnel and policies, maternal or neonatal complications can occur that may make breastfeeding initiation difficult. Therefore prenatal instruction should focus on the basic concepts. In this way the mother will be prepared to request procedures that will facilitate her choice.

If a clinician is unfamiliar with hospital practices in the area, colleagues should be contacted for a tour of the obstetrical area. If this is not possible, clients can describe their hospital experiences. Childbirth education and breastfeeding books and videos can also familiarize clinicians with the variety of childbirth practices (see box on p. 411). Clients

RESOURCES

Ameda/Egnell
755 Industrial Drive
Cary, IL 60013
Breast pumps and other lactation-related equipment

The American Academy of Husband Coached Childbirth-The Bradley Method
Box 5224, Department CB
Sherman Oaks, CA 91413-5224
Childbirth preparation program

American Society for Psychoprophylaxis in Obstetrics, Inc.
(ASPO/Lamaze)
1200 19TH St. NW
Suite 300
Washington, DC 20036-2401
Childbirth preparation program

Best Start
3000 E. Fletcher Avenue, Suite 308
Tampa, FL 33613
Videos and materials for low-income women

Center for Science in the Public Interest
1779 Church Street NW
Washington, DC 20036
Publishes nutritional research

Childbirth Graphics, Ltd.
(A division of WRS Group, Inc.)
PO Box 21207
Waco, TX 76702-1207
http://www.wrsgroup.com
Nutrition and breastfeeding educational materials

Clearinghouse on Infant Feeding and Maternal Nutrition
American Public Health Association
1015 Fifteenth Street, NW
Washington, DC 20005
Literature

Florida Healthy Mothers/Healthy Babies
15 SE 1st Avenue, Suite A
Gainesville, FL 32601
Hospital breastfeeding protocol, in-service training package

Food and Nutrition Information Center
National Agricultural Library Building, Room 304
Beltsville, MD 20705
Literature

Geddes Productions (Kitty Frantz)
10546 McVine Avenue
Sunland, CA 91040
Breastfeeding videos

Georgetown University Hospital
National Capital Lactation Center
3800 Reservoir Road NW
Washington, DC 20007
Professional educational material, continuing education programs, hospital protocols, and nursing care plans

Health Education Associates
8 Jan Sebastian Way
Sandwich, MA 02563
Professional education and lay breast-feeding materials

International Baby Food Action Network (IBFAN)
c/o Action for Corporate Accountability
129 Church St.
New Haven, CT 06510
Promotes breastfeeding worldwide

International Board of Lactation Consultant Examiners
PO Box 2348
Falls Church, VA 22042
Administers annual multilingual worldwide certifying examination

International Lactation Consultant Association
200 N. Michigan Ave.
Suite 300
Chicago, IL. 60601
Professional organization of lactation consultants that distributes the Journal of Human Lactation with membership

Continued.

❖

RESOURCES—*cont'd*

International Childbirth Education Association
PO Box 20048
Minneapolis, MN 55420
Organization of childbirth educators

International Nutrition Communication Service
Education Development Center
55 Chapel Street
Newton, MA 02160
Literature

La Leche League International
1400 Meacham
Schaumburg, IL 60173
Professional and lay materials; also professional workshops on lactation in various U.S. locations annually

Lactation Associates
254 Conant Road
Weston, MA 02193
Professional and consumer educational materials and professional continuing education

Lactation Institute
16430 Ventura Boulevard, Suite 303
Encino, CA 91436
Professional training courses and college credit program in lactation consulting

Medela, Inc.
PO Box 660
McHenry, IL 60051-0660
Breast pumps and other lactation-related equipment

National Health Information Clearinghouse
PO Box 1133
Washington, DC 20013
Literature

UNICEF
United Nations
New York, NY 10017
Promotes breastfeeding worldwide

Weingart Design
4614 Prospect Avenue, #421
Cleveland, OH 44103-4314
Breastfeeding materials, eighth-grade reading level

WELLSTART San Diego Lactation Program
PO Box 87549
4062 First Avenue
San Diego, CA 92138-2045
Professional educational program for multidisciplinary lactation teams (i.e., MD, RN, RD)

World Health Organization (WHO)
Publication Center
49 Sheridan Avenue
Albany, NY 12210
Publications by WHO, especially Baby Friendly Hospital Initiative

---

are often cared for by many different doctors, nurses, and other health care providers. Parents need to know that they may have to state their needs repeatedly throughout obstetrical care. Some clients may deliver their babies in large hospitals, sometimes referred to as tertiary-care centers. Most often found in major medical centers, these centers are designed to provide care to pregnant women whose needs range from an uncomplicated pregnancy to a life-threatening emergency. These institutions are often teaching hospitals, which provide clinical experiences for students in every conceivable health profession. Inevitably, with more care givers, the risk of conflicting information about breastfeeding increases.

Furthermore, if any emergencies arise, breastfeeding preferences may need to be deferred until the mother's and/or baby's condition have stabilized. On the good side, tertiary-care centers often have lactation consultants who can assist your clients, especially in high-risk or complicated breastfeeding situations. In smaller or community hospitals, single-room maternity units, also known as labor-delivery-recovery-postpartum units (LDRs or LDRPs) are becoming more prevalent. In this setting, the number of caregivers is smaller. These obstetrical care facilities are often in hospitals that cater to their community's need for breastfeeding support. However, this is not always the case. Ultimately, it falls to the mother (or her support persons) to make her breastfeeding choice known.

Breastfeeding is more than a physical process. The onset of lactation is related to the fall in **progesterone** following delivery of the placenta.[117] At this time, all the physiologic changes of pregnancy come together so that glandular development, blood supply, and hormonal influences have primed the breasts for lactation. However, the psychosocial and environmental aspects of what is going on around the mother may be the biggest obstacle to establishing lactation and breastfeeding.[67,88,141,168,170] Hospitals and mothers should be aware of these so that they can clearly state their needs in terms with which hospital personnel may already be familiar. Mothers should be prepared to do the following:

1. Clearly state the intention to breastfeed.
2. Clearly state that the baby should not be given water or formula supplements.
3. Clearly state that the baby is not to be given a pacifier.
4. Clearly state she wants to initiate breastfeeding as soon as possible after delivery.
5. Request instruction and help in initiating breastfeeding or breast pumping if she and the baby are separated for any reason.
6. Clearly request 24-hour-a-day rooming-in if the baby is healthy.
7. Insist on feeding the baby at least every 2 to 3 hours.
8. Request referral to a breastfeeding support group before discharge from the hospital.

Rationales for the baby-friendly concepts are documented in the literature as the correct way to initiate lactation and breastfeeding.*

---

*References 38, 62, 82, 88, 90, 134, and 148.

ASSESSMENT OF ADEQUACY OF BREASTFEEDING

Performance and outcome are the breastfeeding concepts that are most important to the mother and baby in the postpartum period. First, the mother may need to be shown basic breastfeeding techniques. She may need a hands-on demonstration to feel comfortable with correct positioning for herself and the baby. She may need assistance with helping the baby latch on over the nipple to the areola for correct suckling and nipple comfort. Some babies do this without help; some do not. These mothers need extra support and instruction.

The mother should also be provided with some tools to evaluate the outcome, such as does she hear swallowing? Is the baby having six to eight wet diapers in a 24-hour period? Is her baby alert when awake? Unfortunately, she also needs this information to ward against well-meaning but ill-informed doctors, nurses, dietitians, husbands, mothers, in-laws, neighbors, friends, and others. Many individuals say and do things to undermine the mother's confidence in her ability to breastfeed. As in the prenatal period, these breastfeeding concepts need to be kept to a minimum so that the mother can focus on what's important and not be confused or turned off by a rigid, extensive list of dos and don'ts. The most important concepts to be shared in the immediate postpartum period are assessment of feeding adequacy, positioning of mother and baby, latching on, and nursing frequency.

The clinician should instruct the mother to listen to her baby. This helps her tune in to her infant, which is sometimes difficult for the first-time breastfeeding mother to do. Television, roommates, telephones, and various hospital personnel are distractions to the first-time breastfeeding mother. There is also the general excitement and disorientation that comes with being hospitalized. The experience of having just gone through a vaginal or cesarean delivery is usually accompanied by both relief and elation, along with the discomforts of intravenous (IV) lines, stitches, fatigue, and bruising. The effect of medications can sedate or decrease the ability of the mother to focus. Finally, there is the gradual realization that the baby is truly here, real, and in need of attention.[126,142]

Listening to the baby provides a mother with an opportunity to learn about the normal variety of infant reflexes that make noise, such as breathing, swallowing, hiccupping, and sneezing. Many new parents are so unfamiliar with babies that they think that the only noise a baby makes is crying.

The most important reason to tell a mother to listen to audible breathing and swallowing is to give her immediate feedback about breathing and feeding. For instance, contrary to breast-feeding instruction in the past, it is not necessary for the mother to press her breast away from the baby's nose for it to breathe, and if she learns to listen to her baby, she will be able to hear that. The infant nose was designed to stick out just enough to push the breast back to create an adequate air passage. When the mother listens for swallowing sounds, she hears her milk going into the baby's esophagus. It tells her that there is something in her breast. Far too many women have been told there is no milk, that the milk does not "come in" for a certain number of days, or worst of all, that they do not have enough milk. This negative thinking is often reinforced by the size of the infant formula bottles used in the hospital. The formula industry packages newborn formula in 3-oz bottles because it is convenient and cost-efficient for the manufacturer to do so. This volume is too much for any newborn to consume. However, for inexperienced parents it becomes a measure of feeding need. If the baby nurses frequently, both his fluid and nutritional requirements will be met by the breast milk alone.[162] Folding the baby's hand into a fist demonstrates to the parents the size of their baby's stomach and provides them with a better understanding of the small volume needed to satisfy the baby's needs at a given feeding. The box below shows how to calculate the amount of breast milk a baby needs each day.

Some mothers have been told they will feel a **let-down,** also known as the milk ejection reflex during breastfeeding. All mothers will experience let-down; but some mothers may not feel it physically. Let-down is a term, borrowed from the dairy industry and used to describe the process by which milk from sinuses higher up in the breast is moved down to those surrounding the areola and nipple, where the baby can milk it out. As the baby's mouth massages the areolar tissue around the nipple, it stimulates the mother's body to release oxytocin, which in turn stimulates the muscles surrounding the alveoli and milk ducts to contract. This sends the milk forward in the breast. Sometimes the only way a mother knows her milk is letting down is when she hears her baby swallowing faster. Other mothers will feel a tingling sensation, or will feel pressure inside of the breast. Mothers with a particularly strong let-down may notice the baby rearing his or her head back until the initial gush subsides. All of these activities are normal.[86]

FEEDING FREQUENCY

The baby needs frequent access to the breast so the mother will be able to build a milk supply that will provide the fluids and kcalories needed for the infant's growth. For almost this entire

---

CALCULATION OF NEWBORN CALORIC REQUIREMENTS

To calculate the number of ounces of breast milk needed per day by the baby, use the following calculation:

$$\frac{\text{weight (kg)} \times 110 \text{ kcal/kg}}{20 \text{ kcal/oz}} = \frac{\text{total}}{\text{oz/day}}$$

Fluid requirements must also be calculated to ensure adequate hydration. The baby needs about 150 ml/kg (70 ml/lb) of fluid per day. This is calculated as follows:

$$\text{weight (kg)} \times 150 \text{ ml} = \text{total ounces/day}$$

To convert milliliters to ounces, divide by 30 (30 ml = 1 oz). Therefore, a 3-kg (6 lb 5 oz) baby will require 16.5 oz of milk and fluid.

century, instructions from physicians and nurses on all infant feeding, but especially breastfeeding, has included regimented timing of feedings.[40] This attempt to schedule breastfeeding was motivated, in part, by a wish to prevent nipple damage.[88] But what it has in fact done, is untold damage to the willingness of mothers to continue breastfeeding. It is now known that human newborns need to nurse a minimum of 10 to 12 times in 24 hours, for at least the first month of life to receive adequate nutrition. This means the infant must nurse about every 2 to 3 hours around the clock.[86,90]

This is a departure from the concept of **demand feeding,** which represents the opposite end of the spectrum from scheduled feeding. Nursing every 2 to 3 hours around the clock represents a reasonable compromise, which allows the baby to meet his nutritional needs while the mother meets her comfort needs by moving milk through her breasts frequently. For new parents this translates into a departure from clock watching to baby watching, the bottom line of which is, "When in doubt, feed the baby!"

New parents need guidelines, not rules. They need to know that not all feedings will last the same length of time, nor will the baby nurse an equal number of minutes from each breast at each feeding. Generally speaking though, both breasts should be offered at each feeding to facilitate the mother's comfort with her milk supply. Encouraging frequent unlimited breastfeeding produces increased milk output, which leads to greater infant weight gain, decreased nipple and breast problems and increased duration of breastfeeding.[38,82] Assure the mother that as the baby grows older the time between feedings will lengthen. This is especially important for mothers who are hesitant to begin breastfeeding because of limited maternity leave policies, or for mothers who fear that breastfeeding will prevent them from pursuing other activities.

Finally, new parents can be told that after awhile, they will begin to observe a pattern to their baby's feedings. The baby will then have a **growth spurt,** and the pattern will change. Growth spurts occur at regular intervals during the first year of life and can be identified by a day when all the baby wants to do is nurse. If the baby is allowed to nurse liberally for the next 24 hours or more, the mother's milk supply will increase and the baby will settle down into a new pattern. However, if the mother gives formula to "fill the baby up," she will start a pattern of insufficient milk supply that can be devastating to her continued breastfeeding.[61]

ASSESSMENT OF OUTPUT AS A MEASURE OF ADEQUACY

If the baby is exclusively breastfeeding, then everything the baby excretes will be the end products of breast milk metabolism. Generally, new parents have equally unrealistic ideas about the output as they do about the input. Television commercials for disposable diapers go to great lengths to explain the need to control wetness. The children used for these commercials are not newborns. So parents have no idea how much to expect in a newborn's diaper. However, urine and stool output are good measures of breast milk input.

For a newborn who is nursing every 2 to 3 hours around the clock, parents can expect about six to eight wet diapers and a minimum of one stool per day for the first few weeks. The measurement of "wetness" can be problematic for new parents. Total urine excretion is about 200 to 300 ml per 24 hours in the first weeks of life. The newborn bladder involuntarily empties when filled by approximately 15 ml. This can result in 15 to 20 voidings per day.[162]

To help parents assess these small amounts of wetness in diapers, A tissue or paper towel can be placed inside the diaper. The tissue or towel will be wet while the paper diaper, which is so absorbent, will not. This proves that the baby is urinating. Breastfed babies are known to pass stools often. A normal breastfed baby's stool is very liquid. This pattern should not be mistaken for diarrhea. Normal stool frequency in a breastfed baby varies widely. A minimum of one to three stools a day in the first month of life is considered a baseline indicator of minimal intake. Conversely, many newborns have a bowel movement with each feeding. However, older infants can pass a stool either more or less often and still be normal. Some older babies even go days between bowel movements.[88] The color of the stools of breastfed babies is also important information for the new parents. Newborn stool goes through several color changes in the first few days of life as the colostrum pushes the meconium stool out of the body and the infant's bowels adapt to oral feeding. The normal stool changes are from black to greenish to bright yellow.[126] A yellow mushy stool is normal for a totally breastfed baby. Finally, the baby should begin to show readily visible signs of growth. A return to birth weight by about 2 weeks of age and outgrowing of newborn sleepers, is considered a good measure. Over the long term, a gain of 4 oz per week or 1 lb per month is considered satisfactory growth for a breastfeeding baby.[148]

Pediatrician Ruth Lawrence has reiterated the American Academy of Pediatrics guidelines, which state that all infants should be seen by their practitioner within 7 days of discharge from the hospital because all infants are at risk for complications in the early weeks regardless of feeding mode. She goes on to say that in the event of early discharge from the hospital (24 hours after delivery or less) the pediatrician should provide within 3 days of discharge in the office or in the home a weight check, observation of the infant for physical status, jaundice, hydration and successful breastfeeding. She goes on to list the following criteria for a healthy infant.

- By the third day, the infant should:
  - Stop losing weight
  - Have lost no more than 7% of birth weight
  - Be passing milk stool (yellow)
  - Have at least three stools (minimum) per day
  - Wet at least six diapers per day (cloth diapers are preferred for accurate assessment in the first 6 weeks)
  - Latch onto breast well
- The mother should:
  - Experience some breast engorgement
  - Notice dripping of milk from opposite breast
  - Expect the infant to feed every 3 hours or a minimum of 8 times a day[91]

IMPORTANCE OF POSITIONING: COMFORT FOR MOTHER

Correct positioning has everything to do with continued breastfeeding. If the mother is not comfortable she will not feel encouraged to continue. In short, if the mother looks uncomfortable, she probably is, even if she is unaware of her discomfort or denies it for the sake of the baby. Advice about chairs, pillows, a footstool, or rocking chairs is relevant in relation to the size of the mother and the size of the baby. Therefore positioning of the mother and baby will have to be adapted to what works best for each mother-baby couple. The mother may either sit up or lie down.

The important anatomical structures involved in positioning for breastfeeding are the relationship of the nipple/areola of the mother to the mouth of the baby. The baby's mouth must approach the nipple in correct geometric alignment or the mother is at risk for nipple trauma. When breastfeeding in a seated position, the mother's body should be upright. This aspect of positioning is crucial if the baby's mouth and the mother's nipple/areola are to be in correct alignment (Fig. 13-9). The baby can now be positioned at the breast in a variety of ways depending on the comfort and needs of the mother. The important thing to do when assisting with positioning for breastfeeding is to look carefully at the mother for signs of stress, such as bending, leaning, or tension in the neck or forehead (Fig. 13-10).

For side-lying, the mother needs a pillow behind her to keep her from rolling backward. Some mothers are comfortable nursing with their arms down, and some are more comfortable with their arms up. In any position, the mother's comfort is the most important factor.

IMPORTANCE OF POSITIONING: CORRECT FOR BABY

The importance of having an alert baby who is interested in nursing also is critical to continued breastfeeding. Darkening the room to help the newborn open his or her eyes is very important. Inexperienced parents do not realize that normal room lighting often is too bright for a newborn and that sometimes the baby's eyes are

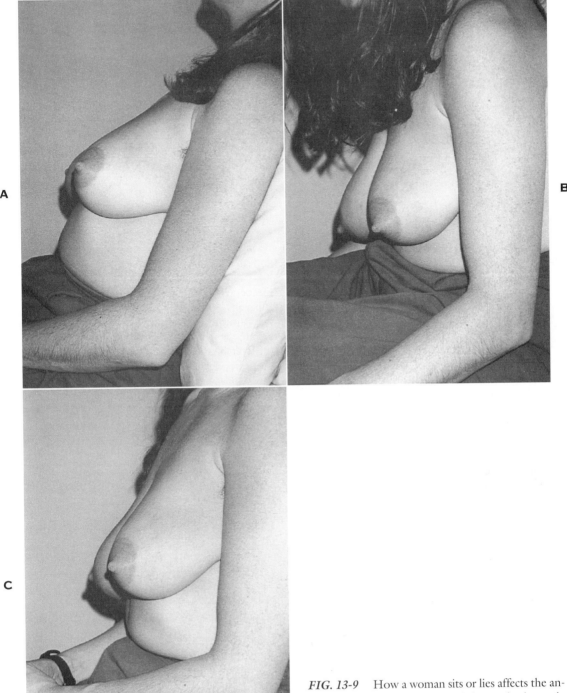

FIG. 13-9 How a woman sits or lies affects the angle of the breasts and how the baby can latch on. **A,** When the woman leans back her nipples point upward. **B,** When she leans forward her nipples point downward. **C,** With the woman's back straight, her breasts are in the most accessible position for the baby.

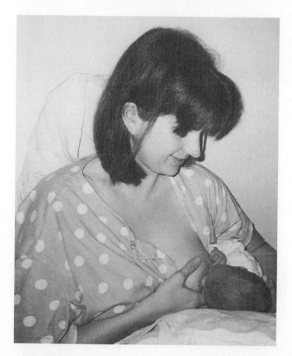

FIG. 13-10   Proper positioning for breastfeeding avoids strain on the mother's shoulders and back.

closed only because the lighting in the room needs to be dimmed. In a few days when the baby is more skilled at breastfeeding, the mother can nurse with or without the lights on. She will know that the baby is nursing properly because it feels comfortable at the breast, regardless of whether the baby's eyes are open or the lights are on or off. Unwrapping the baby so that she or he awakens from sleep before beginning a feeding is another way to help the newborn be alert and ready to learn how to nurse. However, a newborn who has been given a bottle of water or artificial baby milk and is nipple-confused may require patience on the part of the mother as well as readiness on the part of the baby to learn to latch on correctly in the first days of life.

The baby must be positioned at the breast so that the geometry of the baby's mouth and mother's nipple/areola are maintained. This is best accomplished with the baby's entire body rotated toward the mother (tummy to tummy). The baby's head must be facing forward, and not turned to either side with the baby's ears di-

rectly over each shoulder and not tilted back. Maureen Minchin calls this "chest to chest, chin to breast, lips flanged out and back."[114] The mother's hand or the bed should be supporting the baby's body in a neutral alignment. With the baby comfortably supported by a combination of pillows and mother's arm, the baby's mouth should be at the level of the nipple.

IMPORTANCE OF CORRECT LATCHING ON

The mother should tickle the baby's upper lip lightly with the her nipple until the baby opens his or her mouth very wide to teach it how to open wide enough to engage both the nipple and the areola (Fig. 13-11). This activity may take a considerable amount of time and patience. Most babies should know what to do intuitively. Some babies respond in a matter of a few minutes to gentle training. However, if they are sleepy from medication given during labor, a difficult birth, or are not hungry because hospital policy required that they be given a feeding, the process may take more time and patience. This is where a lactation consultant or maternity nurse who is experienced with proper breastfeeding management becomes invaluable. The end result of these efforts should be a well-latched baby. Only recently have studies investigated what the baby's mouth is doing during breastfeeding.[114] Older diagrams were inaccurate and led to erroneous ideas about what the baby's tongue did during breastfeeding (Fig. 13-12). Dr. Michael Woolridge has conducted ultrasound studies of babies at the breast that clearly identify the sequence of events in the baby's mouth during well-latched breastfeeding. Tongue movements can be felt using gloved finger (Fig. 13-13).

Some babies will be able to go easily to the breast within the first day of life. Other babies need more practice to learn the correct movements of lips and tongue. When a baby is having trouble, it is essential to consult a professional who can correctly assess the problem and recommend techniques to overcome it. Lactation consultants and specialized physical and occupational therapists are able to assess sucking problems and suggest ways to get the baby to latch

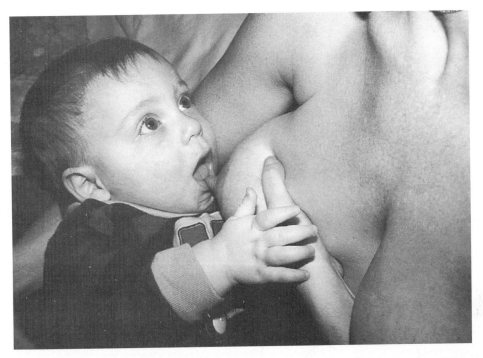

FIG. 13-11   Proper position for the baby to engage both the nipple and the areola.

on. Marmet recommends a simple evaluation process with suggestions for remediation that can be used to help babies to overcome a variety of sucking difficulties.[103]

It is vital to teach both the mother and her baby correct techniques for positioning and latching from the beginning. So much of the dissatisfaction and early abandonment of breastfeeding that occurs because of sore nipples and other problems could be avoided if every feeding was initiated properly so that correct techniques were reinforced and problems avoided.[106,167] The responsibility for modeling the correct techniques is clearly the responsibility of the nursing staff who care for the mother and baby during the intrapartum period.[114,136] However, the lack of breastfeeding knowledge on the part of medical and nursing staff in United States hospitals is an unfortunate reality.[5,18] Furthermore, current short hospital stays, outdated hospital policies mandating complementary water/formula before or after nursing,[85,167] extended delays between birth and initiation of first feeding,[84] time

limitations at breast,[151] and commercial formula discharge packs[48] all contribute to early weaning from breast to bottle. Hospital policies that support early initiation of breastfeeding after birth,[63] feeding on demand, rooming-in,[170] prohibition of complements or supplements unless ordered by the physician for a specific reason, and encouragement from a lactation consultant (see box on p. 421) can contribute to increased breast-feeding duration.*

MOST FREQUENT BREASTFEEDING CONCERNS
Self-Care for Mother

One of the most important things a new mother can do to get breastfeeding to work for her, is to take care of herself. This is not easy under the current system of health care and life in America. Information about and access to pre-

---

*References 14, 18, 49, 75, 76, and 98.

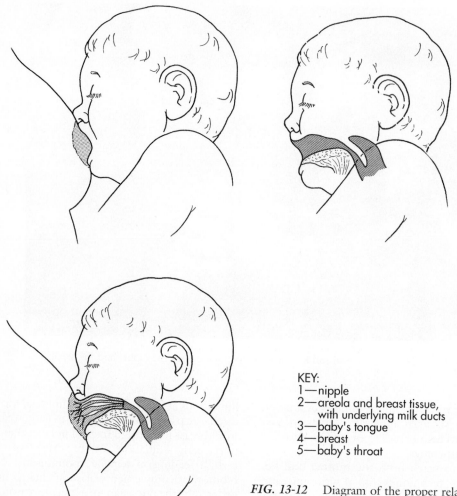

KEY:
1—nipple
2—areola and breast tissue,
 with underlying milk ducts
3—baby's tongue
4—breast
5—baby's throat

FIG. 13-12   Diagram of the proper relationship of the nipple to the baby's mouth.

natal care are not available to American women the way they are in the rest of the western world. Hospital care during the intrapartum period is brief, and more than half of all new mothers must return to employment outside the home within 6 to 8 weeks after delivery. Furthermore, routine home visiting and well-baby care are also not available to many American children, resulting in morbidity and mortality statistics that compare unfavorably in a study of 10 European countries.[164]

Time to provide guidance for the new breast-feeding mother is limited. Therefore it is impor-tant to emphasize the basics before she returns home from the hospital: to continue to eat a well-balanced diet, to drink fluids to satisfy thirst, and to sleep when the baby sleeps.

New mothers also usually are unaware that life with a new baby will be tiring for at least the first month, regardless of how they are fed. The idea of napping during the day sounds foreign to modern women who think they are going to bounce right back from delivery to their usual routine.

As for nutritional counseling, the adage that she can "eat anything in moderation" serves the

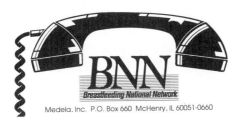
new mother well. Reports of breastfed infants becoming **colicky** from ingestion of certain gas-forming foods have been largely disproved. However, repeated reference to such outdated ideas in grocery store tabloids and other lay literature work to perpetuate such mythology. The limited number of foods that remain exceptions because they seem to have a proven relation to colicky behavior are caffeine, chocolate, and cow's milk.[110,111] That does not mean an individual newborn might not react to other foods that the mother might eat, but this seems to be the exception. The cycle of feeding, fussing, and crying in babies is part of a larger picture of accepted child-rearing practices in a multicultural society and of practices within each family.

Perceived Insufficient Milk Supply

One of the main reasons mothers cite for giving up breastfeeding is a perception of insufficient milk. Insufficient milk supply is defined as a mother's perception that the quantity or quality of her milk is unable to satisfy the baby and/or was not adequate for anticipated weight

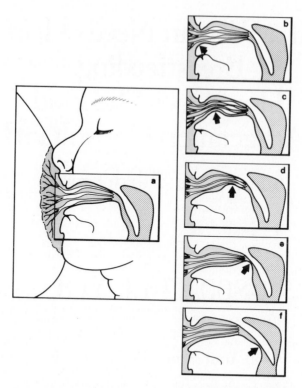

FIG. 13-13 A complete "suck" cycle. Baby is shown in median section, and exhibits good feeding technique with the nipple drawn well into the mouth, extending back to the junction of the hard and soft palate. (Lactiferous sinuses are depicted within the teat, though these cannot be visualized on scans.) **A,** "Teat" is formed from the nipple and much of the areola, with lacteal sinuses (which lie behind the nipple) being drawn into the mouth with the breast tissue. Soft palate is relaxed and nasopharynx is open for breathing. Shape of tongue at the back represents its position at rest, cupped around the tip of the nipple. **B,** Suck cycle is initiated by welling up of the anterior of the tongue. At the same time, the lower jaw, which had been momentarily relaxed (not shown) is raised to constrict the base of the nipple, thereby "pinching off" milk within the ducts of the teat. (These movements are inferred, as they lie outside the sector viewed in ultrasound scans.) **C,** Wave of compression by tongue moves along underside of nipple in posterior direction, pushing against hard palate. This roller-like action squeezes milk from the nipple. Posterior position of tongue may be depressed as milk collects in the oropharynx. **D, E,** Wave of compression passes back past tip of the nipple, in posterior direction, pushing against soft palate. As tongue impinges on soft palate levator muscles of palate contract, raising it to seal off nasal cavity. Milk is pushed into the oropharynx and is swallowed if a sufficient quantity has collected. **F,** Cycle of compression continues and ends at posterior base of tongue. Depression of back portion of tongue creates negative pressure, drawing nipple and its milk contents back into mouth. This is accompanied by lowering of jaw, which allows milk to flow back into the nipple. In ultrasound scans it appears that compression by tongue and negative pressure with the mouth maintain tongue in close conformation to nipple and palate. Events are portrayed here rather more loosely to aid clarity.

From Royal College of Midwives, based on Woolridge M: *Successful breastfeeding,* 1991, Churchill Livingstone.

gain.[64] This is a complex phenomenon, which is receiving increased attention by researchers.[65] A mother's perception of insufficient milk involves factors such as maternal confidence, paternal support, maternal health, mother-in-law disapproval, infant birth weight, baby behavior, solid foods, and formula.[64] The reasons stated most often by mothers for believing they had insufficient milk were a fussy baby, crying after a feeding, and poor weight gain. As a result, mothers begin to believe that their breast milk is inadequate to satisfy their infant's needs. In an attempt to satisfy their infants, the mothers turn to artificial baby milk, which begins a cycle of less demand for the breast, which leads to less frequent nursing, which leads to decreased supply and a self-fulfilling prophecy of insufficient milk for the baby. This cycle is very real and prevalent in U.S. culture. It is reported as the main reason why mothers abandon breastfeeding for bottle feeding.[55,58] Successful intervention to change this pattern of premature weaning to artificial babymilk involves teaching the mother how successful lactation works. Reinforce the concept of frequent nursing (every 2 to 3 hours around the clock for the first month) as a way to balance infant need with maternal supply. Increased support for breastfeeding in the early postpartum period has to come from family and friends who are committed to supporting breastfeeding. Health care providers must make a commitment to learn about correct breastfeeding management techniques, so that when new mothers turn to them for advice and support they are given accurate information.

PHYSICAL DISCOMFORTS WHEN BEGINNING BREASTFEEDING
Nipple Problems

Among the many concerns new mothers have about breastfeeding, one of the most distressing is the fear of pain. Breastfeeding instruction in nursing textbooks and many infant care books would be incomplete without a discussion of sore nipples, cracked nipples, engorgement, and mastitis. These concepts are so thoroughly ingrained in the medical, nursing, and lay childbirth literature that they have come to be considered an expected part of breastfeeding.[90,126]

However, many of the initial problems mothers have with breastfeeding are iatrogenic in nature, stemming from hospital policies and old wives' tales, resulting in practices harmful to successful initiation of breastfeeding.

The great majority of these problems can be prevented by prenatal nipple assessment, intervention to evert nipples when necessary, and correct instruction in breastfeeding techniques that suit the individual mother-baby couple.

Despite these interventions, some mothers still experience nipple problems. The old techniques, such as prenatal nipple "toughening," limiting time at the breast, and the use of soaps, nipple creams, and nipple shields, must be abandoned in favor of techniques that have proved to provide relief and healing to damaged nipple tissue.[141]

Using soaps, creams, and ointments on the nipple is of particular concern for a number of reasons. Current management of nipple trauma is best treated by air drying of the nipples, with or without use of breast shells. This treatment should be accompanied by applying the mother's own breast milk, which contains natural lanolin as well as antibodies to fight infection and promote healing.[141] Also, of the nine most commonly recommended nipple creams, five are listed as "for external use only" and the others all contain instructions to remove the product before nursing. Yet these preparations are routinely recommended for consumption by human neonates as they breastfeed, without regard for the implications for feeding this chemical cocktail to newborn babies.[70] (See Table 13-2.)

Mothers also need to know that a certain amount of tenderness may occur when beginning breastfeeding. This is related to the compression of the infant's mouth on the breast tissue. Most mothers will report the sensation passes as soon as the milk is flowing and the baby settles at breast. This can take anywhere from 30 to 60 seconds or longer for new mothers, and it disappears as the baby gets older.

Two other frequently used breastfeeding products can be hazardous for the mother—breast pads and nipple shields. Wearing breast pads is akin to leaving a bandage on while taking a shower. The moisture collects under the pad,

TABLE 13-2 Products Used on Nipples

Name	Description	Ingredients	Comments
A&D ointment (Schering Corp., Kenilworth, NJ)	Ointment in a tube	Andydrous lanolin, petrolatum, fragrance, mineral oil, fish liver oil, and cholecalciferol	For *external use* only. In case of ingestion, contact a poison control center. There are no vitamins in this ointment.
Bag Balm (Dairy Association, Inc., Lyndonville, VT)	Stiff yellow ointment	Petrolatum, lanolin, 8-hydroxyquinoline sulfate, sanitas, and water	A fungistat and bacteriocide for farm use. *Not for internal use* since 1969, because it causes cancer in laboratory animals.
Eucerin cream (Beiersdorf, Norwalk, Conn)	Cream in a jar	Petrolatum, mineral oil, mineral wax, wool wax alcohol, methylchloroisothiazolinone, methylisothiazolinone	For *external use* only.
Mammol Ointment (Abbott Laboratories, Pharmaceutical Products Division, North Chicago, Ill)	Ointment	Bismuth subnitrate, castor oil, anhydrous lanolin, ceresin wax	Advertised as a dressing for nipples of nursing mothers. However, instructions advise washing and drying nipples before and after use. *Warning:* Subnitrate may be reduced by bacteria in the bowel of infants to yield nitrite, which causes methemoglobinemia after absorption.
Massé Cream (Ortho Pharmaceutical Corp., Raritan, NJ)	Cream in a tube	Glyceryl stearate, glycerin, cetyl alcohol, peanut oil, sorbitan stearate, stearic acid, polysorbate-60, sodium benzoate, propylparaben, methylparaben, potassium hydroxide	Advertised for prenatal and postnatal nipple care. However, instructions advise to cleanse the breasts before and after each nursing with a clean cloth and water. Contraindicated in mastitis and breast abscess. While most of the ingredients are innocuous, the glycerin is rapidly metabolized and can cause hyperglycemia. The cetyl alcohol is a laxative, and aspiration of peanut oil can cause severe and fatal bronchitis in small children.

TABLE 13-2 Products Used on Nipples—cont'd

Name	Description	Ingredients	Comments
Moist towelettes, generic (Although not "an agent for nipple soreness," some hospital staffs ask mothers to wipe their nipples with these.)	Premoistened towelettes	Benzalkonium chloride 1:750, alcohol 20%	A germicide and sanitizer for surface cleaning. Toxic to laboratory animals. For preoperative disinfection of unbroken skin. Rinse thoroughly after use. For *external use* only.
Rotersept (Fair Laboratories, Ltd., United Kingdom)	Antiseptic spray	Chlorhexidine gluconate, propellant gas, alcohol, acetone	Persistent antimicrobial effect against gram-negative and gram-positive bacteria. *Warning:* Avoid contact with eyes, ears, and mucous membranes. Effect of acetone is similar to anesthetic effect of ethyl alcohol. For *external use* only.
USP Lanolin (Merck "Lanum") [Merck Sharp & Dohme, West Point, Pa)	Cream in a tube or jar	Hydrous lanolin	Highly allergenic wool derivative. Analysis of a range of lanolin creams revealed all contained organo-phosphorus pesticide residue including diazinon.
Vaseline Petroleum Jelly [Cheseborough-Ponds, Inc., Trumbull, Conn)	Gel in a jar	White petrolatum	Not meant for puncture wounds, serious burns or cuts. If redness or swelling develops, consult physician promptly.
Vitamin E (generic)	Vitamin capsules, oil, gelatin, or cream	Vitamin E in suspension. Capsules = 400 IU each.	Recommended RDA for vitamin E in infants is 5 IU/day. Effect of increased serum concentrations of vitamin E is unknown.

Riordan J, Auerbach KG: *Breastfeeding and human lactation*, Boston, 1992, Jones & Bartlett.

fostering infection. A new mother may also experience leaking of milk from the breasts in the early days of lactation. However, pressing the heel of her free hand against her nipple can hold back the flow of milk until the sensation of letdown and/or the leaking passes.

Nipple shields are another example of a well-intentioned bad idea. They can be found in the historical literature dating back a century to when they were made out of wood and lead.[110] They are responsible not only for decreased milk production,[88] but can also limit the baby's intake to only 20% of the available milk. They cause an extensive list of problems that only make an already jeopardized breastfeeding experience all the more likely to fail. A far better tool for treating nipple problems is breast shells with ample holes for air circulation. Breast shells also serve as an acceptable alternative tool for nurses who feel the need to use some piece of equipment to relieve the mother's problem.

Breast Problems

New mothers also fear **engorgement.** This is another example of antiquated practices creating a problem.[126] In breastfeeding situations in which the baby has unlimited access to the breast from birth, engorgement is a rare or nonexistent problem. The baby stimulates milk production and is able to freely move the milk through the breast so that the delicate balance of mother's supply and infant need are in harmony.[141] This is the ideal. It is certainly attainable in situations of normal birth with rooming-in and even early discharge from the hospital. However, engorgement can become a problem when breastfeeding initiation is delayed or early feedings are irregular. When engorgement occurs, there are several interventions that can minimize the problem before it leads the mother to abandon breastfeeding out of frustration. Initial engorgement should be an indicator that the baby needs to go to breast more often. If that is not possible, then the milk needs to be moved before tension in the breast becomes so severe that the baby cannot latch on.[141]

Sometimes just manually expressing milk from the areolar area of the breast will make enough room for the baby to latch. If the baby is unavailable, then have the mother use a breast pump to relieve the congestion, move the milk, and maintain the milk supply.

Applying warm moist compresses to the breast before nursing or pumping can help ease the problem. Another technique is for the mother to shower, letting warm water run over her breasts while she either manually expresses or pumps the milk. Another technique is to use warm, moist compresses before nursing or pumping, and cold compresses afterward. The cold eases discomfort and reduces swelling.

Finally, Australian midwives report good results with the application of fresh washed cabbage leaves directly on the engorged breasts, under the bra. The history and mechanism for how and why it works is unknown, but both the Australians and Chinese are familiar with the use of cabbage leaves for sprains and other wounds. The treatment provides rapid relief, sometimes just one 2-hour application will relieve the congestion. The treatment can also be used to suppress lactation completely when rapid delactation is necessary, as in the case of the death of a premature infant for whom the mother was pumping. The only identified contraindications for the use of cabbage leaves in this way would be history of cabbage allergy, and maternal objection to the idea.[140] The technique has been used by American lactation consultants with encouraging results. However, further reports and scientific studies need to be conducted to validate the use of cabbage leaves as a treatment for engorgement.

Infections in the Breast: Mastitis, Herpes, Candidiasis

Any time there is nipple trauma, there is a risk of infection. Therefore it is hoped that a reduction in initial nipple trauma would lead to a reduction in nipple and breast infections. One study puts the incidence of mastitis at under 3%.[77] However, regardless of its low incidence, it is a serious complication of breastfeeding that needs immediate attention to prevent unnecessary weaning to bottle-feeding. The rule of thumb with mastitis is, influenza-like symptoms in a breastfeeding mother should be considered mastitis until proven otherwise. The immediate treatment is to increase the frequency of movement of the milk either by nursing or by pumping more often. The mother should also be counseled to increase her intake of fluids and go to bed. If the symptoms are not improved in 24 hours, a physician must be consulted for a course of antibiotics.[148] Mastitis is not dangerous to the baby, the milk is not infected and breastfeeding should not be stopped or the breasts can become abscessed.[141] A plugged milk duct frequently precedes a case of mastitis and can be treated in the same manner as for mastitis. Other infections seen during breastfeeding include herpes and candidiasis (thrush). These infections involve the nursing couple, because the infectious agent can go back and forth from mother to baby and may even include other family members. Infections of this nature need consultation with a lactation consultant and physician together to recommend modifications of the nursing techniques as well as medications.[4,39,73,171]

Jaundice

Jaundice is a common finding in newborn infants during the first weeks of life. It is a symptom of delayed excretion of the byproducts from the breakdown of fetal hemoglobin called **bilirubin.** The fetal hemoglobin is not needed after birth, and the bilirubin is excreted primarily in the infant stool. Jaundice is important because historically researchers connected jaundice with a severe form of brain damage called kernicterus.[90] After that time, the phenomenon of neonatal jaundice was given a name, hyperbilirubinemia, and a treatment.

Initially, the treatment for severe hyperbilirubinemia was an exchange blood transfusion of the infant. It was a serious and sometimes risky procedure, but then a new treatment was devised, based on the observations of nurses in an English nursery that the babies on the sunny side of the nursery experienced less jaundice.

For approximately the past 20 years, hospital nurseries have used a special fluorescent light box placed over the baby in a technique called *phototherapy* or *bililights.* Much like the sunlight, the fluorescent lights work to assist in removal of jaundice from the skin of newborns and therefore prevent kernicterus. Over the years there have been various schools of thought as to the causes and treatment of jaundice and hyperbilirubinemia. For this discussion, what is important about jaundice is its relationship to breastfeeding. The treatment for jaundice in American hospitals has involved placing the baby in the nursery under phototherapy, and discontinuing breastfeeding either permanently or until the bilirubin levels were acceptable.[126] However, research into hyperbilirubinemia has led to some rethinking of these policies, especially in babies for whom the risks of severe hyperbilirubinemia are very low.[124,155] This is not to say that there are not certain infants who are at higher risk for severe hyperbilirubinemia and even kernicterus.[101] These risk factors include a different blood type or Rh factor than the mother, prematurity, and excessive birth trauma with bruising.[124] However, for the majority of normal newborn infants, increased frequency of breastfeeding in the first days of life will lead to an increase in the passing of stools, which is the physiologically correct outcome of the treatment of jaundice.[141,148] Dr. Lawrence Gartner, a leading expert on neonatal jaundice, has gone on record as saying that for the majority of infants, neonatal jaundice is benign and transient and requires no intervention.[56] However, current hospital policies have yet to catch up with this revised thinking, which has led to researchers looking into the psychological aftereffects of having separated the mother and baby, incurring extra hospitalization and expense, and discontinuing breastfeeding. Both Kemper et al.[80] and Newman and Maisels[124] have expressed concern that further damage is being incurred by overly aggressive treatment of physiological jaundice in the normal newborn who has no risk factors for severe hyperbilirubinemia. This topic is still very controversial and more research needs to be conducted to begin to change treatment methods.

However, early initiation of breastfeeding, and more frequent feeding, usually leads to increased passing of stools, minimized weight loss, and avoidance of reabsorption of the bilirubin from the infant's intestine, which may avoid the occurrence of newborn jaundice.[156]

BEYOND BIRTH: MAINTAINING LACTATION DURING SEPARATIONS AND ILLNESS
Maintaining a Milk Supply

If the mother and baby will be separated for any reason, steps should be taken to keep the milk moving, or the supply will diminish. This can be done by hand or pump expression. There is no one method of expressing milk that is right for everyone. Some women prefer **manual expression** whereas others prefer a particular type of pump. Table 13-3 provides guidelines for breast pump selection. Many women accept and use whatever is made available to them, regardless of whether it is convenient, be-

TABLE 13-3 *Counseling Summary: Helping a Mother Maintain Her Milk Supply when Mother and Baby Are Separated*

Mother's Concern	Suggestions for Mother
Overfullness, leaking	Pump during absence
	Wear breast pads or milk cups
	Nurse directly before and after separation
Low milk supply	Pump regularly during missed feedings
	Drink to thirst
	Nurse frequently when with baby
Nourishment for baby	Offer expressed breast milk or formula
Nipple confusion	Offer supplement in spoon or eyedropper
Baby not accepting bottle	Have another person offer bottle periodically before separation occurs
Baby's behavior	Realize developmental causes of behavior changes
Ability to empty breasts	Practice milk expression before returning to work
Timing of separation	Delay until milk supply is established (2 months)
Difficulty obtaining milk	Establish routine to condition let-down
	Improve milk expression technique (i.e., practice hand expression or acquire more efficient pump)
Avoiding missed feedings	Arrange for mother and baby to be together for feedings: (i.e., bring baby to mother or mother go to baby)

From Lauwers J, Woessner C: *Counseling the nursing mother: a reference handbook for health care providers and lay counselors,* Garden City Park, NY, 1989, Avery Publishing Group, Inc. Reprinted with permission.

cause they are motivated to provide milk for their babies.

When counseling a mother about pumping, a clinician should first assess the mother's goals and the baby's needs (Table 13-4). This will help to determine the techniques best suited to the situation. For a long separation, she should be provided with the best pump she can afford. The mother of a hospitalized or premature infant has very little time or emotional energy for pumping, so the most effective and least stressful option is to rent a double-electric pump. The same is true for a sick or hospitalized mother (Fig. 13-14).

Babies usually are older by the time their mothers return to work or school, and pumping need only be done once or twice per separation. In this situation, the mother usually has more time to weigh price vs. convenience, and can choose between a variety of battery or hand pumps or manual expression. See Fig. 13-15 for information on the correct positioning of the arm and hand during hand pumping.

Pumping for a Premature or Sick Baby

Providing breast milk is something tangible that the mother of a premature or sick baby can do. Ideally, a mother should receive extra support from the lactation consultant from whom she rents the electric breast pump, as well as the nurses at the hospital. [11] Even if the mother is recovering from a high-risk pregnancy or cesarean birth, pumping should begin as soon as the mother is physically able. Ideally, she should pump every 2 to 3 hours during the day and at least once a night. This should total a minimum of seven or eight pumpings in 24 hours, each of which should last for about 10 to 15 minutes.

Guidelines vary for the timing and frequency of pumping, however, the rule of supply and need still applies. The more the mother pumps the more she will stimulate her prolactin levels, which will help keep up her milk supply.[119] A falling milk supply can be helped in a number of ways, not the least of which is support from family, friends, and health care providers.

TABLE 13-4 Guidelines for Breast Pump Selection

Type of Breast Pump	Uses	Reasons	Special Considerations
Hand pump	Short-term separation from baby (1-3 days), except the cylindrical pumps, which may be suitable for longer intervals Regular missed feedings Build milk supply Collect milk	Mother or baby hospitalized Mother working or attending school Mother's milk supply low Mother wishes to provide milk for occasional relief bottle	Portable, easy to carry Inexpensive Can be purchased by mother Can be purchased in bulk by organization and sold to mothers Pump should be used by *one* mother only to avoid passage of bacteria Many ineffective pumps on market
Electric pump	Long-term separation from baby (more than 3 days) Maintain milk supply when baby not nursing Collect milk	Premature baby Birth complications, i.e., prolonged ruptured membranes, infection, etc. Baby has cleft palate Jaundice (when baby not allowed to nurse) Mother on medication Mother or baby hospitalized	Heavy to carry Can be rented by mother. Parents sign rental agreement and pay deposit when picking up pump Rental cost high over long period of time. Cost may be covered by insurance company; mother should pursue this possibility. Can be purchased or leased by organization and rented to individual mothers. Needs 3-hole electrical receptacle or adapter. Adapter must be grounded by inserting grounding wire under screw on wall plate. Pump packets should be used only by *one* mother to avoid passage of bacteria.

From Lauwers J, Woessner C: *Counseling the nursing mother: a reference handbook for health care providers and lay counselors,* Garden City Park, NY, 1989, Avery Publishing Group, Inc. Reprinted with permission.

Mothers can use a variety of techniques to enhance milk production. Sipping water or juice, pumping in a quiet place, using gentle breast massage, looking at a picture of the baby, deep breathing and relaxation techniques, and music have all been known to help milk production.[43,88] Pumping instructions for a hospitalized newborn may be more stringent that those for a working mother of an older healthy baby. It is important for the mother to follow

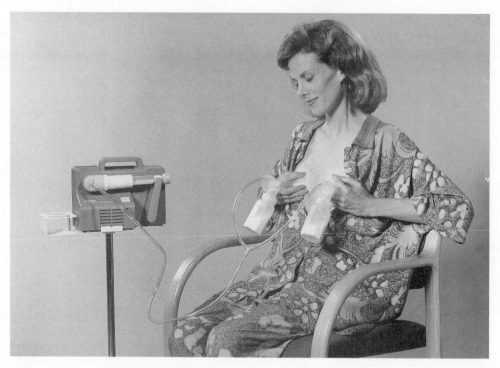

FIG. 13-14   Double pumping saves time and energy when a mother must provide milk for a baby from whom she is separated.

From Medela Breast Pump Company, McHenry, Illinois.

instructions supplied by the hospital about washing and sterilizing the pump equipment, and storing, transporting, and freezing the milk.[119]

Breast milk can be stored in nursing bags, glass, or plastic bottles, or hospital-provided containers (Fig. 13-16). A recent study suggests that ideally, expressed breast milk should be used within 7 hours of refrigerator storage for maximum antibody and cellular function. This research also suggests that glass containers offer a slight advantage over other containers for cellular integrity and efficiency.[166]

Breast milk that will not be fed to the baby within 24 to 48 hours should be frozen (Fig. 13-17, *A*). Frozen breast milk can be kept frozen for weeks or months. Since breast milk changes as the baby grows the frozen milk should be dated so the first pumped is used first. Breast milk should be defrosted using tap water;

it should not be boiled or heated in the microwave (Fig. 13-17, *B*).

Neonatologists' opinions differ about the merits of adding artificial milk fortifiers to the breast milk given to very-low-birth-weight babies. This subject is controversial and deserves further study by dieticians and neonatologists with expertise in the care of these extremely premature infants.[149,174] Most important for the mother and premature or sick newborn is that the baby be given the opportunity to go directly to breast as soon as he or she is physically able to do so. Research studies show that premature infants stay warmer and suck better at a breast than on a rubber nipple. They also have better oxygenation during breast-feeding, and grow well on breast milk at an earlier age and size than was formerly thought possible.[107]

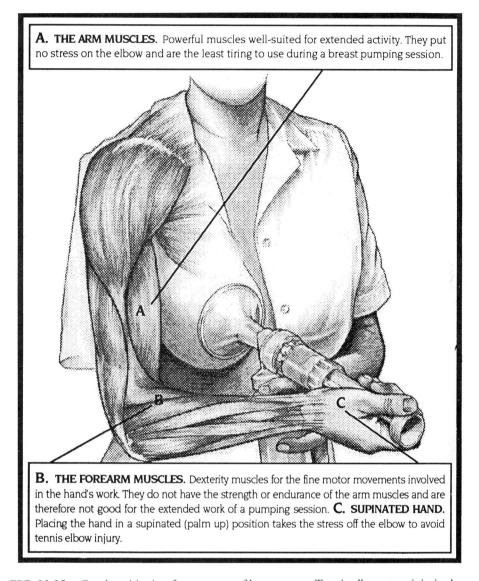

A. THE ARM MUSCLES. Powerful muscles well-suited for extended activity. They put no stress on the elbow and are the least tiring to use during a breast pumping session.

B. THE FOREARM MUSCLES. Dexterity muscles for the fine motor movements involved in the hand's work. They do not have the strength or endurance of the arm muscles and are therefore not good for the extended work of a pumping session. **C. SUPINATED HAND.** Placing the hand in a supinated (palm up) position takes the stress off the elbow to avoid tennis elbow injury.

FIG. 13-15   Good positioning for one type of breastpump. Tennis-elbow–type injuries have been a problem with some kinds of pumps.

From Medela, Inc: Printed with permission of James M. Williams, Ph.D., Assistant Professor of Anatomy, Rush University College of Medicine.

Other Medical or Surgical Conditions in the Baby

Early initiation or resumption of breastfeeding is just as important when the breastfeeding has been delayed or interrupted by a medical or surgical condition in the baby. A study conducted by Weatherly-White et al. of early repair of cleft lips with breastfeeding in the immediate postoperative period demonstrates advantages, not only for babies who have undergone cleft re-

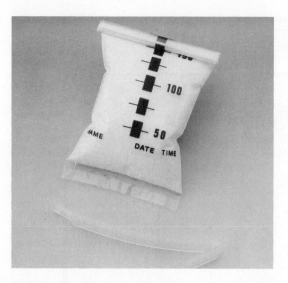

FIG. 13-16 Mother's milk collection bags; useful for storing expressed breast-milk.

From Ameda/Egnell Corporation, Cary, Illinois.

pair, but also for babies receiving general anesthesia for other surgeries.[161] The stresses to both the mother and baby who must experience a hospitalization during infancy are ameliorated to a great extent by staff support for maintaining a milk supply and resuming breastfeeding as soon as possible. It is important to use a team approach to identifying appropriate feeding techniques for infants with craniofacial defects, keeping provision of breast milk in the foreground.[17,31] Physicians, dietitians, lactation consultants, and physical or occupational therapists can each provide essential input to clinical case conferences on the management of hospitalized breastfed infants.

Nursing Supplementer

Infants with medical conditions that cause them to be poor feeders can be assisted with a nursing supplementer—a feeding-tube device that can be used to give supplemental feedings at the breast. These devices can be valuable when dealing with premature infants, infants

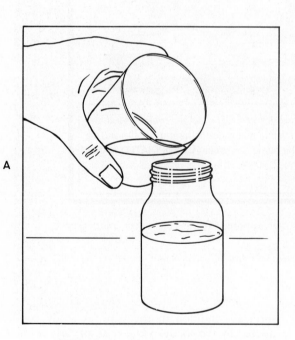

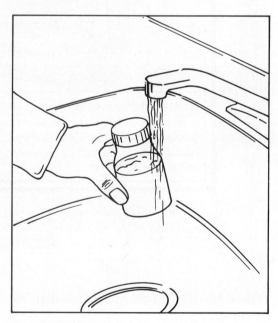

A

B

FIG. 13-17 Storing and thawing frozen breast milk. **A,** Cooled breast milk can be added to frozen milk. **B,** Breast milk can be warmed under running water.

From Lauwers J, Woessner C: Counseling the nursing mother, Garden City Park, NY, 1989, Avery. Reprinted with permission.

with Down syndrome, weak or ineffective nursers, babies who tire easily (such as those with congenital heart defects), low-weight-gain babies, or those with failure to thrive.[90,96] Nursing supplementers are easy for the mother to use but should be used only under the supervision of a lactation consultant who is familiar with their use (Fig. 13-18). A team of specialists may be needed to evaluate and support neurologically impaired breastfeeding infants.

Neurodevelopmental and occupational therapists, who are trained to assess sucking disorders, can often assist the lactation consultant and dietitian to help a mother continue breastfeeding a baby who previously would have been tube fed. These babies especially can benefit from the closeness and comfort afforded by breastfeeding, as well as from the immunological benefits of the breast milk.[90]

Nursing supplementers also can be useful in breastfeeding adopted babies and in relactation. Relactation is a situation in which there has been a fall in milk production for some reason, and the mother wishes to resume breastfeeding. Lactation consultants are useful resources in both situations.

Maternal Illness

Maternal illness can delay breastfeeding initiation. Three major medical problems account for most cases of maternal perinatal morbidity: hemorrhage, infection, and hypertensive disorders of pregnancy (preeclampsia is the old name for one of the hypertensive disorders of pregnancy).[126] These complications can occur with either vaginal or cesarean birth. Recovery from any of these complications is compounded when the mother is recovering from surgery as well. Historically, hospital policies kept these mothers

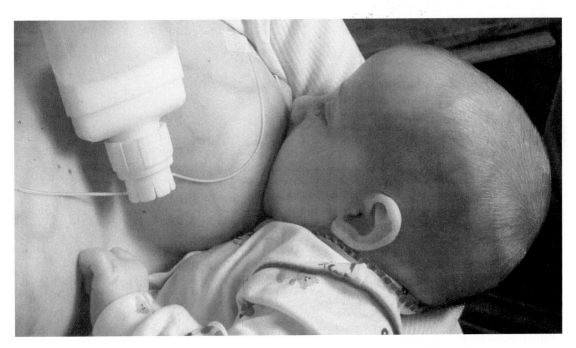

FIG. 13-18 Mother and infant using nursing supplementer, which helps keep baby nursing when supplementation is needed. These devices are useful in relactation situations, for weak or ineffective nursers, premature babies, induced lactation, and for mothers whose milk supply is low.

From Medela Breast Pump Company, McHenry, Illinois.

and babies separated. Certainly if a mother is too ill to care for her baby, it is appropriate that the baby be cared for by the nursing staff. However, babies should be brought in for visits, and infant care can be performed in the mother's room by family members if they wish. Initiating breastfeeding or pumping as soon as the mother is able to sit up is important to begin to stimulate her milk supply. The decision as to whether the infant can consume the milk is a secondary consideration, and should not be used as an excuse to delay the initiation of pumping to build a supply. The milk can be frozen in the nursery freezer for later use by the baby if there is a question about the safety of milk because of the prescription of an unusual medication or because of the nature of the maternal illness.

There are very few situations in which an ill mother cannot maintain a milk supply. Many mothers with chronic illnesses have successfully breastfed a baby, due, in no small part, to their courage in insisting they want to breastfeed. They have actively encouraged the health care community to research the safety of doing so. Historically, women with physically debilitating conditions or chronic diseases that required extensive medication were told not to bear children. However, with improved treatment regimens, not only are these women having children, they are also breastfeeding them. Women can breastfeed with a variety of conditions, including diabetes,[26,72,131] systemic lupus erythematosus,[135] and multiple sclerosis.[120] Certainly mothers with these conditions and their infants need to be monitored closely, but these motivated mothers and babies can breastfeed. Maternal cystic fibrosis[16,100,152] and maternal phenylketonuria,[104] although reported in the literature as being compatible with breastfeeding, need to be carefully monitored for milk composition and infant well-being. The nature of these diseases leads to altered milk composition, which may affect growth and development as the baby gets older.

The question of whether the baby can consume the milk during other maternal illness remains controversial, but is certainly open to case conferences and consultation to see if it is compatible with the mother's treatment. Maternal postpartum depression is a good ex-

ample. There is considerable controversy over the role played by maternal hormones in the onset and severity of postpartum depression. One school of thought believes lactation would prolong the effect and production of the offending hormones, the other school believes the chance to maintain a mother-baby connection is therapeutic.[10] In postpartum depression there is also the question of home management or hospitalization. Here again a team approach in evaluating the mother's condition and safety of the milk are important. A pharmacologist skilled in drug evaluation, in consultation with the baby's pediatrician, is best able to answer questions about maternal milk contamination by medication.[132]

In situations of infectious disease you may need to consult a specialist who can evaluate the literature and assess the risk to the infant. New research is changing our outlook on the safety of breastfeeding with such diseases as hepatitis,[156] where breastfeeding has been shown actually to enhance the clearance of hepatitis surface antigen and thereby decrease the chance of chronic hepatitis in babies born to hepatitis-infected mothers.[156] Infants born to mothers infected with human immunodeficiency virus (HIV) are the group most at risk for HIV infection and acquired immunodeficiency syndrome (AIDS). There is much controversy over whether an HIV-positive mother should be allowed to breastfeed her baby.[128] Breast milk is living tissue, with almost the same number of live cells as blood.[113] Blood contamination is the most common way known of spreading the HIV virus, and infants born to mothers with HIV infection often initially test positive for the virus. AIDS or AIDS-related complex (ARC) will develop in 30% to 60% of these infants.[90] The virus can be acquired in utero, during the birth process, or after birth through the exchange of bodily fluids such as blood. The question is, can it be transmitted through breast milk? There is some evidence that, under certain conditions and in a small percentage of cases, it can.[123]

However, one study shows that heating human breast milk will inactivate the infectivity of HIV-1-infected cells.[127] The same research indicates the possibility of one or more components in human breast milk that may inactivate HIV-1 but that are not toxic to the cells used to replicate the virus. However, more research is needed here.

Current practice around the world varies, most HIV-infected mothers in the United States are advised not to breastfeed their babies,[13,90] but those in developing countries, where the risk of diarrheal and other infections from contaminated water sources is great, are encouraged to do so.[163] The American Academy of Pediatrics Committee on Pediatric AIDS has determined that at this time, the potential for infection (with AIDS) through human milk exists, and must be examined in the context of the prevalence of HIV in women of childbearing age, the low incidence of breastfeeding in populations with the highest incidence of HIV infection, and the known general benefits of human milk. They go on to state the following:

Women who are known to be HIV-infected must be counseled not to breastfeed or provide their milk for the nutrition of their own or other infants. However, the Academy also recognizes that the World Health Organization has developed recommendations for breastfeeding in the developing world . . . where infectious diseases and malnutrition are major causes of infant mortality and where safe alternatives to breastfeeding may not be available.[33,169]

In summary, when it comes to a separation of the mother and baby through illness or surgery, increasingly consultations with physicians, surgeons, anesthesiologists, nursing staff, lactation consultants, dietitians, pharmacists, and patients have reached an amicable and workable resolution to the problem of separation for a breastfeeding mother and baby. These have included instances of maternal surgery for a variety of conditions such as emergency appendectomy, knee arthroscopy, thyroidectomy, cholecystectomy, heart surgery for correction of a maternal ventricular defect and lobectomy to remove a cancerous lung. Progressive medical centers make electric breast pumps available immediately after surgery for the mother's comfort. Provisions for visiting-in by the baby under the supervision of a family member, who also handles infant care such as diaper changing, have been allowed, provided the mother is in a private room. Families respond positively when these needs are met. There are even reports in the literature of successful breastfeeding after extensive surgical procedures, such as maternal renal transplantation. The maternal immunosuppressive drugs were not found to be problematic, and two babies were breastfed for 3 to 4 months each by mothers who had undergone transplantation.[55] Mothers on renal dialysis are also breastfeeding with extensive support and encouragement from the dietitians at a dialysis center in Chicago.

Nutritional problems such as a history of anorexia or bulimia also have been overcome, and these women have gone on to become pregnant and breastfeed well.[19] A Danish study that involved a long-term follow-up of 50 women with a history of anorexia, reported pregnancy rates to be the same as the general population, an unexplained elevated rate of prematurity, but breastfeeding rates and durations that were similar to the country as a whole.[23]

Maternal medication. The crux of the issue in many of the situations involving maternal illness is not so much the pathophysiology of the mother's disease, but the medications the mother is consuming, either temporarily or on a long-term basis. Historically, research into the safety of maternal medications and the breastfeeding infant involved only laboratory confirmation that the drug was present in the milk. More sophisticated techniques for assessment of drug bioavailability have revised the thinking about the safety of breastfeeding while the mother takes medication.

It is also important to keep in mind that it is not the decision of the mother's physician, surgeon, obstetrician, nurses, or any other health care provider as to what the infant can consume. The parents and the pediatrician are those ultimately responsible for infant-feeding decisions. Other health care providers, in particular dietitians, can and should do all they can to facilitate consultations with pharmacologists who are familiar with the literature on pharmacology and breastfeeding. There are several fine resources, such as *Drugs in Pregnancy and Lactation* by

❖ ❖ ❖

CASE STUDY

Maria and Her Baby*

If you already wrote a case outcome for Maria as an earlier assignment, then you can continue to follow her case and determine what you can do to maximize her breastfeeding experience using the material found in this chapter. Otherwise, pick up her story here and do the same thing.

You are working in a large city hospital. The Lactation Consultant position is currently unfilled. You already have many responsibilities, however, you have been asked to make rounds on the newly delivered mothers and give lactation support, instruction and referral.

On your rounds today you visit Maria. She is listed as a breastfeeding mother. Although she is thin, her hands and face are puffy from the preeclampsia she experienced in the last week of her pregnancy. Last night, she had a vaginal delivery of a 36-week gestation, 4 lb 7 oz (2,013 gm) baby girl.

When you ask Maria about breastfeeding she begins to cry. She tells you that the nutritionist at the health department showed videos about the benefits of breastfeeding and about how good it was for the baby, but she was told by someone in the delivery area that the medicine that she was given for the preeclampsia (magnesium sulfate) was bad for the baby. So when the nursery nurses asked her about feeding the baby, she told them to give her baby a bottle.

Write a case report about Maria and her baby. Make a plan for her so that she can meet

her goal of breastfeeding her baby. Identify the resources you will need to use to solve the problem of the roadblock to breastfeeding posed by the information given about magnesium sulfate. Is this information accurate? If not, what is the accurate information about magnesium sulfate and breastfeeding? Where can you go to get accurate information on the safety of magnesium sulfate in breastfeeding?

Outline a plan of care to get Maria's milk supply established. How will you do this if her baby is too ill to come out of the nursery? How will you do this if she can breastfeed, but the baby is nipple confused? How will you do this if Maria is discharged but the baby has to remain for antibiotics or other treatments?

What community resources can you give to Maria? Where can she go to rent a breastpump? Where can she go to learn hand expression of milk? Where can she go for support from other breastfeeding mothers? Where can she get information on nutritional support for herself while breastfeeding? List resources available in your local area. Include phone numbers and pamphlets if possible.

Complete your case report with a description of the length of time Maria breastfed and the pattern of her baby's growth. Describe what you have learned about the role of the Lactation Consultant in the hospital setting.

*Refer to the case study of Maria from Chapter 1, *Nutrition Assessment and Guidance in Prenatal Care.*

Briggs, that should be available to every hospital nursery, dietitian, and pediatrician for quick reference in issues regarding maternal medications.[6,22]

CONTRAINDICATIONS TO BREASTFEEDING

Unfortunately, there are still a few situations in which breastfeeding is contraindicated and would not be in the best interests of the mother or baby. Mothers who are active substance

abusers should not breastfeed, both out of a concern for infant safety while a mother is under the influence of drugs, and for the drug effects themselves. Cocaine is particularly dangerous, not only when ingested by the mother but also in the case of direct application of cocaine to sore nipples.[29,30,47]

Another rare but unfortunate situation is that of maternal cancer. Maternal chemotherapy and radiation are incompatible with breastfeeding.

However, use of diagnostic radioisotopes for use in one-time procedures such as a thyroid scan or lung scan should be evaluated on a case-by-case basis. The radiologists can often find an alternative isotope, or the dosage can be controlled so that breastfeeding need only be suspended for a short time. Furthermore, with planning, a mother can pump and store her milk in advance of the test for the time during which she cannot nurse and resume nursing when it is safe again. The other option when time is of the essence, is for the mother to "pump and dump" her milk until the contamination period has passed. The baby will, out of necessity, need to be fed either artificial baby milk or donated breast milk during the interim.

Contamination of breast milk by various toxins in the environment has also raised safety questions. These situations are also best evaluated on a case-by-case basis. Research into the aftereffects of the Chernobyl nuclear accident has yet to pick up levels of radioactivity in breast milk that exceed those in the environment in general, and no warnings have been noted in the literature coming out of Europe.[57,92] The consensus among radiation oncologists in Chicago is that there is no radiation danger from the breast milk to infants born to mothers who have immigrated from the Chernobyl area to Chicago. However, cases of cerebral palsy in Minamata, Japan, from contaminated fish and in Iraq from contaminated seed have been documented. Cases have also been documented resulting from contamination of fish in Sweden, which has adopted a policy of discouraging breastfeeding in women from contaminated areas despite the inability of researchers to identify a clear link between methylmercury and cerebral palsy.[153]

Working and Nursing

One of the other commonly cited reasons pregnant women give for not breastfeeding is a mistaken notion that breastfeeding and return to employment are not compatible. At a time when more than half the mothers of young children are employed outside the home, those who choose to continue breastfeeding find that they continue to save time as well as money by pumping milk at work and continuing to breastfeed when they are together with the baby.[8,9] Numerous studies speak to the need to advertise the long-term benefits of continued breastfeeding during employment and to support the mothers who choose to do so.[60,159] See Table 13-3 for suggestions for counseling mothers when they are separated from their infants. One recently published study documents the decreased incidence and severity of infant illness and decreased maternal absenteeism in employed breastfeeding mothers who are actively supported in their breastfeeding.[32] One way an employer can demonstrate a commitment to mothers of young children is to provide a lactation station or pump room so that mothers of breastfed infants can have a clean quiet environment in which to pump and store their milk.[8,52,79] The Indiana Breast-feeding Promotion Project prints a pamphlet targeted at employers that explains how promoting breastfeeding can increase workforce productivity (Fig. 13-19).

BREASTFEEDING MULTIPLES

Although giving birth to multiple infants is not inherently prohibitive to breastfeeding, mothers of multiples have not been encouraged to breastfeed with the same enthusiasm as their peers with singleton births. The human body does provide for easy access to the breast for two babies, so availability itself is not the issue. The risk for preterm birth is increased with multiples, whereas the benefits of breast milk for preterm infants is well-established.

However, breastfeeding triplets or quadruplets has been considered by most to be out of the question. One case study reports the success of breastfeeding in a family with quadruplets who went all the way from the neonatal intensive care unit to baby-led weaning.[106] As with breastfeeding in general, one of the most important components of this success with breastfeeding was family support. Scientific research has documented the volume of milk production possible when breastfeeding multiples (Fig. 13-20).[145]

WEANING

The term for the end of lactation and breastfeeding is *weaning*. It signals the end of one phase and the beginning of another. Ideally, it

What Does Your Business Have In Common With A Breastfed Baby?

You Both Rely On A Working Mother

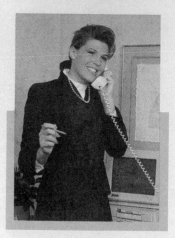

Just as you rely on your female employees to come to work each day and perform their job, a breast-feeding baby relies on his or her mother for a continual supply of fresh breastmilk.

Until recently, many employers didn't realize that only a small amount of time, equipment and space are necessary to support their female employees wishing to breastfeed their infants. Employers all across the country are also realizing that the benefits of providing this supportive environment are tremendously outweighing the costs.

Due to the increased awareness of the nutritional and economical benefits of breastfeeding, more and more women are electing to do so. By working with employers like yourself, we can help support and encourage this decision in which we all can truly benefit.

FIG. 13-19 Promoting working and breast feeding. Target employers to support their breast-feeding employees.

From Indiana Breast-Feeding Promotion Project, Indiana State Board of Health.

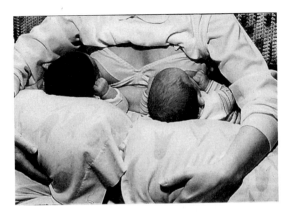

FIG. 13-20 Multiples can be fed in a variety of comfortable positions.

should be a nonevent. Many cultures and La Leche League support the idea of baby-led weaning. Actually, the minute the baby begins eating something other than breast milk, weaning has begun, even if nursing continues for months or years after that. Weaning is a term that connotes a certain maturity on the baby's part, which allows him or her to move from the breast to other foods and beverages. This is rarely the case in current American culture. Far too often the mother weans prematurely for any one or more of the reasons discussed in this chapter.[21,95,165] Certainly there comes a time when a baby needs to move on to other foods for proper growth and development, but all in good time. The U.S. Surgeon General, as well as the American Academy of Pediatrics, and the American Dietetic Association and others recommend that babies be breastfed exclusively for the first 6 months of life, after which weaning should begin with the introduction of solids. How weaning progresses should be up to each mother-baby couple in consultation with their pediatrician and with correct information from dietitians.

It is the responsibility of those most interested in human nutrition to encourage breastfeeding. Breast milk is an environmentally sound, ecologically friendly natural resource. Its properties include the possibility of significantly reducing infant morbidity and mortality, here and in the rest of the world. Its method of delivery goes a long way in promoting the mother-child closeness that is so important to a child's development and self-esteem. Breast milk is nature's most important resource for the continuation of our species.

Summary

There is no doubt that breastfeeding is best for both mother and baby. To encourage more mothers to breastfeed their infants, clinicians must be prepared to support mothers with education and practical information. This requires that health care professionals understand the process of lactation, as well as the cultural differences that affect a woman's decision to breastfeed. The mother's nutritional requirements must be adapted to the foods easily available and culturally acceptable to her. Free and low-cost promotional materials need to be identified and used. Hospital and clinic staff also need to be taught to promote breast-feeding and support families who make this choice.

REVIEW QUESTIONS

1. Discuss breastfeeding trends in the United States and worldwide in this century.
2. Discuss the rise of artificial infant feeding in the industrialized world; in developing countries.
3. List the advantages of breastfeeding for the mother; for the baby.
4. Describe low-cost strategies for breastfeeding promotion.
5. List the breastfeeding concepts that should be shared in the prenatal period; the postpartum period.
6. List the most frequently cited breastfeeding concerns.
7. Describe methods of prevention, management, and evaluation for the most frequently cited breastfeeding concerns.
8. Identify the essential strategies for maintaining lactation during short-term infant separation.
9. Identify the essential strategies for maintaining lactation during prolonged separation.
10. List the most important concepts in maintaining lactation when returning to work or school.
11. Identify sources of support for breastfeeding and promotion on the local, national, and international levels.
12. Describe how you were fed as an infant.

13. List your major concerns (biases) about breast-feeding.
14. Consider how you could encourage change and promote breastfeeding in an environment that was unsupportive of breastfeeding.
15. Comparison shop the prices of various brands, types, and packaging of infant formulas in grocery, discount, and convenience stores.
16. List all the equipment needed to use artificial baby milk. Shop for and price all these items.

LEARNING ACTIVITIES

1. Observe a woman breastfeeding from beginning to end of one feeding experience.
2. Assess the marketplace to determine what breastfeeding accessories are available and attempt to evaluate their usefulness.
3. Survey the breastfeeding literature in local clinics and bookstores to evaluate the quality of the materials.
4. Question local hospital personnel about the breastfeeding support services available to new mothers in the hospital and in a follow-up situation.
5. Talk with a mother who is breastfeeding with the intent of developing a personal feeling for the benefits and disadvantages.

REFERENCES

1. Agras W et al: Does a vigorous feeding style influence early development of adiposity? *J Pediatr* 110:799, 1987.
2. Akre J: Infant feeding: the physiological basis, *Bull World Health Organ* 67:Suppl, 1989.
3. American Academy of Pediatrics: Practice parameter: management of hyperbilirubinemia in the healthy term Newborn, *Pediatrics* 94, (4):558-565, 1994.
4. Amir L and Lawlor-Smith L: Thrush in the ducts? *Med J Aust* 155:853, 1991.
5. Anderson EA, Geden : Nurses knowledge of breastfeeding, *J Obstet Gynecol Neonatal Nurs* 20:58, 1991.
6. Anderson PO: Drug use during breast-feeding, *Clin Pharm* 10:594, 1991.
7. Apple RD: *Mothers and medicine, a social history of infant feeding 1890-1950*, Madison, 1987, University of Wisconsin Press.
8. Auerbach KG: Assisting the employed breastfeeding mother, *J Nurse Midwifery* 35:26, 1990.
9. Auerbach KG: Breastfeeding management for the midwife, *Midwifery Today* 1:26, 1988.
10. Auerbach KG, Jacobi AM: Postpartum depression in the breastfeeding mother. *Clin Issues Perinat Women's Health Nurs* 1:375, 1990.
11. Barnes LP: Lactation consultant in the neonatal intensive care unit, *Med Care Nurs* 16:167, 1991.
12. Barness LA: Cholesterol and children, *JAMA* 256:256, 1986.
13. Bastin N et al: Postpartum care of the HIV positive woman and her newborn, *J Obstet Gynecol Neonatal Nurs* 21:105, 1992.
14. Bernard-Bonnin A, Stachtchenko S, Girard G, et al: Hospital practices and breastfeeding duration: a meta-analysis of controlled trials, *Birth* 16:65, 1989.
15. Beske EJ, Garvis MS: Important factors in breastfeeding success, *Med Care Nurs* 7:174, 1982.
16. Bitman J et al: Lipid composition of milk from mothers with cystic fibrosis, *Pediatrics* 80:927, 1987.
17. Blinkhorn AS, Attwood D: A congenital epulis interfering with feeding in a day-old baby girl, *Dental Update* 17:346, 1990.
18. Bono BJ: Assessment and documentation of the breastfeeding couple by health care professionals, *J of Hum Lact* 8:17, 1992.
19. Bowles BC, Williamson BP: Pregnancy and lactation following anorexia and bulimia, *J Obstet Gynecol Neonatal Nurs* 19:243, 1989.
20. Bradley MW: Breast feeding and necrotizing enterocolitis, *Indiana Med* 10:859, 1986.
21. Brakohiapa LA et al: Does prolonged breastfeeding adversely affect a child's nutritional status? *Lancet* 2:416, 1988.
22. Briggs GG, Freeman RK, Yaffe SJ, editors: *Drugs in pregnancy and lactation*, Baltimore, 1991, Williams & Wilkins.
23. Brinch M, Isager T, Tolstrup K: Anorexia nervosa and motherhood: reproduction pattern and mothering behavior of 50 women, *Acta Paediatr Scand* 77:611, 1988.
24. Broadbent JB, Sampson HA: Food hypersensitivity and atopic dermatitis, *Pediatr Allergic Dis* 35:1115, 1988.
25. Bryant CA: A new strategy for promoting breastfeeding among economically disadvantaged women and adolescents, *AWHONN* formerly *NAACOG*, in press.

26. Butte NF et al: Milk composition of insulin-dependent diabetic women, *J Pediatr Gastroenterol Nutr* 6:936, 1987.

27. Canterbury RJ et al: Postpartum psychosis induced by bromocriptine, *South Med J* 80:1463, 1987.

28. Chandler CG, Roush RE: Training allied health professionals to deliver breast-feeding services to women in the pre- and postnatal periods, *J Allied Health* 5:124, 1982.

29. Chaney NE, Franke J, Wadlington WB: Cocaine convulsions in a breast-feeding baby, *J Pediatr* 112:134, 1988.

30. Chasnoff IJ, Lewis DE, Squires L: Cocaine intoxication in a breast-fed infant, *Pediatrics* 80:836, 1987.

31. Clarren SK, Anderson B, Wolf LS: Feeding infants with cleft lip, cleft palate, or cleft lip and palate, *Cleft Palate J* 24:244, 1987.

32. Cohen R, Mrtek MB, Mrtek RG: Comparison of maternal absenteeism and infant illness rates among breast-feeding and formula-feeding women in two corporations. *Am J Health Promotion* 10(2), 1995, 148-153.

33. Committee on Pediatric AIDS: Human milk, breastfeeding, and transmission of human immunodeficiency virus in the United States. *Pediatrics.* 96 (5), 1995, 997-979.

34. Cross KP: *Adults as learners,* San Francisco, 1988, Jossey-Bass.

35. Cunningham AS: Breastfeeding is protective, *Pediatrics* 114:1052, 1987.

36. Cunningham AS, Jelliffe DB, Jelliffe EFP: Breast-feeding and health in the 1980s: a global epidemiologic review, *J Pediatr* 118:659, 1991.

37. Davis M et al: Infant feeding and childhood cancer, *Lancet* 2:365, 1988.

38. DeCarvalho M et al: Effect of frequent breast-feeding on early milk production and infant weight gain, *Pediatrics* 72:307, 1983.

39. Dekio S, Kawasaki Y, Jidoi J: Herpes simplex on nipples inoculated from herpetic gingivostomatitis of a baby, *Clin Exp Dermatol* 11:664, 1986.

40. DeLee JB: *Obstetrics for nurses,* ed 4, Philadelphia, 1913, WB Saunders.

41. Dewey KG, Lonnerdal B: Infant self-regulation of breast milk intake, *Acta Paediatr Scand* 75:893, 1986.

42. DeZoysa I, Rea M, Martines J: Why promote breastfeeding in diarrhoeal disease control programmes? *Health Policy Plann* 6:371, 1991.

43. Feher SD et al: Increasing breast milk production for premature infants with a relaxation/imagery audiotape, *Pediatrics* 83:57, 1989.

44. Fergusson DM et al: Eczema and infant diet, *Clin Allergy* 11:325, 1981.

45. Fildes V: Breastfeeding and wet nursing, *Midwife Health Visitor* 22:241, 1988.

46. Fomon SJ: Reflections on infant feeding in the 1970s and 1980s, *Am J Clin Nutr* 46:171, 1987.

47. Frank DA et al: Cocaine and marijuana use during pregnancy by women intending and not intending to breast-feed, *J Am Diet Assoc* 92:215, 1992.

48. Frank DA, Wirtz SJ, Sorenson JR, et al: Commercial discharge packs and breastfeeding counseling: effects on infant feeding practices in a randomized controlled trial, *Pediatrics* 80:845, 1987.

49. Gardiner J, Lauwers J, Woessner C, et al: *Relationships and roles: the lactation consultant and lay breastfeeding groups,* unit 7 of the lactation consultant series, Garden City Park, NY, 1986, Avery Publishing Group.

50. Gartner L: Jaundice and the breastfeeding infant. In *Breastfeeding topics: a communication of the breastfeeding promotion taskforce,* Springfield, Spring 1991, Illinois Department of Public Health.

51. Gaskin IM: *Babies, breastfeeding and bonding,* South Hadley, Mass, 1987, Bergin & Garvey.

52. Gielen AC et al: Maternal employment during the early postpartum period: effects on initiation and continuation of breast-feeding, *Pediatrics* 87:298, 1991.

53. Glass RI et al: Estimates of morbidity and mortality rates for diarrheal diseases in American children, *J Pediatr* 118:s27, 1991.

54. Greenberg CS, Smith K: Anticipatory guidance for the employed breast-feeding mother, *J Pediatr Health Care* 5:204, 1991.

55. Grekas D, Tourkantonis A: Serum and human milk IgA and zinc concentrations after successful renal transplantation, *Biol Res Preg* 7:118, 1986.

56. Hartmann PE: Lactation and reproduction in Western Australian women, *J Reprod Med* 32:543, 1987.

57. Haschke F et al: Radioactivity in Austrian milk after the Chernobyl accident, *N Engl J Med* 316:409, 1987.

58. Hawkins LM et al: Predictors of duration of breastfeeding in low-income women, *Birth* 14:204, 1987.

59. Helsing E, King FS: *Breastfeeding in practice: a manual for health workers,* Oxford, 1982, Oxford University Press.

60. Henry FJ, Bartholomew MS: Epidemiology and transmission of rotavirus infections and diarrhoea in St. Lucia, West Indies, *West Indies Med J* 39:205, 1990.

61. Hill PD: The enigma of insufficient milk supply, *Med Care Nurs* 16:313, 1991.

62. Hill PD: Effects of education on breastfeeding success, *Maternal Child Nurs J* 16:145, 1987.

63. Hill PD: Predictors of breast-feeding duration among WIC and non-WIC mothers, *Public Health Nurs* 8:46, 1991.

64. Hill PD, Aldag J: Potential indicators of insufficient milk supply syndrome, *Res Nurs Health* 14:11, 1991.

65. Hill PD, Humenick SS: Insufficient milk supply, *Image* 21:145, 1989.

66. Horton M, Freire P: *We make the road by walking: conversations on education and social change,* Philadelphia, 1990, Temple University Press.

67. Houston MJ, Field PA: Practices and policies in the initiation of breastfeeding, *J Obstet Gynecol Neonatal Nurs* 23:418, 1988.

68. IOCU/IBFAN: *Protecting infant health, a health workers' guide to the international code of marketing of breast milk substitutes,* Penang, Malaysia, February 1987, IOCU/IBFAN.

69. Jackson RL: Ecological breastfeeding and child spacing, *Clin Pediatr* 27:373, 1988.

70. Jacobi AM: Commonly used agents for nipple soreness, In Riordan J and Auerbach KG, editors: Breastfeeding and human lactation, Boston, MA, 1992, Jones and Bartlett.

71. Jakobsson I, Lindberg T, Benediktsson B, et al: Dietary bovine B-lactoglobulin is transferred to human milk, *Acta Paediatr Scand* 74:342, 1985.

72. Jefferis SC, Gagne MP, Leff EW: Having diabetes shouldn't prevent you from sharing this experience, breastfeeding, *Diabetes Forecast* August 28, 1991.

73. Johnstone HA, Marcinak JF: Candidiasis in the breastfeeding mother and infant, *J Obstet Gynecol Neonatal Nurs* 19:171, 1990.

74. Jones DA: The choice to breast feed or bottle feed and influences upon that choice: a survey of 1525 mothers, *Child Care Health Dev* 13:75, 1987.

75. Jones DA, West RR: Effect of a lactation nurse on the success of breastfeeding: a randomized controlled trial, *J Epidemiol Commun Health* 40:45, 1986.

76. Jones DA, West RR: Lactation nurse increases duration of breastfeeding, *Arch Dis Child* 60:772, 1985.

77. Kaufmann R, Foxman B: Mastitis among lactating women: occurrence and risk factors, *Soc Sci Med* 33:701, 1991.

78. Kearney MH: Identifying psychosocial obstacles to breastfeeding success, *J Obstet Gynecol Neonatal Nurs* 13:99, 1988.

79. Kearney MH, Cronenwett L: Breastfeeding and employment. *J Obstet Gynecol Neonatal Nurs* 20:471, 1991.

80. Kemper K, Forsyth B, McCarthy P: Jaundice, terminating breast-feeding and the vulnerable child syndrome, *Pediatrics* 84:773, 778, 1989.

81. Kistin N, Dublin P, Abramson R: Effect of peer counselors on breastfeeding incidence, exclusivity, and duration among low-income urban women, *AWHONN* formerly *NAACOG,* in press.

82. Klaus MH: The frequency of suckling: a neglected but essential ingredient of breast-feeding, *Obstet Gynecol Clin North Am* 14:623, 1987.

83. Kolata G: Wet nursing boom in England explored, *Science,* 2335:745, 1987.

84. Kurinij N, Shiono PH: Early formula supplementation of breastfeeding, *Pediatrics* 88:745, 1991.

85. Kurinij N, Shiono PH, Rhoads GG: Breastfeeding incidence and duration in black and white women, *Pediatrics* 81:365, 1988.

86. La Leche League International: *The womanly art of breastfeeding* 35th Anniversary ed, Franklin Park, Ill, 1991, La Leche League.

87. Lake CR et al: Cyclothymic disorder and bromocriptine: predisposing factors for postpartum mania? *Can J Psychiatry* 32:693, 1987.

88. Lauwers J, Woessner C: *Counseling the nursing mother: a reference handbook for health care providers and lay counselors,* Wayne NJ, 1989, Avery Publishing Group.

89. Lawrence RA: *Clinics in perinatology [breast-feeding]*, vol 14, Philadelphia, 1987, WB Saunders.

90. Lawrence RA: *Breastfeeding: A guide for the medical profession*, ed 4, St Louis, 1994, Mosby.

91. Lawrence RA: Early discharge alert, *Pediatrics* 96(5): 966-657, 1995, 966-967.

92. Lechner W et al: Radioactivity in breast milk after Chernobyl, *Lancet* 2:1326, 1986.

93. Lemons PK, Sharda JK, Lemons JA: Lactation. In Hay WW, editor, *Neonatal nutrition and metabolism*, St Louis, 1991, Mosby.

94. Leventhal JM et al: Does breast-feeding protect against infections in infants less than 3 months of age? *Pediatrics* 78:896, 1986.

95. Lindenberg CS, Artola RC, Estrada VJ: Determinants of early infant weaning: a multivariate approach, *Int J Nurs Stud* 27:35, 1990.

96. Lucas A: Breast milk and subsequent intelligence quotient in children born preterm, *Lancet* 339:261, 1992.

97. Lukefahr JL: Underlying illness associated with failure to thrive in breastfed infants, *Clin Pediatr* 29:468, 1990.

98. Lynch S, Koch A, Hislop T et al: Evaluating the effect of a breastfeeding consultant on the duration of breastfeeding, *Can J Public Health* 77:190, 1986.

99. Machtinger S, Moss R: Cow's milk allergy in breast-fed infants: the role of allergen and maternal secretory IgA antibody, *J Allergy Clin Immunol* 77:341, 1986.

100. MacMullen NJ, Brucker MC: Pregnancy made possible for women with cystic fibrosis, *Med Care Nurs* 14:196, 1989.

101. Maisels MJ and Newman TB: Kernicterus in otherwise healthy breastfed newborns. *Pediatrics.* 96 (4), 730-733.

102. Maki M: Changing pattern of childhood coeliac disease in Finland, *Acta Paediatr Scand* 77:408, 1987.

103. Marmet C, Shell E: Training neonates to suck correctly, *Med Care Nurs* 9:401, 1984.

104. Matalon R, Michals K, Gleason L: Maternal PKU: strategies for dietary treatment and monitoring compliance, *Ann N Y Acad Sci* 477:223, 1987.

105. Matthews MK: Mothers' satisfaction with their neonates breastfeeding behaviors, *J Obstet Gynecol Neonatal Nurs* 21:49, 1991.

106. Mead LJ et al: Breastfeeding success with preterm quadruplets, *J Obstet Gynecol Neonatal Nurs* 21:221, 1992.

107. Meier P: Bottle and breast-feeding: effects of transcutaneous oxygen pressure and temperature in preterm infants, *Nurs Res* 37:36, 1988.

108. Meier P and Anderson GC: Responses of small preterm infants to bottle- and breast-feeding, *Med Care Nurs* 12:97, 1987.

109. Meier P, Pugh E: Breast-feeding behavior of small preterm infants, *MCH* 10:396, 1985.

110. Minchin M: *Breastfeeding matters: what we need to know about infant feeding*, Sydney, Australia, 1985, Alma Publications.

111. Minchin M: *Food for thought: a parents guide to food intolerance*, ed 2, Sydney, Austrlaia, 1986, Alma Publications.

112. Minchin M: Infant feeding, *Med J Aust* 148:604, 1988.

113. Minchin M: Infant formula: a mass uncontrolled trial in perinatal care, *Birth* 14:25, 1987.

114. Minchin M: Positioning for breastfeeding, *Birth* 16:67, 1989.

115. Miskelly FG et al: Infant feeding and allergy, *Arch Dis Child* 63:388, 1988.

116. Montague A: *Touching*, New York, 1971, Harper & Row.

117. Neifert M, McDonald S, Neville M: Failure of lactogenesis associated with placental retention, *Am J Obstet Gynecol* 140:478, 1981.

118. Neifert MR, Seacat JM: Medical management of successful breast-feeding, *Pediatr Clin North Am* 33:749, 1986.

119. Neifert M, Seacat J: Practical aspects of breastfeeding the premature infant, *Perinatol Neonatol* 12:24, 1988.

120. Nelson LM et al: Risk of multiple sclerosis exacerbation during pregnancy and breast-feeding, *JAMA* 259:3441, 1988.

121. Neville MC: Secretion and composition of human milk. In Hay WW, editor: *Neonatal nutrition and metabolism*, St Louis, 1991.

122. Neville MC, Neifert MR: *Lactation: physiology, nutrition, and breast-feeding*, New York, 1983, Plenum Press.

123. Newell ML et al: Risk factors for mother-to-child transmission of HIV-1, *Lancet* 339:1007, 1992.

124. Newman TB, Maisels MJ: Evaluation and treatment of jaundice in the term newborn: a kinder, gentler approach, *Pediatr* 89:809, 1992.

125. *Nutr Rev* 45:236, 1987.

126. Olds SB, London MA, Ladewig PA: *Maternal newborn nursing,* ed 3, Menlo Park, Calif, 1988, Addison-Wesley.

127. Orloff SL, Wallingford JC, McDougal JS: Inactivation of human immunodeficiency virus type 1 in human milk: effects of intrinsic factors in human milk and of pasteurization, *J Hum Lact,* in press.

128. Oxtoby MJ: Human immunodeficiency virus and other viruses in human milk: placing the issues in broader perspective, *Pediatr Infect Dis* 7:825, 1988.

129. Palmer G: *The politics of breastfeeding,* London, 1988, Pandora Press.

130. Petrakis N et al: Influence of pregnancy and lactation on serum and breast fluid estrogen levels: implications for breast cancer risk, *Int J Cancer* 40:587, 1987.

131. Picciano MF: Insulin-dependent diabetes and lactational performance, *Pediatr Gastroenterol Nutr* 6:838, 1987.

132. Poole SR et al: Hospitalization of a psychotic mother and her breast-feeding infant, *Hosp Commun Psychiatr* 31:412, 1980.

133. Popkin BM et al: Breast-feeding and diarrheal morbidity, *Pediatrics* 86:874, 1990.

134. *Protecting, promoting and supporting breastfeeding: the special role of maternity services: a joint WHO/UNICEF statement,* Geneva, Switzerland, 1989, World Health Organization.

135. Ramsey-Goldman R: Pregnancy in systemic lupus erythematosus, *Rheum Dis Clin North Am* 14:169, 1988.

136. Reiff MI, Essock-Vitale SM: Hospital influences on early infant-feeding practices, *Pediatrics* 77:357, 1985.

137. *Report of the Surgeon General's workshop on breastfeeding and human lactation.* Rockville, Md, 1984, Department of Health and Human Services, (DHHS Publ No HRS-D-MC84-2.)

138. Rickitt CW: A study in nipple care, *Midwives Chron* 99:131, 132, 1986.

139. Riordan J, Auerbach: *Breastfeeding and human lactation,* Boston, 1992, Jones and Bartlett.

140. Rosier W: Cool cabbage compresses. *Breastfeeding* Rev 11:28, 1988.

141. Royal College of Midwives: *Successful breastfeeding,* ed 2, Edinburgh, Scotland, 1991, Churchill Livingstone.

142. Rubin R: *Maternal identity and the maternal experience,* New York, 1984, Springer.

143. Ryan AS et al: Recent declines in breast-feeding in the United States, 1984 through 1989, *Pediatrics* 88:719, 1991.

144. Saini AS et al: Human milk in infant nutrition, *Indian Pediatr* 27:681, 1990.

145. Saint L, Maggiore P, Hartmann PE: Yield and nutrient content of milk in eight women breastfeeding twins and one woman breast-feeding triplets, *Br J Nutr* 56:46, 1986.

146. Sarett HP, Bain KR, O'Leary: Decisions on breast-feeding or formula feeding and trends in infant-feeding practices, *Am J Dis Child* 37:720, 1983.

147. Saunders EW: Infant feeding, *Med Rec* 33(1888), 421. Cited in *Mothers and medicine, a social history of infant feeding 1890-1950,* p 54.

148. Saunders S, Carroll JM, Johnson CE: *Breastfeeding: a problem-solving manual,* ed 2, Amityville, NY 1988, Essential Medical Information Systems.

149. Schanler R, Garza C, Nichols B: Fortified mother's milk for very low birth weight infants: results of growth and nutrient balance studies, *J Pediatr* 107:437, 1987.

150. Schneider AP: Risk factor for ovarian cancer, *N Engl J Med* 317:508, 1987.

151. Scrimshaw SCM: The cultural context of breastfeeding in the United States. In *Report of the Surgeon General's workshop on breastfeeding and human lactation,* (DHHS Publ No #HRS-D-MC 84-2.) 1984, Department of Health and Human Services, p 23.

152. Shiffman ML et al: Breast-milk composition in women with cystic fibrosis: report of two cases and a review of the literature, *Am J Clin Nutr* 49:612, 1989.

153. Skerfving S: Mercury in women exposed to methylmercury through fish consumption and in their newborn babies and breast milk, *Bull Environ Contam Toxicol* 41:475, 1988.

154. Strimas JH, Chi DS: Significance of IgE level in amniotic fluid and cord blood for the prediction of allergy, *Ann Allergy* 61:133, 1988.

155. Tudehope D et al: Breastfeeding practices and severe hyperbilirubinaemia, *J Paediatr Child Health* 27:240, 1991.

156. Vajro P, Fontnella A: Breast feeding and hepatitis B, *J Pediatr Gastroenterol Nutr* 12:141, 1991.

157. van den Bogaard et al: The relationship between breast-feeding and early childhood morbidity in a general population, *Fam Med* 23:510, 1991.

158. Virden SF: The relationship between infant feeding method and maternal role adjustment, *J Nurse Midwifery* 33:31, 1988.

159. Walker E, Best MA: Well-being of mothers with infant children: a preliminary comparison of employed women and homemakers, *Women Health* 17:71, 1991.

160. Walker M: Why aren't more mothers breast-feeding? *Childbirth Instr,* Winter 19, 1992.

161. Weatherly-White RCA et al: Early repair and breast-feeding for infants with cleft lip, *Plast Reconstr Surg* 79:879, 1987.

162. Whaley LF, Wong DL: *Nursing care of infants and children,* St Louis, 1979, Mosby-Year Book.

163. WHO/UNICEF Consensus Statement from the consultation on HIV transmission and breastfeeding, *JHL* 8:173, 1992.

164. Williams BC, Miller CA: Preventive health care for young children: findings from a 10-country study and directions for United States policy, *Pediatrics* 89:983, 1992.

165. Williams KM, Morse JM: Weaning patterns of first-time mothers, *Med Care Nurs* 14:188, 1989.

166. Williamson MT, Murti PK: Effects of Storage, time, temperature, and composition of container on biologic components of human milk. *J Hum Lact* 12(1):1996, 31035.

167. Winikoff B et al: Dynamics of infant feeding: mothers, professionals, and the institutional context in a large urban hospital, *Pediatrics* 77:357, 1986.

168. Winikoff B et al: Overcoming obstacles to breast-feeding in a large municipal hospital: applications of lessons learned, *Pediatrics* 80:423, 1987.

169. World Health Organization: *Consensus statement from the WHO/UNICEF Consultation on HIV Transmission and breastfeeding.* April 30-May 1, 1992, Geneva, Switzerland.

170. Yamauchi Y, Yamanouchi I: The relationship between rooming-in/not rooming-in and breast-feeding variables, *Acta Paediatr Scand* 79:1017, 1990.

171. Yates Sealander J, Kerr CP: Herpes simplex of the nipple: infant-to-mother transmission, *Am Fam Physician* 39:111, 1989.

172. Young SA, Kaufman M: Promoting breastfeeding at a migrant health center, *Am J Public Health* 5:523, 1988.

173. Yuan JM: Risk factors for breast cancer in Chinese women in Shanghai, *Cancer Res* 48:1929, 1988.

174. Ziemer MM, George C: Breastfeeding the low-birthweight infant, *Neonatal Network,* Dec:33, 1990.

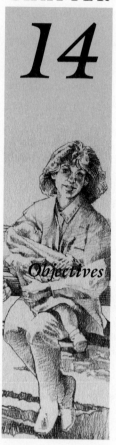

14

Nutrition Education: A Support for Reproduction

Alicia Dixon Docter
Jane Mitchell Rees
Bonnie S. Worthington-Roberts

Objectives

✦✦✦

After completing this chapter, the student will be able to:

✓ *Define the distinct types of nutrition education.*

✓ *Discuss the spectrum of nutrition education needs.*

✓ *Define important content areas for nutrition education related to reproduction.*

✓ *Define the important characteristics of available modes of nutrition education.*

Introduction

To influence the outcome of pregnancy and lactation, knowledge about the role of nutrition in reproduction as described in this book must be put into practice. Education is the communication link that will connect these theoretical concepts to the real world. Education is also one of the most challenging processes in the field of nutrition. There are many unanswered questions about how to provide it. Some of the questions are about how people learn; others are about how to establish programs that can make such learning possible. The skills of many disciplines are being combined in an effort to answer these questions and develop effective education

techniques specific to the field of nutrition. Nutrition professionals interested in improving the reproductive life of people will find that it is essential to consider these education issues.[92,114]

The need to focus on nutrition education has been recognized at various times. By the time of the 1969 White House Conference on Food, Nutrition, and Health,[116] sufficient knowledge and interest had been generated that comprehensive guidelines as to what needed to be done were published. An upsurge of interest in preventive health care issues added impetus in the 1970s. Twenty years later, at an anniversary symposium of the 1969 conference, participants recognized past accomplishments and present and future challenges. Although hunger was and continues to be an issue in America, two other urgent needs in the diet and health areas were noted. These included better health education, with nutrition as a component, from kindergarten through college and as a mandatory part of the curricula in medical, dental, and allied health schools. The second is for continuing, innovative involvement of children in informal nutrition education.[37]

In 1979, the U.S. Surgeon General published *Healthy People,* a report on health promotion and disease prevention.[111] In this report, nutrition was identified as one of 15 areas in which improvements could contribute to better health. In 1980, specific objectives for 1990 were presented, with implementation plans published in 1983.[100] Several of these objectives are directly related to nutrition during pregnancy and lactation and nutrition education. The current version, *Healthy People 2000,* a decade-long strategy to improve the nation's health profile through an emphasis on prevention, includes better nutrition as one of its 21 objectives. Two of the implementation activities that link with the year 2000 objectives include: to increase to at least 75% the proportion of mothers who breastfeed their babies in the early postpartum period and to at least 50% the proportion who continue breastfeeding until their babies are 5 to 6 months old; and to increase to at least 75% the proportion of the nation's schools that provide nutrition education from preschool through twelfth grade, preferably as part of comprehensive school health education.[14]

Political and economic climates have not been favorable for the progress necessary to educate the U.S. population about nutrition during the latter part of the twentieth century.[108] Meanwhile research and knowledge have increased as nutrition education has become a specialized area of study in educational institutions and among practicing health care professionals. The challenge to improve nutrition education remains in two areas: designing effective nutrition education strategies and conducting research to determine the behavioral and health effects of the best available interventions.[35]

The number of techniques that must be studied and perfected is large. It is a fascinating range of topics that requires a unique combination of science and creativity made possible by the interdisciplinary technologic advances of today.

THE NUTRITIONAL ENVIRONMENT

The diet a woman chooses during pregnancy and lactation is a result of the many influences on her feeding pattern since infancy. The building of dietary patterns can be described as pyramidal in nature (Fig. 14-1). The lower part of the pyramid represents factors such as culture and individual family patterns that provide the basis in any family setting for the establishment of food preferences and eating habits of the children. Onto these basic food habits is added the multitude of individual feeding experiences in which every child participates. Finally, the apex of the triangle represents the special food-related experiences of a person at the time of pregnancy. Health professionals who expect to change dietary patterns of the pregnant woman are concerned about the nutritional aspects of the environment in which we all live.

For animals and plants, nourishment in the environment follows fairly simple patterns revolving around the availability of food. Changes are affected by variations and manipulations of the food supply. For humans the nutritional environment is a complex mix of the foods to be eaten; the ideas, beliefs, and knowledge about food and nourishment; and the patterns of managing foods inside and outside the home.[83] To upgrade the quality of the nutritional environment, programs and strategies must affect the various components that make up the whole system.

Altering the Nutritional Environment

Altering the nutritional environment to promote successful reproduction depends on communicating effectively about nutrition to persons in all stages of life. Increased knowledge and changing attitudes about nutrition among the population, its professionals, and business and political leaders will enable society to devise improved systems to control the food supply so that nourishing food in appropriate amounts is

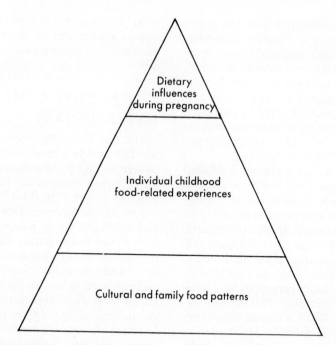

FIG. 14-1   Factors influencing dietary practices in pregnant women.

made available to all. This will be possible through establishment of governmental regulations and cooperation by business and private citizens[12,37,61,116] and approval of a national nutrition policy.[64] All areas represented by the pyramid will be affected by such strategies so that the woman who is pregnant will have an opportunity to develop healthful dietary habits as a result of living in a nutritionally sound environment.

Traditional nutritional counseling provided in the prenatal period promotes minor changes in dietary patterns and may lead to correction of certain acute nutritional deficiencies the woman manifests. Motivation of expectant parents to change may temporarily be great so that nutritional counseling of a short-term nature may be more effective than in situations in which there is no pressing impetus. However, depending on short-term measures alone to promote significant changes and prepare the woman adequately for successful reproduction is naive. Rather, educators should direct their messages about nutritional support of the fetus to potential parents

well before conception. The obvious goal for a woman who wants to bear a child successfully is to conceive when her nutritional status and other controllable environmental factors provide for optimal fetal development.[90,119]

Attention should therefore be given to the development of high-quality nutrition education materials and programs for children and adults.[12] Getting required nourishment is a survival skill today that demands education. Therefore appropriate nutrition education justifiably deserves a position of priority in the U.S. educational and health care systems.[37,116] Increased emphasis should also be placed on the improvements of programs and materials for all professionals in the health sciences. Interdisciplinary relationships among professionals working in fields related to nutrition and human behavior need to be strengthened.[11] The nutritional information system must address the problems of people who need an understanding of how to nourish themselves; this system should aid people in sorting out scientifically sound information from that based on rumor and speculation.[12] Formal and informal techniques can be coordinated to transmit information from the fields of study in which it is generated to the environment in which it can improve the nutritional aspects of health and reproduction.

THE PROCESS OF NUTRITION EDUCATION

The need for nutrition education during the prenatal period has been justified by data throughout this book. Once need has been established, the next step to development of a nutrition education program is to establish program objectives.

Objectives

Basic to an understanding of strategies to alter the nutritional environment is the knowledge that different types of programs meet different objectives within the broad range of processes commonly grouped under the heading "nutrition education." Programs that make up nutrition education are of four distinct types:

1. *Informative nutrition education*—communicates factual information
2. *Attitudinal nutrition education*—focuses attention on and motivates change in attitudes, or personal feelings about nourishment
3. *Behavioral nutrition education*—motivates change in behavior related to nutrition; may include components addressing attitudes and knowledge
4. *Therapeutic nutrition education*—facilitates change in behavior related to a specific nutritional problem; must include components addressing attitudes and knowledge

This principle has been recognized in research in nutrition education, with attention focused on cognitive (knowledge), attitudinal, and behavioral components of programs.[7]

The type of nutrition education in a particular program must be specific to the situation in which it will be used. For example, nutrition education can be transmitted in most classroom settings, as well as in community meetings. Short television and radio messages are most often informative or attitudinal nutrition educa-

tion, directed at changing attitudes. Behavioral nutrition education programs use group interaction and one-to-one counseling; they are of necessity complex and often demand considerable time. Even when persons' attitudes are compatible with change and they have the knowledge base that is required, learning and practice over time are necessary to change behavior. Therapeutic nutrition education programs are actually specialized behavioral nutrition education and are appropriately found in clinical settings.[38]

Examples of nutrition education for the pregnant woman include the following:

1. *Informative*—high school class in which the role of nutrients such as iron and calcium in reproduction is taught
2. *Attitudinal*—radio spots urging the pregnant woman to be concerned about nutrition
3. *Behavioral*—classes presented by a clinician during pregnancy discussing methods for substituting nourishing foods for those popularized by peer group and advertising
4. *Therapeutic*—counseling of the patient by a clinical nutritionist related to increasing the iron content of her diet to ameliorate an iron deficiency diagnosed early in pregnancy

The need for intervention strategies to deal with people's eating habits increases along a continuum (Fig. 14-2). Strategies should be chosen and developed carefully to match the needs of a particular group.[22] Although simpler methods, such as brochures or audiovisuals, work for the highly motivated individual, increasingly complex strategies that incorporate simpler methods within the framework of a comprehensive treatment protocol are necessary for the individual who is anticipating having a "normal" or lower-risk pregnancy. A comprehensive treatment protocol would require use of sophisticated psychosocial counseling techniques to promote a change in eating behavior and would be appropriate for pregnant women in any of the high-risk categories discussed below. Although cognitive, affective, and behavioral components can to some degree be present in all strategies, only the most complex can be expected to significantly address all three aspects of nutrition education.

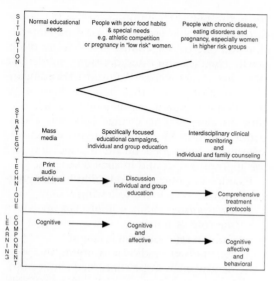

FIG. 14-2 Spectrum of nutrition education needs.

Objectives, techniques, and evaluation are congruent in well-designed programs.[91] Programs that are clearly designed to perform one function while the evaluation is focused on an inappropriately intended outcome may fail,[124] as in the following examples:

Education regarding the role of specific nutrients—testing whether students have changed eating behavior

Radio and television messages directed toward the importance of nutrition in physical fitness—evaluating the intake of certain nutrients

Session of dietetic counseling lasting 20 minutes—evaluating by loss of pounds of weight[124]

Other factors contributing to failure in nutrition education include: (1) attempting programs of a type inappropriate to the setting, (2) designing programs that attempt to perform too many functions and/or basing evaluations on functions not addressed by the program, (3) using materials not designed for reading and comprehension level of audience, (4) cultural bias, and (5) using materials designed for one audience on another.

Evaluation

To ensure that objectives are being accomplished, an evaluation procedure is an integral component of each nutrition education project. In addition, evaluation documents the effectiveness of a program. With such documentation, a program may more confidently share its success, thereby maintaining visibility and financial support within the plethora of commercially produced programs.

Evaluation is a process and must be considered from the beginning of the development of any nutrition education program. The process consists of designing clear program objectives, developing program elements or techniques, and evaluating the program.[91]

Because the educational process is complex, evaluation of nutrition education has become a specialized area of study. Existing instruments from the behavioral sciences and from successful nutrition education efforts can often be adapted for new purposes; new ones need not be developed for each study. Instruments must be statistically reliable, valid, and specific to each situation.[93] Reliability may be defined as the extent to which the measure gives the same results on repeated applications to avoid assessing chance or random error. Validity refers to the extent to which an instrument measures what it purports to measure. Its concern is with systematic error—that is, changes that are part of the natural variation in the phenomenon under study.[91]

GROUPS IN NEED OF NUTRITION EDUCATION

In implementing strategies to alter the nutritional environment in support of reproduction, certain groups that are not commonly addressed should be included. Although not all these groups are actually pregnant or lactating, it is apparent that they influence the nutritional aspects of reproductive life.

High-Risk Groups

The improvement of maternal health and fetal well-being may be partially achieved by dietary counseling and nutrition education to subgroups with unique health beliefs and food habits or economic disadvantages, as well as those at high risk for complications during pregnancy.[81,116] Significant risk factors in reproduction include poverty, lack of education, very young or old age (<17 or >35 years), first pregnancy or high parity, prior obstetrical complications or fetal wastage, and lack of supportive spouse or family. Counseling and educating pregnant adolescents requires a knowledge of human development and adolescent lifestyles and a flexible communication style acquired through specialized training and experience.[78]

Working effectively with other high-risk groups generally requires counseling as well as education.[75] Groups such as Southeast Asians or Hispanics who are faced with a changing cultural food pattern require specific support.[105] Having an understanding of the eating practices, foods, symbolism of foods, values, and health beliefs is essential.[110] Nutrition educators should also attend to the use and meaning of verbal and nonverbal language in a culture and be aware of ethnospecific communication patterns so as to enhance the efficacy of nutritional counseling or program planning.[31] Well-designed studies can provide information useful in pregnant, as well as nonpregnant people, with resulting recommendations that high priority should be given to nutrition education focusing on dietary needs during pregnancy and on the encouragement of breastfeeding. Additional information gleaned from the study can help a clinician understand why a particular group, the Hmong women in one case, are reluctant to take supplements during pregnancy.[45]

The homeless should be considered at risk because of a lack of adequate kitchen facilities, mental illness, and substance abuse (prevalent among some groups of homeless people). These, along with physical conditions that alter or increase nutritional needs (such as growth, pregnancy, lactation, and chronic diet-related diseases), may increase the chances for dietary inadequacy.[115]

Children

Along with nutrition education programs for children in the schools (discussed later in this chapter), parents need to be encouraged to teach their children, in the setting of home and family life, how to use foods. Although skill related to buying and preparing foods and making appropriate food choices and planning menus can be learned by following adult models, learning to manage foods ought not to be left to chance or to the influence of advertising.[3] Traditional patterns of food experience are no longer strong. For example, young women may not learn about food for survival and strength through participation in food preparation and preservation at home, and young men may not learn about food through experiences in tightly knit family units whose members regularly eat together.

Children, however, when properly prepared, take the responsibility for maintaining a healthful diet in the same way that they assume management of money or any other aspect of life. The process can begin gradually in the early school years with children being given simple tasks such as choosing the vegetables for a particular menu or the fruits that the family will buy at the grocery store. Emphasis needs to be placed on choosing foods to be eaten outside the home so that these foods fit into the overall pattern. By the adolescent years, children can develop a feeling of control over their own dietary intake so that food will not become an issue in the rebellion that often characterizes teenage behavior. Habits that have grown out of thoughtful teaching by a family become the basis for a healthful life through the reproductive years and will be passed on to future generations.

Males

It should be recognized that both males and females are candidates for educational efforts[87]; both have significant influence on dietary habits of young women, as well as on reproduction. Consequently, it is essential to plan programs that address both genders when any topic related to health, nutrition, and reproduction is covered. Strangely enough, the simple logic and obvious need of preparing the male for a normal and happy experience with pregnancy have largely been ignored in health and nutrition education programs.

The influence of males on nutritional patterns of females begins in the teen and young adult period, when eating becomes a part of the social behavior and decisions about what to eat are made jointly by males and females. Although some trends indicate that men are assuming greater responsibility for planning, shopping, and preparing meals as part of the lifestyle of the typical family, other studies indicate that food-related activities are clearly still the domain of women.[87] However, the idea of nutrition education directed at males should not be put aside. While narrow targeting of women may be helpful for the cost-benefit ratio, nutrition education efforts targeted at males may actually enhance impact by bringing a supporting actor onto the stage of family food activities and broadening food-related interests among family members.[87]

The sharing of influence on dietary habits alone is sufficient reason to include an appeal to men and/or significant others in nutritional counseling and educational campaigns.[22] Although they may not always accompany their partners on clinic visits during pregnancy, a consideration of their food patterns and related behaviors is imperative for a clinician who intends to be effective in counseling individual women and in educational materials and techniques that are used.

Community Leaders

If nutrition education is to reach people in our society effectively, those who understand its importance must help politicians, bureaucrats, and decision makers in academic and health care institutions incorporate it into their programs.[9,28,61,64,121] Thus leaders of each community, state, and nation are a group that must be the target of more meaningful information about the relationship of optimal nourishment to successful reproduction to increase the distribution of that information to the population as a whole. Influencing community leaders requires organization, cooperation, and the establishment of effective relationships, as well as a scientific knowledge of nutrition and its effect on people. Nutrition educators work through professional organizations such as the Society for Nutrition Education and the American Dietetic Association to promote nutrition education. Other organizations are established primarily to act in an advocacy role. Their newsletters[5,19,21] and sections of professional journals are published to keep interested people informed and to organize their efforts to influence decisions. Young professionals must develop their skill as advocates as they develop other professional skills.

CONTENT OF EDUCATION TO IMPROVE REPRODUCTION

In addition to the aforementioned strategies to upgrade the nutritional environment of the pregnant woman, certain closely related issues deserve greater emphasis in nutrition education and counseling. Along with information on normal nutrition and its relationship to reproduction, these topics should be incorporated into the following total health education process.

Infant Feeding

The advantages of breastfeeding should be clearly presented to the population as a whole, ideally before and during adolescence, when attitudes begin to solidify. By a vigorous effort at education of the total population, health professionals can take advantage of opportunities within the health care system to build interest in breastfeeding and establish this option as a viable practice for the young family today. As part of this effort nutrition educators need to monitor the advertising of formula producers and the attempts to control their practices. Critics accuse them of unfairly influencing women here and abroad to use commercial products instead of breastfeeding.[66] It is the kind of issue about which active professionals develop theories and support solutions that will maintain and improve health. In general, the principles of providing adequate nourishment for infants and young children and the simple methods of carrying them out are quite basic in nature and can become a part of the fund of knowledge passed from one generation to another.

In program planning, educational efforts to increase breastfeeding by improving knowledge about it will be effective only to the extent that the information influences beliefs underlying the maternal attitude. Also, concentrating more on the value of attitudes and subjective norms and less on surveying demographic factors such as age, education, or economic status should be emphasized in planning.[22,54,71] Furthermore, considering the impact a significant other (baby's father or maternal grandmother) has on infant feeding practices has been shown to be important.[48]

Interconceptional Replenishment of the Nutritional State

Another issue that has received minimal attention in the past is the need for women to replenish their nutritional state after childbirth. The usual postpartum guidance in clinic settings is directed toward infant feeding and care without regard for the needs of the mother unless she breastfeeds. Attention should be given to the nutritional status of the mother after childbirth, with emphasis on a nourishing diet and weight adjustment by reasonable diet/exercise planning. If this type of program is instituted, the new mother can more rapidly gain strength and maintain energy to devote to the bonding process and other demands of parenting. In addition, she will be better prepared to support future pregnancies should these occur.

Weight Management

An aspect of total preconceptual and interconceptual care that influences the course of pregnancy is the successful management of body weight. As pointed out previously, the state of obesity is a hazard to the pregnant woman. Since it is inappropriate to attempt weight reduction during pregnancy,[119] the problem of being overweight or obese requires attention on a long-term basis.

Effective weight management should begin in childhood and be supported throughout the life cycle. Although a large percentage of the population is overweight, rational education and care have not been developed to bring the problem under control. Although research indicates that a variety of physical and psychological factors foster the overweight state, most messages to the public focus on quick weight loss rather than reasonable weight management. Messages are also generally authoritarian and directed only toward restricting food.[70] New approaches and reasonable programs concerned with the total physical and emotional well-being of the individual are required if weight management is to be successful.[43,53,59]

Because of the complexity of the condition, therapeutic programs ideally are interdisciplinary, with professionals of the psychosocial sciences working with physicians and nutritionists. In the initial assessment the team should screen patients to determine the likelihood of their losing weight based on dietary parameters, growth, history of adiposity, physical activity, and attitude. The physician should evaluate overall physical health. The psychological and social aspects of the obese patient's situation will best be assessed by psychologists and social workers who focus especially on feelings of self-worth, body image, and family and social interactions.

The course of further management is based on the results of initial assessments. Appropriate therapists come from the ranks of social workers, psychologists, or nurses who have specialized training; experts in behavior modification programs also make important contributions.[73]

The overall goal of the team endeavor should be to attend to all aspects of the nutritional, physical, and emotional patterns of the patient's life, using the skills of team members most suited to the particular problems of the individual. The objective in terms of nutrition is to improve the dietary intake regardless of the probability of weight loss. Intervention strategies to bring about changes in food habits to lose weight, decrease the rate of gain, or eliminate weight gain, proceed in conjunction with therapy directed toward the psychosocial aspects of the problem. The nutritionist aids the patient in developing a nutritionally adequate dietary intake at the appropriate energy level to gradually lose and maintain weight, with the patient assuming full responsibility for nutritional management on a long-term basis. An individually designed physical fitness program is an integral part of a successful therapeutic regimen. If the probability of success in maintaining a normal weight is slight, intervention is nevertheless planned, with the objective of helping the patient take control of energy intake and output, gain an increased sense of self-worth, improve skills in coping with relationships and social situations, and improve his or her overall physical health and well-being.

Although such programs are not currently common, the increase in numbers of nutritionists establishing private practices can lead to a more realistic approach. When such professionals establish liaisons with medical specialists and counselors to treat obesity and other eating disorders, an interdisciplinary team is formed. The development is overdue. The amount of money spent on inappropriate weight loss schemes can be turned by strong educational efforts to support realistic professional programs. In the absence of organized interdisciplinary programs for weight management, the health professional can be very helpful in guiding patients away from the potential harm of short-term measures in which the emphasis is on quick weight loss without consideration for maintenance of adequate nutritional status. These programs can be hazardous to one's health, as well as ineffective.

Healthful Nutrition Habits as Part of Total Fitness

People active in sports or personal exercise are often motivated to learn to nourish themselves adequately to reach their full physical potential. Teaching them to develop dietary habits to support physical activity is a positive approach that is more rewarding to both the educator and the patient than the use of traditional negative messages about limiting certain foods.

Nutritionists and health educators can encourage the upsurge of interest in total fitness and bring to those involved the nutrition information they appear to want. Since many of these people are of reproductive age, total fitness programming becomes both a message and an intervention strategy supporting reproduction.

Basic Nutrition

Leading nutrition educators have developed a set of concepts (see box) that are seen as basic to an understanding of nutrition.[98] Using these concepts helps to systematize teaching. Incorporating these concepts ensures that the content of lessons is organized, inclusive, and sequential. Presentation of the concepts, printed in the box on p 455, will be varied to suit the unique characteristics in each situation.

Another aid to nutrition education is the Food Guide Pyramid, designed to teach people to choose a nutritious diet. The pyramid scheme and variations on it have all but replaced the Four Food Groups Guide as a primary teaching tool.[1,41] This system should be combined with innovative techniques, since overuse can produce boredom among a sophisticated population.

A more controversial educational resource was developed by the Departments of Health and Human Services (formerly Health, Education and Welfare) and Agriculture as the U.S. Dietary Guidelines.[68] Although there has been debate over the scientific interpretations that served as the basis for the guidelines, efforts have been made to clear up some of the controversial or ambiguous wording in the 1990 and 1995 editions.[72] Nevertheless, many educators have found the Dietary Guidelines to be an effective way of presenting the concept that food must be used in moderation.

Alcohol may be related to decreased dietary intake, impaired metabolism and absorption of nutrients, and altered nutrient activation and utilization.[33] Therefore effective materials and counseling should contain discussion of alcohol and drugs and their effects. These should be available to women early in the pregnancy or before. Examples in which alcohol and drugs are discussed include *Inside My Mom*,[74] *Great Beginnings*,[63] and *Outside My Mom*.[76]

TECHNIQUES

No single mode of presentation is adequate for all situations encountered in the effort to improve nutritional readiness for the reproductive experience. Consequently, nutritionists and nutrition educators need to be skilled communicators[44,67,92,114] to meet the demands of any audience. Professionals in the field of nutrition benefit by active working relationships with those involved in education, psychology, social work, and anthropology to keep abreast of developments in communication methods.[11,93] Moralistic admonishments related to "good" and "bad" foods or food habits should be replaced by communication centering on the relationship of food intake to health, fitness, and optimal body functions, thereby avoiding the creation of guilt feelings the public may expect from nutrition education.[23] Use of the prenatal weight gain grid and an illustration of the components of weight gain (Fig. 14-3) provides concrete factual information that allows the woman to un-

CONCEPTS FOR FOOD AND NUTRITION EDUCATION

Nutrition

Nutrition is the process by which food is selected and becomes part of the human body.

Food and its handling

1. Food contains nutrients that work together and interact with body chemicals to serve the needs of the body.
2. No one food, by itself, contains all the nutrients in the appropriate amounts and combinations needed for optimal growth and health.
3. Many different combinations of food can provide the needed nutrients in appropriate amounts.
4. Food contains important nonnutritive components, such as dietary fiber, which are needed for healthy functioning of the body.
5. Toxicants, additives, contaminants, and other nonnutritive factors in food affect its safety and quality.
6. The way food is grown, processed, stored, and prepared for eating influences the amount of nutrients in the food and its safety, appearance, taste, cost, and waste.
7. Food requires varying amounts of energy and other resources to produce, process, package, and deliver to the consumer.

Nutrients and dietary components

1. Nutrients in the food that we eat enable us to live, to grow, to keep healthy and well, and to be active.
2. Each nutrient—carbohydrates, protein, fats, vitamins, minerals, and water—has specific functions in the body.
3. Nutrients must be obtained from outside the body on a regular basis because the body cannot produce them in sufficient amounts.
4. Most healthy people can obtain all the nutrients, in the amounts needed, from a variety of foods.
5. Nutrients are distributed to and used by all parts of the body.

6. Nutrient interactions may affect the amounts of nutrients needed and their functioning.
7. The body stores some nutrients and withdraws them for use as needed.
8. Nutrients are found in varying amounts, proportions, and combinations in the plant and animal sources that serve as food.
9. Ongoing scientific research determines nutrients, their functions, and the amounts needed.
10. Both dietary excesses and nutrient deficiencies affect health.
11. Optimum intakes of nutrients and dietary components have both upper and lower limits.
12. All persons throughout life have need for the same nutrients, but the amounts of nutrients needed are influenced by age, sex, size, activity, specific activity, specific conditions of growth, state of health, pregnancy, lactation, and environmental stress.

Nutrition and physical activity

1. Balancing energy intake and energy expenditure is important for achieving and maintaining desirable body weight.
2. There is a synergistic relationship between nutrition and physical activity that affects health and well-being.

Food selection

1. Food, that is, what people consider edible, is culturally defined.
2. Physiological, cultural, social, economic, psychological, and geographical factors influence food selection.
3. Knowledge, attitudes, and beliefs about food and nutrition affect food selection.
4. Food availability and merchandising influence food choices.

National and international food policy

1. Food plays an important role in the physical, psychological, and economic health of a society.

Continued.

❖

CONCEPTS FOR FOOD AND NUTRITION EDUCATION—*cont'd*

2. Food production, distribution, and merchandising systems have economic, social, political, and ecological consequences.
3. Effective utilization of individual and community resources is beneficial for the economic and nutritional well-being of the individual, family, and society.
4. The availability of food and maintenance of nutritional well-being is a matter of public policy.

5. Knowledge of food and nutrition combined with social consciousness enables citizens to understand and participate in the development and adoption of public policy affecting the nutritional well-being of societies.

From Society for Nutritional Education: Society for Nutrition Education concepts for food and nutrition education, *J Nutr Educ* 14:1, 1982. © Society for Nutrition Education.

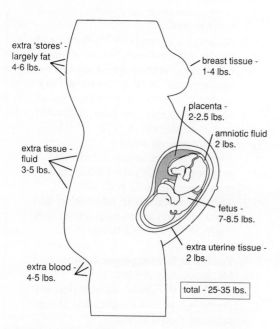

extra 'stores' - largely fat 4-6 lbs.

breast tissue - 1-4 lbs.

placenta - 2-2.5 lbs.

amniotic fluid 2 lbs.

extra tissue - fluid 3-5 lbs.

fetus - 7-8.5 lbs.

extra uterine tissue - 2 lbs.

extra blood - 4-5 lbs.

total - 25-35 lbs.

FIG. 14-3   Distribution of extra maternal weight at 40 weeks.

derstand more fully the reasons for an adequate weight gain.

The nutrition educator may, in part, help to empower or support people in making their own analyses so they can decide themselves what is good for them. Hence, at least some aspects of

nutrition education should help people to understand why they do not eat well and support them in deciding what they can do about it.[47]

Counseling

Dietitians and nutritionists, as well as other health professionals, need to be familiar with advanced techniques in counseling.[44,75,95] The therapeutic process involves establishing a dialogue with the patient so that a meaningful exchange of information can take place. A couple, for example, who is coping with an unexpected pregnancy, financial problems, and a recent move to a strange city may accept nutritional guidance only if the opportunity is provided for discussing the solutions to a variety of problems with the clinician. This approach to nutrition counseling allows recommendations for modifications to be given in line with the ability of the patient to receive and utilize new ideas. The success of the interchange depends largely on the communication skills of the clinician.[124] In direct opposition to this method is the rigid approach in which the professional has a fixed agenda and presents information in formal fashion without regard for the patient's input or ability to assimilate information that is provided.

When intensive intervention is necessary, behavioral scientists can assist in improving the abilities of nutritionists in a counseling setting to facilitate changes in the behavior of patients.

Persons often express the desire to alter their habits but are unable to do so without aid. The obese adolescent near the age of reproduction, who knows her eating habits are unhealthful but is powerless to resist the energy-laden foods in her social milieu, is a striking example of a situation in which nutritionists require the use of special techniques developed by other professionals to assist in changing human behavior.

Public Speaking

In many situations nutritionists are required to project information and influence attitudes through public meetings and the broadcast media. Examples include a prenatal nutrition class for women in their first trimester and a nutrition class to help support lactation while a new mother is simultaneously hoping to fit into prepregnancy clothing. A nutrition educator may also be involved in a radio call-in program or television talk show to discuss practical advice or instruction on maternal nutrition during breastfeeding or introduction of infant feeding.

Credibility is the ultimate goal of the professional in public speaking. Caring about your topic is essential. Preparing for a speech helps build confidence. A conversational approach helps establish direct and immediate contact with the audience, lends a sense of immediacy and spontaneity, and sets the audience at ease.[17,51] Competencies that enable a professional to communicate effectively in public forums are gained by conscious study of the subject, continued progress through practice, and self-awareness in evaluation of the results.

The overriding aim in preparing for public speaking is to learn how to establish positive and active two-way communication with the audience.[52] Consideration must be given to matching the intellectual level of the message to the audience so that its delivery is neither too difficult to understand nor, at the other extreme, demeaning of the audience's intelligence; avoidance of technical jargon will help establish rapport. Developing a dynamic style of delivery, learning how to use auxiliary materials, and becoming knowledgeable about interaction with groups are exercises that enhance the nutritionist's effectiveness in communicating with the public.[57] Evaluation generally requires accurate self-assessments of performance (Fig. 14-4) and of audience reaction without formal testing. In rare instances critiques by colleagues may be available.

Motivating Large Population Groups

Motivating entire populations of people to change established eating habits in relation to a changing food supply is a difficult task requiring innovative methods. Social marketing may provide an effective conceptual system for thinking through the problems of bringing about changes in the ideas or practices of a target public.[57,85] **Social marketing** is defined as "the design, implementation, and control of programs seeking to increase the acceptability of a social idea or cause (e.g., behavioral change) in a target group."[50]

The Expanded Food, Nutrition, and Education Program of the U.S. Department of Agriculture (USDA), which makes use of a special training technique involving the preparation of qualified lay persons to act as conveyors of updated information to members of their own communities, has been successful.[113] Since the establishment of this system in 1968, many trained homemakers have taught other homemakers to improve their skills in providing for the nutritional needs of their families. This technique takes advantage of the superior communication that exists between persons of the same culture and socioeconomic groupings. There is a special need for such peer consultation techniques when significant differences in native language or basic cultural values exist. A specific example of one effort at such consultation was conducted among the Hmong population in central California.[45]

The expertise and historical perspective of anthropologists are invaluable in designing additional programs that will be suitably comprehensive to achieve informative, attitudinal, and behavioral objectives related to the improvement of dietary patterns in large segments of the population. The relationships that have been established between nutrition and anthropology to this point[11,113] should be strengthened by increasing the energy and resources devoted to maintaining such linkages.

	Rating				
	Excellent ←			→ *Unsatisfactory*	
	5	4	3	2	1
Material Presented					
Accuracy	☐	☐	☐	☐	☐
Interest to audience	☐	☐	☐	☐	☐
Clarity of main points	☐	☐	☐	☐	☐
Match of level of presentation and vocabulary to audience	☐	☐	☐	☐	☐
Communication with the Audience					
Interchange/interaction	☐	☐	☐	☐	☐
Control of the audience	☐	☐	☐	☐	☐
Provoking interest	☐	☐	☐	☐	☐
Preventing domination by vociferous members	☐	☐	☐	☐	☐
Use of auxiliary materials	☐	☐	☐	☐	☐
Audiovisual aids	☐	☐	☐	☐	☐
Handouts	☐	☐	☐	☐	☐
Motivating techniques	☐	☐	☐	☐	☐
Management of questions and comments	☐	☐	☐	☐	☐
Overall response of audience	☐	☐	☐	☐	☐
Manner of Presentation					
Quality of voice	☐	☐	☐	☐	☐
Eye contact	☐	☐	☐	☐	☐
Posture	☐	☐	☐	☐	☐
Attitude	☐	☐	☐	☐	☐
Mannerisms	☐	☐	☐	☐	☐
Composure	☐	☐	☐	☐	☐
Sense of timing	☐	☐	☐	☐	☐
Sense of purpose	☐	☐	☐	☐	☐

FIG. 14-4   Evaluation of public presentations.

Television and Radio

At present, broadcast media use has been co-opted by commercial interests, with the result that the influence of radio and television on dietary patterns is heavily weighted in favor of foods with low nutrient density in relation to energy value. The latter is especially true in the case of television. For a variety of reasons it is appropriate to claim that television advertising at this time is a distinct detriment to promoting healthful food habits in both children and adults.[3,25,30,69,101]

For adults references to food are pervasive, both in prime-time programs and in accompanying commercials. The **"prime-time diet"** primarily consists of foods low in nutritional quality, such as low-nutrient beverages, sweets, and salty snack foods. Foods are typically consumed as snacks rather than meals.[101] Continuous exposure to this type of food alone creates for the participant a feeling of familiarity with less valuable foods, promotes positive feelings about them, and as a result supports their continued use.[123]

Not only are less valuable foods heavily emphasized but also an effort is made to convince adults that today's lifestyle provides limited time for food preparation and that it is necessary to depend on convenience foods. This idea has become so ingrained that the public fails to notice advertising time is not generally devoted to foods of a highly nourishing nature, such as fruit, milk, or cheese, which require no more preparation than products usually classified as "fast" foods, which are of less nutritional value.

The trends toward increasing expenditures for food eaten out of the home and the large percentage of space in grocery stores given over to a range of processed foods partially reflect the widespread habits of Americans who eat foods that are advertised as easy to prepare or already prepared.

Health care workers can and should be effective advocates for change in the commercial media, in which **saturation techniques** are most often used by promoters of unhealthful food habits. Professionals must first perceive the sizable influence of mass media on living patterns in comparison with their own sphere of influence. They must then recognize the legitimate need for attention to this problem and allocate professional time to its solution.[26,116] Groups of professionals with similar goals can work together for common results. Media can be important in creating social norms and promoting healthy eating practices. With television shows, there is an opportunity to present health-promoting messages by having characters model good dietary practices. Health professionals should work with the television industry to encourage the inclusion of healthy eating patterns in programming.[101]

In the clinical setting an alert professional should make specific inquiry into the influence of media advertising on food habits and counsel patients about sound strategies for coping with the imbalances inherent in this source of messages about food.

In a positive sense, nutrition educators recognize the potential of using mass media in a comprehensive manner to reach millions of persons in all stages of the reproductive cycle.[12,26] A campaign could be based on an issue related to maternal nutrition, such as need for iron-rich foods in the diet, and could be planned specifically for the population to whom the messages would be aired. Time would be arranged for the selected broadcasts through the station manager who accept a certain number of public service announcements. An effective educational campaign of this sort requires a great deal of careful planning and a commitment to competence in fields beyond those in which nutritionists normally have expertise. It would also be likely to require monetary support, since laws requiring free public service announcements have been repealed. Nevertheless, television is an effective medium and should not be overlooked as a potential method of providing worthwhile nutrition information for all age groups.[116]

Telecourses are a well-established type of programming. A course on nutritional considerations in human reproduction could be developed and distributed widely, increasing appreciation for the role of nutrition in supporting a healthy pregnancy.

Radio campaigns are less expensive than those designed for the television medium and are more accessible for people with a busy lifestyle. Radio messages reach large numbers of people throughout the day and should not be overlooked as potentially powerful tools of nutrition education.[20,116] Talk shows and "magazine-of-the-air" formats allow for greater depth in discussion of complex and controversial subjects. Nutritionists are more often being asked to host or at least be the resource person for radio talk shows. Time should be set aside for discussion of preparation of women for reproduction (or women's health and nutrition), prenatal nutrition, lactation and child-feeding issues. It is clear that health educators in developing countries have made significantly more use of radio presentations than similar educators in the United States.[71]

Audiovisual Aids to Education

People in the modern world are accustomed to sophisticated audiovisual (AV) communication and, in fact, expect it in any high-quality educational production. Nutritionists must therefore contribute their share of such productions to be effective in gaining audience attention.[116] Concepts that are acquired through visual perception are effectively incorporated into the human mind and may appeal to various learning styles. The combined auditory and visual experience is concrete and participatory. It presents the audience with specific models to which they can relate.[88,111] Packages of materials employing AVs, graphics, and printed matter lend versatility to projects that extend one theme.[74]

Differences in the various types of AV media make it necessary to match the characteristics of a particular format to the special demands of a particular educational project. Table 12-1 provides guidance for comparing functional aspects of the various formats. AVs that are thoughtfully produced should be widely distributed because of the need for aids to communication. The format that is most appropriate to the purpose and affords the widest distribution should be used. A plan for distribution should be incorporated into the overall project plan.[116]

Slide/sound presentations. Presentations consisting of a series of slides or a filmstrip with audio accompaniment have great potential adaptability for nutrition education, although in the late 1990s, production on a commercial basis is being limited as a result of expense and popularity of other dissemination formats (see Table 12-1). The presentations and simple playback equipment can easily be carried by one person and shown in a variety of settings. Compared with the motion-picture format, this method is less expensive, entailing, in the simplest form, still photographs and a script that is read by the presenter as the photographs change. A more sophisticated form of slide presentation is the programmed slide or filmstrip show with equipment that changes the photographs automatically in coordination with the recorded audio portion.[82] Flexibility can be achieved with the slide format by revising the slides and the script as appropriate. Multiprojector slide/sound presentations are effective but expensive to produce and inflexible to use.

A study of the process of making a slide/sound presentation provides a model for producing educational aids in various media. One needs to develop a precise plan, such as that presented in the box at right. Even the simplest forms require a significant expenditure of funds. An assessment of all resources, including funding, personnel, equipment, and distribution system,[82] should be accomplished early in the project. Explicit objectives based on the intended use of the

❖

PROCEDURE FOR PRODUCING AN AUDIOVISUAL TEACHING AID

Preliminary processes
  Ascertaining the need for an audiovisual program
  Defining the message
  Assessing the characteristics of the target population
  Selecting the approach
  Preproduction planning
  Assessing available resources (including personnel)
  Acquiring project consultants

Producing a pilot presentation
  Field testing
  Securing monetary support
  Planning distribution
  Defining responsibilities
  Finalizing production plans

Production
  Setting up the production schedule
  Writing the script
  Designing graphics and modeling any cartoon characters
  Creating the story board
  Planning photographs
  Casting the actors and voices
  Executing the cartoon graphics and live scenes
  Producing the sound track
  Reviewing and revising periodically
  Assembling the audiovisual
  Developing the teaching manual

Evaluation
  Formative evaluation
  Surveying the educator/user as to the perceived effectiveness
  Summative evaluation

NOTE: Each process in the series requires attention, although several may be carried out simultaneously and not necessarily in the order above.

Developed by Rees J and Doan R: *Producing an audio-visual aid for nutrition education*, Seattle, 1980, University of Washington.

final product for transmitting information, changing attitudes, or stimulating discussion provide an overall guide to organization. Analysis of the character of the audience is an important preliminary step. The resulting information largely determines the manner in which the material will be presented—the **"approach."** The approach includes the theme or story in which the nutrition information will be embodied, the type of visual material, and the emotional tone to be communicated.

Choosing appropriate consultants is an important task. Few people have the skills to produce their own educational materials; they must work closely with those who have the technical skill to implement the plan.[40] Members of the **target audience** and professionals familiar with them will serve in advisory roles, ensuring that characteristics that appeal to the intended audience will be incorporated into the production. The slide/sound presentation, *Inside My Mom*[74] and the prenatal calendar, *Great Beginnings*[63] are excellent examples of the collaboration involved in production of a successful nutrition education tool. Professional or amateur specialists in photography, art, and sound recording can be assembled to do the work of production if a comprehensive media group cannot be employed.[116] It is appropriate to try out ideas during the decision-making phases, using materials produced by amateurs, until it is certain that the scope of the project requires professional involvement. Colleges, universities, and even high schools often have media groups that can provide resources; local television and radio stations may also be supportive. A complex presentation necessitates the preparation of projected budgets, production schedules, actors, sets, field testing, legal coverage, and supplementary instructional materials. It is advisable to consult professional media personnel and consider contracting for the work with a professional public or private organization if a comprehensive project is planned or if extensive distribution is proposed. Agreements are drawn up between various persons participating in the project to clarify responsibilities in formulating the materials, costs to each party, and rights to the finished project.

With defined objectives and audience analysis

as background, the story idea and specific plans are formulated. The main pitfalls to avoid in planning the content are a delivery that is "preachy" in tone, material that is dry and uninteresting, inclusion of a broad range of nutrition topics in one script, and use of material that is removed from reality in the lives of the audience. (Use of an affluent set design in a project directed toward low-income persons is an example of the latter.)[116]

A combination of photographs and graphics is used to achieve the desired visual result, a distinct and lasting image to enhance communications.[116] The ratio of graphics to photographs depends on the approach and on the availability of funds for the project. Visuals move the presentation toward the desired end, not being mere accessories to the audio portion. The visuals, including characters and sets, are planned so that the specific target audience will identify with them. An effort is made to avoid projecting bias or to alienate members of the target audience by stereotyping. For example, if the target audience is adolescents in general, the material should appeal to all racial groups and both sexes.[82]

Decisions related to the final revisions are made only after gathering opinions from a full range of consultants so that a maximum of objectivity is built into the process.[82] Testing preliminary materials and concepts with the target audience during the process of production allows the producers to observe the audience responses and to make alterations to enhance the effect of the AV as it is being assembled. Periodic review by those responsible for funding is scheduled after each major step in the process to ensure that they are satisfied with the material. Summative evaluation of the AV assesses its value as a communication agent with the target audience. User questionnaires gather information from educators about the effectiveness of the tool and their intent to use it in a specific situation.[116] Results of these evaluations guide the producers in future work with AV projects.

A fresh approach can often be achieved in a slide show with themes that are simple but attractively presented. This format is well-suited to the needs of the individual nutritionist or educator who can analyze the audience and organize the material into a presentation that appeals specifically to the defined group. The images that can be employed to enhance the effectiveness of a message are virtually unlimited when photographs and drawings are used.[116] Under all circumstances in which monetary support for minimal media assistance is available, slide show preparation should be seriously considered as a useful mechanism of improving the quality of communication in the area of nutrition.

An example of an organized slide presentation (transferred to videotape in the latest revision) is *Inside My Mom*,[74] featuring the cartoon character illustrated in Fig. 14-5. In this presentation a light approach to the subject of fetal dependence on maternal nutrition provides a stimulant for discussing the relationship of nutrition to reproduction appropriate for a classroom or clinic, with individuals or groups. It appeals to people in a variety of socioeconomic, ethnic, and age categories. An accompanying flyer provides information about use of the program.

Evaluation shows that the material successfully improves attitudes of both males and females about the role of nutrition in reproduction. Posters and take-home pamphlets reinforce and expand the message for an audience that does not usually acquire knowledge by reading. The follow-up, *Outside My Mom: The Story of a Breast-Fed Baby*, emphasizes the advantages of breastfeeding.[77]

Videotapes. Videotapes[122] offer a versatile format that is used to prepare programmed teaching, provide observations of live scenes, or present educational programs for distribution either in the commercial broadcast medium or for use by institutions or individuals.[116] The cost of editing is moderate, and there is no need for professional production facilities, making videotapes especially useful for recording naturally occurring or minimally staged events that transmit realistic images from one setting to another. For example, a videotape of mothers successfully breastfeeding can be shown to a group of women who are discussing alternatives in child feeding prenatally. Then, in the postpartum period, a tape of actual techniques of breastfeeding or of preparing infant formula can be a great boon for a new mother struggling with the day-to-day realities of "how to." Also, videotapes demonstrating "the feeding relationship" between infant and parent are available.[85] The cost of the project is kept low because neither script nor editing is necessary. The low cost of copying keeps distribution costs down.

Effective videotaped programs include plenty of action to hold the attention of a population that has experienced modern media productions. A scene depicting eating in an interesting way constitutes appropriate action when food habits are the theme of the discussion. Lecturing and simple interviewing are uninteresting and do not merit being taped, except in unique circumstances in which the personalities involved provide an interest in themselves. Still graphics should be used sparingly on videotapes.

With the proliferation of home videotape recorders, videotapes are becoming more versa-

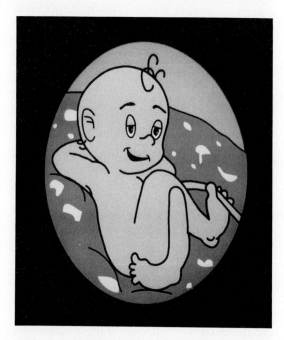

FIG. 14-5 Cartoon depicting healthy uterine environment—example of humorous approach to subject of fetal dependence on maternal nutrition.

Slide, audiotape or videocassette, *Inside My Mom*, available from March of Dimes, Birth Defects Foundation, National Offices. Provided courtesy of J. Rees.

tile and accessible in most settings, though equipment is difficult to transport if unavailable. Furthermore, 16-mm movie formats are currently being transferred to videotape.

Current video uses in nutrition education are for specifically planned purposes: to train professionals, to provide continuing education, to bring education to hospitalized patients on closed-circuit systems, and to offer an alternative choice of formats when teaching aids are made for use in public health programs. Expanded use of home video playback equipment will allow programs to be purchased or rented for personal use. Foresighted nutrition educators will take advantage of such capability by planning exciting material for the videotape format, keeping abreast of the latest trends in the communication equipment and its capabilities.[28] Production follows a plan like that described in the section on slide/sound presentations.

Motion pictures. Motion pictures, of course, are highly effective in assisting in a variety of educational efforts.[116] As the capabilities of nutritionists for working with the media improve and their familiarity with AV production becomes more expert, the expenditure of time and funds for working in this medium is justified. Several interesting films are available that provide information related to issues in pregnancy and child feeding.[62,73] Because of the combination of sound, movement, clear imagery, and nearly limitless settings, films are capable of creating a mood more completely than other media formats. The comprehensive nature of motion pictures allows for exploration of subject matter in depth so that supplementary materials may be unnecessary and persons without any background of dealing with the subject matter can use them as tools. Many of the principles described in the previous section on making slide shows apply to producing motion pictures.

Certain pitfalls, however, in the use of films for nutrition education are apparent. There is a tendency because of the relative length of motion pictures to fill them with more material than an audience can grasp during one showing. Extraneous material and complex detail that are not supportive of the central message clutter films.

Videodisk and multimedia. Distribution formats that show potential are the videodisk

and CD-ROM, on which materials produced by traditional means (16-mm film, slides, videotape) are reproduced in a format that can be integrated with computers in a way that may allow for interaction (see Table 14-1).[2,27,42,99]

Innovative Techniques

Nutrition educators have made use of computers, the fastest-growing educational technique of modern times, to educate specific patient and professional groups, as well as the general public.[68] What could be more useful to a pregnant woman than a quick computer analysis of her current eating habits coupled with a specific plan for enhancing her intake to support reproduction and then breastfeeding? They have also used direct mail, pension-check inserts,[34,89] campaigns, songs, games, and stories and have been urged to consider folklore as a vehicle. In addition, trained peer counselors have been found to have a positive effect on breastfeeding practices.[49] The basic principles for development and use of new techniques are the same as described for more traditional methods. The necessary specialized skills may be provided by professionals within the related field or nutrition educators who have trained themselves by working with the other discipline. Results are not positive when nutrition educators attempt to practice a specialized skill without help from that field unless specially trained themselves.

Printed Materials

Printed materials are the most commonly used educational aid available at present. This aid generally takes the form of short printed pamphlets or inexpensively reproduced sheets. In actuality, however, a tremendous range of different formats exists. Popular magazines provide one possible forum for health education, including nutrition.[116] Indeed, relevant topics in nutrition are often covered in articles and advertising in a variety of magazines, but trained health professionals are seldom involved in their preparation. The overall effect can be detrimental when erroneous or poorly justified recommendations are made. Opportunities to reach millions of readers are lost when this source of communication with the public is neglected. It seems justifiable, in fact necessary, that health

*TABLE 14-1 Comparison of Functional Characteristics of Educational Audio-visual Media Formats**

	16-mm Film†	Videotape‡	Slide-Tape§ Sound-Filmstrip	Videodisk	Multimedia‖	CD-Rom¶
Production						
1. Investment in production equipment	Medium $	High $	Low $	High $	High $	Medium-high
2. Time required for production	Medium-long	Short-medium	Short-medium	Long	Long	Medium
3. Cost of production per minute	Thousands $	Hundreds-thousands $	Hundreds-thousands $	Thousands $	Thousands $	Hundreds-thousands
Technical						
1. Full animation	Yes	Yes	No	Yes	Yes	Yes
2. Cost of special effects	High	Low-medium	Low	Medium	Low-medium	Low-high
3. Running time limits	None	1 hr	Less than 20 min	?	Varies	Up to 74 min.
4. Cost of editing/mixing	High	Medium-high	Low-medium	High	Medium-high	Medium-high
Distribution						
1. Cost of copies (typical costs)	High $ (100s of $)	Low $ (under 200 $)	Low-medium $ (100 $)	Low $	Low $	Low $
2. Playback availability and compatibility	Fair	Excellent	Good (filmstrips only fair outside schools)	Poor-fair	Poor	Fair-good (depends on location)
3. Cost of playback equipment	Medium	Low	Low-medium	Medium-high	High	Low-medium
4. Portability of equipment	Fair	Fair	Fair-good	Fair	Poor	Fair-good

*Certain nonstandardized media formats are available for use with particular brands of media equipment. They are typically variations of the above.

†Super 8 film and ‡ Home video may be acceptable for "in-house" use. Production in usually limited to the original recording and not generally of sufficient quality for mass duplication and distribution.

‖Integration of videodisk and computer for the purpose of student-directed learning of a potentially complex body of information.

§Included, but no longer produced on a commercial basis due to expense. Other drawbacks include lack of animation.

¶CD-ROM is considered a dissemination format that utilizes other technologies for production.

Developed by Ross A and Rees J: Producing an audiovisual aid for nutrition education, University of Washington, 1980, revised 1988, 1992, 1996.

educators focus more attention on this important mechanism of educating both children and adults. An article, for example, about the dangers of weight loss during pregnancy could be extremely interesting and effective if written in popular style. Such an article could be developed specifically for magazines that appeal to readers in groups at high risk for complications in pregnancy. Preparing themselves to communicate in written form to any population group[32] is vital to professionals interested in nutrition education.[39]

Periodicals bring interesting nutrition and health information to adults and supply guidance in applying the principles of nutrition to an everchanging living situation.[29,107,109] The opportunity for gaining current information is essential and cannot be provided as well in other formats.

Nutritionists are infrequently involved in the preparation of books that are interesting and understandable to lay persons. Most popular books on nutrition topics have been written by persons without valid qualification who are seeking to exploit the market by promoting spectacular but unfounded ideas about dietary prevention or cures. Usually these special diets or ideas have not been subjected to the traditional scientific process of evaluation, and their bases are at variance with the widely accepted body of scientific information.

One publication, *Eating Expectantly: Essential Eating Guide and Cookbook for Pregnancy*,[101] is a source of nutrition information for pregnant women in a style suited to the general public. *Child of Mine: Feeding With Love and Good Sense*[84] is a practical guide to nutrition during pregnancy and for infant feeding. *How to Get Your Kid to Eat . . . But Not Too Much* is the sequel, covering various aspects of feeding and eating from birth through teenage years.[86]

Newspapers publish an abundance of material about food but very little about nutrition. The few articles that are written often represent dubious interpretations of poorly trained "science editors." Welcome exceptions are the nationally syndicated column written by Mayer and Goldberg[56] and the work of Brody[15] and Burros[16] in New York City, which deal with contemporary nutrition issues and questions from the public in a practical and authoritative way. There is a need for additional columns or presentations of this

---

❖

THE GUNNING FOG INDEX

1. Randomly select passages of 100-125 words. Determine the average number of words per sentence in this passage. Treat independent clauses as separate sentences. Example: "I came. I saw. I conquered." This would be counted as three sentences, even if semicolons or dashes were used instead of periods.

2. Count the number of words of three syllables or more per 100 words. Omit from this count all capitalized words, combinations of short, easy words like "manpower" and "butterfly," and verbs made into three syllables by adding "-es" or "-ed" (Examples: "trespasses," "created").

(To get the percentage, divide the number of long words in the passage by the total number of words. Fourteen long words divided by 115 words = 12 percent when rounded.)

3. Add the average sentence length (from 1) and the percentage of long words (from 2). Multiply the sum by 0.4. Ignore digits following the decimal point. And because few readers have more than 17 years' schooling, any passage that tests higher than 17 is given a Fog Index of "17-plus," hard reading for college graduates. The result is the number of years of schooling needed to read the passage with ease.

Adapted from *The Technique of Clear Writing* by Robert Gunning. New York: McGraw-Hill, rev ed, 1968. Used with permission of the copyright owner, Gunning-Mueller Clear Writing Institute, Inc, Santa Barbara, California. "Fog Index" is a service mark of Gunning-Mueller.

type in local newspapers.[116] Until a well-informed public encourages such a service, professionals will need to be assertive in taking advantage of opportunities to disseminate nutrition information through this popular form of communication. Nutrition professionals should be encouraged to prioritize areas on which to focus.

Photographs, posters, and graphics can be used in various settings to promote nutrition-related ideas to the general public.[116] At present, budgets of most nutrition education programs do not allot sufficient funds for such projects. The lack of attention to graphics in many circumstances is short-sighted, since this form of communication is often employed in preventive campaigns, which save the public's money in the long run by decreasing the need for costly crisis-oriented treatment. One example of such a project is a calendar that becomes a vehicle for nutritional messages.[63] Material utilizing specialized print and graphics has been developed and disseminated for use by both educators and consumers in prenatal education.[18]

Evaluating the production of AV and print educational aids. Evaluation of an AV product is a unique undertaking because of the complex art of communication involved. This exercise judges whether the needs of the audience have been met; it also provides feedback to the producers, who stand to improve with criticism.[26,46,103,116] A combination of objective tests and attitudinal scales are often developed as instruments to test whether cognitive and affective objectives have been met. Short-term AVs are seldom appropriate tools to elicit behavior change. Printed media are somewhat easier to test with traditional paper and pencil techniques. The aspect that cannot be overlooked is whether AV or print material is *interesting* and *attractive* to the target population. The content will be lost if it does not appeal to the audience.

Choosing Materials for a Particular Use

When making decisions about the use of auxiliary materials to enhance the effectiveness of the nutrition education whether for one occasion or to have available on an ongoing basis, various attributes of the available material should be considered (Table 14-2). The factual

content, the technical manner in which the content is presented, the format, and the evidence that the material is a successful aid to communication of information or change in attitudes or behaviors should be considered.[118] In addition, numerous tips for effective teaching of literate, as well as semiliterate, audiences have recently been suggested.[65,81,94]

Tailoring a nutrition education message to the literacy limitations and the information preferences of client groups is essential in preparing effective instructional materials. Literacy limitations are more common among adults who live in poverty, live in inner-city locations, are recent immigrants, belong to racial and ethnic minorities, and terminate their education before completing high school. In addition, poor health, unemployment, large families, isolation, immobility, inadequate housing, low self-esteem, and a high degree of dependency are more common among people with low literacy skills than in the general population.

Health care instructional materials are typically written at a level that requires ninth- or tenth-grade reading skills, while patients and clients often have reading abilities at the sixth-grade level or lower.[65]

An important element of printed material is that it be the appropriate **reading level** for the audience.[39,40] This can be estimated by use of the formula presented in the box. However, again it should be emphasized that the appeal of the presentation to the audience is of prime importance in addition to the traditional focus on technical correctness. The topic must be perceived by clients as interesting and relevant to their needs and problems or they will not bother to decipher the message.[65]

Assessments are carried out by more than one professional; more important, the material is subjected to testing (however informal) with the population for which it is intended. A decision-making process is not dependable when one person far removed from the population to be served retains total responsibility.

Sources of Educational Materials and Techniques

Various agencies make available lists of materials that become resources to nutritionists and

TABLE 14-2 *Guide for Evaluation of Nutrition Education Materials*

Identification: Title	Format	Cost (Loan/Rent/Purchase)	Length, Company, Date
Audiovisual		**Print**	

Technical aspects

Audiovisual	Print
Quality of sound track (e.g., voice quality, appropriateness of music, sound effects)	Clarity of layout (title, headings, margins, type, illustrations)
Quality of visuals (color, settings, animation, graphics, timeliness)	Attractiveness of layout
Appropriateness of sound track to visuals	Quality of accompanying visuals (color, timeliness)
Effectiveness of approach (theme, emotional tone, motivational component)	Appropriateness of visuals
Appropriateness of length	Quality of physical characteristics in relation to intended purpose (elaborateness, durability, size)
Overall technical quality	Effectiveness of approach (e.g., theme, emotional tone, motivational component)
	Appropriateness of length
	Overall technical quality

Content

Audiovisual	Print
Accuracy of material	Accuracy of material
Timeliness of material	Timeliness of material
Possibility of material becoming rapidly outdated	Possibility of material becoming rapidly outdated
Presence of inappropriate bias (overt or covert)	Presence of inappropriate bias
Clarity of major points	Clarity of material
Relevancy of all material to main points	Relevancy of all material to main points
Appropriateness of organization of the material	Organization of material
Appropriateness of pace of presentation	Realism of material to user
Necessity for supplemental materials	Appropriateness for the intellectual and reading level of the intended user group
Appropriateness for the intended audience	Appropriateness for the intended user group
Effectiveness in holding interest	Effectiveness in holding interest
	Necessity for supplemental materials

Accompanying information

Audiovisual	Print
Identifies intended audience	Identifies intended audience
Identifies objectives	Identifies objectives
Identifies consultants and references	Identifies consultants and references
Includes teaching manual	Includes suggestions for use
Helpfulness of manual	Helpfulness of suggestions
Includes evidence of evaluation or endorsement by creditable groups/individuals	Includes evidence of evaluation or endorsement by creditable groups/individuals

Overall qualities

Audiovisual	Print
Accomplishment of stated objectives	Accomplishment of stated objectives
Effectiveness of the material	Effectiveness of the material
Usefulness to the agency	Usefulness to the agency
Cost effectiveness	Cost effectiveness
Ready availability (with or without purchase)	Ready availability
Ready availability of equipment needed	Chief function of the material (motivator, information giving, stimulant to discussion)
Ease of use of format (portability)	

Continued.

TABLE 14-2 *Guide for Evaluation of Nutrition Education Materials—cont'd*

Identification: Title	Format	Cost (Loan/Rent/Purchase)	Length, Company, Date
Audiovisual			Print

Chief function of the material (motivator, information giving, stimulant to discussion)	Specific audiences/settings in which material would be most effective
Specific audiences/settings in which material would be most effective	Estimate of amounts needed
Relative need for the material within the agency	Relative need for the material within the agency
Results of testing materials with clients served by agency	Results of testing materials with clients served by agency

(Factors to be considered: Actual evaluation forms should be designed to meet the needs of each specific agency.)

health educators. National sources of information regarding nutrition education materials for use with the public are listed in the box on p. 469. To date most of the sources do not contain objective evaluations. Journals of both the Society for Nutrition Education and the American Dietetic Association publish lists and reviews of educational materials and techniques that have become important resources for nutrition educators.

OPPORTUNITIES FOR NUTRITION EDUCATION

Opportunities for nutritional counseling and education present themselves throughout the life cycle.[26,96] The idea of nutrition education is an exciting prospect at the present time because of expressed desires on the parts of many people to know about this aspect of their lives. Table 14-3 provides a summary of the kind of situations in which such programs can be included, expanded, or improved if they now exist. Increased coordination in already-existing systems is as important as adding new programs.[12]

In particular, for teenagers approaching the reproductive years, the typical high school home economics curriculum (in which nutrition information is only briefly presented and the baking of pastries takes up the major portion of time) can be redesigned to meet present-day needs. The initial course for all students would include basic cooking skills combined with nutrition information. For example, one component would be vegetable selection, preparation, and cookery, coupled with study of nutritional contribution of vegetables to the diet. Consideration of each type of food (vegetables, vegetable proteins, fruits, meats, dairy products, carbohydrates, and fats) in turn would contribute to a comprehensive understanding of nutrition and food. Following the basic course, three optional courses could be provided. Weight management, child feeding, and nutrition for fitness/athletics would provide nutrition education that would be applicable to the concerns of young males and females near the stage of reproduction. The weight management course should be informational as opposed to therapeutic in nature. It should appeal to high school students, who have great concern over the composition of their bodies, and establish a knowledge base that has lifelong utility. Nutrition for fitness/athletics has appeal for males; a child feeding course would fit well with the child development component of curriculum.

In many respects persons in *community colleges* and *vocational schools* may be more accepting of guidance about nutrition than traditional university students, motivated by a limitation of funds, time, and facilities for preparation of meals. The need for nutrition information may be especially great in the inner-city schools, where students are often "nontraditional" in

❖

SOURCES OF NUTRITION EDUCATION MATERIALS

Food and Nutrition Information Center (FNIC).
National Agricultural Library, Rm. 304
10301 Baltimore Blvd.
Beltsville, MD 20705-2351
(301) 504-5719
    Lending center for books, catalogs, AVs and specific catalogs relating to pregnancy, lactation, and nutrition education:
Nutrition Education Resource Guide: An Annotated Bibliography of Educational Materials for the WIC and CSF Programs
Promoting Nutrition Through Education, A Guide to the Nutrition Education and Training Program
Nutrition and Adolescent Pregnancy—A Selected Annotated Bibliography
Food and Consumer Service
U.S. Department of Agriculture
3101 Park Center Dr., Rm. 609
Alexandria, VA 22302-1594
    Booklets available:
Cross-cultural Counseling—A Guide for Nutrition and Health Counselors
Working with the Pregnant Teenager: A Guide for Nutrition Educators.

March of Dimes, Birth Defects Foundation
National Office
1275 Mamaroneck Ave.
White Plains, NY 10605
(914) 428-7100
Numerous educational materials relating to various aspects of pregnancy and lactation including nutrition
National Maternal and Child Clearinghouse
2070 Chain Bridge Road
Vienna, VA 22182-2536
(703) 821-8955
Publications on maternal and child health topics
Penn State Nutrition Center
417 East Calderway
The Pennsylvania State University
University Park, PA 16802
(814) 865-6323
Answers individual written and telephone requests for information about materials for a particular use
Society for Nutrition Education
2001 Killebrew Dr., Suite 340
Minneapolis, MN 55425-1882
    Publishes journal that includes reviews of nutrition education material
    (800) 235-6690

---

terms of age, ethnic background, lifestyle, and degree of responsibility.

In *university settings* the typical health service for students is an appropriate opportunity to reach young women and men close to the age of reproduction. Personnel in these clinics need the specific communication skills that foster a relationship of trust in which information provided by the "counselor" can be meaningful in the life of a busy, often newly independent individual.

For persons receiving *advanced education in professions,* such as dentistry, medicine, nursing, occupational therapy, and dental hygiene, study of nutrition is of prime importance if the public is to have access to holistic care.[12,116] Health

care workers must recognize nutrition as a basic aspect of the environment, understand its relationship to their area of expertise, and be able to teach their patients how to apply basic principles of nutrition in the maintenance of physical well-being.[26,58,116]

Although proper education of physicians regarding nutrition is needed, progress toward such education has not been rapid.[24] Concern for the apparent lack of nutrition education provided in training programs for physicians is documented in both the professional and lay literature.[6] However, it appears, from one study, that obstetricians play a significant role as sources of nutrition information for women. Nevertheless,[60] it is not surprising that many people have

TABLE 14-3 *Opportunities for Bringing Nutrition Education to Persons at All Stages in the Life Cycle Leading to Reproduction*

Schools

Day care and preschool	Meaningful, nutritious food experiences included
	Non-nourishing food excluded; food reinforcement excluded
Public schools, K through 12	Appropriate school lunches provided along with accompanying education
	Nutrition education specifically planned for all educational levels and integrated into various classes
University, community college, and vocational schools	Nutrition counseling and educational campaigns made available through campus health services
	Basic nutrition courses made available without prerequisite
	Nutrition education provided to the community through "adult education" classes
	Appropriate nutrition information included in training for vocations that will influence food habits of others
Professional training and advanced education in medicine, nursing, occupational therapy, dentistry, dental hygiene	Complete education in the principles of nutrition provided along with interdisciplinary experience in utilizing the capabilities of nutritionists
	Techniques in counseling patients and disseminating information emphasized

Clinical settings

Pediatrician, adolescent specialist, nutritionist, nurse, and other clinicians	Professional knowledge and skill to disseminate nutrition education mandated
	Prevention rather than acute care emphasized
	Nutritional aspect of health care included with time given to answer questions of parents and/or children
	Relationship of nutritional health to successful future life including reproduction stressed

Government agencies

Public (federal, state, local) and private (commercial, voluntary) organizations combating disease and disability	Nutrition education and consulting services provided
	Nutrition emphasized in programs dealing with family planning and reproduction
	Nutritionists employed in sufficient numbers to act as impetus for expanded programs
Juvenile institutions including group homes and detention facilities	Nutrition education and consultation regarding quality of food served
Point-of-purchase food markets	Education about food and nutrition made available

turned to unorthodox sources of nutrition information.

One recommendation is that the ultimate objective of medical education in human lactation is not only to inform medical students about physiologic and nutrition principles, but also to motivate them when they enter medical practice to recommend breastfeeding. It has also been suggested that instruction to improve medical students' endorsement of lactation must be derived from highly authoritative references (e.g., the American Academy of Pediatrics) and must be openly supported by the professional staff involved in educational delivery.[55] As well as studying nutrition in a didactic format, health care professionals should be provided with opportunities to work with capable nutritionists for the purpose of comprehending their functions more fully. Such experiences improve the skills of health care workers to assess problem situations and make appropriate referrals. Professionals who will ultimately be responsible for planning health care programs and facilities require experience with effective nutritionists to become committed to the provision of adequate resources for such services in their institutions.

Clinical Settings

When professionals practice preventive rather than curative medicine,[58,116] a great deal of nutrition information and influence on attitudes can be communicated to the public by health professionals who also see patients for therapeutic management of specific problems in a clinical setting. Private patients from higher income families are in need of the same nutrition services that are built into programs for the low-income population, especially since many nutritional programs in this era are reflective of patterns of overconsumption that persons with greater financial resources may be inclined to develop. The clinic is a setting in which nutrition information can be incorporated into a total fitness program,[116] as described earlier in this chapter. The rapport inherent in the one-to-one clinical relationship makes it conducive to the successful communication of nutrition information with a unique combination of attitudinal and behavioral components. Each clinician's effectiveness can be magnified if various professionals are sufficiently attuned to providing nutrition information so that they support the messages others deliver.[58] Sufficient time should be allocated to present the nutritional aspects of health and to answer questions of parents and children.

Health-Related Agencies: General

Comprehensive medical care plans offer an optimum setting for nutrition education. It is one focus in the effort to prevent illness, its complications, and the need for costly hospital care. Nutritionists should provide not only nutrition education but also ongoing consultation throughout the system to parents and patients, with special attention to the area of reproduction.[116]

Health insurance companies have a vested interest in supplying consumers with information such as written materials to help them maintain their health.[58] Newspaper, radio, and television campaigns on behalf of improving nutritional status would be effective, and use of funds allotted for communication and education should be considered for this purpose.

Labor unions and businesses recognize the importance of health education for their members and employees.[58] Seminars, lectures, and films provide personnel with another opportunity to improve their understanding of alternatives in lifestyle that maintain health.

Privately financed voluntary organizations, such as the International Childbirth Education Association* and LaLeche League,† have continuous contact with persons involved in reproduction. Significant community benefit can be realized from the nutrition education activities of these and all voluntary organizations concerned with family health.[116]

State Agencies

State governments have a special responsibility to establish communication among their population, their health professionals, and their governing agencies with the goal of providing a health care system that includes health education. A network of health care in many cases can be designed to use existing facilities to deliver improved health care to a greater number of the population. At present, however, many needy persons are virtually unserved.

---

*International Childbirth Education Association, Inc., an organization devoted to educating persons about childbearing, P.O. Box 20048, Minneapolis, MN 55420.

†LaLeche League International, Inc., an organization devoted to educating persons about breast-feeding, 1400 North Meachum Rd., Schaumburg, IL 60173, (708) 519-7730. LaLeche League Hotline for mothers: 1-800-LaLeche (9am-3pm) Central Standard Time.

Nutritional services are an integral part of community health care systems. Advisory groups can act as liaison between legislative bodies and health agencies to examine decisions that will have an impact on the nutritional environment of the state. Nutritionists at the state level plan programs and provide consultation to the networks of nutritionists throughout the state in individual county and city health departments.[116] Local-level nutritionists have the responsibility for surveillance, consultative, and educational functions, as well as delivery of health care to the population.

Federal Agencies

In any discussion of how health education, including nutrition, can be realistically integrated into the system of health care, it is generally accepted that the federal government plays at least an advisory role.[26] The Food and Drug Administration initiated nutritional labeling as part of a policy that regulatory bodies should take an energetic hand in the education of the public. The USDA funds a network of personnel and a wide range of materials that provide nutritional information to the public. The Expanded Food, Nutrition, and Education Program is part of this agency's educational program.

The federally sponsored, USDA-managed food supplementation program for Women, Infants, and Children (WIC) is designed to upgrade the nutritional status of high-risk individuals in the population during pregnancy, lactation, and infancy.[106] Through this program a nationwide network of health workers provides food and nutritional guidance to people at risk for malnutrition to support an optimal nutritional environment during early development. A basic level of nutritional training is provided to the staff involved with WIC so that project workers are valuable consultants to the patients who receive health assessment and food vouchers.

In addition to the programs presently originating from the federal government, innovative nutrition programs are needed. Because the private health care system has not incorporated comprehensive nutrition services, it may be a governmental responsibility to allocate (often through state and local agencies) sufficient resources to assure that the population receives adequate nutrition information from competent professionals.[12,116]

Governments, from the federal to local levels, and healthcare professionals must become more active as policymakers, role models, and agenda setters in implementing dietary recommendations.[101]

Point of Purchase

To influence the choices consumers make and to reach a broad cross section of the public, educational campaigns have been designed for retail food outlets.[32,68] Although a great deal more must be learned about how to do this effectively, the potential benefits warrant the attention necessary for nutrition educators to develop this technique.

Worksite

Nutrition education efforts in the workplace have taken hold and are increasing. The worksite provides some advantages over more traditional routes for implementing nutrition education programs. These include potential for social support and influence, availability of a dining situation, and opportunities for follow-up, monitoring, and reinforcement of messages.[4,36]

These efforts can have an impact on the health of the pregnant or lactating woman. With increased numbers of women in the workforce, pregnancy, lactation, and work are no longer considered socially or medically incompatible. Nutrition educators need to focus their energies in this area.[8] Design of worksite programs should incorporate program design principles discussed earlier in this chapter.

Academic Preparation

The process of nutrition education may be part of many nutrition professionals' job responsibilities. Some may even specialize in nutrition education. Guidelines developed by the Society for Nutrition Education (SNE) provide a good outline of the very specific training one needs to be an effective nutrition educator.[97] As defined by SNE, a nutrition education specialist is "a professional who is trained in the fundamental principles of human nutrition, learning theory, and educational methods including behavior change strategies. This professional nutrition educator designs, implements, and evaluates nutrition education programs that focus on developing and maintaining positive food and nutrition behavior."[97]

Summary

There are several distinct kinds of nutrition education. Needs for nutrition education cover a wide spectrum. Content of nutrition education programs must therefore vary. Only with continuous appropriate nutritional support throughout childhood and adolescence can the mature woman enter pregnancy in optimal nutritional condition to provide for the development of a healthy infant without undue stress to herself. Informative nutrition education efforts within schools can be accompanied by the continual support of community organizations, clinics, mass media, and family environment and directed toward attitudes and behaviors. A variety of educational tools and techniques can be employed by well-prepared professionals to arouse and maintain active interest in health status from early childhood through maturity. Where health-oriented climates of this type are created in communities in the world today, unnecessary maternal and infant mortality are greatly reduced and overall complications of reproduction are minimized.

❖ ❖ ❖
CASE STUDY

You are now in your new job—you love it. You have access to lots of media material or at least assistance in developing what you need. The phone rings and you are asked to provide a day-long seminar on nutrition for expecting mothers. What do you do?

1. What pieces of information do you want to convey?
2. How can I organize this information to be interesting and sequentially relevant?
3. How can you encourage the participants to get to know each other?
4. Can the women in the group support each other - can you help them?

REVIEW QUESTIONS

1. Describe the distinct types of nutrition education.
2. Diagram the spectrum of nutrition education needs.
3. Define the important content areas related to nutrition education.
4. Describe the advantages and disadvantages of each mode of nutrition education.

LEARNING ACTIVITIES

1. Review available nutrition education materials found in a WIC setting.
2. Carry out the same process in a private Ob/Gyn setting that focuses on middle- and upper-class women.
3. Develop a brochure for pregnant women focused on a specific population and a specific topic.
4. Familiarize yourself with the International Childbirth Association and its resources.
5. Evaluate several audiovisual materials focused on nutrition and designed for pregnant adults or pregnant teens.

REFERENCES

1. Achterberg C, McDonnell E, Bagby R: How to put the Food Guide Pyramid into practice, *JADA* 94:1030, 1994.
2. Achterberg C, Miller C: Should nutrition be launched into hyperspace? *Nutr Today* 30:186, 1995.
3. Adler RP, Lesser GS, Ward S: *The effects of television advertising on children: review and recommendations,* Lexington, Mass, 1980, DC. Heath.
4. Alford MM: A guide for nutrition educators at the worksite, *J Nutr Educ* 18(Suppl):S19, 1986.
5. American Dietetic Association, Legislative newsletter, 1988.
6. American Dietetic Association: *Position statement: Nutrition:* essential component of medical education, 87:642, 1987.
7. Anderson AS, Shepherd R: Beliefs and Attitudes toward "healthier eating" among women attending maternity hospital. *J Nutr Educ* 21:208, 1989.
8. Barber-Madden R et al: Nutrition for pregnant and lactating women: implications for worksite health promotion, *J Nutr Educ,* 18(Suppl):S72, 1986.

9. Bass MA, Wakefield L, Kolasa K: *Community nutrition and individual food behavior,* Minneapolis, 1979, Burgess Publishing.

10. Batten S, Hirschman J, Thomas D: Impact of the special supplemental food program on infants, *J Pediatr* 117(Suppl):S101, 1990.

11. Bleibtreu HK: An anthropologist views the nutrition professions, *J Nutr Educ* 5:11, 1973.

12. Board of the National Nutrition Consortium: Statement of nutrition education policy, *J Nutr Educ* 12:138, 1980.

13. Brillinger MF: Helping adults learn. *J Hum Lact* 6:171, 1990.

14. Britt EC: Healthy people 2000, *J Nutr Educ* 22:239, 1990.

15. Brody J: Nutrition column, *New York Times.*

16. Burros M: Nutrition column, *Washington Post.*

17. Campbell JA: *Speech communication, Modules in speech communication,* 1981, Science Research Associates.

18. Center for Science in the Public Interest, Breast milk is best (poster), undated.

19. Center for Science in the Public Interest: *Nutrition action health letter* (newsletter), Washington, DC, current edition.

20. Chicci AHM, Guthrie H: Effectiveness of radio in nutrition education, *J Nutr Educ* 14:99, 1982.

21. Community Nutrition Institute: *Nutrition week* (newsletter), Washington, D.C., current edition.

22. Contento I et al: Nutrition education for pregnant women and caretakers of infants (Chapter 6) in Nutrition Education and Implications, *J Nutr Educ* 27:329, 1995.

23. Crockett SJ: Adult attitudes about attending classes on healthy eating, *J Nutr Educ* 19:101, 1987.

24. Cyborski CK: Nutrition content in medical curricula, *J Nutr Educ* 9:17, 1977.

25. Dietz WH, Gortmaker SL: Do we fatten our children at the television set?: obesity and television viewing in children and adolescents, *Pediatrics* 75:807, 1985.

26. Dwyer J, editor: National conference on nutrition education, *J Nutr Educ* 12(Suppl):79, 1980.

27. Edmunds G, Wyse BW, DeBloois M: Using videodisc technology and the index of nutritional quality to teach dietary guidance to young adults, *J Am Diet Assoc* 87(Suppl):519, 1987.

28. Eide WB: The nutrition educator's role in access to food—from individual orientation to social orientation, *J Nutr Educ* 14:14, 1982.

29. Environmental Nutrition Incorporated: *Environmental Nutrition Newsletter,* New York, current edition.

30. Falciglia GA, Gussow JD: Television commercials and eating behavior of obese and normal-weight women, *J Nutr Educ* 12:196, 1980.

31. Farkas CS: Ethno-specific communication patterns implications for nutrition education, *J Nutr Educ* 18:99, 1986.

32. Fjeld CR, Sommer R: Ideas for point-of-purchase nutrition education, *J Nutr Educ* 13:135, 1981.

33. Food and Nutrition Board. Institute of Medicine: *Nutrition during pregnancy,* Washington, DC, 1990, National Academy Press.

34. Gillespie AH, Yarbrough JP, Roderuck CE: Nutrition communication program: a direct-mail approach, *J Am Diet Assoc* 82:254, 1983.

35. Glanz K, Damberg CL: Meeting our nation's health objectives in nutrition, *J Nutr Educ* 19:211, 1987.

36. Glanz K, Seewald-Klein T: Nutrition at the worksite: an overview, *J Nutr Educ* 18 (suppl):S1, 1986.

37. Goldberg J, Mayer J: The White House Conference on Food, nutrition and health twenty years later: where are we now? *J Nutr Educ* 22:49, 1990.

38. Guild PB, Garger S: Marching to different drummers, 1985, ACSD.

39. Gunning R: *The technique of clear writing,* New York, 1952, McGraw-Hill.

40. Guthrie HA: The many faces of nutrition education, *J Nutr Educ* 21:226, 1989.

41. Haughton B, Gussow JD, Dodds JM: An historical study of the underlying assumptions for U.S. food guides from 1917 through the basic four food group guide, *J Nutr Educ* 19:169, 1987.

42. Hawthorne DL: Eliminating interactive barriers, *E-ITV* 9:15, 1986.

43. Hoerr SLM, Nelso RA, Essex-Sorlie D: Treatment and follow-up of obesity in adolescent girls, *J Adolesc Health Care* 9:28, 1988.

44. Holli BB, Calabrese RJ: *Communication and education skills—the dietitian's guide,* ed 2, Philadelphia, 1991, Lea and Febiger.

45. Ikeda JP, et al: Food habits of the Hmong living in Central California, *J Nutr Educ* 23:168, 1991.

46. Joint Committee on Standards for Education Evaluation: *Standards for evaluations of educational programs, projects and materials,* New York, 1981, McGraw-Hill.

47. Kent G: Nutrition education as an instrument of enpowerment, *J Nutr Educ* 20:193, 1988.

48. Kessler LA et al: The effect of a woman's significant other on her breastfeeding decision, *J Hum Lact* 11:103, 1995.

49. Kistin N, Abramson R, Dublin P: Effect of peer counselors on breastfeeding initiation, exclusivity, and duration among low-income urban women, *J Human Lact* 10:11, 1994.

50. Kotler P: *Marketing for non-profit organizations,* Englewood Cliffs, NJ, 1982, Prentice-Hall.

51. Kroger M: Communicating science to the public, *J Nutr Educ* 18:274, 1986.

52. Lucas DR: Getting the message across, *J Hum Nutr* 33:371, 1979.

53. Mahan KL: Family-focused behavioral approach to weight control in children, *Ped Clin North Am* 34:983, 1987.

54. Matheny RJ, Picciano MF, Birch L: Attitudinal and social influences on infant feeding preference, *J Nutr Educ* 19:21, 1987.

55. Matheny RJ, Picciano MF, Bowermaster J: What to teach medical students about human lactation, *J Nutr Educ* 22:35, 1990.

56. Mayer J, Goldberg A: *Nutrition,* Washington, DC, current edition, Washington Post Co.

57. McCullough WJ: *Hold your audience,* Englewood Cliffs, NJ, 1978, Prentice-Hall.

58. McNerney WJ: The missing link in health services, *J Med Educ* 50:11, 1975.

59. Mellin LM, Slinkard LA, Irwin CE: Adolescent obesity intervention: validation of SHAPE-DOWN program, *J Am Diet Assoc* 87:333, 1987.

60. Mitchell MC, Lerner E: Nutrition knowledge, attitudes and practices of pregnant middle-class women, *J Nutr Ed* 23:239, 1991.

61. Mosio M, Eide WB: Broadening the scope of nutrition education, *J Nutr Educ* 17:173, 1985.

62. *Breastfeeding—a practical guide,* pts I and II (Film, video tape, home video tape), Washington, DC, Motion, Inc., 1982.

63. National Dairy Council: *Great beginnings calendar,* ed 2, Rosemont, IL, 1991, National Dairy council.

64. Nestle M: National nutrition monitoring policy: the continuing need for legislative intervention, *J Nutr Educ* 22:141, 1990.

65. Nitzke S: Improving the effectiveness of nutrition education materials for low literacy clients, *Nutr Today,* September, October:17, 1989.

66. Oace SM: WHO marketing code, *J Nutr Educ* 14:70, 1982.

67. Olson CM, Gillespie AH, editors: Proceedings of the workshop on nutrition education research/applying principles from the behavioral sciences, *J Nutr Educ* 13(Suppl 1):51, 1981.

68. O'Malley DT et al: Computerized nutrition education in the supermarket, *J Nutr Educ* 19:159, 1987.

69. Palumbo FM, Dietz WH: Children's television: its effect on nutrition and cognitive development, *Pediatr Ann* 14:793, 1985.

70. Parham ES, Frigo VS, Perkins AH: Weight control as portrayed in popular magazines, *J Nutr Educ* 14:153, 1982.

71. Parlato MB: The use of mass media to promote breastfeeding, *Int J Gynecol Obstet* 31(Suppl 1):105, 1990.

72. Peterkin BB: What's new about the 1990 dietary guidelines for Americans? *J Nutr Educ* 23:183, 1991.

73. Rees JM: *Eating disorders.* In Mahan LK, Rees JM, editors: *Nutrition in adolescence* St Louis, 1984, Mosby–Year Book.

74. Rees JM: *Inside my mom* (slide/tape, sound/filmstrip or video), Mamaroneck, NY, 1990, March of Dimes, Birth Defects Foundation, National Office.

75. Rees JM: *Nutritional counseling for adolescents.* In Mahan LK, Rees JM, editors: *Nutrition in adolescence,* St Louis, 1984, Mosby–Year Book.

76. Rees J, Doan R: *Producing an audio-visual aid for nutrition education,* Seattle, 1980, University of Washington. (Unpublished).

77. Rees JM, Murphy S: *Outside my mom* (slide/sound or sound/filmstrip, pamphlet, poster), Mamaroneck, NY, 1984, March of Dimes, Birth Defects Foundation, National Office.

78. Rees JM, Worthington-Roberts B: *Adolescence, nutrition, and pregnancy: interrelationships.* In Mahan LK, Rees JM, editors: *Nutrition in adolescence,* St Louis, 1984, The CV Mosby Co.

79. Ross A, Rees J: Producing an audiovisual aid for nutrition education, Seattle, 1980, University of Washington (revised 1988 and 1992).

80. Robbins GE: Ten-state nutrition survey: educational implications, *J Nutr Educ* 4:157, 1972.

81. Ruud J, Betts NM, Dirkx J: Developing written nutrition information for adults with low literacy skills, *J Nutr Educ* 25:11, 1993.

82. Ryan M: *Preparing a slide-tape program: a step-by-step approach,* pts. I and II, Audiovisual Instruction 20:36 (Sept.) and 20:36, (Nov.), 1975.

83. Sanjur D: *Social and cultural perspectives in nutrition,* Englewood Cliffs, NJ, 1981, Prentice-Hall.

84. Satter E: *Child of mine: feeding with love and good sense,* Palo Alto, CA, 1983, Bull Publishing.

85. Satter E: *Feeding with love and good sense* (set of 4 videotapes), Palo Alto, CA, 1989, Bull Publishing.

86. Satter E: *How to get your kid to eat . . . but not too much,* Palo Alto, CA, 1987, Bull Publishing.

87. Schafer RB, Schafer E: Relationship between gender and food roles in the family, *J Nutr Educ* 21:119, 1989.

88. Schramm W: The researcher and the producer in ETV, *Pub Telecommunications Rev* 5:11, 1977.

89. Shannon B, Pelican S: Nutrition information delivered via pension-check envelopes: an effective and well-received means of providing nutrition education, *J Am Diet Assoc* 84:930, 1984.

90. Sharbaugh CS, ed: *Call to action: better nutrition for mothers, children, and families,* Washington, DC, 1991, National Center for Education in Maternal and Child Health.

91. Shortell SM, Richardson WC: *Health program evaluation,* St Louis, 1978, Mosby.

92. Sims LS: Identification and evaluation of competencies of public health nutritionists, *Am J Public Health* 69:1099, 1979.

93. Sims L: Nutrition education research: reaching toward the leading edge, *J Am Diet Assoc* 87:S10, 1987.

94. Smith SB, Alford BJ: Literate and semi-literate audiences: tips for effective teaching, *J Nutr Educ* 20:238B, 1988.

95. Snetsalaar LG: *Nutrition counseling skills: assessment, treatment and evaluation,* 1983, Aspen Systems Corporation.

96. Society for Nutrition Education, Nutrition education research: Announcement of a grant program, *J Nutr Educ* 19:268, 1987.

97. Society for Nutrition Education, Recommendations of Society for Nutrition Education on the academic preparation of nutrition education specialists, *J Nutr Educ* 19:209, 1987.

98. Society for Nutrition Education: Society for Nutrition Education concepts for food and nutrition education, *J Nutr Educ* 14:1, 1982.

99. Starr M: A dollars and sense approach to the interactive videodisc, *E-ITV* 9:27, 1986.

100. Stephenson MG: The 1990 national objectives for improved nutrition, *J Nutr Educ* 19:155, 1987.

101. Story M, Faulkner P: The prime time diet: a content analysis of eating behavior and food messages in television program content and commercials. *Am J Public Health* 80:738, 1990.

102. Swinney B: *Eating expectantly: the essential eating guide and cookbook for pregnancy,* Fall River Press, Colorado Springs, Colo, 1993.

103. Talmage H, Rasher SP: Design issues in developing and selecting measurement instruments, *J Nutr Educ* 14:54, 1982.

104. Thomas PR: Improving America's diet and health: from recommendations to action, *J Nutr Educ* 23:128, 1991.

105. Tong A: Refugees and the need to understand their problems, *J Home Econ* 73:21, 1981.

106. Torillo AD et al: Four views of WIC: a unique environment for nutrition education, *J Nutr Educ* 8:156, 1976.

107. *Tufts University diet and nutrition letter,* Tufts University, New York, William H. White.

108. Ulrich HD: Legislative and administrative policy—a historic perspective, *J Nutr Educ* 15:1, 1983.

109. University of California, Berkeley: *University of California, Berkeley, wellness letter,* New York, Health Letter Associates.

110. U.S. Department of Health and Human Services: *Cross-cultural counseling: a guide for nutrition and health counselors,* Washington, DC, 1986, Government Printing Office.

111. U.S. Department of Health and Human Services, Public Health Service: *Promoting health, preventing disease: objectives for the nation*, Washington, DC, 1980, Government Printing Office.

112. Wager W: Media selection in the affective domain: a further interpretation of Dale's cone of experience for cognitive and affective learning, *J Educ Tech* 15:9, 1975.

113. Wang VL, Ephross PH: EFNEP evaluated, *J Nutr Educ* 2:148, 1971.

114. Wardlaw JM: Preparing the nutrition education professional for the 1980's, *J Nutr Educ* 13:6, 1981.

115. Weicha JL, Dwyer JT, Dunn-Strohecker M: Nutrition and health services needs among the homeless, *Public Health Rep* 106:364, 1991.

116. White House Conference on Food, Nutrition and Health: Recommendations of White House panels on nutrition education, *J Nutr Educ* 1:24, 1970.

117. Wilson C: Call for liaison with nutritional anthropologists, *J Nutr Educ* 11:170, 1979.

118. Wilson C, Maretzke A, Talmage H: *Profiling nutrition education materials*, Oakland, Calif, 1983, Society for Nutrition Education.

119. Worthington-Roberts B: Nutrition support of successful reproduction: an update, *J Nutr Ed* 19:1, 1987.

120. Worthington-Roberts B: Distribution of extra maternal weight at 40 weeks (figure). *Contemporary developments in nutrition*, St Louis, 1981, Mosby–Year Book, p 456.

121. Wright HS, Sims LS: *Community nutrition: people, policies and programs*, Belmont, Calif, 1981, Wadsworth.

122. Wurtzel A: *Television production*, New York, 1979, McGraw-Hill.

123. Zajonc RB: Attitudinal effects of mere exposure, *J Pers Soc Psychol* 9:1, 1968.

124. Zifferblatt SM, Wilbur CS: Dietary counseling: some realistic expectations and guidelines, *J Am Diet Assoc* 70:591, 1977.

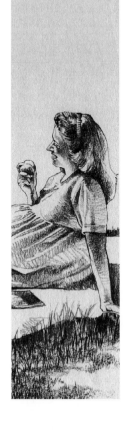

Vitamins and Minerals and Pregnancy Outcome

Vitamin and Mineral Deficiencies and Excesses and Human Pregnancy Course and Outcome

Deficiency	Excess

Vitamin A

Indian woman, blind from vitamin A deficiency, gave birth to premature infant with microcephaly and anophthalmia

Prenatal vitamin A deficiency has been related in several instances to eye abnormalities and impaired vision in children

Congenital renal anomalies in infant whose mother consumed high doses of vitamin A during pregnancy.

Multiple malformations, esp. involving CNS, in infant whose mother consumed 150,000 IU of vitamin A from day 19 through day 40 of pregnancy

Higher concentrations of vitamin A found in blood of mothers of infants with CNS anomalies vs. mothers of normal infants. Liver vitamin A levels from aborted and/or malformed fetuses were higher than in normal fetal liver

Amniotic fluid concentrations of vitamin A in second trimester were significantly higher in mothers of infants with neural tube defects vs. controls

Prominent frontal bossing, hydrocephalus, microphthalmia, and small, malformed, low-set, undifferentiated ears in two infants whose mothers had taken isotretinoin (a vitamin A analogue) in the first trimester of pregnancy. Also microcephaly, hypertelorism, small ear canals, cleft palate, small mouth, and congenital heart disease. One child did not survive

FDA reported many cases of birth defects and instances of spontaneous abortions in women receiving isotretinoin

Boston researchers report that risk of birth defects associated with neural crest-derived tissues increases significantly with intakes of preformed vitamin A as low as 10,000 IU

Vitamin D

Fetal rickets: mother had low serum vitamin D, developed osteomalacia some months after delivery

Neonatal rickets: mother suffered from osteomalacia during pregnancy

Low levels of 25-OH-D seen in hypocalcemic premature infants and their mothers

Enamel hypoplasia of the teeth seen in infants with neonatal tetany; maternal vitamin D deficiency was associated

Babies with vitamin D-resistant or vitamin D-dependent rickets demonstrate growth failure, convulsions, and rickets in the neonatal period

Infants of mothers treated with high doses of vitamin D for hypoparathyroidism show no evidence of cardiovascular or craniofacial abnormalities, although mothers do not develop hypercalcemia

Excessive intake of vitamin D or unusual sensitivity to the vitamin might be related to mild idiopathic hypercalcemia in infants

Supravalvular aortic stenosis with elfin facies and mental retardation appeared in Gottingen, Germany, where rickets prophylaxis (consisting of huge doses of vitamin D) was begun

Deficiency	Excess

Vitamin D—cont'd

Vitamin D supplementation of pregnant Asian women was associated with improved maternal weight gain, normal 25-OH-D levels in mothers and infants at term, reduced incidence of SGA babies and neonatal hypocalcemia

Neonatal hypocalcemia is more common during months when daily sunlight is least

Vitamin E

Correlation noted between birth weight and cord blood levels of vitamin E, but gestational age and other variables not controlled for

Comparison of 50 spontaneously aborting women with 50 women with normal pregnancies showed a significantly higher percentage of aborting women with serum α-tocopherol above normal limits; a causal association was not proposed.

Vitamin K

Some evidence that use of dicumarol during pregnancy is associated with increased fetal mortality and morbidity. Cases reported of fetal abnormalities in infants of mothers treated with anticoagulants. Prenatal vitamin K deficiency caused by dicumarol drugs known to produce coumadin syndrome unless dosage properly controlled

Parenteral administration of menadione to the mother has been associated with hyperbilirubinemia and kernicterus of premature infants and severe hyperbilirubinemia in term infants

Thiamin

If severe deficiency, congenital beriberi. If mild to moderate deficiency, no reported complications

Riboflavin

In study of 900 pregnant women, 190 were riboflavin deficient. These women had higher incidence of vomiting during pregnancy, premature delivery, stillbirths. No increased incidence of malformations seen. Unsuccessful lactation more common

Among middle-class European women, biochemical evidence of riboflavin deficiency not associated with abortion, hydroamnios, preeclampsia, stillbirth or low birth weights

Vitamin and Mineral Deficiencies and Excesses and Human Pregnancy Course and Outcome—cont'd

Deficiency	Excess
Ascorbic acid	
Vanderbilt study more than 2,000 pregnant women assessed diet and serum vitamin C; frequency of congenital malformations no higher in women with lowest serum levels, but increased frequency of premature births in women with lowest intake; these women also had lowest serum concentrations of vitamin C	In one study, women took large doses (6 gm/day for 3 days) of ascorbic acid to terminate suspected pregnancies; each had 10- to 15-day delay in onset of menstrual period. In 16 of 20, menstrual bleeding occurred within 1 to 3 days after starting the treatment. Results interpreted as indicating that large doses of ascorbic acid interrupted pregnancies. Since pregnancies were not initially confirmed, conclusion must be questioned.
Similar findings reported by others	Several infants have been reported to develop "conditioned scurvy" in neonatal period as a result of excessive ascorbic acid catabolism following high prenatal exposure
Several reports indicate low serum vitamin C levels associated with threatened abortion or history of previous abortions	
Other studies found no relation	
Folate	
Humans treated with folate antagonists (methotrexate, aminopterin, chlorambucil) during early pregnancy often suffer spontaneous abortion	
Some cases reported of severe congenital anomalies in term infants associated with use of these drugs during pregnancy	
Although naturally occurring folate deficiency in pregnant women has not been *proven* to have an adverse effect on pregnancy outcome, correlations have been reported between red cell folate level and incidence of congenital malformations, small-for-gestational-age (SGA) babies, and third trimester bleeding	
Observation questioned by others and relationship between folate deficiency and abruptio placentae is equally controversial	
Most folate supplementation studies report no effect on pregnancy outcome but several reports from Africa and India indicated that rate of prematurity was significantly reduced	
Prospective study of 800 women indicated low red cell folate level associated with increased incidence of SGA infants and congenital malformations	
Large prospective study showed significantly lower levels of red-cell folate in mothers who subsequently bore infants with neural tube defects vs. controls	

Deficiency	Excess

Folate—cont'd

Several reports from northern Europe showed that women previously delivering babies with neural tube defects showed reduced incidence of same problem when multiple-vitamin supplementation (rich in folic acid) or pure folic acid supplementation was provided instead of no supplement at all.

A large multicenter study of periconceptional vitamin supplementation showed a very significant reduction in recurrence of neural tube defects when folic acid was included in the supplement

A large prospective study in Hungary indicated that periconceptional vitamin supplementation significantly reduced the *occurrence* of neural tube defects in a population of women attempting to conceive

Periconceptional vitamin supplementation has been reported to significantly reduce the occurrence of orofacial clefts and congenital urinary tract abnormalities

A number of observational studies have shown that periconceptional use of folic acid or multivitamins is associated with reduced risk of neural tube defects

Government agencies in several developed countries have advised that all women who have previously delivered a baby with a neural tube defect take 4 mg/day folic acid periconceptionally

The U.S. Public Health Service has advised all women who are capable of conceiving take 0.4 mg/day of folic acid

Vitamin B$_{12}$

Pernicious anemia is rare in women of childbearing age but generally is accompanied by infertility

Human fetus with vitamin B$_{12}$ dependency successfully treated by feeding high doses of vitamin B$_{12}$ to mother

Vitamin B$_6$

Low maternal blood levels of B$_6$ have not generally been associated with neonatal clinical sequelae. Several studies reported that women with low dietary and/or serum levels of B$_6$ produced more babies with low Apgar scores than comparable mothers with good B$_6$ status

Vitamin and Mineral Deficiencies and Excesses and Human Pregnancy Course and Outcome—cont'd

Deficiency	Excess

Vitamin B6—cont'd

Supplementation of pregnant women with B_6 has not been found to reduce any clinical complication of pregnancy except pregnancy sickness

Maternal serum levels of B_6 were inversely correlated with degree of pure pregnancy depression

Pregnant women in low socioeconomic group showed biochemical evidence of B_6 deficiency and orolingual lesions (e.g., glossitis, angular stomatitis); both responded positively to B_6 supplementation

Pyridoxine supplementation of nonsupplemented pregnant women during labor (100 mg IM) appeared to favorably influence oxygen transport to newborn

Iron

Mean hemoglobin level of fetus is unaffected by maternal iron levels, unless deficiency is severe

Infants of anemic mothers showed reduced iron stores and greater tendency to develop anemia in first year of life

Effect of maternal iron deficiency on birth weight of infant is controversial

Increased incidence of prematurity reported with maternal iron deficiency

No evidence links iron deficiency with congenital malformations

Calcium

Mean bone densities of malnourished mothers and their neonates were lower vs. well-nourished counterparts

Study of Indian women with low daily intake (~400 mg/day) indicated that daily supplementation during the third trimester was associated with increased bone density in infants

Deficiency	Excess

Calcium—cont'd

Calcium deficiency proposed to be major etiologic factor in pregnancy-associated hypertension. Data indicate that in populations with low intake, incidence of eclampsia is higher. Supplementation of pregnant women also associated with reduced incidence of preeclampsia. Also noted that individuals with high intake have lower blood pressure and rats with restricted intake develop hypertension that is reversible with calcium administration. Furthermore, eclampsia syndrome is quite similar to that of tetany caused by hypocalcemia.

Iodine

Cretinism first described in sixteenth century; associated with goiter was recognized in nineteenth century although cretinism does not always occur where there is a high incidence of endemic goiter. Cretinous children show mental and physical retardation with potbelly, large tongue and facial characteristics like Down syndrome. Iodine prophylaxis has reduced the incidence of cretinism and goiter dramatically

New Guinea reported the most recent outbreak of cretinism, related to substituting imported rock salt low in iodine for local iodine-rich salt. Intramuscular iodized oil injections to women before pregnancy were later shown to markedly reduce incidence of cretinism. In addition offspring of injected women were significantly faster and more accurate in tests of manual function than children without cretinism from non-injected mothers.

Women provided large amounts of iodides during pregnancy (often as treatment for asthma or bronchitis) have had infants with congenital goiter and hypothyroidism. Neonatal mortality was high; infants were mentally retarded. Radioactive sodium iodide use during pregnancy is associated with the same outcome

Sodium

Hyponatremia has been reported in offspring of women who rigorously restricted sodium during pregnancy

Sodium restriction does not help prevent or alleviate pregnancy-associated hypertension

Potassium

Human embryonic kidney development in culture is abnormal. Suggests that potassium insufficiency in fetal plasma may cause abnormal development of the kidney in humans

Vitamin and Mineral Deficiencies and Excesses and Human Pregnancy Course and Outcome—cont'd

Deficiency	Excess

Copper

Menkes kinky hair syndrome demonstrates impact of prenatal copper deficiency in humans. Abnormalities seen in development of brain, hair, bones, and blood vessels

Women treated with penicillamine during pregnancy bore infants with connective tissue defects including lax skin, hyperflexibility of joints, fragility of veins, varicosities, impairment of wound healing. Copper deficiency proposed to be of possible etiologic importance

Excess: Small amounts of metallic copper from intrauterine devices (IUDs) can prevent mammalian embryogenesis; teratogenicity not established

Zinc

Epidemiologic data may support relationship between zinc deficiency and CNS malformations; significant zinc deficiency found in Egypt, Turkey, and Iran where high rates of CNS anomalies are seen

Women with acrodermatitis enteropathica (a genetic disorder of zinc metabolism now treated with supplemental zinc) have shown very poor pregnancy outcome in the past when zinc therapy was not used; miscarriage and malformations were much higher than in general population

Alcohol-abusing mothers show reduced serum levels of zinc and are known to demonstrate higher than normal incidence of poor pregnancy outcome. Relationship proposed but not proven

Among 272 pregnant adolescent women in Belfast, Northern Ireland, two aborted spontaneously; these two women had serum zinc levels in the lower range and hair zinc values in the higher range

Leukocyte zinc levels were significantly lower in mothers giving birth to SGA babies vs. mothers of normal babies or mothers of infants who were small but appropriate for gestational age

Plasma zinc concentration was significantly lower in the maternal blood of 54 mothers of congenitally abnormal babies either within 24 hours or 24 months previously when compared with control mothers

Zinc supplementation in a group of low income women in the southern part of the United States has been associated with improved birthweight

Excess: Zinc supplements given to pregnant women (100 mg zinc sulfate, three times daily) during third trimester; in four consecutive subjects, three delivered prematurely and one gave birth to a stillborn infant

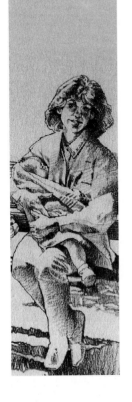

Glossary

abortion Expulsion of a fetus before it is viable

abruptio placenta Premature separation of a normally situated placenta

acetoacetic acid Ketone body

acetonuria Presence of acetone in the urine

achondroplasia Skeletal disease that produces a form of dwarfism

acidosis Condition in which excess hydrogen ions or lowered bicarbonate causes a marked lowering of pH

acinar structures Lobular, epithelial masses in the breast that are components of the milk-producing system; most numerous during pregnancy and lactation

acrodermatitis enteropathica Genetically transmitted eczematous disease linked to malabsorption of zinc

active transport Movement of substances across a membrane against the concentration gradient, requiring energy expenditure

adenohypophysis Anterior portion of the pituitary

adipose tissue Fatty tissue

adrenal glands Suprarenal glands; glands located at the upper end of each kidney. The cortex produces estrogen, androgen, progesterone, aldosterone, and cortisone; the medulla produces epinephrine and norepinephrine

adrenergic Pertaining to or causing stimulation of the sympathetic nervous system

adrenocortical hormones Hormones of the adrenal cortex: aldosterone and cortisone

adsorption Attachment of a substance to the surface of another substance

aflatoxin Potent and sometimes lethal fungal toxin

affective learning component Related to attitudes, feelings, or emotions

agnathia Congenital absence of the lower jaw

aldosterone Adrenocortical hormone that acts on the distal tubules of the kidney to resorb sodium and water and to excrete potassium

aliquot Known fraction of a sample

allergen Any agent capable of producing an allergic response

allergy Exaggerated response to a substance that is harmless in similar amounts to most people

alveolar tissue Terminal glandular tissue made up of lobules leading to the lactiferous ducts of the mammary gland

amenorrhea Absence or abnormal stoppage of menses

amino acids Fundamental structural units of protein

amylophagia Abnormal craving for starch; a type of pica

anencephaly Absence of a brain

angiotensinogen Precursor of angiotensin which is a vasoconstrictor substance found in the blood

anophthalmia Congenital absence of the eyeballs

anorexia Lack of or loss of appetite

anorexia nervosa Disease state characterized by rejection of food, extreme weight loss, and low basal metabolic rate

anovulation Absence of ovulation

antiemetics Agents that relieve vomiting

antigenic agents Proteins that stimulate antibody production

aortic stenosis Obstruction to the outflow of blood from the left ventricle into the aorta

Apgar scale Method for determining an infant's condition at birth by scoring the heart rate, respiratory effect, muscle tone, reflex irritability and color

apnea Transient cessation of breathing

apocrine Descriptive of cells that lose part of their protoplasm while secreting their particular product

arachidonic acid An unsaturated 20-carbon fatty acid that is a precursor of prostaglandin synthesis and is a component of lecithin and cephalin

areola Circular pigmented area surrounding the nipple of the breast

arrhymia Abnormal rhythm of the heartbeat

aspartame Dipeptide sweetener composed of phenylalanine and aspartic acid

ataxia Loss of muscle coordination

atrophy Wasting of a cell, tissue, or part

auscultory Pertaining to auscultation, which is the process of listening to sounds produced within the body by various organs as they perform their functions

basolateral membrane Lower part of the membrane between mucosal epithelial cells

behavioral learning component Related to behavior

betahydroxybutyric acid Ketone body

bioavailable nutrient Amount of nutrition that is actually absorbed, as opposed to that which is described in food tables

Bitot's spot Small, triangular silvery patch of epithelial degeneration, sometimes with a foamy surface, on the conjunctiva; may be found in persons with vitamin A deficiency

blastocyst Stage in the development of the embryo in which cells are arranged in a single layer to form a hollow sphere; a modified blastula

bonding Strong interaction between mother and child that develops through physical, visual, and aural contacts soon after birth

bradycardia Abnormal slowness of the heart rate and pulse

breast milk jaundice Physiological hyperbilirubinemia produced in the newborn after the first week; origin unknown

brown adipose tissue Type of storage fat that produces much heat; important in hibernating animals

bulimia Food bingeing followed by self-induced vomiting

calyx (calyces) Cuplike segments of the renal pelvis

cardiomyopathy Subacute or chronic disorders of the heart muscle

cardiorespiratory arrest Sudden cessation of heart and lung functions

casein Phosphoprotein; the principle protein of milk. The enzyme rennin, in the presence of calcium, converts milk proteins to curds and whey. Casein remains in the curds; the protein in the clear residual fluid is lactalbumin.

cephalopelvic disproportion Undesirable maternal pelvic shape for properly carrying a fetus.

cerebral palsy Partial paralysis and lack of muscle coordination resulting from a defect, injury or disease of the nervous tissue contained within the skull

cheilosis Angular cracks and fissures at the corners of the mouth characteristic of riboflavin deficiency. Lesions begin with redness and denudation along the line of closure or as pale macerations at the corners. Lips look dry and cracked; nonnutritional factors may also cause cheilosis.

cholestasis Retention and accumulation of bile in the liver due to factors within or outside the liver

cholesterol Chief steroid in the body; found in all tissues, especially the brain, nerves, adrenal cortex, and liver. It is a constituent of bile and serves as a precursor of vitamin D. Cholesterol within the body comes from two sources: (1) exogenous, or dietary, cholesterol, chiefly from egg yolk, liver, and other organ meats and dairy products; and (2) endogenous cholesterol, synthesized by the liver and other organs, such as the adrenal cortex, skin, and intestines. Cholesterol circulates in the blood as lipoprotein in combination with protein and other blood lipids. Total cholesterol, low-density lipoproteins (LDL), and high-density lipoproteins (HDL) are often reported. LDL fractions are strongly related to incidence of coronary heart disease; HDL fractions are inversely related to this disease.

chondrodystrophy Rickets in the fetus

chorea Nervous disease in which there are involuntary and irregular movements

chorionic gonadotropin Gonad-stimulating substance in human urine during pregnancy, commonly abbreviated as β-HCG

chromatography Measurement of color perception

cleft palate Congenital fissure of the palate

clonus Spasms in which rigidity and relaxation succeed each other

cobalamin Vitamin B_{12}, a cobalt-containing complex

cognitive learning component Related to the process of knowing and learning; mental processes of thinking and remembering

cognitive restructuring Process by which a person learns to challenge and replace harmful thoughts, beliefs, and attitudes

colic Abdominal pain

colostrum First liquid secreted by the mammary gland a few days after parturition. Compared with later milk secretion, it is higher in protein content and immunoglobulins, which contain antibodies responsible for immunity in the newborn. It is also higher in β-carotene, riboflavin, and niacinamide content but has less fat and carbohydrate than true milk.

computed tomography Measurement of selected internal planes or structures determined by serial roentgenogram (x-ray)

condom Rubber sheath worn over the penis in coitus, to prevent impregnation or infection

congenital lactase deficiency Condition present at birth in which the enzyme that breaks down lactose is absent

conjunctive Delicate membrane that lines the eyelids

corpus luteum Yellow mass in the ovary that is formed by the graafian follicle after it has matured and discharged the ovum

cortisol Major adrenal cortical steroid influencing carbohydrate metabolism. It increases the release of glucose from the liver, stimulates gluconeogenesis from amino acids, and decreases peripheral utilization of blood glucose. It is released into the blood and transported to the tissues in combination with a globulin as transcortin.

counseling Discussion between a person with expertise in solving particular problems and a person or persons with problems, within a relationship established for the purpose of solving these problems

cretinism Chronic condition occurring in fetal life or early infancy caused by deficient thyroid activity; characterized by arrested physical and mental development, dry skin, and low basal metabolic rate. Related to adult myxedema

cuboidal epithelium Epithelial tissue consisting of cells of cuboidal shape, like those that line the alveoli and ducts of the mammary tissue

cyclamate Artificial sweetener that has been banned from use in the United States

cyclophosphamide Anticancer drug

cystic acne Very severe acne characterized by the eruption of papules and pustules

cystic fibrosis Fatal disease in young children characterized by general dysfunction of the exocrine glands; the pancreas, respiratory system, salivary glands, gastrointestinal tract, biliary system, and paranasal glands may be involved. Sweat, when tested, contains abnormal amounts of sodium and potassium. Abnormal mucus secretion results in obstruction of mucus-producing cells or organ passages. Lack of pancreatic enzymes interferes with utilization of protein, fat, and carbohydrate. Vitamin and mineral deficiencies occur because of digestive defects.

decidua Membranous lining of the uterus shed after childbirth or at menstruation

dementia Any psychosis characterized by serious mental impairment or deterioration

demography Statistical study of populations

Denver Development Test Standardized screening device to assess developmental progress in children between 1 month and 6 years of age

deoxycorticosterone Hormone of the adrenal cortex very similar in structure to corticosterone

desensitization Abolition of sensitivity to a particular antigen

diaphragm Contraceptive device of molded rubber or other soft plastic material fitted over the cervix to prevent entrance of spermatozoa

dioxin Pesticide

diuretics Agents promoting urine secretion

diplopia Double vision

Down's syndrome Congenital condition characterized by specific chromosomal translocations or mosaics; mongolism. Various degrees of mental retardation have been described.

dysmature Infants born postterm, generally considered to be after 42 weeks' gestation

dysplasia Abnormal development or growth

dyspnea Difficult or labored breathing

dystocia Difficult parturition

eclampsia Combination of edema, hypertension, and proteinuria that may occur in late pregnancy (preeclampsia) and is sometimes followed by convulsions and coma

ectoderm Outermost of the three primitive germ layers of the embryo

ectopic pregnancy Pregnancy in which the fertilized ovum becomes implanted outside the uterus

electrophoresis Method used to analyze the plasma protein content; involves the movement of charged particles suspended in a liquid on various media

embolus Mass of clotted blood carried in the bloodstream

embryonal sarcoma Tumor made up of tissue looking like embryonic connective tissue; often highly malignant

emphysema Lung disorder in which the terminal bronchi become plugged with mucus

enamel hypoplasia Underdevelopment of tooth enamel

encephalography Roentgenographic photography of the brain

endoderm Innermost of the three primitive germ layers of the embryo

endometrium Mucous membrane lining the uterus

enteropathogenic organism Any organism, usually bacterial, that causes intestinal disease or disturbance

enzootic Present in an animal community at all times but associated with disease in only small numbers of cases

EPH-gestosis Edema-proteinuria-hypertension of pregnancy; preeclampsia

epicanthal fold Fold of skin projected over the inner angle of the eye at the junction of the eyelid

epidemiologic studies Examination of the factors that influence the frequency and distribution of infectious diseases in humans

epilepsy Disorder of the nervous system in which the major symptom is a convulsive seizure that results from a temporary disturbance of nerve impulses

epistaxia Hemorrhage from the nose; nosebleed

erythropoiesis Process of synthesizing red blood cells

esterification Formation of a compound from an alcohol and an acid by elimination of water

estrogen Collective term for natural and synthetic female sex hormones. Natural estrogens (estradiol, estrone, and estriol) are produced by maturing follicles in the ovary, placenta, and adrenal cortex. They are responsible for development of female sex organs, growth of genitalia and mammary glands, and development of secondary characteristics such as alteration in body contour and growth of axillary and pubic hair. In addition, estrogenic hormones have profound effects on calcium and phosphorus metabolism and are probably related to bone and lipid metabolism.

etiology Study and theory of causes of disease

exocytosis Excretion of a substance by pinching off of an out-pouching of the cell membrane after the membrane has changed shape to surround the substance

external rectus palsy Neuropathy or paralysis of the muscle that controls adduction or inward motion of the eye

extrinsic Originating outside the body. The length of the gastrointestinal tract, including the mouth, is considered extrinsic because it is essentially open from the mouth to the anus.

eustachian tube Narrow tube between the ear and the pharynx

facilitated diffusion Movement of molecules across membranes by a carrier molecule to equalize concentrations

failure to thrive (FTT) Descriptive of infants demonstrating growth failure with no clear pathological cause, such as inadequate intake of food, unusually high energy requirement, excessive losses from diarrhea or vomiting, or any two or more of these factors; FTT frequently affects the child who has been deprived of adequate maternal love and attention.

fecal impaction Confinement of feces in the bowel

fecundity Ability to reproduce

fetal alcohol syndrome (FAS) Combination of fetal anomalies, including microcephaly, the presence of epicanthal folds, micrognathia, and other less constant features that may be found in offspring of women who consume various levels of alcohol during pregnancy

fibrinolytic activity Process of clot dissolution

flatulence Excessive formation of gases in the intestines or stomach

fluorosis Mottling of tooth enamel that arises from excessive intake of fluorine, usually from water with concentrations over 2.5 ppm. Incidence and severity of the condition increase as levels approach 10 to 20 ppm

fontanelle Any one of the unossified spots on the head of an infant

formative evaluation Testing of preliminary materials and concepts with the target audience during the process of production to allow the authors or producers to make alterations to enhance the effectiveness of a program or audiovisual

formulogenic disease Disease resulting from any aspect of use or misuse of infant formulas

furosemide (Lasix) Potent diuretic, which if given in excess, can lead to profound diuresis with water and electrolyte depletion

galactopoietic factors Factors associated with milk production

galactorrhea Excessive flow of milk

galactosemia Inborn error of metabolism resulting in the presence of lactose in the blood. An inability to convert galactose to glucose is caused by the absence of the enzyme galactose-1-phosphate uridyl transferase. Symptoms are varied and may include jaundice, enlarged liver and spleen, anorexia, weight loss, vomiting, diarrhea, cataract formation, and mental retardation. Treatment consists of elimination of all galactose-containing foods from the diet.

geophagia Type of pica specific to eating of dirt

gestosis Any toxic manifestation occurring in pregnancy

gingival hypertrophy Overgrowth of the gums

glossitis Inflammation of the tongue, possibly caused by deficiency of one or more of the B vitamins. It may also occur with gastrointestinal tract disorders or from biting, burning, or injuring the tongue

glucocorticoid Term applied to those steroid hormones of the adrenal cortex that affect carbohydrate metabolism; cortisone and corticosterone

gluten-free diet Restrictive eating pattern in which foods containing the protein gluten are eliminated; these foods include wheat, rye, barley and oats

glycolipids Compound containing an alcohol, fatty acids and a carbohydrate

glycosylated hemoglobin Laboratory test estimating glucose association with hemoglobin; used to examine how well a diabetic is controlling her blood glucose level

gravida Pregnant woman; primigravida denotes a first pregnancy

growth retarded Length of weight measures below the third percentile on standard growth charts usually identify growth retardation; however, recognition of parent size must be included in such an evaluation

Guthrie test Microbiological assay for phenylalanine that can be performed on blood from a baby's heel; used in screening for phenylketonuria during the first week of life. Levels greater than 1 to 2 mg/100 ml of plasma mandate additional testing.

gynecological age Number of years that have passed since menstruation began

hematoma Tumor-like mass produced by coagulation of blood in a tissue or cavity

hemoconcentration Increase in the proportion of formed elements in the blood

hemodialysis Removal of certain elements from the blood by virtue of differences in rates of their diffusion through a semi-permeable membrane while the blood is being circulated outside the body

hemodilution Increase in the fluid content of blood, resulting in diminution of the proportion of formed elements

hemolytic anemia Anemia caused by the increased destruction of red blood cells

hemorrhoid Enlarged vein in the mucous membrane inside or just outside the rectum

herniation Abnormal protrusion of an organ or other body structure through a defect or natural opening in a covering membrane, muscle or bone

human chorionic somatomammotropin (HCS) Hormone of pregnancy, also called human placental lactogen (HPL); similar in structure and function to growth hormone, but, at term, this hormone reaches maternal circulating levels 1000 times that of growth hormone. Secretion occurs mainly during the third trimester of pregnancy. Functions are to stimulate protein metabolism-

anabolism and alter carbohydrate metabolism by diminishing insulin action and increasing mobilization of free fatty acids from maternal peripheral fat depots. In addition, it has a lactogenic effect on mammary glands, ensuring nutrition for the newborn infant.

human placental lactogen (HPL) *See* human chorionic somatomammotropin

hydrogen breath test Clinical test used to estimate degree of gas release in the lower bowel from undigested sugar

hydroscopic effect Water-holding tendency

hyper- Prefix denoting excess

hyperalimination Administration of higher than normal amounts of nutrients either orally or intravenously. In parenteral hyperalimentation an indwelling catheter is passed into the superior vena cava through which a hypertonic solution of glucose, amino acids, vitamins, and minerals can be administered continuously. Up to 4,000 kcal/day can be given by this method.

hyperbilirubinemia Excess bulirubin in the blood

hypercalcemia Excess calcium in the blood

hyperemesis gravidarum Severe nausea and vomiting in pregnancy

hyperemia Excess of blood in a part of the body

hyperlipidemia Excess of lipids in the blood

hyperlipoproteinemia Excess of lipoproteins in the blood, often a specific type

hyperphagia Excessive appetite/overeating

hyperplasia Term applied to rapidly increased cell numbers; describes both the interval of cell replication that occurs immediately after conception and before cell growth begins and also the increased cell numbers in tumor growth

hypertrophy Describes increased cell size or growth as opposed to increased cell numbers

hyperventilation Increase in air in the lungs above the normal amount

hypo- Prefix indicating reduced; lower than normal

hypoalbuminemia Low blood albumin level

hyponatremia Low blood sodium level

hypoperistalsis Low intestinal smooth muscle contraction leading to slow movement of food and feces through the intestinal tract

hypophysectomy Excision of the pituitary gland

hyporeninemic hypoaldosteronism Reduced activity of both renin-angiotension and aldosterone hormones, which results in electrolyte imbalance and edema

hypotonia Reduced muscle tone

hypovolemia Abnormally decreased volume of circulating fluid

hypoxia Diminished availability of oxygen to body tissues

immunogenic Producing immunity

immunoglobin Antibodies; specialized proteins with a capacity to combine chemically with the specific antigens stimulating their production

intra- Prefix signifying within, such as intracellular (within the cell) and intravenous (within the vein)

intrinsic Inherent; belonging to the real nature of a thing

intrinsic factor Chemical substance present in normal gastric juice that facilitates absorption of vitamin B_{12}; its secretion is impaired in pernicious anemia and often following gastrectomy

intubation Insertion of a tube (into a variety of sites)

involution Reduction in size, such as the return of the uterus to normal size after delivery of an infant

isotretinoin Drug containing a vitamin A analogue, used to treat a variety of skin conditions

jaundice (icterus) Yellowish discoloration of skin, mucous membranes, and certain body fluids caused by an accumulation of bile pigments in the blood either from reduced excretion resulting from failure of the liver or from increased production of bile pigments from hemoglobin

jejunoileal bypass Surgical procedure for shortening the small intestine by linking the jejunum with the ileum and thereby reducing its total absorptive area; used for some persons with gross obesity

juxtaglomerular apparatus Component of the kidney, located near the glomerulus, responsible for sensing the level of sodium in the bloodstream

kaliuresis Excessive elimination of potassium (kalium) in the urine

karyotype Map of the chromosomes of a cell

keratomalacia Softening and necrosis of the cornea of the eye. The earliest sign is dryness of the conjunctiva, which may lead to ulceration and blindness; associated with vitamin A deficiency

keto- Prefix denoting the presence of a ketone or carbonyl group

ketoacidosis Metabolic acidosis with markedly increased production of ketoacids; breath may have a fruity or acetone odor. Alkali reserves in plasma are decreased, hyperventilation may occur, carbon dioxide tension in alveolar air is reduced, urinary ammonia is increased, and blood pH falls.

ketogenesis Synthesis of ketone bodies

ketone bodies Term given to intermediate products of fatty acid degradation. These are acetoacetic acid, β-hydroxybutyric acid, and acetone, believed to stem from acetoacetyl CoA.

ketosis Clinical condition in which ketone bodies accumulate in the blood and appear in the urine; acetone odor is apparent in breath

koilonychia Spoon-shaped nails; nail deformity in which the outer surface of the nail is concave

lactalbumin Protein found in the whey component of milk

lactase Enzyme that splits lactose to glucose and galactose

lactiferous ducts Mammary ducts that extend radially from the nipple toward the chest wall and that transport milk toward the nipple or store milk that has been produced by lobular epithelial masses (acinar structures)

lactogenesis Production of milk by the mammary glands

lacunae Small pit, hollow, or depression

lanolin Wool fat or wool grease that is refined and incorporated into many commercial preparations

let-down reflex Neurohormonal mechanism regulated in part by central nervous factors; the primary stimulus is sucking on the nipple, which triggers discharge of oxytocin from the posterior pituitary. Oxytocin is then transported in the blood to the myoepithelial cells around the alveoli, causing them to contract, thereby pushing the milk out of the alveoli and along the ductal system to the nipple.

linoleic acid Essential fatty acid; a polyunsaturated fatty acid with two double bonds and 18 carbon atoms found in linseed, safflower, cottonseed, soybean, corn, and fish oils and in animal tissues. Infantile eczema, with leathery skin and desquamation and oozing, may occur when formulas lacking in essential fatty acids are used.

linolenic acid Polyunsaturated fatty acid with growth-promoting effect; contains three double bonds and 18 carbon atoms and can be synthesized in the body with linoleic acid

lipase Fat-splitting enzyme occurring in the pancreas, stomach, and certain plants. It hydrolyzes fats into fatty acids and glycerol.

lipolysis Breaking down of fat

lipoprotein Compound protein formed by union of a simple protein with a lipid; involved in lipid transport. Four types that circulate in blood are chylomicrons, α-lipoproteins (high-density lipoproteins [HDL]), pre-β-lipoproteins (very-low-density lipoprotein [VLDL]), and β-lipoproteins (low-density lipoprotein [LDL])

lipoprotein lipase Enzyme that catalyzes the hydrolysis of fats present in chylomicrons and lipoproteins; found in various tissues and important in mobilization of fatty acids from depot fats

lithium Chemical element, atomic number 3

Lofenalac Proprietary milk substitute useful in dietary management of phenylketonuria. It is prepared by enzymatic digestion of casein, which is then followed by treatment to destroy phenylalanine and supplementation with methionine, tryptophan, tyrosine, corn oil, sugar, minerals, and vitamins (Mead Johnson).

luteinizing hormone (LH) One of the gonadotropic hormones. It provokes ovulation and the formulation of the corpus luteum; stimulates the interstitial cells of the ovary and testicle.

lyophilization Freeze-drying under vacuum; useful in biochemistry for protein fractionization and stabilization of tissue samples

macrocytosis Presence of abnormally large red blood cells in the blood

macrosomia Great bodily size; in this text, refers to a very large baby at birth

malocclusion Distortion of the bony structures of the oral cavity such that teeth do not demonstrate optimum alignment

mammogenesis Development of the mammary glands

marasmus Form of extreme undernutrition primarily caused by lack of calories and protein. Atrophy in infants that occurs as a sequel to acute disease, especially diarrhea; characterized by weight loss, subcutaneous fat loss, and wasting of muscle tissue. The term is also used by social scientists to describe the failure to thrive syndrome seen in infants who receive minimum care and no warm interaction with the caregiver.

mastitis Inflammation of the breast, particularly the mammary glands

maxillofacial Pertaining to the relationship of the jawbone and the face

meconium Dark green mucilaginous material in the intestine of the full-term fetus; it constitutes the first stools passed by the newborn infant

media Intermediate processes or carriers that permit communication through space and time

megablastic anemia Type of anemia characterized by larger than normal red blood cells (macrocytosis); symptomatic of folacin and/or vitamin B_{12} deficiency

megaloblastosis Presence in the bloodstream of very large red blood cells

menarche Time when menstruation begins

meningocele *See* spina bifida

meningomyelocele *See* spina bifida

menopause Time when menstruation ends permanently

mesoderm Intermediate layer of cells developing between the ectoderm and endoderm of the embryo

metalloenzymes Enzymes containing some mineral

methotrexate Poisonous compound used as an anti-cancer agent

methylxanthines Classification of compounds into which caffeine falls

microcephaly Small size of the head in relation to the rest of the body

mineralocorticoid Term applied to adrenocortical hormones that regulate electrolyte balance. Aldosterone is the most potent.

miscarriage Spontaneous interruption of pregnancy before the seventh month

monovalent ions Having a valence of one, like Na^+ and Cl^-

morbidity Pertaining to disease

mortality Pertaining to death

mutagenic Capable of producing changes in DNA or chromosomal structure, resulting in permanent alteration in the genetic information carried by DNA

myelination Production of myelin (a fatty-like substance) around the axons

myoepithelial tissue Muscle layer of the lining of vessels and small cavities and other coverings of the body

necrotizing enterocolitis Disease seen in infants that involves degeneration of a part of the intestinal tract

neonatal Period of early infancy within 28 days following birth

neoplasia Condition characterized by the presence of new growths (tumors)

nephrotic syndrome Set of symptoms applied to renal diseases characterized by marked edema and heavy proteinuria

neurotransmitter Classification of chemical compounds in the nervous system responsible for the transfer of information

normochromic Normal color

normocytic Normal size

nystagmus Continuous movement of the eyeball

ocular fundi Back portions of the interior of the eyeballs

oliguria Decreased urinary output or volume

organohalides Organic compounds containing a halogen (bromide, chlorine, fluorine, iodine)

orthopnea Inability to breathe except in an upright position

osmolality Measure of solute per solvent as opposed to osmolarity, which is the measure of solute to solution

osmolarity Total ionic solute concentration of a solution

otitis media Inflammation of the middle ear

ovarectomy Removal of an ovary

oxytocin (Pitocin) Hormone synthesized in the hypothalamus and transported to the posterior pituitary as a larger peptide, neurophysine. It stimulates uterine contractions and promotes "let-down." Muscular walls of the intestine, gallbladder, and urinary bladder are also stimulated by this hormone. Pitocin is used clinically to induce labor.

pallor Absence of skin coloration

palpebral fissure Eyelid opening

papillae Small nippleshaped elevations on various organs. The term is usually preceded or followed by a locating term, such as mammary papillae.

para When followed by a number, para describes the number of viable births in a woman's obstetrical history. Primipara denotes the previous birth of one child.

parity Condition of a woman with respect to her having borne viable offspring

parturition Delivery of the fetus from the body of the maternal organism

pelvimetry Measurement of the capacity and diameter of the pelvis, either internally or externally or both

penicillamine Amino acid obtained from penicillin by treatment with hot mineral acids; used in the treatment of diseases characterized by copper deposition in the body

peptide Small compound with two or more amino acids

periductal structures Structures surrounding a duct; the fibrous and fatty tissues responsible for the increasing size of the adolescent female mammary gland

perinatal period Interval overlapping the last half of pregnancy and the neonatal period of 28 days after birth

peripartum Around the time of delivery of the fetus

Peyer's patches Whitish patches of lymphatic follicles in mucous and submucous layers of the small intestine

phagocytosis Process of ingestion of a foreign particle across the cell membrane in which a portion of the cell membrane develops the foreign body and then pinches it off from the surface, creating an intracellular vacuole

Phenyl-free Phenylalanine-free beverage for individuals with PKU

phenylketonuria (PKU) Inborn error of metabolism transmitted as a simple mendelian recessive trait. The absence of the liver enzyme phenylalanine hydroxylase results in failure to convert phenylalanine to tyrosine. Buildup of phenylpyruvic acid in the blood results in mental retardation, reduced growth and head size, reduced pigment production, eczematous dermatitis, and poor muscle coordination. Treatment by dietary restriction of phenylalanine intake to no more than the minimum required for growth and function can prevent mental retardation when instituted shortly after birth.

physiological adjustment Clinical and/or physiological changes observed during altered conditions such as pregnancy for which standard norms are no longer applicable. Norms may or may not be available for specific altered conditions.

pinocytosis Uptake of fluid material by a living cell, particularly by means of invagination of the cell membrane and vacuole formation

PKU-3 Beverage product for individuals with PKU

placenta previa Condition in which the placenta is located in the lower uterine segment instead of in the proper position higher on the uterine wall

placental lactogen *See* human placental lactogen

ploidy Chromosome status; usually either diploid, with a full complement of chromosomes from both parents, or haploid, as in the gamete with only half the number of chromosomes found in somatic cells

Polycose Commercial product providing glucose (in solution) in the form of glucose polymers, short glucose chains that are easily digested

ponderal index Index of normality of body composition; height/cube root of weight (H/W1/3)

postneonatal period Interval in infancy between the end of the first 28 days and the end of the first year of life

postprandial After a meal

preeclampsia Hypertension, proteinuria, and edema occurring during the latter half of pregnancy. (*See* eclampsia)

prelacteal Before the beginning of milk production

primipara Woman who has had one pregnancy that resulted in a viable offspring

protocolitis Inflammation of the colon and rectum

progesterone Hormone produced by the corpus luteum in preparation for the reception and development of the fertilized ovum by glandular proliferation of the endometrium; also produced by the placenta during pregnancy

progestogen General term for any of a variety of progesterone derivatives; often contained in contraceptive agents

prolactin Luteotropic hormone (LTH). A hormone secreted by the anterior lobe of the pituitary that helps in development of the mammary gland and initiates milk secretion. It stimulates the corpus luteum to synthesize progesterone and estrogens.

prophylaxis Prevention of disease

point-of-purchase Location, or point in a store, at which a consumer makes a purchase, and where educational or promotional material may be available to the consumer

prostaglandins Hormones composed of 14 fatty acids with 20 carbons, of which carbons 8 to 12 are involved in a five-membered ring. Polyunsaturated fatty acids serve as precursors for these compounds. They may function as blood pressure depressants, smooth muscle stimulants, and/or antagonists to several other hormones.

proteolytic enzymes Enzymes that digest proteins

prothrombin time (PT) Length of time required for blood to clot; useful in measuring amounts of prothrombin and assessing vitamin K sufficiency

puerperal infection Infectious disease of childbirth

puerperium Period between parturition and the time the mother's womb or uterus returns to normal, usually about 6 weeks

pyelonephritis Inflammation of the kidney and renal pelvis

reflex Involuntary response to a given stimulus

relactation Reinstatement of lactation without pregnancy and following an interval of nonlactation. Sucking is the primary stimulus for prolactin secretion, and adequate stimulation will often produce milk flow

reliability May be defined as the extent to which the measure gives the same results on repeated applications to avoid assessing chance or random error

renal solute load Dissolved molecules that enter the kidney for excretion and/or reabsorption

renin-angiotensin-aldosterone system Interactive system whereby kidney production of renin-angiotensin promotes sodium and water retention with resultant increases in aldosterone synthesis and secretion by the adrenal cortex, which in turn promote sodium retention and potassium excretion

reserpine Drug used as an antihypertensive, sedative, or tranquilizer

respiratory quotient Expression of the ratio of the carbon dioxide produced to the oxygen consumed by the organism

retrognathia Receding jawbone

rooting reflex Automatic turn of an infant's face toward the source of a stimulus to the cheek

saccharin Noncaloric artificial sweetener, approved for use in the U.S. food supply

septicemia Presence of bacteria or their toxins in the blood

spermicides Chemical agents that kill spermatozoa

spina bifida Cleft spine; this condition may be accompanied by a protruding fluid-filled sac formed solely from the membrane of the spinal cord (meningomyelocele) or including local herniation of the spinal cord into the protruding sac (meningomyelocele)

splenic atrophy Deterioration of the spleen

stasis Stoppage of the flow of body fluid in its compartment

sterilization Process of rendering an individual incapable of reproduction

stomatitis Inflammation of the oral mucosa or soft tissues of the mouth

stroma Tissue that forms the ground substance or matrix of an organ; supporting framework

suck Reflexive response of neonate in which sucking, swallowing, and breathing are rhythmically coordinated; different in process from the true sucking that develops later

sucking Acquired feature of orofacial muscles. It is a discontinuous process in which both sucking and breathing are interrupted by swallowing, as opposed to the reflexive suck of the neonate.

suckling Pattern of milk expression that occurs intermediate to reflexive suck and true sucking in which milk is apparently squirted directly into the lateral food channels, bypassing a need for alternation between breathing and swallowing

summative evaluation Assessment of program outcomes

supine Lying with the face upward

syndactyly Most common congenital anomaly of the hand, marked by the persistence of the webbing between adjacent digits; the anomaly may also occur in the foot

synergism Joint action of agents such that the combined effects are greater than the sum of the individual effects

tachycardia Rapid heartbeat. The term is usually applied to a pulse rate above 100 beats per minute.

tachypnea Very rapid respiration

taurine Bile acid

teratogen Agent or disease state capable of causing congenital malformations, monstrosities, and other serious deviations from normal fetal development

thermogenesis Production of heat in organisms

therapeutic nutrition education Facilitates change in behavior related to nutrition, must include components addressing attitudes and knowledge

thromboembolism Obstruction of a vessel by a plug found at its point of origin

thrombosis Development of a blood clot

toxemia General term historically given to disorders of late-pregnancy in which hypertension, proteinuria, and edema occur and convulsions and coma may occur. The terms preeclampsia and eclampsia are generally used, and neither is related to toxins in the blood as the term appears to indicate.

transaminases Enzymes that catalyze the transfer of an amino group from one compound to another

triglyceride Fat molecule with three fatty acids attached to a glycerol backbone

trophoblast Extraembryonic ectodermal tissue on the surface of the cleaving, fertilized ovum, which is responsible for contact with the maternal circulation and supply of nutrients to the embryo. It contributes to the syncytium of maternal-embryonic tissues of the placenta

tympanic membranes Thin, semitransparent membranes that stretch across the ear canal separating the middle ear from the outer ear; also called the eardrum

ultrasonography Noninvasive nonradiologic method of examining internal structures by means of reflected sound waves; commonly used to assess fetal growth

urogenital anomalies Conditions in which the reproductive and urinary systems failed to develop normally

uteroplacental perfusion Passage of fluids between the uterus and the placenta

validity Refers to the extent to which an instrument measures what it purports to measure. Its concern is with systematic error, that is, changes that are part of the natural variation in the phenomenon under study

vasopressin Hormone of the posterior pituitary that exerts both pressor and antidiuretic action. The pressor effect is the result of peripheral vasoconstriction in the systemic arterioles and capillaries. There is constriction of the coronary and pulmonary vessels and dilation of cerebral and renal vessels. The antidiuretic effect is exerted in the collecting tubules of the kidney, accelerating the rate of water reabsorption and causing an increase in urine volume with high concentrations of sodium, chloride, phosphate, and total nitrogen.

vasopressor agent Compound that stimulates contraction of the muscular tissue of capillaries and arteries

vegans Subgroup of vegetarians who subsist entirely on plants

vegetarian Person who consumes no animal tissue protein and who may or may not use eggs and dairy products

venipuncture Puncture of a vein for therapeutic purposes or for collection of blood specimens

videodisc Distribution format on which materials produced by traditional means (16-mm film, slides, video) are reproduced in a format that can integrate computers in a way that may allow for interaction

villous atrophy Degeneration of the lining of the small intestine

Wernicke's encephalopathy Disease caused by an acute biochemical lesion in the brain resulting from thiamin deficiency. Wernicke first described the syndrome in alcoholics. It is characterized by paralysis or weakness of eye muscles, ataxia, and mental disturbances.

whey Liquid that remains after curd and cream are removed from milk; contains lactose and lactalbumin

xerosis Abnormal dryness of the skin, mucous membranes, or conjunctiva

Yom Kippur Jewish holiday observed from Tishri in accordance with rights described by Leviticus 16

Index

A

Abdominal disorder, 64
Abortion
    maternal death and, 5
    neural tube defect and, 146
    spontaneous, 59
Abuse, substance, 52-53; *see also* Alcohol
Acetone, calorie restriction and, 139
Acid
    amino; *see* Amino acid
    fatty
        in breast milk, 347t, 356, 357-358
        essential, 142-143
Acne, cystic, 159
Acquired immunodeficiency syndrome, 380-382, *382,* 434-435
Acrodermatitis enteropathica, 374
ACTH, 333t
Active transport, 86
A&D Ointment, 424t
Adipose tissue
    brown
        carnitine and, 359
        energy and, 131
    deposition of, in pregnancy, 70
    malnutrition and, 107
    volume of, 81, *84*
Adolescent
    anorexia nervosa in, 282-283
    bulimia in, 283-284
Adolescent pregnancy, 292-316
    demographics of, *293,* 293-294, 296
    expectations versus reality as, 295t
    infant of, 297-298
    international perspective of, 312-313
    maternal health and, 8-9
    mortality in, 297, 297t
    nutrition in, 215, 302-312
        assessment of, 308-309
        calcium and, 307-308
        dietary patterns in, 309-310
        energy and, 305-306
        factors influencing, 303
        folate and, 308
        improvement of, 310-312
        iron and, 306-307
        protein and, 306
        Recommended Dietary Allowance and, 304t, 304-305
    outcome of, 32-33, 298-302, *300, 301,* 302t

Adolescent pregnancy—cont'd
    rates of, 2-3
    special programs concerning, 313-315
    weight gain and, 75
    weight-related disorders in, 311-312
Adrenocortical steroid, 324
Adverse pregnancy outcome; *see* Pregnancy outcome
Advertising, 458-459
Aflatoxin, 206
Age, maternal
    adolescent pregnancy and, 292-316; *see also* Adolescent pregnancy
    birth rate and, 2t, 2-3, 7t
    hypertension and, 261
    low-birth-weight infant and, 9t
    maternal death and, 5-6
    nutrition assessment and, 231-232
    pregnancy outcome and, 8-9, 33-34
    smoking and, 208
Agent Orange, 205
AIDS, 380-382, *382,* 434-435
Alanine, 68
Albumin, 230, 263
Alcohol
    in breast milk, 377, *379,* 380
    fertility and, 37
    fetal effects of, 52-53, 195-203, *196,* 197t, *198, 200-202*
    nutrition assessment and, 233-234
    pregnancy outcome and, 12
Aldosterone, 66
Allergy
    breastfeeding and, 396-397
    nutrition assessment and, 233
Alphatocopherol, 161
Aluminum phosphate salt, 177
Alveolar cell of breast, 326, *326,* 328
Amenorrhea
    breastfeeding and, 399
    hypercarotenemia and, 37
    postpartum, 35
American Academy of Pediatrics
    drugs in breast milk and, 375
    office visits and, 416
    phenylketonuria and, 274
    weaning and, 439
American College of Obstetricians and Gynecologists, 211-212
American Diabetes Association, 264, 269
Amino acid
    in breast milk, 347t, 351

Amino acid—cont'd
  oral contraceptives and, 41
  phenylketonuria and, 277
  total parenteral nutrition, 286
Amniocentesis, 155
Amylophagia, 194-195
Anemia, 256t, 256-258, 257t, 258t
  in breastfed infant, 363
  folate deficiency, 258
  hemolytic, pica and, 195
  iron deficiency, 171-172, 256-258, 257t
  megaloblastic, 258
    folic acid and, 145
    vitamin B$_{12}$ and, 156
  pernicious, 152
Anencephaly, *145,* 145-146
Anorexia nervosa, 282-283, 311-312
  breastfeeding and, 435
  drug abuse and, 234
Anovulation
  breastfeeding and, 399
  in postpartum period, 34-35
Anterior axillary line, 319
Anthropometric data in nutrition assessment, 223, 225-226
Antigen, 373
Antihypertensive therapy, 264
Antiinfective properties of breast milk, 370, 370t, *372,* 372-374, *373,* 395-396
Arachidonic acid
  in breast milk, 358
  pregnancy and, 142
Areola of breast, 321
Artificial infant feeding
  breastfeeding versus, 393, 394, 395
  promotion of, 400-401
  volume of, 414
Artificial sweetener; *see* Aspartame
Ascorbic acid (vitamin C), 368, *369, 371*
Aspartame
  breast milk and, 351, 354
  fetal effects of, 53
  pregnancy and, 204
Assessment, nutrition; *see* Nutrition assessment
Atopic disease, 396-397
Attachment, 398
Attitudinal nutrition education, 449
Audience for nutrition education, 461
Audiovisual aid to education, 459-463, 4464t
Autoimmune disease, hypertension and, 261
Aversion, food, 193-194, 242
Axillary line, anterior, 319

B

"Baby-friendly" hospital, 410, 412-413
Background personal data, 233-234
Bacteria, resistance to, 370, 370t, *372,* 372-374, *373*
Bag Balm, 424t
Banked milk, HIV infection and, 382
Basal energy expenditure, 285-286
Basal metabolic rate, 130, *131,* 133
  adolescent and, 305

Basolateral membrane of alveolar cell, 328
Behavior
  new, 239
  nutrition education and, 449
Belief, food, 193-194
Bifidus factor, 350-351
Bile acid, taurine and, 354
Bile-salt-stimulated lipase, 359, 395
Bilights for jaundice, 427
Bilirubin, 427
Binge drinking, 197
Binge eating disorder, 282, 283-284, 311-312
Biological immaturity of adolescent, 298-302, *300, 301,* 302t
Birth, diabetes and, 270-271
Birth control
  breastfeeding and, 35
  counseling about, 46-47
  intrauterine device for, 46
  nutrition and, 38-39
  oral contraceptives and, 39-46, 40t, 43t, *44, 45,* 46t
Birth defect
  folic acid and; *see* Folic acid/folate
  phenylketonuria and, 271-272, 272t
  vitamin A causing, 158t
Birth rate, 2t, 2-3
Birth spacing, 34-35, 36t
Birth weight
  low; *see* Low-birth-weight infant
  malnutrition and, 107
  maternal, 32, 33
  nutrition assessment and, 232
  nutritional correlates of, 108-110, *109, 110*
  phenylketonuria and, 273
  smoking and, 206-208
  supplementation and, 111
  WIC program and, 120
  zinc and, 180
Blacks; *see* Racial/ethnic factors
Blastogenesis, 103
Bleeding, vitamin K and, 162
Blood cells
  anemia and, 256t, 256-258, 257t, 258t
  folate in, 150t
  iron-binding capacity and, 230
  pregnancy and, 60
Blood level
  glucose, 265-266
  hemoglobin, 172-173
  phenylalanine, 272-273
Blood pressure
  birth weight and, 110
  hypertension and, 259-264; *see also* Hypertension
  pregnancy and, 59
Blood test for genetic disorder, 155
Blood volume in pregnancy, 59-63, *60, 61*
Blood-forming nutrient, 229-231
Body, ketone, 134, 138-139
Body mass index, *78, 79*
  obesity and, 280
  underweight and, 282

Body mass index—cont'd
  weight problems and, 279
Body water, 69t
Body weight; *see* Birth weight; Weight *entries*
Bone
  calcium and, 174
  vitamin D and, 161
Bottle-feeding of infant
  breastfeeding versus, 393, 394, *394,* 395
  promotion of, 400-401
  volume of, 414
Bowel movement of infant, 415-416
Brain
  fetal, 103
    fatty acids and, 142
  iodine and, 178
Breast
  anatomy of, 319, *320,* 321
  development of, 321-324, *322, 324*
Breast cancer, protection against, 399
Breast cup, 408, *409*
Breast milk; *see* Milk, human
Breastfeeding; *see also* Lactation; Milk, human
  adequacy of, 413-414, 415-416
  anovulation and, 35
  assessment of, 413-414
  benefits of, 393-405
    allergy and, 396-397
    cognitive, 397-398
    gastrointestinal, 395
    immunologic, 395-396
    nutritional, 397
    protective, 398-405
  case study about, 340, 436
  concerns about, 419-421, 423
  contraindications to, 436-437
  cost of, 341, 399-400
  discomfort with, 423-424, 424t-425t, 425-427
  duration of, 334
  frequency of, 414-415
  illness or separation and, 427-436, 428t, 429t, *430-433*
  latching on and, 418-419, *419*
  of multiple infants, 437, *439*
  nutrition education and, 452-453
  positioning for, 416, *417, 418,* 418
  in postpartum period, 409-410, 412-413
  preconceptual and prenatal period and, 405-406, 407t-
    408t, 408-409, *409*
  promotion of, 400-405
  resources about, 411-412
  successful, 334
  suck cycle in, *422*
  weaning from, 437, 439
  working and, 437
Breathing of breastfeeding infant, 414
Bromocriptine, 399
Brown adipose tissue
  carnitine and, 359
  energy and, 131
Bulimia, 283-284, 311-312

C

Cabbage leaves for breast engorgement, 426
Cadmium, 205
Caffeine, 203
  in breast milk, 380
  fertility and, 37
  fetal effects of, 52-53
  nutrition assessment and, 234
Calcium, 173-177, 174t, *175, 178*
  adolescent pregnancy and, 307-308
  in breast milk, *362*
  hypertension and, 264
  lactation and, 339-341
  vitamin D and, 161
Calcium-phosphorus balance, 176-177
Calories; *see also* Energy
  infant requirement of, 414
  protein and, 141
  restriction of, 136, 138-139
  supplementation and, 116
Cancer
  maternal, 436-437
  protection against, 398, 399
Candidiasis, 426-427
Carbohydrate
  in breast milk, 328-329, 359-360
  diabetes and, 268
  as energy source, 134
  obesity and, 281
  oral contraceptives and, 40-41
  total parenteral nutrition and, 286
Carbon monoxide, 206-207
Cardiac output, 59
Cardiovascular system in pregnancy, 59
Caries, fluoride and, 184
Carnitine, 359
Carotene, amenorrhea and, 37
Casein, 350-351
Catheter, central line, 285
Cell
  blood; *see* Blood cells
  lipid deposition in, 103
  mammary gland, *325*
Cell growth, 99-100
Centers for Disease Control and Prevention
  folic acid recommendations and, 50, 51
  HIV infection and, 381
Central line catheter, 285
Central nervous system
  iodine and, 178
  vitamin B_{12} and, 156-157
Cessation, smoking, 209
Chart, weight gain, 76, *77-80,* 81
Chemicals in breast milk, 376-377, 437
Chemotherapy, 436-437
Child, nutrition education for, 451
Chlorinated dioxin derivatives, 205
Chlorinated hydrocarbons in breast milk, *377*
Cholesterol
  in breast milk, 356, 358-359

Cholesterol—cont'd
  pregnancy and, 62-63
Chorionic gonadotropin
    lactation and, 323-324, 333t
    placenta and, 88-89
Chorionic somatomammotropin, 89, 173
Chorionic villus sampling, 155
Chromium, 365
Chronic disease, 53-54
Cigarette smoking; *see* Smoking
Clay ingestion, 194-195
Cocaine, 209-210
  in breast milk, 376
  nutrition assessment and, 234
Coffee, breast milk and, 380
Cognitive development of breastfed infant, 397-398
Cognitive restructuring, 311
Colic, 421
Coliform, 370, 372
Colostrum, 349-350, 372
Commercial factors in nutrition, 458-459
Commodities Distribution Program, Supplemental, *250,* 251
Community leaders, nutrition education for, 452
Community nutrition services, 245, 251-252
Compliance with PKU diet, 278
Compress, for breast, 426
Conception, interval between, 34-35, 36t, 399
  nutrition education and, 453
Congenital disorder
  lactase deficiency as, 360
  malnutrition and, 107
  rate of, 18t
Constipation, 244
Consultant, lactation, 393
Contaminant
  in breast milk, 375-380, 376t, 378t, *379,* 379t, 437
  in food, 204-206
Contraceptive, oral, 39-46, 40t, 43t, *44, 45,* 46t
  lactation and, 330
Copper, 182-183
Cortisol, lactation and, 329-330
Cortisone, 67-68
Cost of breastfeeding, 341, 399-400
Cost-benefit analysis of nutritional services, 121, 122t-123t, 124-125
Counseling
  for adolescent, 310-312
  breastfeeding and, 402-403
  contraception and, 46-47
  nutrition, 448-449, 456-457
  phenylketonuria and, 274-275
Cow's milk
  amino acid content of, 353t
  fatty acids in, 356
  minerals in, 361
  vitamin E and, 367
  whey proteins in, 350-351
Cramp, leg, magnesium and, 177-178
Cranial neural crest defect, 159, *160*
Craving, 193-194

Creatinine, 231
Crest, neural, 159, *160*
Crohn's disease, 398
Crystal, lead, 205
Cup, breast, 408, *409*
Cyanide, in cigarette smoke, 206-207
Cyclamate, 204
Cycle
  menstrual, breast and, 323
  suck, *422*
Cyclophosphamide, 375
Cystic acne, 159

D

Daily food plan, 246t-249t
Day-care program for child of adolescent, 315
DDT in breast milk, 377, 378t
Death
  fetal; *see* Fetus, death of
  infant; *see* Infant mortality
  maternal, 3-8, *4,* 4t, 5t, *6,* 6t
    adolescent, 297, 297t
Demand feeding, 415
Dentition, fluoride and, 184
Deoxycorticosterone, 110
Deoxyribonucleic acid
  cell growth and, 99
  folic acid and, 144
Dermatitis, atopic, 396-397
Development, fetal; *see* Growth, fetal
Diabetes mellitus, 255, 264-271, 287-288
  classification of, 266t
  energy metabolism and, 265-267, 266t
  management of, 266-270
  postpartum care in, 270-271
  preconception assessment of, 53-54
  protection against, 398
Diarrhea
  in breastfed infant, 395
  resistance against, 374
Dichlorodiphenyltrichloroethane in breast milk, 377, 378t
Diet
  adolescent pregnancy and, 309-310
  diabetes and, 269
  for nursing mother, 335, 335t, *336,* 337-342, *338, 340*
  phenylketonuria and, 275, 276t, 277-279
  prime-time, 458
  sodium-restricted, 184-185, *185, 186*
  for woman of child-bearing age, 153t-154t
Diet analysis, 236, 238t
Diet history, 234-236, 235t
Diet history questionnaire, 237
Dietary Guidelines, 454
Dieting, 136, 138-139
  breastfeeding and, 338-339
Dioxin derivatives, 205
Dirt ingestion, 194-195
DNA
  cell growth and, 99
  folic acid and, 144

Docosahexaenoic acid, 142, 358
Drug
  in breast milk, 375-376, 376t, 435-436
  bromocriptine, 399
  copper deficiency and, 183
  nutrition assessment and, 233
Drug abuse; *see also* Alcohol
  asking about, 199, 201
  fetal effects of, 52-53
  nutrition assessment and, 234
Duct, lactiferous, 321

E

Early fetal period, 13, 14
Eating disorder, 282-284
  adolescent and, 311-312
Eclampsia, 260t
Ectoderm, 103
Ectopic pregnancy, 4
Edema, 223
  hypertension and, 261, 262
Education
  about breastfeeding, 403-405
  birth control and, 38
  folic acid and, 152
  nutrition; *see* Nutrition education
  obstetrical history and, 10
  sex, 294
Ejection reflex, 414
  milk, 331
Electric breast pump, 429t, 429-430, *430*
Electrolytes
  hyperemesis gravidarum and, 259
  hypertension and, 262-263
  total parenteral nutrition, 286
Embryology, 103
Emotional stress, 312
Emulsion, fat, 286
Enamel hypoplasia, 161
Endoderm, 103
Endometrium, 259
Endoplasmic reticulum, rough, 324
Energy
  adolescent pregnancy and, 305-306
  daily food plan and, 247t
  diabetes and, 265-267, 266t, 268
  expenditure of, in pregnancy, 129-131, *130, 131,* 131t
  five-country studies of, 132t, 132-133, 133t
  food restriction and, 136, 138-139
  hypertension and, 263
  lactation and, 337, 339
  obesity and, 281
  pregnancy and, 68, 133-134, *137*
  protein and, 139-142
  requirement for, 129t, 129-131, *130*
  sources of, 134, 138-139
  total parenteral nutrition, 285-286
  weight gain and, 226
Engorgement, breast, 426
Enterocolitis, necrotizing, 374
Environment, nutritional, 242, 447-449, *448*

Environmental factors in neural tube defect, 147
Environmental pollutant in breast milk, 376-377, 378t-379t
Environmental stress in adolescent pregnancy, 298-302
Enzyme
  in breast milk
    lipase, 359
    proteolytic, 351
  lactation and, 328
  nutrition assessment and, 231
Epidemiological study, of malnutrition, 106-107
Epithelium of breast, 321
Erythrocyte; *see* Red blood cells
Erythropoiesis, 167-168
Escherichia coli, 370, 372, 374
Essential fatty acid, 142-143
Estrogen
  breast and, 323
  calcium and, 173
  function of, 332t
  hyperemesis gravidarum and, 259
  lactation and, 330
  mechanism of action of, 41t
  in oral contraceptive, 39
  pregnancy and, 64-65, 65
Ethanol in breast milk, 377, *379,* 380
Ethnic factors; *see* Racial/ethnic factors
Etretinate, 159
Eucerin cream, 424t
Euglycemia, 266
Everted nipple, 408, *409*
Exchange, food, 269
Excretory exchange, placental, 88
Exercise
  breastfeeding and, 339
  nutrition assessment and, 234
  weight gain and, *227*
Exocytosis, 326, 328
Expanded Food, Nutrition, and Education Program, 457
Expectations of pregnant adolescent, 295t
Expression of milk, 426
  manual, 427-428
  for preterm or sick infant, 428t, 428-430, 429t, *430, 431*
Extrinsic growth failure, 100

F

Facial characteristics of fetal alcohol syndrome, 195-196, *196*
Facial dysmorphology, 272
Famine, 106-107, 136, 138
Fasting, 136, 138-139, *140*
Fasting blood glucose, 265-266
Fat; *see also* Obesity
  in breast milk, 354, *355,* 356-357, *357*
  brown, 131, 359
  deposition of, 133
  diabetes and, 269
  energy cost and, 129t
  milk synthesis and, 328
  in pregnancy, 69-70

Fat—cont'd
total parenteral nutrition and, 286
Fat cell, 107
Fatty acid
in breast milk, 347t, 356, 357-358
essential, 142-143
Fecal impaction, pica and, 195
Federal governmental agency, 472
Feeding of infant
artificial, 393, 394, 395, 400-401, 414
breastfeeding; *see also* Breastfeeding
Ferritin, *170,* 230
breastfed infant and, *363*
Fertility
adolescent pregnancy and, 32-33
birth spacing and, 34-35, 36t
caffeine and, 37
control of, 38-47; *see also* Birth control
diet and, 36-38
maternal age affecting, 33-34
preconception assessment and, 47-54, 49t, 51t, *52*
Fetal alcohol syndrome, 52-53, 195-203, *196,* 197t, *198, 200-202*
Fetal hemoglobin, 427
Fetal period, definition of, 12-14
Fetal tobacco syndrome, 207-208
Fetus
caffeine effects on, 203
calcium and, 173-174
cocaine effects on, 209-210
death of
fetal death ratio, 14
high hemoglobin levels and, 172-173
interconceptional interval and, 35
malnutrition and, 107
WIC program and, 120, 121
exercise and, 211-212
folic acid deficiency and, 49-51
growth of, 98-125; *see also* Growth, fetal
iodine and, 178
kilocalorie requirement of, 68
marijuana effects on, 209
maternal diabetes and, 265
pica effects on, 195
placenta and, 85-90, *86, 87,* 89t, *90*
smoking effects on, *206,* 206-209, *207, 208*
vitamin A and, 51t, 51-52, 157-160
vitamin A excess and, 51t, 51-52, *52*
vitamin D and, 161-162
zinc deficiency and, 52
Financial aspects of breastfeeding, 341, 399-400
Fish oil, *358*
Fitness, total, 454
Flat nipple, *409*
Fluid and electrolytes
hyperemesis gravidarum and, 259
hypertension and, 262-263
total parenteral nutrition, 286
Fluid retention, 66
Fluoride, 184
in breast milk, 360, *361*

Fluorine, 365
Folacin, 370, *371*
Folic acid/folate
adolescent pregnancy and, 308
anemia and, 258
in breast milk, *368*
deficiency of, 49-51
neural tube defect and, 143-152, *145,* 147t, 148t, 149t, 150t, *151,* 154
oral contraceptives and, 44
recommendations for, 146
sources of, 144t
Folk remedies, herbal teas as, 203-204
Food; *see also* Nutrition *entries*
additives to, 204
allergy to, 233
beliefs about, 193-194
contaminants of, 204-205
folate-rich, 258
restriction of, 136, 138-139
Food and Drug Administration
caffeine and, 203
herbal teas and, 203-204
pollutants in breast milk, 377
vitamin A and, 158
Food frequency questionnaire, 235
Food group, nutrient check by, 236
Food intake record, 234, *235*
Food plan, personal, 245, 246t-249t, *250*
Formula, total parenteral nutrition, 286-287
Formula feeding, 393, 394, 395
history of, 400-401
promotion of, 400
volume of, 414
Fourth trimester of pregnancy, lactation as, 399
Freezing of milk, 374, 430

G

Galactopoietic factors, 329
Galactose, fertility and, 37
Gallbladder, 64
Gastric pressure, 244-245
Gastroenteritis, 396
Gastrointestinal system
breastfed infant and, 395
disorder of, 244-245
hyperemesis gravidarum and, 244, 258-259
pregnancy effects on, 64
General Accounting Office analysis of WIC program, 119-120
Genetics
hypertension and, 261
of neural tube defect, 147
testing and, 155
Geographic differences
in birth rate, 2
in death rate, 5, 6-7
infant, 14, 14t, 21
Geophagia, 194-195
Gestation, duration of, 25, 58

Gestational diabetes, 266t, 287-288; *see also* Diabetes mellitus
Gingival hypertrophy, 223
Gland, mammary
    anatomy of, 319, *320*, 321
    development of, 321-324, *322, 324*
Glomerular function, 63
Glucocorticoid, breast development and, 324
Glucose
    diabetes and, 53-54, 265-267, 268
    nutrition assessment and, 231
    pregnancy and, 68
Glucose tolerance test, 267
Glycosylated hemoglobin, 270
Golgi apparatus, 326, 328
Gonadotropin, chorionic
    lactation and, 323-324, 333t
    placenta and, 88-89
Governmental agency, 471-472
Growth; *see also* Growth, fetal; Growth retardation
    of adolescent mother, 299
    of breastfed infant, 397
    fat content in milk and, 356-357
Growth, fetal, 98-125
    animal experiments on, 98-102
    human studies on, 102
    malnutrition affecting, 106-108
    nutritional effects on
        birth weight and, 108-110, *109, 110*
        cost-benefit studies of, 121, 122t-123t, 124-125
        malnutrition and, 106-107
        organ studies of, 107-108
        supplementation and, 111, 112t-115t, 116-119
        WIC program and, 119-121
    retardation of, 103, 106
    stages of, 102-103, *104-105*
Growth hormone
    lactation and, 329-330, 333t
    pregnancy and, 67-68
Growth retardation
    animal studies of, 100-102, 101t
    fatty acids and, 143
    human, 103, 106
    tobacco causing, 206-208
Growth spurt, 415
Gunning fog index, 465

H

Hand breast pump, 429t, 429-430, *431*
Head circumference, in PKU, 274
Health and Human Services, 255
Health promotion, 1-28
    for adolescent, 313-315
    birth rate and, 2t, 2-3
    challenges to, 26-27
    epidemiologic factors in, 8-21
        age as, 8-9, 9t
        infant death rates and, 12, 14t, 14-21, *15*, 17t, 18t, *19, 20*, 21t, 22t
        medical risk factors as, 9-10

Health promotion—cont'd
    epidemiologic factors in—cont'd
        parity as, 9
        past obstetrical history, 10-12, *11*, 12t, 13t
    low-birth-weight infant infant and, 9t, 21-25
    maternal mortality and morbidity and, 3-8, *4*, 4t, 5t, *6*, 6t, 7t
    programs for, 25-26
Health-related agency, 472
Healthy People 2000, 296, 447
Heart, 59
Heartburn, 244
Heavy metal contamination, 204-205
Heavy metals, 380
Height, 225
    weight gain and, *79*
Hemoconcentration, hypertension and, 263
Hemodynamics
    birth weight and, 110
    pregnancy and, 59
Hemoglobin
    in breastfed infant, *363*
    fetal, 427
    glycosylated, 270
    iron and, 167-168, 171-173, 257
    nutrition assessment and, 230
    placenta, 88
Hemolytic anemia, pica and, 195
Hemorrhage, 162
Hemorrhoid, 244
Herbal teas, 203-204
Herbicide, 205
Hereditary disorder
    hypertension and, 261
    neural tube defect as, 147
    testing for, 155
Herpes infection, 426-427
High density lipoprotein, 62
High-risk pregnancy, 254-288
    anemia and, 256t, 256-258, 257t, 258t
    diabetes mellitus and, 264-271; *see also* Diabetes mellitus
    general health care and, 254-256
    hypertension and, 259-264, 260t; *see also* Hypertension
    nutrition in, 215-216
        education about, 450-451
    phenylketonuria and, 272t, 272-279, 273t, 276t, 278t
    total parenteral nutrition in, 284-287
    weight-related, 279-284
Hispanics
    infant mortality rate for, 18t
    low-birth-weight infant and, 10
    medical complications rate in, 9-10
History
    diet, 234-236, 235t
    in nutrition assessment, *231*, 231-232, 235t
    obstetrical, 10
    prenatal nutrition, 96-98
Homocysteine, 151
Hormone
    breast development and, 323-324
    in breast milk, 374t, 374-375

Hormone—cont'd
  hypertension and, 261
  lactation and, *329,* 329-330, 332t-333t
  parathyroid, 87
  placental, 88-89
  pregnancy and, 64-68, 65t, *67*
Hospital practices on breastfeeding, 410, 412-413
Human chorionic gonadotropin
  hyperemesis gravidarum and, 259
  lactation and, 333t
  placenta and, 88-89
Human chorionic somatomammotropin, 173, 333t
Human immunodeficiency virus
  breastfeeding and, 380-382, *382,* 434-435
  as sexually transmitted disease, 296
  vitamin A and, 157
Human milk; *see* Milk, human
Human placental lactogen, 89
25-Hydroxyvitamin D, 365-367, *366*
Hyperbilirubinemia, 427
Hypercarotenemia, 37
Hyperemesis gravidarum, 244, 258-259
  bulimia versus, 312
  total parenteral nutrition for, 284
Hypernatremia in breastfed infant, 364-365
Hyperolfaction, 259
Hyperphagia, 131
Hyperplasia of breast, 323
Hypertension, 259-264, 260t
  adolescent and, 297
  calcium and, *175,* 175-176
  fetal, 172-173
  incidence of, 259-260
  nutrition and, 287
  oral contraceptives and, 39
  protein and, 141-142
Hyperthyroidism, 178-179
Hypertrophy
  of brown fat, 131
  cardiac, 59
  gingival, 223
Hyperventilation, 88
Hypoalbuminemia, 263
Hypochromic anemia, microcytic, 256
Hypophysectomy, 323
Hypoplasia, enamel, 161
Hypothyroidism, 178
Hypovolemia, 263

I

Illness, lactation during, 427-436, 428t, 429t, *430-433*
Immaturity of adolescent, 298-302, *300, 301,* 302t
Immigrant, infant death rate for, 20
Immunoglobulin
  atopic disease and, 397
  in breast milk, 351, 370, 370t, *372,* 372-374, *373*
  milk synthesis and, 328
Immunologic rejection, placenta and, 89-90
Impaction, fecal, pica and, 195

Index
  body mass, *78, 79*
    obesity and, 280
    underweight and, 282
    weight problems and, 279
  gunning fog, 465
  ponderal, 208
Induced lactation, 334-335
Infancy, definition of, 14
Infant; *see also* Infant mortality
  of adolescent mother, 297-298
  anemia in, 363
  birth weight of; *see* Birth weight
  cocaine-exposed, 376
  docosahexaenoic acid and, 358
  fat content in milk and, 356-357
  feeding of
    artificial, 393, 394, 395, 400-401, 414
    breastfeeding; *see* Breastfeeding
  growth of; *see* Growth *entries*
  health promotion for, 1-28; *see also* Health promotion
  hypernatremia in, 364-365
  hyponatremia in, 185
  infection in, 426-427
  jaundice in, 427
  phenylketonuria and, 273-274
  preterm
    breast milk for, 383-384
    docosahexaenoic acid and, 358
    risks to, 21-25, 23t, 24t
  vitamin B$_6$ and, 156
  vitamin D and, 161
  vitamin E and, 161
  vitamin K and, 162, 368
Infant health paradox, 27
Infant mortality
  breastfeeding and, 400-401
  interconceptional interval and, 35
  rates of, 14, 14t, *15,* 16-21, 17t, 18t, *19, 20,* 21t, 22t
    WIC program and, 120, 121
  smoking and, 208-209
  undernutrition and, 32
  weight gain and, 226-227
Infection
  breast, 426-427
  in breastfed infant, 395
  HIV, 380-382, *382*
  immunoglobulins in breast milk and, 370, 370t, *372,* 372-374, *373*
  maternal, 434
  total parenteral nutrition and, 285
Infertility; *see* Fertility
Inside My Mom, 462
Insulin
  fetus and, 265
  management of, 269-270
  pregnancy and, 66-67
Insulin-dependent diabetes mellitus, 265-271
  preconception assessment of, 53-54
  protection against, 398
Intake, food, 234, *235*

Interconceptional interval
    fetal death and, 35
    nutrition assessment and, 232
International Center for Research on Women, 312-313
Interview, diet history, 236-237
Intrauterine device, 46
Intrauterine growth retardation; *see* Growth retardation
Intrinsic growth failure, 100
Inverted nipple, 408, *409*
Involution of breast, 321, 328
Iodine, 178-179
    in breast milk, 365
IQ of breastfed infant, 398
    DHA and, 358
Iron
    adolescent pregnancy and, 306-307
    in breast milk, 361, 363
    nutrition assessment and, 230
    supplementation of, 167-168, 168t, *169, 170,* 171-173
        effects of, 245
Iron deficiency anemia, 171-172, 256-257, 257t
Isoretinoin, 159

J

Jaundice, 427

K

Kernicterus, 427
Ketoacidosis, 270
Ketogenesis, carnitine and, 359
Ketone body, 134, 138-139
Ketosis, 266t
    starvation, 269-270
Kidney, 63
Kilocalorie, 68
    fatty acids in breast milk and, 357
    intake of, 130
    pregnancy and, 68
    total parenteral nutrition, 285-286

L

La Leche League, 393
α-Lactalbumin, 351
Lactation, 319-343; *see also* Breastfeeding; Milk, human
    breast anatomy and, 319, *320,* 321
    breast development and, 321-324, *322, 324*
    diet and, 335, 335t, *336,* 337-342, *338, 340*
    during illness or separation, 427-436, 428t, 429t, *430-433*
    induced, 334-335
    nutrition assessment and, 232
    physiology of, *324-326,* 324-335
        hormones and, 332t-333t
        induction and, 334-335
        maintenance of, 331, 334
        milk synthesis and secretion and, *326,* 326-331, *327*
    preterm, 383-384
Lactation consultant, 393
Lactiferous duct, 321
Lactiferous sinus, 321

Lactobacillus bifidus, 350, 359-360
    resistance factors and, 350-351
Lactoferrin, 351
    in breast milk, 372-373
Lactogen, 67-68, 323-324
    placental, 333t
Lactogenesis, 324
Lactose, 328-329, *329*
    in breast milk, 359
Lanolin, 408, 425t
Latching on, 418-419
Late fetal period, *13, 14*
Late transient hypertension, 260t
Laxative, 375
Lead
    in breast milk, 380
    toxicity of, 204-205
Learning
    about breastfeeding, 407t-408t
    framework for, 239
    motivation for, 239, 241-243
Leg cramp, magnesium and, 177-178
Let-down reflex, 330-331, 414
Leukocyte, zinc deficiency and, 180
Lifestyle concerns, 193-217
    adolescent pregnancy and, 303
    alcohol and, 195-203, *196,* 197t, *198, 200-202*
    caffeine and, 203
    cocaine and, 209-210
    food additives and, 204
    food beliefs and, 193-194
    food contaminants and, 204-205
    herbal tea and, 203-204
    marijuana and, 209
    nutrition and, 213-216, 214t, 215t, *216*
    pica and, 194-195
    rigorous exercise as, 211-212
    tobacco and, *206,* 206-209, *207, 208*
    weight gain as, 212-213, *213; see also* Weight gain
Line, anterior axillary, 319
Lipase
    in breast milk, 359, 395
    lipoprotein, 62
Lipid
    brain cells and, 103
    in breast milk, 354, *355,* 356-357
    essential fatty acids and, 142-143
    hypertension and, 263
    milk synthesis and, 328
    nutrition assessment and, 231
Lipid metabolism
    oral contraceptives and, 40
    pregnancy and, 62-63
Lipoprotein lipase, 62, 328
Liver, hypertension and, 263
Long-chain polyunsaturated fatty acids in breast milk, 357-358
Low density lipoprotein, 62
Low-birth-weight infant
    age and race affecting, 9t
    breast milk for, 383-384

Low-birth-weight infant—cont'd
  fatty acids and, 142
  mother as, 32, *33*
  nutrition related to, 96-97
  risks to, 21-25, 23t, 24t
  smoking and, 207
  supplementation and, 116-117, 118
  WIC program and, 120
Luteinizing hormone, 330
Lymphoblast, 372
Lymphocyte, 373
Lysozyme, 372

M

Macrophage, 373
Magnesium, 177-178
  in breast milk, *362*
Maintaining lactation, 427-436, 428t, 429t, *430-433*
Male, nutrition education for, 451-452
Malignancy, protection against, 398, 399
Malnutrition; *see also* Undernutrition; Underweight
  fertility and, 31-32
  growth failure and, 100-102, 101t
  growth retardation and, 106
  placenta and, 90
  research on effects of, 106-110, *109, 110*
  resistance against infection and, 374
Mammary gland
  anatomy of, 319, *320,* 321
  development of, 321-324, *322, 324*
Mammogenesis, 321
Mammol Ointment, 424t
Manual expression of milk, 427-428
Marijuana, 209
  breast milk and, 380
Massé Cream, 424t
Mastitic breast, 328
Mastitis, 426-427
Maternal Addiction Project, 199
Maternal health promotion, 1-28; *see also* Health
    promotion
Maternal illness, 433-436
Maternal mortality, 3-8, *4,* 4t, 5t, *6,* 6t
Maternal Nutrition and the Course of Pregnancy, 97
Maximum-XP, 275, 276t
Meconium, 350
Media
  audiovisual, 459-463
  broadcast, 458-459
Medical foods for phenylketonuria, 275, 276t, 277-278
Medical history, 232
Medical risk factors, 9
Medication; *see* Drug
Megaloblastic anemia, 258
  folic acid and, 145
  vitamin B$_{12}$ and, 156
Megaloblastosis, 258
Menstrual cycle, breast and, 323
Mental retardation
  aflatoxin and, 206

Mental retardation—cont'd
  phenylketonuria and, 271
Menu for woman of child-bearing age, 153t-154t
Mercury, 205, 380
Mesoderm, 103
Metabolic rate in pregnancy, 130, 131t, 133
  adolescent, 305
Metabolism
  of folate, 150-151
  nutritional status and, 130-131
  oral contraceptives affecting, 39-46, 43t, *44, 45*
  placental, 88
  pregnancy and, 68
  protein, 230-231
  total parenteral nutrition and, 285
Methionine, 151
Methotrexate, 375
Methylmercury, 205
Mexican infant
  death rate for, 20
  low-birth-weight, 24
Micelle, 326
Microcytic hypochromic anemia, 256
Micronutrient; *see* Minerals; Vitamin
Mid-upper-arm muscle circumference, 225-226
Milk, human, 345-384; *see also* Lactation
  animal milk compared with, 345-346, 350-351, 353t
  benefits of, 393-395
  carbohydrate in, 328-329, 359-360
  carnitine in, 359
  cholesterol in, 356, 358-359, 397
  colostrum and, 349-350
  composition of, 347t-349t, 397
  contaminants in, 375-380, 376t, 378t, *379,* 379t
  fatty acids in, 347t, 356, 357-358
  freezing of, 430
  HIV infection and, 380-382, *382*
  hormones in, 374t, 374-375
  immunoglobulins in, 351, 370, 370t, *372,* 372-374, *373*
  insufficient supply of, 421, 423
  lipase in, 359
  lipids in, 354, *355,* 356-357
  manual expression of, 426
  minerals in, 348t, 360-361, *362-364,* 363-365, 397
  nonprotein nitrogen in, 354
  output of, *336, 337*
  preterm, 383-384
  protein in, 347t, 350t, 350-351, *352,* 353t, 354
  pumping of, 429t, 429-430, *430, 431*
  storage of, 430-432, *432*
  synthesis and secretion of, *326,* 326-331, *327, 329-331*
  transitional, 350
  vitamins in, 348t, 365-370, *366, 368, 369,* 370t, *371*
  witch's, 321
Milk bank, HIV infection and, 382
Milk ejection reflex, 331
Milk products in daily food plan, 248t
Minerals
  in breast milk, 348t, 360-361, *362-364,* 363-365
  calcium, 173-177, 174t, *175, 178*
  copper, 182-183

Minerals—cont'd
 in daily food plan, 246t
 determinants of disease and, 186, *187,* 188
 fluoride, 184
 hypertension and, 263
 iodine, 178-179
 iron, 167-168, 168t, *169, 170,* 171-173
 nutrition assessment and, 231
 oral contraceptives and, 45
 phosphorus, 176-177
 Recommended Dietary Allowance for, 188
 total parenteral nutrition and, 285, 286
 zinc, 179-182, 181t; *see also* Zinc
Minipill, contraceptive, 39
Moist compress, for breast, 426
Molybdenum, 365
Monophasic oral contraceptive, 39
Monovalent ion, milk synthesis and, 328
Morbidity, maternal, 3-8, *4,* 4t, 5t, *6,* 6t
Morphogen, 159
Mortality
 fetal; *see* Fetus, death of
 infant; *see* Infant mortality
 maternal, 3-8, *4,* 4t, 5t, *6,* 6t
  adolescent, 297, 297t
Motion picture presentation, 463
Motivation
 of large population groups, 457
 for learning, 239, 241-243
MSAFP test, 155
Multimedia presentation, 463
Multipara, weight and, 83
Multiphasic oral contraceptive, 39
Multiple pregnancy
 breastfeeding and, 437
 hypertension and, 261
 milk output and, *336*
 weight gain and, 76, 77
Muscle, mid-upper-arm, 225-226

N

National Academy of Sciences, 74-75, 76, 229
National Commission to Prevent Infant Mortality, 12
National Institutes of Health, diabetes and, 266-267
Native American infant
 death rate for, 19-20
 low-birth-weight, 24
Nausea and vomiting
 hyperemesis gravidarum, 244
 hyperemesis gravidarum and, 244, 258-259
 phenylketonuria and, 278
 vitamin B_6 and, 157
Necrotizing enterocolitis, 374
Neonatal period, *13,* 14; *see also* Infant *entries*
Nerve cell, fetal, 103
Nervous system
 iodine and, 178
 vitamin B_{12} and, 156-157
Neural crest defect, 159, *160*

Neural tube defect, 143-152, 144t, *145,* 147t, 148t, 149t, 150t, *151,* 154
 folic acid and, 49-51
Neurological status, DHA and, 358
Newborn; *see* Infant
Newspaper articles, 465-466
Niacin, 143
Nickel, 365
Nicotine, 206-207
 in breast milk, 380
Nipple
 applying breast milk to, 399
 discomfort with, 423, 425-426
 everted or inverted, 408, *409*
 products applied to, 424t-425t
 relationship to baby's mouth, 418, *420*
Nitrogen
 adolescent pregnancy and, 306
 in breast milk, 347t, 350
 nonprotein, 354
 protein and, 139, 141, 230-231
 total parenteral nutrition and, 285
Non–insulin-dependent diabetes mellitus, 266t
Nonprotein nitrogen, 354
Norethynodrel, 39
NPH insulin, 269
Nurse, wet, 393
Nursing of infant; *see* Breastfeeding; Lactation
Nursing supplementer, 432-433, *433*
Nutrient
 calculation of, 236
 diabetes and, 268-269
 placental transfer of, *86, 87,* 89t, *90*
 in pregnancy, 240t-241t
 serum levels of, 60-62
Nutrient transfer, placental, 85-90
Nutrition
 in adolescent pregnancy, 302-312; *see also* Adolescent pregnancy, nutrition in
 of breast milk, 397
 diabetes and, 268-269
 education about, 236, 238t, 238-245, 240t-241t
 fertility and
  adolescent pregnancy and, 32-33
  birth spacing and, 34-35, 36t
  diet and, 36-38
  late maternal age and, 33-34
 hyperemesis gravidarum and, 259
 hypertension and, 261, 262-263, 264
 for nursing mother, 335, 335t, *336,* 337-342, *338, 340*
 obesity and, 280-281
 parenteral
  hyperemesis gravidarum and, 259
  total, 284-287
 in phenylketonuria, 272t, 272-279, 273t, 276t, 278t
 prenatal, 94-125; *see also* Prenatal nutrition
 teaching about, 241-243
 underweight and, 282; *see also* Undernutrition; Underweight
Nutrition analysis, 236, 238t

Nutrition assessment
  of adolescent, 308-309
  common functional problems and, 244-245
  education and, 236, 238-239, 240t-241t, 241-245
  obesity and, 280
  preconception, 47-54, 49t, 51t, *52*
  prenatal, 220-236
    anthropometric data in, 223, 225-226
    clinical observation in, 223, 224t-225t
    health status and, 221-222
    individual, 232-236, 235t
    laboratory data in, 229-231
    patient history in, *231,* 231-232, 235t
    risk factors concerning, 222t
    weight gain and, 226-229, *227,* 228t
  total parenteral nutrition and, 284-285
  underweight and, 282; *see also* Undernutrition;
      Underweight
Nutrition counseling, 456-457
Nutrition education, 446-473
  concepts for, 455-456
  content of, 452-454
  diet analysis and, 236, 238-239, 240t-241t, 241-245
  for high-risk groups, 450-451
  motivation for learning and, 239, 241-243
  nutrition environment and, 447-449, *448*
  opportunities for, 468-473, 470t
  process of, 449-450, *450*
  sources for materials about, 469
  techniques for, 454-463, 464t, 465-466, 467t-468t

O

Obesity, 279-281
  assessment of, 280
  definition of, 279
  effects of, 48-49
  hypertension and, 260-261
  incidence of, 279-280
  nutrition in, 280-281
  weight gain in pregnancy and, 75
Obstetrical history, 10
Oral contraceptive, 39-46, 40t, 43t, *45*
  carbohydrate metabolism and, 40-41
  lactation and, 330
  lipid metabolism and, 40
  minerals and, 45, 46t
  nutritional consequences of, 45-46
  protein metabolism and, 41
  side effects of, 39-40
  types of, 39
  vitamins and, 41-45, *44*
Organ, malnutrition and, 107-108
Organohalide in breast milk, 377
Osteomalacia, 161
Outcome, pregnancy; *see* Pregnancy outcome
Output of breast milk, 415-416
Ovarian cancer, 399
Ovarian function, 37
Ovariectomy, 323
Overnutrition; *see* Obesity

Overweight
  definition of, 279
  pregnancy outcome and, 227-228
Ovulation
  lactation and, 330
  in postpartum period, 34-35
  vegetarianism affecting, 37
Oxygen, placenta, 88
Oxytocin, 399
  function of, 332t

P

Palmitoyl-coenzyme A L glycerol-3-phosphate palmitoyl
      transferase, 328
Paracellular pathway of breast, 328
Paradox, infant health, 27
Parathyroid hormone, 87
Parenteral nutrition
  hyperemesis gravidarum and, 259
  total, 284-287
Parity
  hypertension and, 261
  maternal health and, 9
  nutrition assessment and, 232
  weight retention and, 83, 85
Parturition, mammogenesis and, 321
Patch, Peyer's, 374
Paternal factors
  adolescent pregnancy and, 303
  alcohol abuse as, 201, 203
  phenylketonuria as, 271
D-Penicillamine, copper deficiency and, 183
Penicillin, 375
Peptide, 354
Perfusion, uteroplacental, 110
Perinatal period
  definition of, *13,* 14
  diabetes and, 270
Periodicals, 465
Pernicious anemia, 152
Personal background data, 233-234
Personal food plan, 245, 246t-249t, *250*
Pesticide residue in breast milk, 376-377, 378t-379t
Peyer's patches, 374
Phenex 2, 276t
Phenylalanine
  aspartame and, 53, 204
  in breast milk, 351, 354
  phenylketonuria and, 271-279
Phenyl-Free, 276t
Phenylketonuria, 255
  aspartame and, 53, 204
  case study about, 287
  counseling for, 274-275
  identification of, 274
  incidence of, 271-272
  management of, 272t, 272-279, 273t, 276t, 278t
Phospholipid, 356
Phosphorus, 176-177
Phototherapy for jaundice, 427

Physical exercise; *see* Exercise
Physiology of pregnancy, 58-91; *see also* Pregnancy, physiology of
Pica, 172, 194-195
Pinocytosis, 85
PKU-3, 275, 276t
Placenta, 85-90, *86, 87,* 89t, *90*
  breast and, 323-324
  malnutrition and, 107-108
  smoking and, 207
  weight of
    socioeconomic status and, 107
    supplementation and, 111, 116
Placental lactogen, 333t
Plasma proteins, oral contraceptives and, 41
Plasma volume, *61*
Point-of-purchase educational campaign, 472
Pollutants in breast milk, 376-377, 378t-379t
Polybrominated biphenyls, 206, 379t
Polychlorinated biphenyls, 205-206, 378t
Polycose, 275
Polyunsaturated fat, 357
Ponderal index, smoking and, 208
Positioning for breastfeeding, 416, *417, 418,* 418
Postneonatal period
  death rate in, 14, 14t, *15,* 16-21, 17t, 18t, *19,* 21t, 22t
  definition of, *13,* 14
Postpartum period
  breastfeeding in, 409-410, 412-413; *see also* Breastfeeding
  diabetes and, 270-271
  maternal death in, 6, 8
  weight loss or retention in, 81-83, *82-84,* 85
    for adolescent, 311
    breastfeeding and, 337
Potassium, milk synthesis and, 328
Poverty
  maternal effects of, 32
  mortality and, 4
Preconception assessment, 47-54
  breastfeeding preparation and, 405-409, 407t-408t, *409*
Preeclampsia
  characteristics of, 260t, 260-264
  mortality and, 4
  sodium-restriction and, 185
  vitamin B_6 and, 156
Pregnancy; *see also* Pregnancy outcome
  adverse outcome of, low birth weight as, 25
  anorexia nervosa and, 283
  bulimia and, 283-284
  energy needs during, 129-143; *see also* Energy
  health promotion in, 1-28; *see also* Health promotion
  high-risk, 254-288; *see also* High-risk pregnancy
  interval between, 34-35, 36t
  late maternal age and, 34
  physiology of, 58-91
    blood volume and, 59-63, *60, 61,* 61t
    cardiovascular system and, 59
    early pregnancy loss and, 59
    gastrointestinal system and, 64
    hormones and, 64-68, 65t, *67*

Pregnancy—cont'd
  physiology of—cont'd
    length of gestation, 58
    metabolic rate and, 68
    placenta and, 85-91, *86, 87,* 89t, *90*
    renal function and, 63
    respiration and, 63
    weight gain and, 68-85; *see also* Weight gain
  vitamin requirements in; *see also* Vitamin
Pregnancy outcome
  for adolescent, 32-33, 298-302, *300, 301,* 302t
  late maternal age and, 33-34
  nutrition and, 32, 213-216, 214t, 215t, *216,* 221
    assessment of, 232
  phenylketonuria and, 272-275
  smoking and, 208
  vitamin A excess and, 51-52
  weight gain and, 226-228
  WIC program and, 120
  zinc deficiency and, 52
Pregnancy test, negative, 54
Pregnancy-induced hypertension, 259-264, 260t; *see also* Hypertension
Premature infant; *see also* Low-birth-weight infant; Preterm infant
Premature rupture of membranes, zinc and, 180
Prenatal care
  adolescent pregnancy and, 303
  cost-benefit analysis of, 122t-123t
  diabetes and, 270
  maternal death and, 7
  pregnancy outcome and, 10-12, *11,* 12t, 13
  in Sweden, Finland, and U.S., 13t
Prenatal nutrition, 94-125
  assessment of, 220-236; *see also* Nutrition assessment
  early beliefs about, 95
  early research on, 95-96
  fetal growth and, 98-125; *see also* Growth, fetal
  in high-risk pregnancy, 215-216
  history of, 96-98
  pregnancy outcome and, 213-216, 214t, 215t, *216*
Prenatal period
  breastfeeding preparation and, 405-409, 407t-408t, *409*
  definition of, 12, *13,* 14
  nutrition in, 94-125; *see also* Prenatal nutrition
  weight gain in, 68-81; *see also* Weight gain
Prepregnancy weight, 226, 279
Prescription, total parenteral nutrition, 285-286
Pressure, gastric, 244-245
Preterm infant
  docosahexaenoic acid and, 358
  pumping milk for, 428t, 428-430, 429t, *430*
  risks to, 21-25, 23t, 24t; *see also* Low-birth-weight infant
Preterm milk, 383-384
Prime-time diet, 458
Primigravida, weight gain in, 68-69
Printed educational materials, 463, 465-466
Progesterone
  breastfeeding and, 413
  function of, 333t
  gastrointestinal system and, 64

Progesterone—cont'd
  pregnancy and, 64-65, 66
Progestin
  lactation and, 330
  mechanism of action of, 41t
Prolactin, 323-324, 329
  function of, 332t
Prolactin-inhibiting factor, 332t
Promotion
  of breastfeeding, 400-405
  of formula feeding, 400
  health, 1-28; *see also* Health promotion
Prophylaxis
  iron, 169, 171
  sodium-restriction as, 185
Protein
  adolescent pregnancy and, 306
  in breast milk, 328, 347t, 350t, 350-351, *352,* 353t, 354
  daily food plan and, 248t
  deficiency of, 141-142
  diabetes and, 268-269
  energy cost and, 129t
  as energy source, 134
  excess of, 142
  growth failure and, 100-101
  hypertension and, 262
  lactation and, 339
  metabolism of, 230-231
  obesity and, 281
  oral contraceptives and, 41
  phenylketonuria and, 275
  requirement for, 139-141
  serum, 61, 230
  supplementation and, 116
Proteinuria, hypertension and, 260t, 261, 262
Proteolytic enzyme, 351
Protoporphyrin, 230
Protozoan infection, 370, 372
Pseudo-Cushing syndrome, 377, *379*
Pseudoinverted nipple, *409*
Puberty, 321
Public speaking, 457
Puerperal infection, iron deficiency and, 171
Pulmonary embolus, 6
Pumping milk for preterm infant, 428t, 428-430, 429t, *430, 431*

Q

Questionnaire
  diet history, 237
  food frequency, 235

R

Racial/ethnic factors
  in birth rate, 2, 2t, 2-3, 3
  breastfeeding and, 403-404, 406
  infant mortality rate and, 14, 14t, *15,* 16-21, 17t, 18t, *19,* 21t
  in maternal death rate, 3-5, *4, 6*
  medical risk factors and, 9-10

Racial/ethnic factors—cont'd
  nutrition assessment and, 233
  nutrition education and, 451
  obstetrical history and, 10, *11*
  postpartum weight retention and, 82-83
  prenatal care and, *11,* 12t
  weight gain and, 73-74
Radiation therapy, 437
Radio commercials, 458-459
Radioisotope therapy, 436-437
Recommended Dietary Allowance, 189t
  adolescent pregnancy and, 304t, 304-305
    calcium, 308
    iron, 307
    protein, 306
  calcium, 174, 174t
  explanation of, 188
  folate, 258
  folic acid, 152, 258
  iron, 256
  for minerals, 188
  in pregnancy, 240t-241t
  total parenteral nutrition and, 285
  zinc, 182
Red blood cells
  anemia and, 256t, 256-258, 257t, 258t
  folate in, 150t
  iron and, 167-168
  iron-binding capacity and, 230
  pregnancy and, 60
Reflex
  ejection, 414
  let-down, 330-331, 414
  milk ejection, 331
Reinforcement, 239, 241
Rejection, immunologic, 89-90
Renal system
  pregnancy and, 63
  sodium and, 184-185
Renin, 66
Renin-angiotensin-aldosterone system, 184-185
Reproductive counseling, for PKU, 274-275
Research in prenatal nutrition, 94-125; *see also* Prenatal nutrition
Resistance factors in breast milk, 370, 370t, *372,* 372-374, *373,* 395-396
Resources
  on breastfeeding, 411-412
  for nutrition education materials, 469
Respiratory exchange, placental, 88
Respiratory system, 63
Retardation
  growth
    animal studies of, 100-102
    human, 103, 106
    tobacco causing, 206-208
  mental, aflatoxin and, 206
Retention, weight, 81-83, *82-84,* 85
Reticulum, endoplasmic, 324
Retinoid, 159, 160

Retinol
   in breast milk, 367
   teratogenesis of, 51t, 51-52, *52*
Riboflavin, 143
Ribonucleic acid, folic acid and, 144
Rickets, 95
Risk factors
   for alcohol abuse, 201
   nutritional, 221-222, 222t
RNA, folic acid and, 144
Rotavirus infection, 395
Rotersept, 425t
Rough endoplasmic reticulum, 324

S

Saccharin, 204
Saccharomyces fragilis, 360
Screening
   for diabetes, 267
   phenylketonuria and, 274
Secretion, milk, 325-331; *see also* Lactation
Secretory IgA, 372
Sedative, 375
Selenium, 365
Self-care, maternal, 419-421
Self-image, anorexia nervosa and, 282-283
Separation
   breastfeeding and, 427-436, 428t, 429t, *430-433*
   maintaining lactation during, 427-436, 428t, 429t, *430-433*
Sepsis, total parenteral nutrition and, 285
Serum iron level, 257-258
Serum nutrient levels, 60-61, 128-129
Serum protein, 61, 230
Sex education, 294
Sexually transmitted disease, 294, 296
Shigella, 370, 372
Sinus, lactiferous, 321
Skin, atopic dermatitis and, 396-397
Skinfold thickness, *72*
Slide/sound presentation, 460-462
Small for gestational age infant; *see also* Low-birth-weight infant
Smoking
   breast milk and, 380
   cessation programs, 209
   fertility and, 37-38
   fetal effects of, *206,* 206-209, *207, 208*
   nutrition assessment and, 234
   weight gain and, 85
Social marketing, 457
Society for Nutrition Education, 472-473
Socioeconomic status
   of adolescent, 298-299, 312
   birth control and, 38
   breastfeeding and, 402
   maternal effects of, 32
   nutrition and, 222
      assessment of, 232
      teaching about, 242
   obstetrical history and, 10

Socioeconomic status—cont'd
   placental characteristics of, 89t
   placental weight and, 107
   supplementation and, 118-119
Sodium
   in breast milk, 364-365
   hypertension and, 263-264
   milk synthesis and, 328
   pregnancy and, 66
   restriction of, 184-186, *185, 186*
Solution, total parenteral nutrition, 286-287
Somatomammotropin, 89
   human chorionic, 173
Spacing of births, 34-35, 36t
Special programs for adolescent, 313-315
Special Supplemental Food Program for Women, Infants, and Children
   beginning of, 98
   cost-benefit analysis of, 122t-123t
   evaluation of, 124
   pregnancy outcome and, 12
   provisions of, 25-26
   recipients of, *250,* 251
   results of, 119-121
Spina bifida, *145,* 145-146
Spontaneous abortion, incidence of, 59
Starch ingestion, 194-195
Starvation
   effects of, 106-107
   ketosis and, 269-270
State governmental agency, 471-472
Steroid, breast development and, 324
Stillbirth, malnutrition and, 107
Stillbirth ratio, 14
Stool, infant, 415-416
Storage of milk, 374, 430-432, *432*
Stress, in adolescent pregnancy, 298-302, 312
Substance abuse; *see also* Alcohol
   asking about, 199, 201
   fetal effects of, 52-53
   nutrition assessment and, 234
Suck cycle, *422*
Suckling
   anovulation and, 35
   disorders of, 433
   fat content in milk and, 356
   hormones and, 329, *329*
   maintenance of lactation and, 331, 334
Sudden infant death syndrome, 208-209
Supplemental Commodities Distribution Program, *250,* 251
Supplementation
   breast milk and, 354
   calcium, 176
   cost-benefit analysis of, 121, 122t-123t, 124-125
   fat deposition and, 70
   fluoride, 184, 184t
   folic acid; *see* Folic acid/folate
   iron, 169, *170,* 171-172, 257t
      anemia treatment with, 256-258
      effects of, 245
   lactation and, 339

Supplementation—cont'd
    magnesium, 177-178
    neural tube defect and, 147
    nutrition assessment and, 233
    phenylketonuria and, 275, 276t, 277-279
    protein excess and, 142
    research on, 111, 112t-115t, 116-121
    vitamin B₆, 157
    vitamin D, 161, 367
    zinc and, 181-182
Supplementer, nursing, 432-433, *433*
Suppression of lactation, 399
Sweetener, artificial
    breast milk and, 351, 354
    fetal effects of, 53
    pregnancy and, 204
Synthesis, milk, *326,* 326-331, *327, 329-331*

T

Target audience for nutrition education, 461
Taurine, 354
Tea, herbal, 203-204
Teaching, nutrition; *see* Nutrition education
Teenage pregnancy; *see* Adolescent pregnancy
Teeth, fluoride and, 184
Television commercials, 458-459
Teratogenesis
    of alcohol, 195-203, *196,* 197t, *198, 200-202*
    of caffeine, 203
    vitamin A, 51t, 51-52, *52,* 158-160, 159t
    vitamin D, 161-162
Testing for birth defect, 155
Therapeutic nutrition education, 449
Thermogenesis
    brown adipose tissue, 131
    carnitine and, 359
Thiamin, 143
Thiamin pyrophosphate, 143
Thromboembolism, oral contraceptives and, 40
Thrush, 426-427
Thyroid, iodine and, 178-179
Thyroid-stimulating hormone, 66
Thyrotropin-releasing hormone, 333t
Thyroxine
    iodine and, 178
    lactation and, 333t
    pregnancy and, 66
Tissue synthesis, hypertension and, 263
Tobacco; *see* Smoking
Tocopherol, 367-368
Total iron-binding capacity, 230, 257
Total parenteral nutrition, 284-287
    hyperemesis gravidarum and, 259
Toxemia, 261; *see also* Preeclampsia
Toxicity
    heavy metal, 204-205
    pica and, 194-195
Trace minerals; *see* Minerals
Transaminase, 156
Transferrin, 230
Transient hypertension, 260t

Transitional milk, 350
Triceps skinfold thickness, 225
2,3,5-Trichlorophenoxyacetic acid, 205
Triglyceride, 356
Trophoblast, 85
    hyperemesis gravidarum and, 259
Tryptophan, 41
Tube, neural, defect of, 143-152, 144t, *145,* 147t, 148t, 149t, 150t, *151,* 154
Twenty-four-hour recall of food intake, 234-235
Twin gestation
    breastfeeding and, 437
    hypertension and, 261
    milk output and, *336*
    weight gain in, 76, *77*

U

Ultrasound, birth defect and, 155
Undernutrition; *see also* Malnutrition; Underweight
    adult disease and, 186, *187,* 188
    breast milk and, 354
    fetal effects of, 48
    maternal effects of, 32
Underweight
    assessment of, 282
    birth weight correlated to, 109-110
    cardiovascular system and, 59
    definition of, 279
    eating disorder and, 282-284
    fertility and, 48
    incidence of, 281-282
    weight gain in, 75
Unmarried woman, birth rates for, 3
Urea nitrogen, 230
Urine
    acetonuria and, 139
    vitamin B₆ and, 156
U.S. Department of Health and Human Services, 255
Uterine dysfunction, 297
Uteroplacental perfusion, 110

V

Valium, 375
Vascular system
    hypertension and, 261
    vitamin D and, 162
Vaseline Petroleum Jelly, 425t
Vegetarian diet
    lactation and, 339
    nutrition assessment and, 233
    nutrition teaching and, 242-243, 243t
    ovulatory irregularity and, 37
Very low density lipoprotein, 62
Videodisk presentation, 463
Videotape presentation, 462-463
Villus, 85
Villus sampling, chorionic, 155
Virus, human immunodeficiency
    breastfeeding and, 380-382, *382,* 434-435
    as sexually transmitted disease, 296
    vitamin A and, 157

Visuals in nutrition education, 461
Vital statistics
  birth rate, 2t, 2-3
  infant death rate, 14, 14t, *15,* 16-21, 17t, 18t, *19, 20,*
    21t, 22t
  maternal death rate, 3-8, *4,* 4t, 5t, *6,* 6t
Vitamin; *see also* Folic acid/folate
  in breast milk, 348t, 365-370, *366, 368, 369,* 370t, *371*
  in daily food plan, 247t, 249t
  folic acid and, 143-154
  hypertension and, 264
  niacin, 143
  nutrition assessment and, 231
  placenta and, 87
  riboflavin, 143
  thiamin, 143
  total parenteral nutrition and, 285, 286
Vitamin A
  in breast milk, 367
  placenta and, 87-88
  requirement for, 157-158
  teratogenesis of, 51t, 51-52, *52,* 158-160, 159t
Vitamin B$_6$
  in breast milk, 368-369
  oral contraceptives and, 41-44, *44, 45*
  requirements for, 156-157
Vitamin B$_{12}$
  in breast milk, 369-370
  neural tube defect and, 151
  requirements for, 155-156
Vitamin B, placenta and, 88
Vitamin C
  deficiency of, 160-161
  placenta and, 88
Vitamin C (ascorbic acid), 368, *369, 371*
Vitamin D, 161-162
  in breast milk, 365-367, *366*
  placenta and, 87-88
Vitamin E, 161
  in breast milk, 367-368
  for nipples, 425t
Vitamin K, 162
  in breast milk, 368
Vomiting
  hyperemesis gravidarum and, 244, 258-259
  phenylketonuria and, 278
  vitamin B$_6$ and, 157

W

Water
  body, in pregnancy, 69t
  milk synthesis and, 328
Water-soluble vitamin, 368-370
Weaning, 326, *327,* 437, 439
Weight; *see also* Obesity; Weight gain
  anthropometry and, 223, 225
  birth; *see* Birth weight
  breastfeeding and, 337, 338-339
  correlations with
    infant birth weight, 108-109

Weight—cont'd
  maternal birth weight, 32, 33
  high-risk pregnancy and, 279-284
  low-birth-weight infant and; *see* Low-birth-weight infant
  oral contraceptives and, 39
  placental
    socioeconomic status and, 107
    supplementation and, 111, 116
  postpartum, 81-83, *82-84,* 85
    of adolescent, 311
  preconception assessment and, 48-49
Weight gain, 68-95
  of adolescent mother, 299-302, *301,* 302t
    disorders of, 311-312
  amount of, 212, *213*
  body water and, 69t
  breastfeeding and, 399
  charts of, 76, *77-80,* 81
  exercise and, 211
  Gambian study of, 69-71
  hypertension and, 260-261
  initial weight and, 132
  nutrition assessment and, 226-229, *227,*
    228t
  nutrition education and, 453-454
  pattern of, *71-73,* 71-74
  postpartum retention of, 81-83, *82-84,* 85
    breastfeeding and, 337
  racial differences in, 213
  recommendations for, 74t, 74-75, 75t
  seasonally adjusted, *135*
  in special subgroups, 75-76
  supplementation and, 111
  total parenteral nutrition and, 284-285
Weight-for-height measure, 279
Wet nurse, 393
Whey protein, 350-351
White House Conference on Food, Nutrition, and
    Health, 97
WHO recommendations about HIV infection, 381-382
WIC program
  beginning of, 98
  cost-benefit analysis of, 122t-123t
  evaluation of, 124
  pregnancy outcome and, 12
  provisions of, 25-26
  recipients of, *250,* 251
  results of, 119-121
Witch's milk, 321
Working, breastfeeding and, 437, *438*
Worksite educational campaign, 472
World Health Organization recommendations on HIV
    infection, 381-382
Written educational materials, 463, 465-466

Z

Zinc
  in breast milk, *362,* 363-364
  deficiency of, 52, 179-180, 181t
  oral contraceptives and, 45, 46t